# ROITT'S
# ESSENTIAL
# IMMUNOLOGY

NINTH EDITION

# ROITT'S ESSENTIAL IMMUNOLOGY

## Ivan M. Roitt

MA, DSc(Oxon), FRCPath, Hon FRCP(Lond), FRS
*Emeritus Professor, Department of Immunology,*
*University College London Medical School,*
*London WIP 6DB*

*b*

**Blackwell**
**Science**

© 1971, 1974, 1977, 1980, 1984, 1988,
1991, 1994, 1997 by Blackwell Science Ltd
Editorial Offices:
Osney Mead, Oxford OX2 0EL
25 John Street, London WC1N 2BL
23 Ainslie Place, Edinburgh EH3 6AJ
350 Main Street, Malden
  MA 02148 5018,   USA
54 University Street, Carlton
  Victoria 3053, Australia

Other Editorial Offices:

Blackwell Wissenschafts-Verlag GmbH
  Kurfürstendamm 57
  10707 Berlin, Germany

Zehetnergasse 6
A-1140 Wien
Austria

Set by Excel Typesetters Co., Hong Kong
Printed and bound in Italy
by Rotolito Lombarda S.p.A., Milan

The Blackwell Science logo is a
trade mark of Blackwell Science Ltd,
registered at the United Kingdom
Trade Marks Registry

First published 1971
Reprinted 1972 (twice), 1973 (twice)
Second edition 1974, Reprinted 1975
Third edition 1977, Reprinted 1978, 1979
Fourth edition 1980, Reprinted 1982, 1983
Fifth edition 1984
Sixth edition 1988, Reprinted 1988
Reprinted with corrections 1989
Seventh edition 1991
Eighth edition 1994, Reprinted 1996
Ninth edition 1997

Spanish editions 1972, 1975, 1978, 1982,
  1988, 1989, 1993
Italian editions 1973, 1975, 1979, 1986,
  1988, 1990, 1993, 1995
Portuguese editions 1973, 1979, 1983
French editions 1975, 1979, 1990
Dutch editions 1975, 1978, 1982
Japanese editions 1976, 1978, 1982, 1986, 1988
German editions 1977, 1984, 1988, 1993
Polish edition 1977
Greek editions 1978, 1989, 1992
Turkish edition 1979
Slovak edition 1981
Indonesian editions 1985, 1991
Russian edition 1988
Korean edition 1991
ELBS editions 1977, 1982, 1988, Reprinted 1991
Chinese (Taiwan) editions 1991, 1994

DISTRIBUTORS

Marston Book Services Ltd
PO Box 269
Abingdon
Oxon OX14 4YN
(*Orders*: Tel: 01235 465500
       Fax: 01235 465555)

USA
Blackwell Science, Inc.
Commerce Place
350 Main Street
Malden, MA 02148 5018
(*Orders*: Tel: 800 759 6102
       617 388 8250
       Fax: 617 388 8255)

Canada
Copp Clark Professional
200 Adelaide St West, 3rd Floor
Toronto, Ontario M5H 1W7
(*Orders*: Tel: 416 597-1616
       800 815-9417
       Fax: 416 597-1617)

Australia
Blackwell Science Pty Ltd
54 University Street
Carlton, Victoria 3053
(*Orders*: Tel: 3 9347 0300
       Fax: 3 9347 5001)

Catalogue records for this title
are available from the British Library
and the Library of Congress

ISBN 0-86542-729-1

# CONTENTS

# PREFACE

Dear Reader; At last full color has hit *Roitt's Essential Immunology* and I hope that this improves the understanding of the figures and induces a pleasurable aesthetic response. In several instances, I have extended the strategy of incorporating more advanced material in the figure legends. The relative importance of the *Immunological Journals* listed in 'Further Reading' at the end of chapter 2 is based on the *Citation Index*. Attention is drawn to associated electronic publications linked to *Roitt's Essential Immunology*, including an interactive CD Rom tutorial disk.

Increasing focus has been brought to bear on the following areas:
• Apoptosis
• Invertebrate defense mechanisms
• Natural killer (NK) effector mechanisms and inhibitory receptors for the major histocompatibility complex (MHC)
• CD markers; the table in Appendix 1 is bang up-to-date at the time of publication
• Peptide partial agonists and antagonists of T-cell activation
• T-cell recognition of nonpeptides and nonclassical class-I-related MHC
• γδ T-cell recognition of native unprocessed molecules

• Protein tyrosine kinase cascades in intracellular signaling
• The complex world of chemokines
• Further elaboration of $T_H1/T_H2$ polarities
• The ubiquitous roles of heat-shock proteins as chaperones and in nonclassical antigen presentation
• Mucosal immunity and the increasing emphasis on intranasal vaccines
• Epitope-specific and DNA-based vaccines
• New viral escape strategies
• Tolerance induction by oral and intranasal routes
• Further recognition of mutations leading to immunodeficiencies
• Slowly progressing understanding of AIDS pathogenesis
• The emerging subject of psychoimmunology
• Tackling the problems of xenografts
• Identification of tumor antigens and genetic engineering of tumor vaccines
• Mechanisms of epitope spreading within autoantigenic complexes
• Further light on the shared DR epitope hypothesis in rheumatoid arthritis
• At the technological level, the burgeoning use of 'knockout mice' and the expression of antigens, antibodies and defensins in plants.

# ACKNOWLEDGEMENTS

Producing a new edition of a book which attempts to provide a useful view of the whole field of Immunology is not exactly a trival exercise, and I have been helped tremendously by the support of my wife and the very effective secretarial assistance of Christine Griffin. The input of the editorial team of Julie Jones and Edward Wates at Blackwell Science and the illustrations of Mike Rubens and Graeme Chambers have clearly improved the impact of the book and I am especially grateful to them. I am further indebted to my co-editors J. Brostoff and D. Male, the publishers of Mosby-Wolfe and the following individuals for permission to utilize or modify their figures which have appeared in *Immunology*: J. Brostoff and A. Hall for figures 1.15 and 16.7; J. Horton for figure 12.18; G. Rook for figures 13.4 and 13.11 and J. Taverne for figure 13.20 and table 13.2.

A number of other scientists generously provided illustrations for inclusion in this edition, and I have acknowledged my gratitude to them in the relevant figure legends.

# ABBREVIATIONS

| | |
|---|---|
| Ab | antibody |
| ACh-R | acetylcholine receptor |
| ACTH | adrenocorticotropic hormone |
| ADA | adenosine deaminase |
| ADCC | antibody-dependent cell-mediated cytotoxicity |
| Ag | antigen |
| AIDS | acquired immunodeficiency syndrome |
| ANCA | antineutrophil cytoplasmic antibodies |
| APC | antigen-presenting cell |
| ARRE-1 | antigen receptor response element-1 |
| ARRE-2 | antigen receptor response element-2 |
| AZT | zidovudine (3′-azido-3′-deoxythymidine) |
| B-cell | lymphocyte which matures in bone marrow |
| BCG | bacille Calmette–Guérin attenuated form of tuberculosis |
| BCR | B-cell receptor |
| BM | bone marrow |
| BSA | bovine serum albumin |
| BUDR | bromodeoxyuridine |
| C | complement |
| $C\alpha(\beta/\gamma/\delta)$ | constant part of TCR $\alpha(\beta/\gamma/\delta)$ chain |
| CALLA | common acute lymphoblastic leukemia antigen |
| cAMP | cyclic adenosine monophosphate |
| CCP | complement control protein repeat |
| CD | cluster of differentiation |
| CDR | complementarity determining regions of Ig or TCR variable portion |
| CEA | carcinembryonic antigen |

| | |
|---|---|
| cGMP | cyclic guanosine monophosphate |
| $C_{H(L)}$ | constant part of Ig heavy (light) chain |
| CMI | cell-mediated immunity |
| CML | cell-mediated lympholysis |
| CMV | cytomegalovirus |
| Cn | complement component 'n' |
| $C\bar{n}$ | activated complement component 'n' |
| iCn | inactivated complement component 'n' |
| Cna | small peptide derived by proteolytic activation of Cn |
| CR(n) | complement receptor 'n' |
| CRP | C-reactive protein |
| CsA | cyclosporin A |
| CSF | cerebrospinal fluid |
| *D* gene | diversity minigene joining V and J segments to form variable region |
| DAF | decay accelerating factor |
| DAG | diacylglycerol |
| DC | dendritic cells |
| DNP | dinitrophenyl |
| DTP | diphtheria, tetanus, pertussis triple vaccine |
| EAE | experimental allergic encephalomyelitis |
| EBV | Epstein–Barr virus |
| ELISA | enzyme-linked immunosorbent assay |
| EM | electron microscope |
| E$\phi$ | eosinophil |
| ER | endoplasmic reticulum |
| ES | embryonic stem (cell) |
| F(B) | factor (B, etc.) |
| Fab | monovalent Ig antigen-binding fragment after papain digestion |

| | | | |
|---|---|---|---|
| F(ab')$_2$ | divalent antigen-binding fragment after pepsin digestion | | associated with sIgM B-cell receptor |
| FACS | fluorescence-activated cell sorter | IL-1 | interleukin-1 (also IL-2, IL-3, etc.) |
| Fc | Ig crystallisable-fragment originally; now non-Fab part of Ig | iNOS | inducible nitric oxide synthase |
| | | IP$_3$ | inositol triphosphate |
| | | ISCOM | immunostimulating complex |
| FCA | Freund's complete adjuvant | ITP | idiopathic thrombocytopenic purpura |
| FcγR | receptor for IgG Fc fragment | | |
| FDC | follicular dendritic cells | JAK | Janus kinases |
| (sc)Fv | (single chain) V$_H$–V$_L$ antigen binding fragment | J chain | peptide chain in IgA dimer and IgM |
| G | granulocyte | J gene | joining gene linking V or D segment to constant region |
| g.b.m. | glomerular basement membrane | | |
| GM-CSF | granulocyte–macrophage colony-stimulating factor | Ka(d) | association (dissociation) affinity constant (usually Ag–Ab reactions) |
| gp$n$ | $n$kDa glycoprotein | | |
| g.v.h. | graft versus host | kDa | units of molecular mass in kilo Daltons |
| H-2 | the mouse major histocompatibility complex | | |
| | | KLH | keyhole limpet hemocyanin |
| H-2D/K/L | main loci for classical class I (class II) | LAK | lymphocyte activated killer cell |
| | | LATS | long-acting thyroid stimulator |
| (A/E) | murine MHC molecules | LCM | lymphocytic choriomeningitis virus |
| HAMA | human antimouse antibodies | Le$^{a/b/x}$ | Lewis$^{a/b/x}$ blood group antigens |
| HBsAg | hepatitis B surface antigen | LFA-1 | lymphocyte functional antigen-1 |
| hCG | human chorionic gonadotropin | LGL | large granular lymphocyte |
| HEV | high walled endothelium of post capillary venule | LHRH | luteinizing hormone releasing hormone |
| Hi | high | LIF | leukemia inhibiting factor |
| HIV-1(2) | human immunodeficiency virus-1 (2) | Lo | low |
| | | LT(B) | leukotriene (B etc.) |
| HLA | the human major histo-compatibility complex | LPS | lipopolysaccharide (endotoxin) |
| | | Mφ | macrophage |
| HLA-A/B/C | main loci for classical class I (class II) | mAb | monoclonal antibody |
| | | MAC | membrane attack complex |
| (DP/DQ/DR) | human MHC molecules | MALT | mucosal-associated lymphoid tissue |
| HRF | homologous restriction factor | | |
| HSA | heat-stable antigen | MAP kinase | mitogen-activated protein kinase |
| hsp | heat-shock protein | MBP | basic protein of eosinophils (also myelin basic protein) |
| 5HT | 5-hydroxytryptamine | | |
| HTLV | human T-cell leukemia virus | MC | mast cell |
| H-Y | male transplantation antigen | MCP | membrane cofactor protein (C' regulation) |
| IC | interdigitating cell | | |
| ICAM-1 | intercellular adhesion molecule-1 | MCP-1 | monocyte chemotactic protein-1 |
| Id (αId) | idiotype (anti-idiotype) | M-CSF | macrophage colony-stimulating factor |
| IDC | interdigitating dendritic cells | | |
| IDDM | insulin-dependent diabetes mellitus | MDP | muramyl dipeptide |
| | | MHC | major histocompatibility complex |
| IFNα | α-interferon (also IFNβ, IFNγ) | MIF | macrophage migration inhibitory factor |
| Ig | immunoglobulin | | |
| IgG | immunoglobulin G (also IgM, IgA, IgD, IgE) | MLA | monophosphoryl lipid A |
| | | MLR | mixed lymphocyte reaction |
| sIg | surface immunoglobulin | MMTV | mouse mammary tumor virus |
| IgM-α/Ig-β | membrane peptide chains | MS | multiple sclerosis |

| | | | |
|---|---|---|---|
| MSH | melanocyte stimulating hormone | SCG | sodium cromoglycate |
| MuLV | murine leukemia virus | SCID | severe combined immunodeficiency |
| NAP | neutrophil activating peptide | | |
| NBT | nitro blue tetrazolium | SDS-PAGE | sodium dodecylsulfate–polyacrylamide gel electrophoresis |
| NCF | neutrophil chemotactic factor | | |
| NFAT | nuclear factor of activated T-cells | SEA(B etc.) | *Staphylococcus aureus* enterotoxin A (B etc.) |
| NF$\kappa$B | nuclear transcription factor | | |
| NK | natural killer cell | SIV | Simian immunodeficiency virus |
| NO$\cdot$ | nitric oxide | SLE | systemic lupus erythematosus |
| NOD | nonobese diabetic mouse | SRID | single radial immunodiffusion |
| NZB | New Zealand Black mouse | STAT | signal transducer and activator of transcription |
| NZB$\times$W | New Zealand Black mouse $\times$ NZ White F1 hybrid | | |
| | | TAP | transporter for antigen processing |
| $\cdot$O$_2^-$ | superoxide anion | T ALL | T-acute lymphoblastic leukemia |
| OD | optical density | TB | tubercle bacillus |
| ORF | open reading frame | Tc | cytotoxic T-cell |
| OS | obese strain chicken | T-cell | thymus-derived lymphocyte |
| Ova | ovalbumin | TCR1(2) | T-cell receptor with $\gamma/\delta$ chains (with $\alpha/\beta$ chains) |
| PAF(-R) | platelet activating factor (-receptor) | | |
| PCA | passive cutaneous anaphylaxis | TdT | terminal deoxynucleotidyl transferase |
| PCR | polymerase chain reaction | | |
| PG(E) | prostaglandin (E etc.) | TG-A-L | polylysine with polyalanyl side-chains randomly tipped with tyrosine and glutamic acid |
| PHA | phytohemagglutinin | | |
| phox | phagocyte oxidase | | |
| PIP$_2$ | phosphatidylinositol diphosphate | TGF$\beta$ | transforming growth factor-$\beta$ |
| PKC | protein kinase C | T$_{H(1/2)}$ | T-helper cell (subset 1 or 2) |
| PLC | phospholipase C | T$_{HP}$ | T-helper precursor |
| PMN | polymorphonuclear neutrophil | TLI | total lymphoid irradiation |
| PMT | photomultiplier tube | TM | transmembrane |
| PNH | paroxysmal nocturnal hemoglobinuria | TNF | tumor necrosis factor |
| | | Ts | suppressor T-cell |
| PPD | purified protein derivative from *Mycobacterium tuberculosis* | TSAb | thyroid stimulating antibodies |
| | | TSH(R) | thyroid stimulating hormone (receptor) |
| PTK | protein tyrosine kinase | | |
| PWM | pokeweed mitogen | tum- | strongly immunogenic mutant tumors |
| RA | rheumatoid arthritis | | |
| RANTES | regulated upon activation normal T-cell expressed and secreted chemokine | V$\alpha$($\beta$/$\gamma$/$\delta$) | variable part of TCR $\alpha$($\beta$/$\gamma$/$\delta$) chain |
| | | *V* gene | variable region gene for immunoglobulin or T-cell receptor |
| RAST | radioallergosorbent test | | |
| RF | rheumatoid factor | V$_H$ | variable part of Ig heavy chain |
| Rh(D) | rhesus blood group (D) | VIP | vasoactive intestinal peptide |
| ROI | reactive oxygen intermediates | V$_L$ | variable part of light chain |
| SAP | serum amyloid P | V$_{\kappa/\lambda}$ | variable part of $\kappa$($\lambda$) light chain |
| SC | Ig secretory component | VLA | very late antigens |
| SCF | stem cell factor | VNTR | variable number of tandem repeats |
| scFv | single chain variable region antibody fragment (V$_H$ + V$_L$ joined by a flexible linker) | VP1 | virus-specific peptide 1 |
| | | XL | X-linked |

# USER GUIDE

Throughout the illustrations standard forms have been used for commonly-occurring cells and pathways. A key to these is given in the figure below.

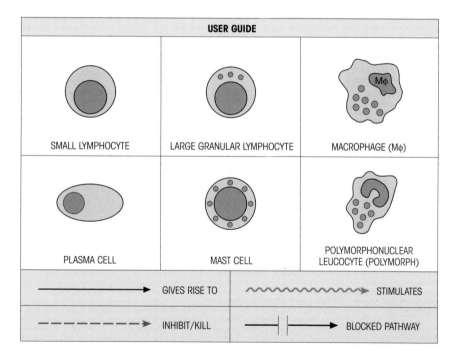

# THE BASIS OF IMMUNOLOGY

This section attempts to provide an introductory broad canvas of immunology upon which the more detailed picture of the subject with its ramifications and widespread impact can subsequently be painted. In essence, immunologic systems have evolved to combat infection but they resemble the nervous system in the sense that we are born with innate functions but acquire more flexible and sophisticated behavior through learning processes. In Chapter 1 we examine the **innate defense mechanisms** which are constitutional and do not improve on repeated contact with the same infectious agent. They rely primarily on the professional phagocytic cells to deal with lower organisms and natural killer cells for viruses, backed up by antimicrobial factors such as complement, acute phase proteins, lysozyme and the interferons. The innate mechanisms, faced with the mutational versatility of the teeming external microbial hordes, do not have universal efficacy and Chapter 2 chronicles the tremendous gains offered by the evolution of the **specific acquired responses**. We describe how large populations of lymphocytes, each with its own individual specificity for a given microbial component, produce effector responses which mesh with the innate mechanisms to provide strong protection against a wide range of both extracellular and intracellular infections. Furthermore, the memory imprinted on the system through the clonal expansion of specific lymphocytes on first contact with the foreign molecule establishes the basis for a more vigorous response on any second contact, this of course being the principle underlying vaccination health programs.

# C H A P T E R 1

# INNATE IMMUNITY

## C O N T E N T S

We live in a potentially hostile world filled with a bewildering array of infectious agents (figure 1.1) of diverse shape, size, composition and subversive character which would very happily use us as rich sanctuaries for propagating their 'selfish genes' had we not also developed a series of defense mechanisms at least their equal in effectiveness and ingenuity (except in the case of many parasitic infections where the situation is best described as an uneasy and often unsatisfactory truce). It is these defense mechanisms which can establish a state of immunity against infection (Latin *immunitas*, freedom from) and whose operation provides the basis for the delightful subject called 'Immunology'.

Aside from ill-understood constitutional factors which make one species innately susceptible and another resistant to certain infections, a number of nonspecific antimicrobial systems (e.g. phagocytosis) have been recognized which are **innate** in the sense that they are not intrinsically affected by prior contact with the infectious agent. We shall discuss these systems and examine how, in the state of **specific acquired immunity**, their effectiveness can be greatly increased.

## EXTERNAL BARRIERS AGAINST INFECTION

The simplest way to avoid infection is to prevent the microorganisms from gaining access to the body (figure 1.2). The major line of defense is of course the skin which, when intact, is impermeable to most

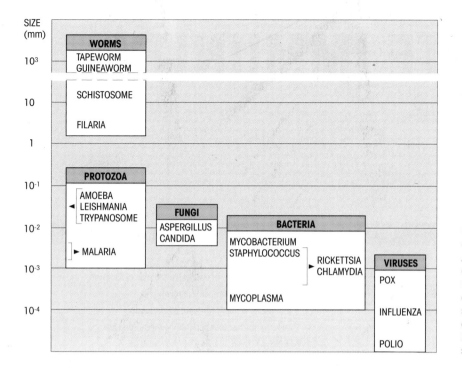

**Figure 1.1. The formidable range of infectious agents which confronts the immune system.** Although not normally classified as such because of their lack of a cell wall, the mycoplasmas are included under bacteria for convenience. Fungi adopt many forms and approximate values for some of the smallest forms are given. ⌐►, range of sizes observed for the organism(s) indicated by the arrow; ◄⌐, the organisms listed have the size denoted by the arrow.

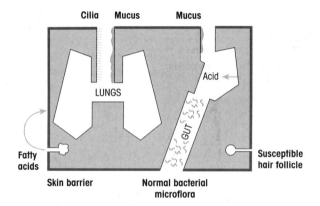

**Figure 1.2. The first lines of defense against infection:** protection at the external body surfaces.

infectious agents; when there is skin loss, as for example in burns, infection becomes a major problem. Additionally, most bacteria fail to survive for long on the skin because of the direct inhibitory effects of lactic acid and fatty acids in sweat and sebaceous secretions and the low pH which they generate. An exception is *Staphylococcus aureus* which often infects the relatively vulnerable hair follicles and glands.

Mucus, secreted by the membranes lining the inner surfaces of the body, acts as a protective barrier to block the adherence of bacteria to epithelial cells. Microbial and other foreign particles trapped within the adhesive mucus are removed by mechanical stratagems such as ciliary movement, coughing and sneezing. Among other mechanical factors which

help protect the epithelial surfaces, one should also include the washing action of tears, saliva and urine. Many of the secreted body fluids contain bactericidal components, such as acid in gastric juice, spermine and zinc in semen, lactoperoxidase in milk and lysozyme in tears, nasal secretions and saliva.

A totally different mechanism is that of microbial antagonism associated with the normal bacterial flora of the body. This suppresses the growth of many potentially pathogenic bacteria and fungi at superficial sites by competition for essential nutrients or by production of inhibitory substances. To give one example, pathogen invasion is limited by lactic acid produced by particular species of commensal bacteria which metabolize glycogen secreted by the vaginal epithelium. When protective commensals are disturbed by antibiotics, susceptibility to opportunistic infections by *Candida* and *Clostridium difficile* is increased. Gut commensals may also produce colicins, a class of bactericidins which bind to the negatively charged surface of susceptible bacteria and insert a hydrophobic helical hairpin into the membrane; the molecule then undergoes a 'Jekyll and Hyde' transformation to become completely hydrophobic and form a voltage-dependent channel in the membrane which kills by destroying the cell's energy potential. Even at this level, survival is a tough game.

If microorganisms do penetrate the body, two main defensive operations come into play, the destructive

# Milestone 1.1 – Phagocytosis

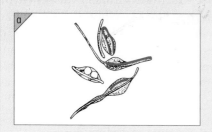
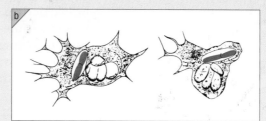
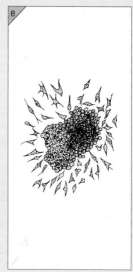
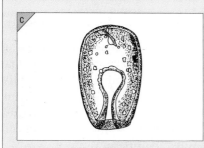
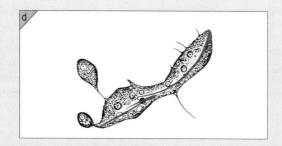

**Figure M1.1.1.** Reproductions of some of the illustrations in Metch-nikoff's book, *Comparative Pathology of Inflammation* (1893). (a) Four leukocytes from the frog, enclosing anthrax bacilli. Some are alive and unstained, others which have been killed have taken up the vesuvine dye and have been coloured; (b) drawing of an anthrax bacillus, stained by vesuvine, in a leukocyte of the frog. The two figures represent two phases of movement of the same frog leukocyte which contains stained anthrax bacilli within its phagocytic vacuole; (c and d) a foreign body (colored) in a starfish larva surrounded by phagocytes which have fused to form a multinucleate plasmodium shown at higher power in (d); (e) this gives a feel for the dynamic attraction of the mobile mesenchymal phagocytes to a foreign intruder within a starfish larva.

The perceptive Russian zoologist, Elie Metchnikoff (1845–1916), recognized that certain specialized cells mediate defense against microbial infections, so fathering the whole concept of cellular immunity. He was intrigued by the motile cells of transparent starfish larvae and made the critical observation that a few hours after the introduction of a rose thorn into these larvae, it became surrounded by these motile cells. A year later, in 1883, he observed that fungal spores can be attacked by the blood cells of *Daphnia*, a tiny metozoan which, also being transparent, can be studied directly under the microscope. He went on to extend his investigations to mammalian leukocytes, showing their ability to engulf microorganisms, a process which he termed **phagocytosis**.

Because he found this process to be even more effective in animals recovering from infection, he came to a somewhat polarized view that phagocytosis provided the main, if not the only, defense against infection. He went on to define the existence of two types of circulating phagocytes: the polymorphonuclear leukocyte, which he termed a 'microphage' and the larger 'macrophage'.

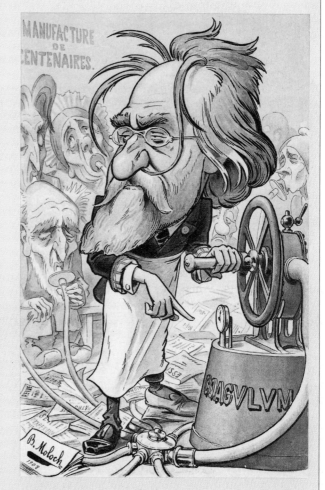

**Figure M1.1.2.** Caricature of Professor Metchnikoff from *Chanteclair*, 1908, No. 4, p. 7. (Reproduction kindly provided by The Wellcome Institute Library, London.)

effect of soluble chemical factors such as bactericidal enzymes and the mechanism of **phagocytosis**—literally 'eating' by the cell (Milestone 1.1).

## PHAGOCYTIC CELLS KILL MICROORGANISMS

### Polymorphs and macrophages are dedicated 'professional' phagocytes

The engulfment and digestion of microorganisms is assigned to two major cell types recognized by Metchnikoff at the turn of the century as microphages and macrophages.

### The polymorphonuclear neutrophil

This cell, the smaller of the two, shares a common hematopoietic stem cell precursor with the other

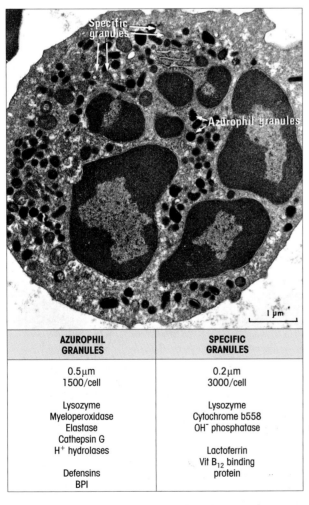

| AZUROPHIL GRANULES | SPECIFIC GRANULES |
|---|---|
| 0.5 μm 1500/cell | 0.2 μm 3000/cell |
| Lysozyme Myeloperoxidase Elastase Cathepsin G H⁺ hydrolases Defensins BPI | Lysozyme Cytochrome b558 OH⁻ phosphatase Lactoferrin Vit B₁₂ binding protein |

**Figure 1.3. Ultrastructure of neutrophil.** The multilobed nucleus and two main types of cytoplasmic granules are well displayed. (Courtesy of Dr D. McLaren.)

formed elements of the blood and is the dominant white cell in the bloodstream. It is a nondividing short-lived cell with a multilobed nucleus and an array of granules which are virtually unstained by histologic dyes such as hematoxylin and eosin, unlike those structures in the closely related eosinophil and basophil (figures 1.3 and 1.4). These neutrophil granules are of two main types: (i) the **primary azurophil granule** which develops early (figure 1.4e), has the typical lysosomal morphology and contains myeloperoxidase together with most of the nonoxidative antimicrobial effectors including defensins, bactericidal/permeability increasing (BPI) factor and cathepsin G (figure 1.3), and (ii) the peroxidase-negative **secondary specific granules** containing lactoferrin, much of the lysozyme, alkaline phosphatase (figure 1.4d) and membrane-bound cytochrome $b_{558}$ which replenishes the plasma membrane enzyme (figure 1.3). The abundant glycogen stores can be utilized by glycolysis enabling the cells to function under anerobic conditions.

### The macrophage

These cells derive from bone marrow promonocytes which, after differentiation to blood monocytes, finally settle in the tissues as mature macrophages where they constitute the **mononuclear phagocyte system** (figure 1.5). They are present throughout the connective tissue and around the basement membrane of small blood vessels and are particularly concentrated in the lung (figure 1.4h; alveolar macrophages), liver (Kupffer cells), and lining of spleen sinusoids and lymph node medullary sinuses where they are strategically placed to filter off foreign material. Other examples are mesangial cells in the kidney glomerulus, brain microglia and osteoclasts in bone. Unlike the polymorphs, they are long-lived cells with significant rough-surfaced endoplasmic reticulum and mitochondria (figure 1.7b) and whereas the polymorphs provide the major defense against pyogenic (pus-forming) bacteria, as a rough generalization it may be said that macrophages are at their best in combating those bacteria (figure 1.4g), viruses and protozoa which are capable of living within the cells of the host.

### Microbes are engulfed by phagocytosis

Before phagocytosis can occur, the microbe must first adhere to the surface of the polymorph or macrophage, an event mediated by some rather primitive recognition mechanism likely to involve

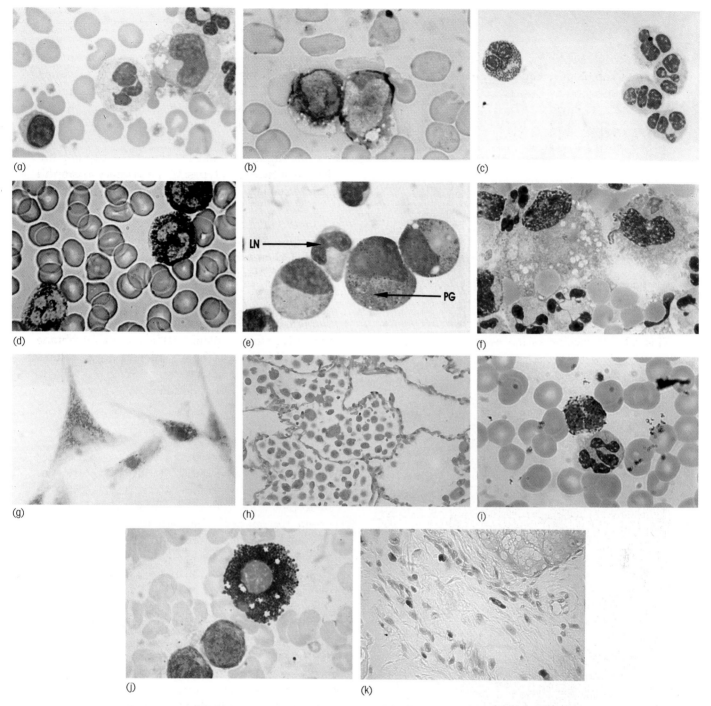

(a)

(b)

(c)

(d)

(e)  LN  PG

(f)

(g)

(h)

(i)

(j)

(k)

**Figure 1.4. Cells involved in innate immunity.** (a) Monocyte, showing 'horseshoe-shaped' nucleus and moderately abundant pale cytoplasm. Note the three multilobed polymorphonuclear neutrophils and the small lymphocyte (bottom left). Romanowsky stain. (b) Two monocytes stained for non-specific esterase with α-naphthyl acetate. Note the vacuolated cytoplasm. The small cell with focal staining at the top is a T-lymphocyte. (c) Four polymorphonuclear leukocytes (neutrophils) and one eosinophil. The multilobed nuclei and the cytoplasmic granules are clearly shown, those of the eosinophil being heavily stained. (d) Polymorphonuclear neutrophil showing cytoplasmic granules stained for alkaline phosphatase. (e) Early neutrophils in bone marrow. The primary azurophilic granules (PG) originally clustered near the nucleus, move towards the periphery where the neutrophil-specific granules are generated by the Golgi apparatus as the cell matures. The nucleus gradually becomes lobular (LN). Giemsa. (f) Inflammatory cells from the site of a brain hemorrhage showing the large active macrophage in the center with phagocytosed red cells and prominent vacuoles. To the right is

a monocyte with horseshoe-shaped nucleus and cytoplasmic bilirubin crystals (hematoidin). Several multilobed neutrophils are clearly delineated. Giemsa. (g) Macrophages in monolayer cultures after phagocytosis of mycobacteria (stained red). Carbol-Fuchsin counterstained with Malachite Green. (h) Numerous plump alveolar macrophages within air spaces in the lung. (i) Basophil with heavily staining granules compared with a neutrophil (below). (j) Mast cell from bone marrow. Round central nucleus surrounded by large darkly staining granules. Two small red cell precursors are shown at the bottom. Romanowsky stain. (k) Tissue mast cells in skin stained with Toluidine Blue. The intracellular granules are metachromatic and stain reddish purple. Note the clustering in relation to dermal capillaries. (The slides from which illustrations (a), (b), (d), (e), (f), (i) and (j) were reproduced were very kindly provided by Mr M. Watts of the Department of Haematology, Middlesex Hospital Medical School; (c) was kindly supplied by Professor J.J. Owen; (g) by Drs P. Lydyard and G. Rook; (h) by Dr Meryl Griffiths and (k) by Professor N. Woolf.)

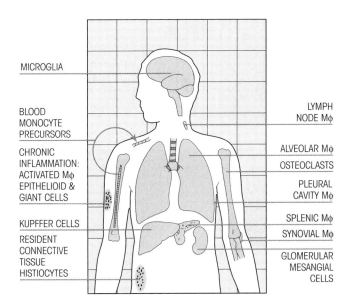

**Figure 1.5. The mononuclear phagocyte system.** Promonocyte precursors in the bone marrow develop into circulating blood monocytes which eventually become distributed throughout the body as mature macrophages (Mφ) as shown. The other major phagocytic cell, the polymorphonuclear neutrophil, is largely confined to the bloodstream except when recruited into sites of acute inflammation.

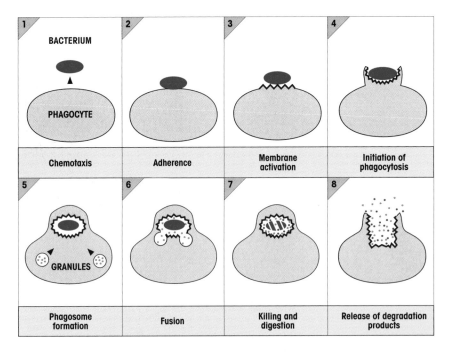

**Figure 1.6. Phagocytosis and killing of a bacterium.** Stage 3/4, respiratory burst and activation of NADPH oxidase; stage 5, damage by reactive oxygen intermediates; stage 6/7, damage by peroxidase, cationic proteins, lysozyme and lactoferrin.

carbohydrate elements. Depending on its nature, a particle attached to the surface membrane may initiate the ingestion phase by activating an actin–myosin contractile system which extends pseudopods around the particle (figures 1.6 and 1.7); as adjacent receptors sequentially attach to the surface of the microbe, the plasma membrane is pulled around the particle just like a 'zipper' until it is completely enclosed in a vacuole (phagosome; figures 1.6 and 1.8). Events are now moving smartly and within 1 minute the cytoplasmic granules fuse with the phagosome and discharge their contents around the imprisoned microorganism (figure 1.8) which is subject to a formidable battery of microbicidal mechanisms.

## There is an array of killing mechanisms

### Killing by reactive oxygen intermediates

Trouble starts for the invader from the moment phagocytosis is initiated. There is a dramatic increase in activity of the hexose monophosphate shunt generating reduced nicotinamide-adenine-dinucleotide phosphate (NADPH). Electrons pass from the NADPH to a flavine adenine dinucleotide (FAD)-containing membrane flavoprotein and thence to a unique plasma membrane **cytochrome (cyt b$_{558}$).** This has the very low midpoint redox potential of $-245\,\text{mV}$ which allows it to reduce molecular oxygen

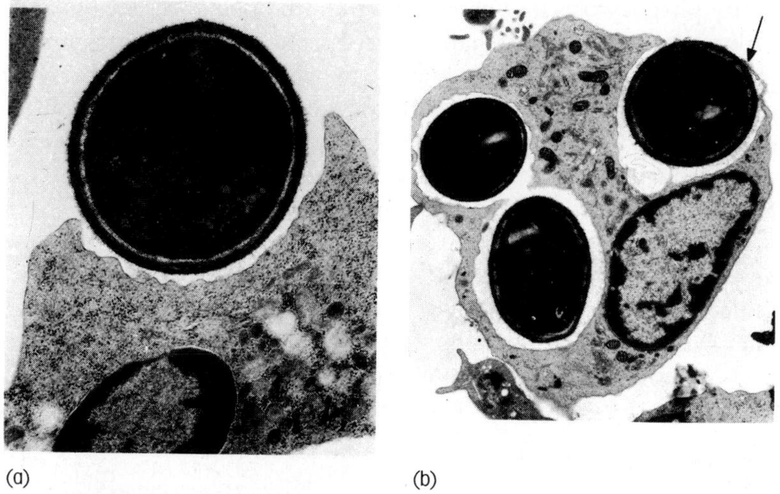

**Figure 1.7. Adherence and phagocytosis.**
(a) Phagocytosis of *Candida albicans* by a polymorpho-nuclear leukocyte (neutrophil). Adherence to the surface initiates enclosure of the fungal particle within arms of cytoplasm. Lysosomal granules are abundant but mito-chondria are rare (× 15 000). (b) Phagocytosis of *C. albicans* by a monocyte showing near completion of phagosome formation (arrowed) around one organism and complete ingestion of two others (× 5000). (Courtesy of Dr H. Valdimarsson.)

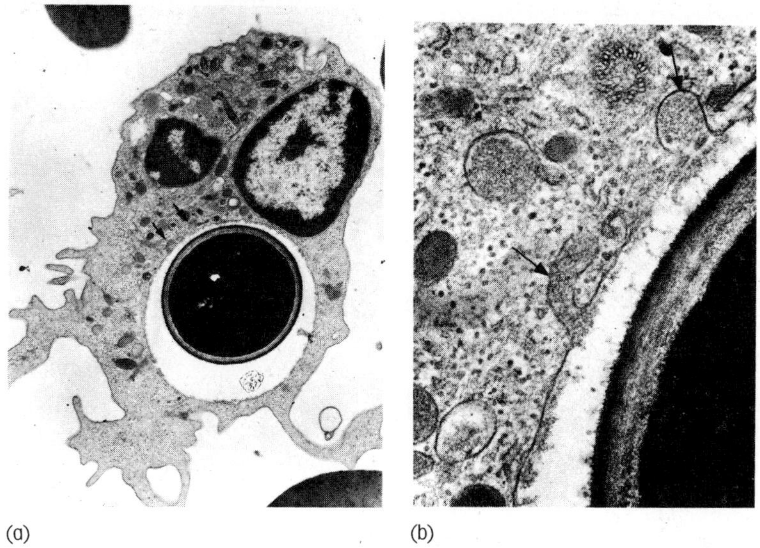

**Figure 1.8. Phagolysosome formation.**
(a) Neutrophil 30 minutes after ingestion of *C. albicans*. The cytoplasm is already partly degranulated and two lysosomal granules (arrowed) are fusing with the phago-cytic vacuole. Two lobes of the nucleus are evident (× 5000). (b) Higher magnification of (a) showing fusing granules discharging their contents into the phagocytic vacuole (arrowed) (× 33 000). (Courtesy of Dr H. Valdimarsson.)

directly to superoxide anion (figure 1.9a). Thus the key reaction catalysed by this NADPH oxidase which initiates the formation of reactive oxygen intermediates (ROI) is:

$$NADPH + O_2 \xrightarrow{\text{oxidase}} NADP^+ + \cdot O_2^-$$
$$\text{(superoxide anion)}$$

The superoxide anion undergoes conversion to hydrogen peroxide under the influence of superoxide dismutase, and subsequently to hydroxyl radicals ($\cdot OH$). Each of these products has remarkable chemical reactivity with a wide range of molecular targets making them formidable microbicidal agents; $\cdot OH$ in particular is one of the most reactive free radicals known. Furthermore, the combination of peroxide, myeloperoxidase and halide ions constitutes a potent halogenating system capable of killing both bacteria and viruses (figure 1.9a). Although $H_2O_2$ and the

halogenated compounds are not as active as the free radicals, they are more stable and therefore diffuse further, making them toxic to microorganisms in the extracellular vicinity.

### Killing by reactive nitrogen intermediates

Nitric oxide surfaced prominently as a physiologic mediator when it was shown to be identical with endothelium-derived relaxing factor. This has proved to be just one of its many roles (including the mediation of penile erection, would you believe it!), but of major interest in the present context is its formation by an inducible NO synthase (iNOS) within most cells but particularly macrophages and human neutrophils thereby generating a powerful antimicrobial system (figure 1.9b). Whereas the NADPH oxidase is dedicated to the killing of extracellular organisms taken up by phagocytosis and cornered within the phagocytic vacuole, the NO mechanism can operate against microbes which invade the cytosol; so, it is not surprising that the majority of nonphagocytic cells which may be infected by viruses and other parasites are endowed with an iNOS capability. The mechanism of action may be through degradation of the Fe–S prosthetic groups of certain electron transport enzymes, depletion of iron and production of toxic ·ONOO radicals. The *N-ramp* gene linked with resistance to microbes such as bacille Calmette–Guérin (BCG), *Salmonella* and *Leishmania* which can live within an intracellular habitat, is now known to express a protein forming a transmembrane channel which may be involved in transporting NO across lysosome membranes.

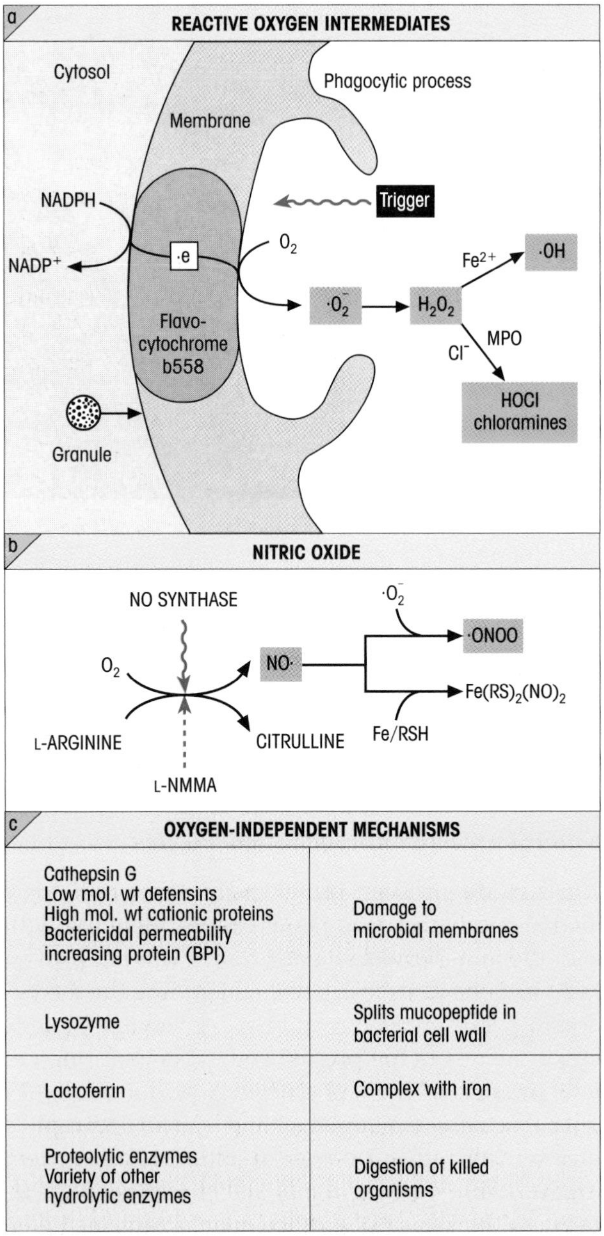


c OXYGEN-INDEPENDENT MECHANISMS

| | |
|---|---|
| Cathepsin G<br>Low mol. wt defensins<br>High mol. wt cationic proteins<br>Bactericidal permeability increasing protein (BPI) | Damage to microbial membranes |
| Lysozyme | Splits mucopeptide in bacterial cell wall |
| Lactoferrin | Complex with iron |
| Proteolytic enzymes<br>Variety of other hydrolytic enzymes | Digestion of killed organisms |

**Figure 1.9. Microbicidal mechanisms of phagocytic cells.** (a) Production of reactive oxygen intermediates. Electrons from NADPH are transferred by the flavocytochrome oxidase enzyme to molecular oxygen to form the microbicidal molecular species shown in the boxes. (*For the more studious*—The phagocytosis triggering agent binds to a classic G-protein linked 7 transmembrane domain receptor which activates an intracellular GTP-binding protein. This in turn activates an array of enzymes: phosphoinositol-3 kinase concerned in the cytoskeletal reorganization underlying chemotactic responses (p. 11), phospholipase-Cγ2 mediating events leading to lysosome degranulation and phosphorylation of p47 phox through activation of protein kinase C, and the MEK and MAP kinase systems which oversee the assembly of the NADPH oxidase. This is composed of the membrane cytochrome $b_{558}$, consisting of a p21 heme protein linked to gp91 with binding sites for NADPH and FAD on its intracellular aspect, to which phosphorylated p47 and p67 translocate from the cytosol on activation of the oxidase.) (b) Generation of nitric oxide. The enzyme, which structurally resembles the NADH oxidase, can be inhibited by the arginine analog N-monomethyl-L-arginine (L-NMMA). Combination of NO with superoxide anion yields the highly toxic peroxynitrite radical ·NOO which cleaves on protonation to form reactive ·OH and $NO_2$ molecules. NO can form mononuclear iron dithioldinitroso complexes leading to iron depletion and inhibition of several enzymes. (c) The basis of oxygen-independent antimicrobial systems.

### *Killing by preformed antimicrobials* (figure 1.9c)

These molecules, contained within the polymorph granules, contact the ingested microorganism when fusion with the phagosome occurs. The dismutation of superoxide consumes hydrogen ions and raises the pH of the vacuole gently so allowing the family of cationic proteins and peptides to function optimally. The latter, known as **defensins**, are approximately 3.5–4 kDa and invariably rich in arginine, and reach incredibly high concentrations within the phagosome, of the order of 20–100 mg/ml. Like the bacterial colicins described above, they have an amphipathic structure which allows them to insert into microbial membranes to form destabilizing voltage-regulated ion channels (who copied whom?). These antibiotic peptides at concentrations of 10–100 μg/ml, act as disinfectants against a wide spectrum of Gram-positive and -negative bacteria, many fungi and a number of enveloped viruses. Many exhibit remarkable selectivity for prokaryotic and eukaryotic microbes relative to host cells, partly dependent upon lipid composition. One must be impressed by the ability of this surprisingly simple tool to discriminate large classes of nonself cells, i.e. microbes from self.

If this were not enough, further damage is inflicted on the bacterial membranes both by neutral proteinase (cathepsin G) action and by direct transfer to the microbial surface of a protein, BP1, which increases bacterial permeability. Low pH, lysozyme and lactoferrin constitute bactericidal or bacteriostatic factors which are oxygen independent and can function under anerobic circumstances. Finally, the killed organisms are digested by hydrolytic enzymes and the degradation products released to the exterior (figure 1.6).

By now, the reader may be excused a little smugness as she or he shelters behind the impressive antimicrobial potential of the phagocytic cells. But there are snags to consider; our formidable array of weaponry is useless unless the phagocyte can (i) 'home onto' the microorganism, (ii) adhere to it, and (iii) respond by the membrane activation which initiates engulfment. Some bacteria do produce chemical substances such as the peptide formyl.Met.Leu.Phe. which directionally attract leukocytes, a process known as **chemotaxis**; some organisms do adhere to the phagocyte surface and some do spontaneously provide the appropriate membrane initiation signal. However, our teeming microbial adversaries are continually mutating to produce new species which may outwit the defenses by doing none of these. What then? The body has solved these problems with the effortless ease that comes with a few million years of evolution by developing the **complement** system.

## COMPLEMENT FACILITATES PHAGOCYTOSIS

### Complement and its activation

Complement is the name given to a complex series of some 20 proteins which, along with blood clotting, fibrinolysis and kinin formation, forms one of the triggered enzyme systems found in plasma. These systems characteristically produce a rapid, highly amplified response to a trigger stimulus mediated by a cascade phenomenon where the product of one reaction is the enzymic catalyst of the next.

Some of the complement components are designated by the letter 'C' followed by a number which is related more to the chronology of its discovery than to its position in the reaction sequence. The most abundant and the most pivotal component is C3 which has a molecular weight of 195 kDa and is present in plasma at a concentration of around 1.2 mg/ml.

### C3 undergoes slow spontaneous cleavage

Under normal circumstances, an internal thiolester bond in C3 (figure 1.10) becomes activated spontaneously at a very slow rate either through reaction with water or with trace amounts of a plasma proteolytic enzyme to form a reactive intermediate, either the split product C3b, or a functionally similar molecule designated C3i or C3($H_2O$). In the presence of $Mg^{2+}$ this can complex with another complement component, factor B, which then undergoes cleavage by a normal plasma enzyme (factor D) to generate $\overline{C3bBb}$. Note that conventionally, a bar over a complex denotes enzymic activity and that on cleavage of a complement component, the larger product is generally given the suffix 'b' and the smaller 'a'.

$\overline{C3bBb}$ has an important new enzymic activity: it is a **C3 convertase** which can split C3 to give C3a and C3b. We will shortly discuss the important biologic consequences of C3 cleavage in relation to microbial defenses, but under normal conditions there must be some mechanism to restrain this process to a 'tick-over' level since it can also give rise to more $\overline{C3bBb}$, that is, we are dealing with a potentially runaway **positive-feedback loop** (figure 1.11). As with all potentially explosive triggered cascades, there are powerful regulatory mechanisms.

### C3b levels are normally tightly controlled

In solution, the $\overline{C3bBb}$ convertase is unstable and factor B is readily displaced by another component, factor H, to form C3bH which is susceptible to attack by the C3b inactivator, factor I (figure 1.12; further discussed on p. 312). The inactivated iC3b is biologically inactive and undergoes further degradation by proteases in the body fluids. Other regulatory mechanisms are discussed at a later stage (see p. 313).

### C3 convertase is stabilized on microbial surfaces

A number of microorganisms can activate the $\overline{C3bBb}$ convertase to generate large amounts of C3 cleavage products by stabilizing the enzyme on their (carbohydrate) surfaces, thereby protecting the C3b from factor H. Another protein, properdin, acts subsequently on this bound convertase to stabilize it even further. As C3 is split by the surface membrane-bound enzyme to nascent C3b, it undergoes conformational change and its potentially reactive internal thiolester bond becomes exposed. Since the half-life of nascent C3b is less than 100 μsec, it can only diffuse a

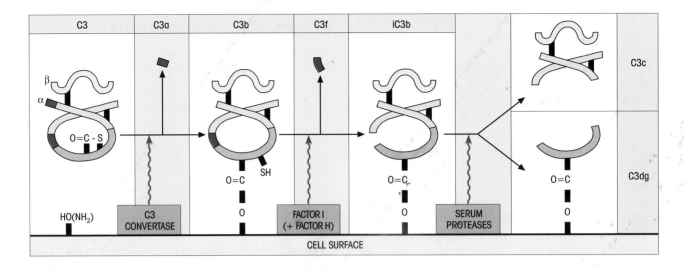

**Figure 1.10. Structural basis for the cleavage of C3 by C3 convertase** and its covalent binding to ·OH or ·NH₂ groups at the cell surface through exposure of the internal thiolester bonds. Further cleavage leaves the progressively smaller fragments, C3dg and C3d, attached to the membrane. (Based essentially on Law S.H.A. & Reid K.B.M. (1988) *Complement*, figure 2.4. IRL Press, Oxford.)

short distance before reacting covalently with local hydroxyl or amino groups available at the microbial cell surface (figure 1.10). Each catalytic site thereby leads to the clustering of large numbers of C3b molecules on the microorganism. This series of reactions leading to C3 breakdown provoked directly by microbes has been called **the alternative pathway** of complement activation (figure 1.12).

### The post-C3 pathway generates a membrane attack complex

Recruitment of a further C3b molecule into the C3bBb enzymic complex generates a C5 convertase which activates C5 by proteolytic cleavage releasing a small polypeptide, C5a, and leaving the large C5b fragment loosely bound to C3b. Sequential attachment of C6 and C7 to C5b forms a complex with a transient membrane binding site and an affinity for the β-peptide chain of C8. The C8α chain sits in the membrane and directs the conformational changes in C9 which transform it into an amphipathic molecule capable of insertion into the lipid bilayer (cf. the colicins, p. 4) and polymerization to an annular **membrane attack complex** (MAC; figures 1.13 and 2.3). This forms a transmembrane channel fully permeable to electrolytes and water, and due to the high internal colloid osmotic pressure of cells, there is a net influx of Na⁺ and water frequently leading to lysis.

## Complement has a range of defensive biological functions

These can be grouped conveniently under three headings:

### 1   C3b adheres to complement receptors

Phagocytic cells have receptors for C3b (CR1) and iC3b (CR3) which facilitate the adherence of C3b-coated microorganisms to the cell surface (discussed more fully on p. 263).

### 2   Biologically active fragments are released

C3a and C5a, the small peptides split from the parent molecules during complement activation, have

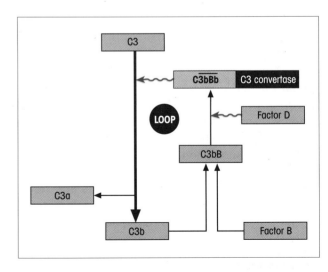

**Figure 1.11. The C3 convertase feedback loop.** ←∿∿ represents an activation process. The horizontal bar above a component designates its activation.

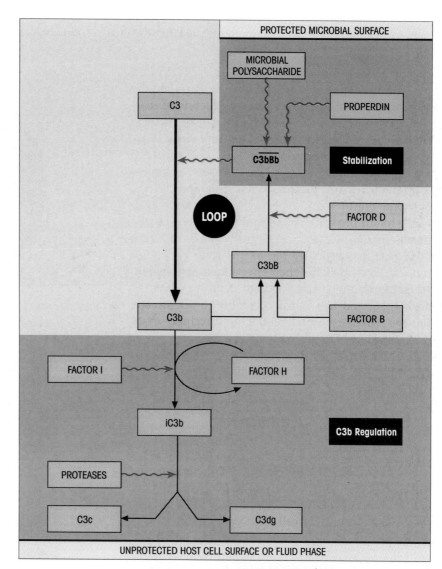

**Figure 1.12. Microbial activation of the alternative complement pathway** by stabilization of the C3 convertase (C3bBb), and its control by factors H and I. When bound to the surface of a host cell or in the fluid phase, the C3b in the convertase is said to be 'unprotected' in that its affinity for factor H is much greater than for factor B and is therefore susceptible to breakdown by factors H and I. On a microbial surface, C3b binds factor B more strongly than factor H and is therefore 'protected' from or 'stabilized' against cleavage—even more so when subsequently bound by properdin. Although in phylogenetic terms this is the oldest complement pathway, it was discovered after a separate pathway to be discussed in the next chapter, and so has the confusing designation 'alternative'.

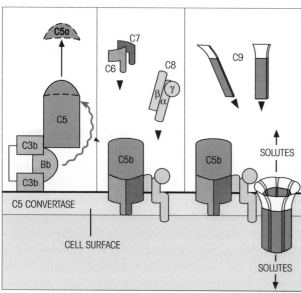

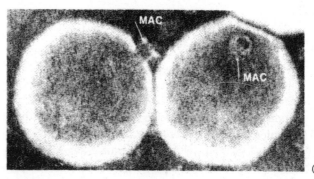

**Figure 1.13. Post-C3 pathway generating C5a and the C5b–9 membrane attack complex (MAC).** (a) Cartoon of molecular assembly. The conformational change in C9 protein structure which converts it from a hydrophilic to an amphipathic molecule (bearing both hydrophobic and hydrophilic regions) can be interrupted by an antibody raised against linear peptides derived from C9; since the antibody does not react with the soluble or membrane-bound forms of the molecule, it must be detecting an intermediate structure transiently revealed in a deep-seated structural rearrangement. (b) Electron micrograph of a membrane C5b–9 complex incorporated into liposomal membranes clearly showing the annular structure. The cylindrical complex is seen from the side inserted into the membrane of the liposome on the left, and end-on in that on the right. Although in itself a rather splendid structure, formation of the annular C9 cylinder is probably not essential for cytotoxic perturbation of the target cell membrane, since this can be achieved by insertion of amphipathic C9 molecules in numbers too few to form a clearly defined MAC. (Courtesy of Professor J. Tranum-Jensen and Dr S. Bhakdi.)

several important actions. Both act directly on phagocytes, especially neutrophils, to stimulate the respiratory burst associated with production of reactive oxygen intermediates and to enhance the expression of surface receptors for C3b and iC3b. Also, both are **anaphylatoxins** in that they are capable of triggering mediator release from mast cells (figures 1.4k and 1.14) and their circulating counterpart the basophil (figure 1.4i), a phenomenon of such relevance to our present discussion that I have presented details of the mediators and their actions in figure 1.15; note in particular the chemotactic properties of these mediators and their effects on blood vessels. In its own right, C5a is a potent neutrophil chemoactic agent and has a striking ability to act directly on the capillary endothelium to produce vasodilatation and increased permeability, an effect which seems to be prolonged by leukotriene B$_4$ released from activated mast cells, neutrophils and macrophages.

### 3   The terminal complex can induce membrane lesions

As described above, the insertion of the membrane attack complex into a membrane may bring about cell lysis. Providentially, complement is relatively inefficient at lysing the cell membranes of the autologous host due to the presence of control proteins (cf. p. 313).

## COMPLEMENT CAN MEDIATE AN ACUTE INFLAMMATORY REACTION

We can now put together an effectively orchestrated defensive scenario initiated by activation of the alternative complement pathway (see figure 1.16).

In the first act, $\overline{C3bBb}$ is stabilized on the surface of the microbe and cleaves large amounts of C3. The C3a fragment is released but C3b molecules bind copiously to the microbe. These activate the next step in the sequence to generate C5a and the membrane attack complex (although many organisms will be resistant to its action).

### The mast cell plays a central role

The next act sees C3a and C5a, together with the mediators they trigger from the mast cell, acting to recruit polymorphonuclear neutrophils and further plasma complement components to the site of microbial invasion. The relaxation induced in arteriolar walls causes increased blood flow and dilatation of

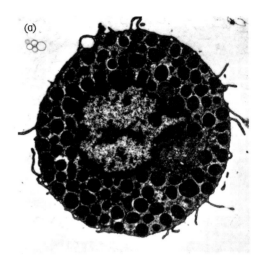

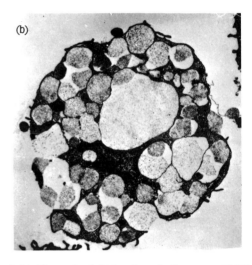

**Figure 1.14.  The mast cell.** (a) A resting cell with many membrane-bound granules containing preformed mediators. (b) A triggered mast cell. Note that the granules have released their contents and are morphologically altered, being larger and less electron dense. Although most of the altered granules remain within the circumference of the cell, they are open to the extracellular space. (Electron micrographs ×5400.) (Courtesy of Drs D. Lawson, C. Fewtrell, B. Gomperts and M.C. Raff from (1975) *Journal of Experimental Medicine* **142**, 391.)

the small vessels, while contraction of capillary endothelial cells allows exudation of plasma proteins. Under the influence of the chemotaxins, neutrophils slow down and the surface adhesion molecules they are stimulated to express cause them to marginate to the walls of the capillaries where they pass through gaps between the endothelial cells (diapedesis) and move up the concentration gradient of chemotactic factors until they come face to face with the C3b-coated microbe. Adherence to the neutrophil C3b-receptors then takes place, C3a and C5a at relatively high concentrations in the chemotactic gradient activate the respiratory burst and, hey presto, the slaughter of the last act can begin!

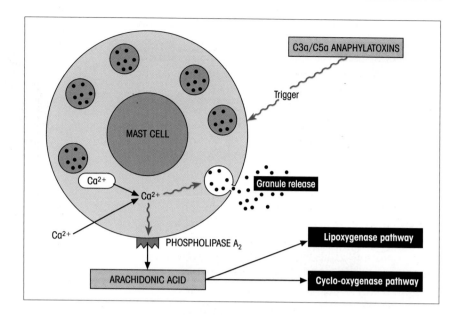

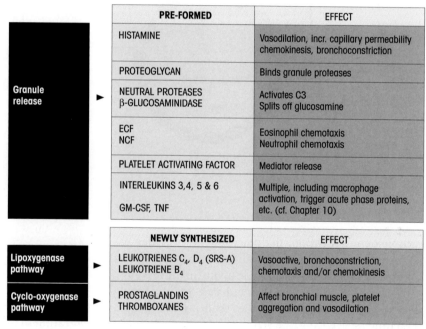

| PRE-FORMED | EFFECT |
|---|---|
| HISTAMINE | Vasodilation, incr. capillary permeability chemokinesis, bronchoconstriction |
| PROTEOGLYCAN | Binds granule proteases |
| NEUTRAL PROTEASES β-GLUCOSAMINIDASE | Activates C3 Splits off glucosamine |
| ECF NCF | Eosinophil chemotaxis Neutrophil chemotaxis |
| PLATELET ACTIVATING FACTOR | Mediator release |
| INTERLEUKINS 3,4, 5 & 6 GM-CSF, TNF | Multiple, including macrophage activation, trigger acute phase proteins, etc. (cf. Chapter 10) |

| NEWLY SYNTHESIZED | EFFECT |
|---|---|
| LEUKOTRIENES $C_4$, $D_4$ (SRS-A) LEUKOTRIENE $B_4$ | Vasoactive, bronchoconstriction, chemotaxis and/or chemokinesis |
| PROSTAGLANDINS THROMBOXANES | Affect bronchial muscle, platelet aggregation and vasodilation |

Granule release ▶

Lipoxygenase pathway ▶

Cyclo-oxygenase pathway ▶

**Figure 1.15. Mast cell triggering leading to release of mediators by two major pathways:** (i) release of preformed mediators present in the granules, and (ii) the metabolism of arachidonic acid produced through activation of a phospholipase. Intracellular $Ca^{2+}$ and cAMP are central to the initiation of these events but details are still unclear. Mast cell heterogeneity is discussed on p. 330. (ECF = eosinophil chemotactic factor; NCF = neutrophil chemotactic factor. Chemotaxis refers to directed migration of granulocytes up the concentration gradient of the mediator while chemokinesis describes randomly increased motility of these cells.)

The processes of capillary dilatation (redness), exudation of plasma proteins and also of fluid (edema) due to hydrostatic and osmotic pressure changes, and accumulation of neutrophils are collectively termed the **acute inflammatory response**.

## Macrophages can also do it

Although not yet established with the same confidence that surrounds the role of the mast cell in acute inflammation, the concept seems to be emerging that the tissue macrophage may mediate a parallel series of events with the same final end result. Non-

specific phagocytic events and certain bacterial toxins such as the lipopolysaccharides (LPS) can activate macrophages, but the phagocytosis of C3b-opsonized microbes and the direct action of C5a generated through complement activation are guaranteed to goad the cell into copious secretion of soluble mediators of the acute inflammatory response (figure 1.17).

These upregulate the expression of adhesion molecules for neutrophils on the surface of endothelial cells, increase capillary permeability and promote the chemotaxis and activation of the polymorphonuclear neutrophils themselves. Thus, under the stimulus of

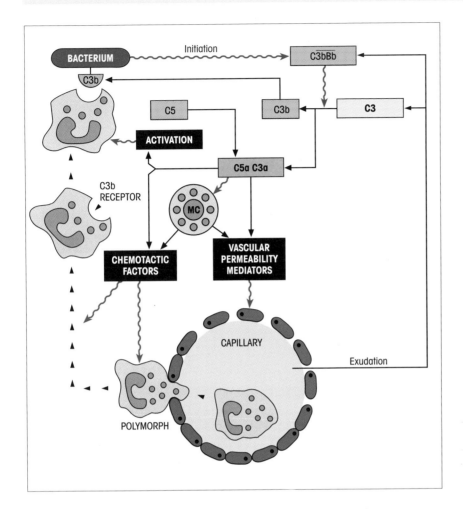

**Figure 1.16. The defensive strategy of the acute inflammatory reaction initiated by bacterial activation of the alternative C pathway.** Directions: start with the activation of the C3bBb C3 convertase by the bacterium, notice the generation of C3b (which binds to the bacterium), C3a and C5a, and recruitment of mast cell mediators; follow their effect on capillary dilatation and exudation of plasma proteins and their chemotactic attraction of polymorphs to the C3b-coated bacterium and triumph in their adherence and final activation for the kill.

complement activation, the macrophage provides a pattern of cellular events which reinforces the mast cell-mediated pathway leading to acute inflammation — yet another of the body's fail-safe redundancy systems (often known as the 'belt and braces' principle).

## HUMORAL MECHANISMS PROVIDE A SECOND DEFENSIVE STRATEGY

Turning now to those defense systems which are mediated entirely by soluble factors, we recollect that many microbes activate the complement system and may be lysed by the insertion of the membrane attack complex. The spread of infection may be limited by enzymes released through tissue injury which activate the clotting system. Of the soluble bactericidal substances elaborated by the body, perhaps the most abundant and widespread is the enzyme lysozyme, a muramidase which splits the exposed peptidoglycan wall of susceptible bacteria (cf. figure 10.1).

## Acute phase proteins increase in response to infection

A number of plasma proteins collectively termed acute phase proteins show a dramatic increase in concentration in response to early 'alarm' mediators such as macrophage-derived interleukin-1 (IL-1) released as a result of infection or tissue injury. These include C-reactive protein (CRP), mannose-binding protein and serum amyloid P component (Table 1.1). Other acute phase proteins showing a more modest rise in concentration include $\alpha_1$-antitrypsin, fibrinogen, ceruloplasmin, C9 and factor B. Overall, it seems likely that the acute phase response achieves a beneficial effect through enhancing host resistance, minimizing tissue injury and promoting the resolution and repair of the inflammatory lesion.

To take an example, during an infection, microbial products such as endotoxins stimulate the release of IL-1 which is an endogenous pyrogen (incidentally capable of improving our general defenses by raising

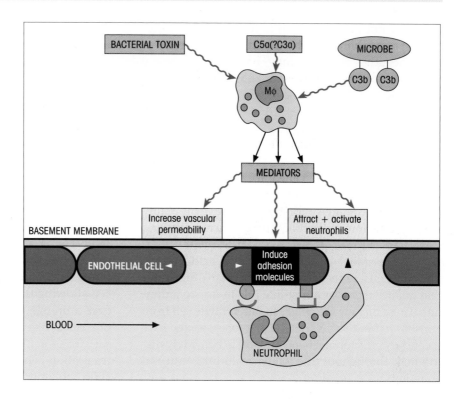

**Figure 1.17. Stimulation by complement components induces macrophage secretion of mediators of the acute inflammatory response.** Blood neutrophils stick to the adhesion molecules on the endothelial cell and use this to provide traction as they force their way between the cells, through the basement membrane (with the help of secreted elastase) and up the chemotactic gradient.

the body temperature) and IL-6. These in turn act on the liver to increase the synthesis and secretion of CRP to such an extent that its plasma concentration may rise 1000-fold.

Human CRP is composed of five identical polypeptide units noncovalently arranged as a cyclic pentamer around a Ca-binding cavity. These **pentraxins** of protein have been around in the animal kingdom for some time since a closely related homolog, limulin, is present in the hemolymph of the horseshoe crab, not exactly a close relative of *Homo sapiens*. A major property of CRP is its ability to bind, in a Ca-dependent fashion, to a number of microorganisms which contain phosphorylcholine in their membranes, the complex having the useful property of activating complement (by the classical and not the alternative pathway with which we are at present familiar). This results in the deposition of C3b on the surface of the microbe which thus becomes **opsonized** (i.e. 'made ready for the table') for adherence to phagocytes.

Yet another member of this pentameric family is the serum amyloid P (SAP) component. This protein can complex with chondroitin sulfate, a cell matrix glycosaminoglycan, and subsequently bind lysosomal enzymes such as cathepsin B released within a focus of inflammation. The degraded SAP becomes a component of the amyloid fibrillar deposits which

accompany chronic infections—it might even be a key initiator of amyloid deposition (cf. p. 391).

A most important acute phase opsonin is the Ca-dependent **mannose-binding protein (MBP)** which

**Table 1.1. Acute phase proteins.**

| Acute phase reactant | Role |
|---|---|
| **Dramatic increases in concentration:** | |
| C-reactive protein | Fixes complement, opsonizes |
| Mannose binding protein | Fixes complement, opsonizes |
| $\alpha_1$-acid glycoprotein | Transport protein |
| Serum amyloid P component | Amyloid component precursor |
| **Moderate increases in concentration:** | |
| $\alpha_1$-proteinase inhibitors | Inhibit bacterial proteases |
| $\alpha_1$-antichymotrypsin | Inhibit bacterial proteases |
| C3, C9, factor B | Increase complement function |
| Ceruloplasmin | $\cdot O_2^-$ scavenger |
| Fibrinogen | Coagulation |
| Angiotensin | Blood pressure |
| Haptoglobin | Bind hemoglobin |
| Fibronectin | Cell attachment |

can react not only with mannose but several other sugars, so enabling it to bind with a wide variety of Gram-negative and -positive bacteria, and some yeasts, viruses and parasites; its subsequent ability to trigger the classical C3 convertase through a novel associated serine protease (MASP), qualifies it as an opsonin. (Please relax, we unravel the secrets of the classical pathway in the next chapter.) MBP is a multiple of trimeric complexes, each unit of which contains a collagen-like region joined to a globular lectin-binding domain. This structure places it in the family of **collectins** (**col**lagen + **lectin**) which have the ability to recognize 'foreign' carbohydrate patterns differing from 'self' surface polysaccharides normally decorated by terminal galactose and sialic acid groups. The collectins, especially MBP, have many attributes that qualify them for a first-line role in innate immunity. These include the ability to differentiate self from nonself, to bind to a variety of microbes, to generate secondary effector mechanisms, and to be widely distributed throughout the body including mucosal secretions.

Interest in the collectin conglutinin has perked up recently with the demonstration first, that it is found in humans and not just in cows, and second, that it can bind to *N*-acetylglucosamine; being polyvalent, this implies an ability to coat bacteria with C3b by cross-linking the available sugar residue in the complement fragment with the bacterial proteoglycan. Although it is not clear whether conglutinin is a member of the acute phase protein family, I mention it here because it embellishes this general idea that the evolution of lectin-like molecules which bind to microbial rather than self-polysaccharides and which can then hitch themselves to the complement system, has proved to be such a useful form of protection for the host. The collectin family has expanded even further to include the surfactant molecules SP-A and SP-D. These are narrower in sugar specificity than MBP but are present in many body fluids. They are particularly prominent in alveolar defense against *Pneumocystis carinii* and *Cryptococcus neoformans*.

For completeness we should also mention scavenger receptors on the macrophage surface, defined by their ability to bind low-density lipoproteins but which can recognize and bind microbial surface molecules and intact bacteria.

### Interferons inhibit viral replication

These are a family of broad-spectrum antiviral agents present in birds, reptiles and fishes as well as the higher animals, and first recognized by the phenomenon of viral interference in which an animal infected with one virus resists superinfection by a second unrelated virus. Different molecular forms of interferon have been identified, all of which have been gene cloned. There are at least 14 different α-interferons (IFNα) produced by leukocytes, while fibroblasts, and probably all cell types, synthesize IFNβ. We will keep a third type (IFNγ), which is not directly induced by viruses, up our sleeves for the moment.

Cells synthesize interferon when infected by a virus and secrete it into the extracellular fluid whence it binds to specific receptors on uninfected neighboring cells. The bound interferon now exerts its antiviral effect in the following way. At least two genes are thought to be derepressed in the interferon-treated cell allowing the synthesis of two new enzymes. The first, a protein kinase, catalyzes the phosphorylation of a ribosomal protein and an initiation factor necessary for protein synthesis, so greatly reducing mRNA translation. The other catalyses the formation of a short polymer of adenylic acid which activates a latent endonuclease; this in turn degrades both viral and host mRNA.

Whatever the precise mechanism of action ultimately proves to be, the net result is to establish a cordon of uninfectable cells around the site of virus infection so restraining its spread. The effectiveness of interferon *in vivo* may be inferred from experiments in which mice injected with an antiserum to murine interferons could be killed by several hundred times less virus than was needed to kill the controls. However, it must be presumed that interferon plays a significant role in the recovery from, as distinct from the prevention of, viral infections.

As a group, the interferons may prove to have a wider biologic role than the control of viral infection. It will be clear, for example, that the induced enzymes described above would act to inhibit host cell division just as effectively as viral replication. The interferons may also modulate the activity of other cells such as the natural killer cells, to be discussed in the following section.

## EXTRACELLULAR KILLING

### Natural killer (NK) cells

Viruses lack the apparatus for self-renewal so it is essential for them to penetrate the cells of the infected host in order to take over its replicative machinery. It is clearly in the interest of the host to find a way to kill such infected cells before the virus has had a chance to reproduce. NK cells appear to do just that when studied *in vitro*.

They are large granular lymphocytes (figure 2.6a) with a characteristic morphology (figure 2.7b). They are thought to recognize structures on high molecular weight glycoproteins which appear on the surface of virally infected cells and which allow them to be differentiated from normal cells. This recognition probably occurs through lectin-like (i.e. carbohydrate binding) receptors on the NK cell surface which bring killer and target into close opposition (figure 1.18a). Activation of the NK cell ensues and leads to polarization of granules between nucleus and target within minutes and extracellular release of their contents into the space between the two cells.

Perhaps the most important of these is a **perforin** or cytolysin bearing some structural homology to C9; like that protein, but without any help other than from $Ca^{2+}$, it can insert itself into the membrane of the target, apparently by binding to phosphorylcholine through its central amphipathic domain. It then polymerizes to form a transmembrane pore with an annular structure, comparable to the complement membrane attack complex (figure 1.18a).

### Target cells are told to commit suicide

Whereas C9-induced cell lysis is brought about through damage to outer membranes followed later by nuclear changes, NK cells kill by activating **apoptosis** (programed cell death), a mechanism present in every cell which leads to self immolation. One sees very rapid nuclear fragmentation effected by a Ca-dependent endonuclease which acts on the vulnerable DNA between nucleosomes to produce the 200 kb 'nucleosome ladder' fragments (figure 1.18b); only afterwards can one detect release of $^{51}Cr$-labeled cytoplasmic proteins through defective cell surface membranes. These nuclear changes are not produced by C9. Thus, although perforin and C9 appear to produce comparable membrane 'pores', there is a dramatic difference in their killing mechanisms.

In addition to perforin, the granules contain tumor necrosis factor β and a family of serine proteases termed **granzymes**, one of which, granzyme B, can function as an NK cytotoxic factor. Another candidate is fully ionized ATP which can cause apoptosis in many different cell types; the effectors themselves are resistant probably due to a lack of ATP receptors on their surface. Each factor alone seems incapable of mimicking the full picture of NK-mediated lysis, but the following seems a likely scenario. Following exo-

cytosis of the granules, perforin precursors are activated and form a membrane pore which acts as a conduit to allow entry of granzyme B and other potential inducers of apoptosis into the target cell. A current view is that granzyme B kills by directly activating an endogenous family of ICE (IL-1β converting enzyme) proteases which subsequently degrade other molecules including the repair enzyme poly (ADP-ribose) polymerase. Chondroitin sulfate A, a protease-resistant highly negatively charged proteoglycan, is also present in the granules and may subserve the function of protecting the NK cell from autolysis by its own lethal agents.

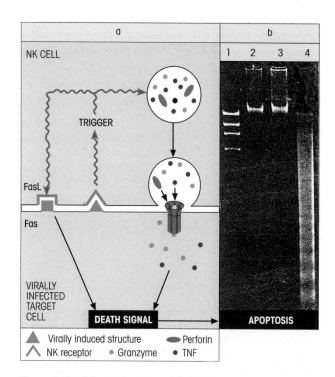

**Figure 1.18. Extracellular killing of virally infected cell by natural killer (NK) cell.** (a) Binding of the NK receptors to the surface of the virally infected cell triggers the extracellular release of perforin molecules from the granules; these polymerize to form transmembrane channels which may facilitate lysis of the target by permitting entry of granzymes, tumor necrosis factor (TNF) and other potentially cytotoxic factors derived from the granules. (Model resembling that proposed by Hudig D., Ewoldt G.R. & Woodward S.L. (1993) *Current Opinion in Immunology* **5**, 90.). Engagement of the NK receptor also activates a parallel killing mechanism which is mediated through the binding of the Fas ligand (FasL) on the effector to the Fas receptor on the target cell thereby delivering a signal for apoptosis. (b) Fragmentation of nucleosome DNA into 200 kb 'ladder' fragments following programed cell death (kindly provided by Dr S. Martin). Lane 1: standards obtained by digestion of λ DNA by *Hind*III; lanes 2 and 3: undegraded DNA from normal control cells; lane 4: characteristic breakdown of DNA from apoptotic cells. The word 'apoptosis' in ancient Greek describes the falling of leaves from trees or of petals from flowers and aptly illustrates apoptosis in cells where they detach from their extracellular matrix support structures. (See figure 12.6 for morphologic appearance of apoptotic cells and figure 7.9 for the detection of apoptosis by flow cytometry.)

Killing by NK cells can still occur in perforin-deficient mice, probably through a parallel mechanism involving **Fas** receptor molecules on the target cell surface. Engagement of Fas by the so-called **Fas-ligand (FasL)** on the effector cell induces an apoptotic signal in the unlucky target.

The various interferons augment NK cytotoxicity and since interferons are produced by virally infected cells, we have a nicely integrated feedback defense system.

### Eosinophils

Large parasites such as helminths cannot physically be phagocytosed and extracellular killing by eosinophils would seem to have evolved to help cope with this situation. These polymorphonuclear 'cousins' of the neutrophil have distinctive granules which stain avidly with acid dyes (figure 1.4c) and have a characteristic appearance in the electron microscope (figure 13.21). A major basic protein (MBP) is localized in the core of the granules while an eosinophilic cationic protein together with a peroxidase have been identified in the granule matrix. Other enzymes include arylsulfatase B, phospholipase D and histaminase. They have surface receptors for C3b and on activation produce a particularly impressive respiratory burst with concomitant generation of active oxygen metabolites. Not satisfied with that, nature has also armed the cell with granule proteins capable of producing a transmembrane plug in the target membrane like C9 and the NK perforin. Quite a nasty cell.

Most helminths can activate the alternative complement pathway, but although resistant to C9 attack, their coating with C3b allows adherence of eosinophils through their C3b receptors. If this contact should lead to activation, the eosinophil will launch its extracellular attack which includes the release of MBP and especially the cationic protein which damages the parasite membrane.

## SUMMARY

A wide range of innate immune mechanisms operate which do not improve with repeated exposure to infection.

### Barriers against infection

• Microorganisms are kept out of the body by the skin, the secretion of mucus, ciliary action, the lavaging action of bactericidal fluids (e.g. tears), gastric acid and microbial antagonism.
• If penetration occurs, bacteria are destroyed by soluble factors such as lysozyme and by phagocytosis with intracellular digestion.

### Phagocytic cells kill microorganisms

• The main phagocytic cells are polymorphonuclear neutrophils and macrophages. Organisms adhere to their surface, activate the engulfment process and are taken inside the cell where they fuse with cytoplasmic granules.
• A formidable array of microbicidal mechanisms then come into play: the conversion of $O_2$ to reactive oxygen intermediates, the synthesis of nitric oxide and the release of multiple oxygen-independent factors from the granules.

### Complement facilitates phagocytosis

• The complement system, a multicomponent triggered enzyme cascade, is used to attract phagocytic cells to the microbes and engulf them.
• The most abundant component, C3, is split by a convertase enzyme formed from its own cleavage product C3b and factor B and stabilized against breakdown caused by factors H and I, through association with the microbial surface. As it is formed, C3b becomes linked covalently to the microorganism.
• The next component, C5, is activated yielding a small peptide, C5a; the residual C5b binds to the surface and assembles the terminal components C6–9 into a membrane attack complex which is freely permeable to solutes and can lead to osmotic lysis.
• C5a is a potent chemotactic agent for polymorphs and greatly increases capillary permeability.
• C3a and C5a act on mast cells causing the release of further mediators such as histamine, leukotriene $B_4$ and tumor necrosis factor (TNF) with effects on capillary permeability and adhesiveness, and neutrophil chemotaxis; they also activate neutrophils.

*SIRS?*

### The complement-mediated acute inflammatory reaction

• Following the activation of complement with the ensuing attraction and stimulation of neutrophils, the activated phagocytes bind to the C3b-coated microbes by their surface C3b receptors and may then ingest them. The influx of polymorphs and the increase in vascular permeability constitute the potent antimicrobial **acute inflammatory response** (figure 2.18).

• Inflammation can also be initiated by tissue macrophages which subserve a similar role to the mast cell, since signalling by bacterial toxins, C5a or by iC3b-coated bacteria adhering to surface complement receptors causes release of neutrophil chemotactic and activating factors.

### Humoral mechanisms provide a second defensive strategy

• In addition to lysozyme and the complement system, other humoral defenses involve the acute phase proteins such as C-reactive and mannose binding proteins whose synthesis is greatly augmented by infection. Mannose-binding protein is a member of the collectin family including conglutinin and surfactants SP-A and SP-D, notable for their ability to distinguish microbial from 'self' surface carbohydrate groups.

• Recovery from viral infections can be effected by the interferons which block viral replication.

### Extracellular killing

• Virally infected cells can be killed by large granular lymphocytes with NK activity through a perforin/granzyme and a separate Fas-mediated pathway leading to programmed cell death (apoptosis) mediated by activation of endogenous ICE (IL-1β converting enzyme) proteases.

• Extracellular killing by C3b-bound eosinophils may be responsible for the failure of many large parasites to establish a foothold in potential hosts.

# SPECIFIC ACQUIRED IMMUNITY

## C O N T E N T S

## THE NEED FOR SPECIFIC IMMUNE MECHANISMS

Our microbial adversaries have tremendous opportunities through mutation to evolve strategies which evade our innate immune defenses. For example, most of the *successful* parasites activate the alternative complement pathway and bind C3b, yet eosinophils which adhere are somehow not triggered into offensive action. The same holds true for many bacteria, while some may so shape their exteriors as to avoid complement activation completely. The body obviously needed to 'devise' defense mechanisms which could be dovetailed individually to each of these organisms no matter how many there were. In other words *a very large number* of **specific immune defenses** needed to be at the body's disposal. Quite a tall order!

## ANTIBODY — THE SPECIFIC ADAPTOR

Evolutionary processes came up with what can only be described as a brilliant solution. This was to fashion an adaptor molecule which was intrinsically capable not only of activating the complement system *and* of stimulating phagocytic cells, but also of sticking to the offending microbe. The adaptor thus had three main regions, two concerned with communicating with complement and the phagocytes (the biological functions) and one devoted to binding to an individual microorganism (the external recognition function). In most biological systems like hormones and receptors, and enzymes and substrates, recognition usually occurs through fairly accurate complementarity in shape allowing the ligands to approach so close to each other as to permit the normal intermolecular forces to become relatively strong. In the present case, each adaptor would have a recognition portion complementary in shape to some microorganism to which it could then bind reasonably firmly. The part of the adaptor with biological function would be constant, but for each of hundreds of thousands of different organisms, a special recognition portion would be needed.

Thus the body has to make hundreds of thousands, or even millions, of **adaptors with different recognition sites.** The adaptor is of course the molecule we know affectionately as **antibody** (figure 2.1).

## Antibody initiates a new complement pathway ('classical')

Antibody, when bound to a microbe, will link to the first molecule in the so-called **classical complement sequence**, C1q, and trigger the latent proteolytic activity of the C1 complex (figure 2.2). This then dutifully plays its role in the amplifying cascade by acting on components C4 and C2 to generate many molecules of **C4b2b**, a new **C3-splitting enzyme** (figure 2.3).

The molecular events responsible for this seem to be rather clear. C1q is polyvalent with respect to antibody binding and consists of a central collagen-like stem branching into six peptide chains each tipped by an antibody-binding subunit (resembling the blooms on a bouquet of flowers). C1q is associated with two further subunits, C1r and C1s, in a $Ca^{2+}$ stabilized trimolecular complex (figure 2.2). Both these molecules

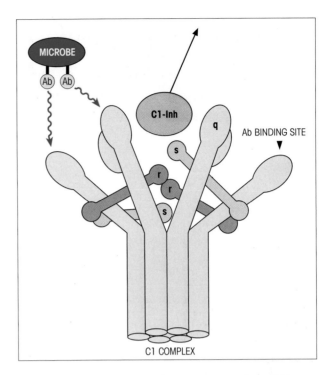

**Figure 2.2. Activation of the classical complement pathway.** C1 is composed of C1q associated with the flexible rod-like Ca-dependent complex, $C1r_2–C1s_2$ (s and r indicate potential serine protease active sites), which interdigitate with the six arms of C1q, either as indicated or as 'W' shapes on the outer side of these arms. The C1-inhibitor normally prevents spontaneous activation of $C1r_2–C1s_2$. If the complex of a microbe or antigen with antibodies attaches two or more of the globular Ab-binding sites on C1q, the molecule presumably undergoes conformational change which releases the C1–Inh and activates $C1r_2–C1s_2$.

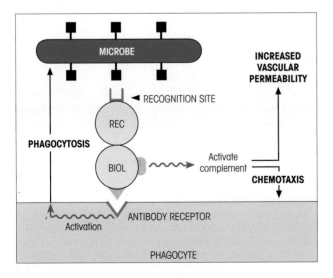

**Figure 2.1. The antibody adaptor molecule.** The constant part with biological function (BIOL) activates complement and the phagocyte. The portion with the recognition unit for the foreign microbe (REC) varies from one antibody to another.

contain repeats of a 60 amino acid unit folded as a globular domain and referred to as a complement control protein (CCP) repeat since it is a characteristic structural feature of several proteins involved in control of the complement system. Changes in C1q consequent upon binding the antigen–antibody complex bring about the sequential activation of proteolytic activity in C1r and then C1s.

The next component in the chain C4 (unfortunately components were numbered before the sequence was established) now binds to C1 through these CCPs and is cleaved enzymically by C1s. As expected in a multi-enzyme cascade, several molecules of C4 undergo cleavage, each releasing a small C4a fragment and revealing a nascent labile internal thiolester bond in the residual C4b like that in C3 (cf. figure 1.10) which may then bind either to the antibody–C1 complex or the surface of the microbe itself. Note that C4a, like C5a and C3a, has anaphylatoxin activity, although feeble, and 4b resembles C3b in its opsonic activity. In the presence of $Mg^{2+}$, C2 can complex with the C4b

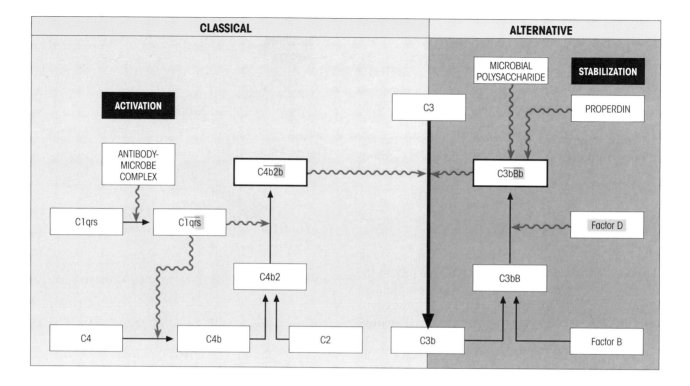

**Figure 2.3. Comparison of the alternative and classical complement pathways.** The classical pathway, with odd exceptions such as C-reactive protein, is antibody dependent, the alternative pathway is not. The molecular units with protease activity are highlighted, the enzymic domains showing considerable homology. Beware confusion with nomenclature; the large C2 fragment which forms the C3 convertase is often labeled as C2a but to be consistent with C4b, C3b and C5b, it seems more logical to call it C2b.

to become a new substrate for the C1s; the resulting product C4b2b now has the vital C3 convertase activity required to cleave C3.

This classical pathway C3 convertase has the same specificity as the C3bBb generated by the alternative pathway likewise producing the same C3a and C3b fragments. Activation of a single C1 complex can bring about the proteolysis of literally thousands of C3 molecules. From then on things march along exactly in parallel to the post-C3 pathway with one molecule of C3b added to the C4b2b to make it into a C5-splitting enzyme with eventual production of the **membrane attack complex** (figures 1.13 and 2.4). Just as the alternative pathway C3 convertase is controlled by factors H and I, so the breakdown of C4b2b is brought about by either a C4 binding protein (C4bp) or a cell surface C3b receptor (CR1) in the presence of factor I.

The similarities between the two pathways are set out in figure 2.3 and show how antibody can supplement and even improve on the ability of the innate

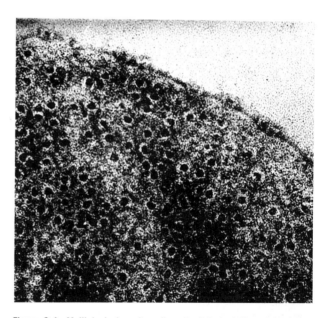

**Figure 2.4. Multiple lesions in cell wall of *Escherichia coli* bacterium caused by interaction with IgM antibody and complement.** (Human antibodies are divided into five main classes: immunoglobulin M (shortened to IgM), IgG, IgA, IgE and IgD, which differ in the specialization of their 'rear ends' for different biological functions such as complement activation or mast cell sensitization.) Each lesion is caused by a single IgM molecule and shows as a 'dark pit' due to penetration by the 'negative stain'. This is somewhat of an illusion since in reality these 'pits' are like volcano craters standing proud of the surface, and are each single 'membrane attack' complexes. Comparable results may be obtained in the absence of antibody since the cell wall endotoxin can activate the alternative pathway in the presence of higher concentration of serum (× 400 000). (Courtesy of Drs R. Dourmashkin and J.H. Humphrey.)

immune system to initiate **acute inflammatory reactions**. Antibody provides yet a further bonus in this respect; the class known as immunoglobulin E (see legend to figure 2.4) can sensitize mast cells through binding to their surface so that combination with antigen triggers mediator release independently of C3a or C5a, adding yet more flexibility to our defenses. The major proteins involved in the complement system are summarized in table 2.1.

## Complexed antibody activates phagocytic cells

I drew attention to the fact that many C3b-coated organisms adhere to phagocytic cells yet avoid provoking their uptake. If small amounts of antibody are added the phagocyte springs into action. It does so through the recognition of two or more antibody molecules bound to the microbe, using specialized receptors on the cell surface.

A single antibody molecule complexed to the microorganism is not enough because it cannot cause the cross-linking of antibody receptors in the phagocyte surface membrane which is required to activate

the cell. There is a further consideration connected with what is often called **the bonus effect of multivalency**; for thermodynamic reasons, which will be touched on in Chapter 5, the association constant of ligands which use several rather than a single bond to react with receptors is increased geometrically rather than arithmetically. For example, three antibodies bound close together on a bacterium could be attracted to a macrophage a thousand times more strongly than a single antibody molecule (figure 2.5).

## CELLULAR BASIS OF ANTIBODY PRODUCTION

### Antibodies are made by lymphocytes

The majority of resting **lymphocytes** are small cells with a darkly staining nucleus due to condensed chromatin and relatively little cytoplasm containing the odd mitochondrion required for basic energy provision. Figures 2.6 and 2.7 compare the morphology of these cells with that of the minority population of

**Table 2.1.** Proteins of the complement system.

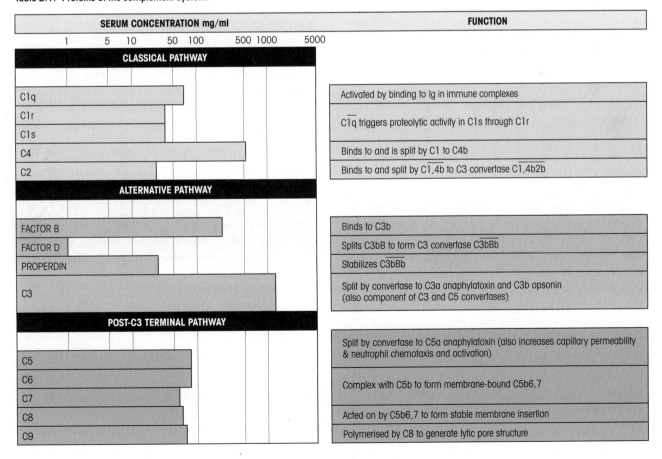

| SERUM CONCENTRATION mg/ml | FUNCTION |
|---|---|
| **CLASSICAL PATHWAY** | |
| C1q | Activated by binding to Ig in immune complexes |
| C1r | C̄1q triggers proteolytic activity in C1s through C1r |
| C1s | |
| C4 | Binds to and is split by C1 to C4b |
| C2 | Binds to and split by C̄1,4b to C3 convertase C̄1,4b2b |
| **ALTERNATIVE PATHWAY** | |
| FACTOR B | Binds to C3b |
| FACTOR D | Splits C3bB to form C3 convertase C̄3bBb |
| PROPERDIN | Stabilizes C3bBb |
| C3 | Split by convertase to C3a anaphylatoxin and C3b opsonin (also component of C3 and C5 convertases) |
| **POST-C3 TERMINAL PATHWAY** | |
| C5 | Split by convertase to C5a anaphylatoxin (also increases capillary permeability & neutrophil chemotaxis and activation) |
| C6 | Complex with C5b to form membrane-bound C5b6,7 |
| C7 | |
| C8 | Acted on by C5b6,7 to form stable membrane insertion |
| C9 | Polymerised by C8 to generate lytic pore structure |

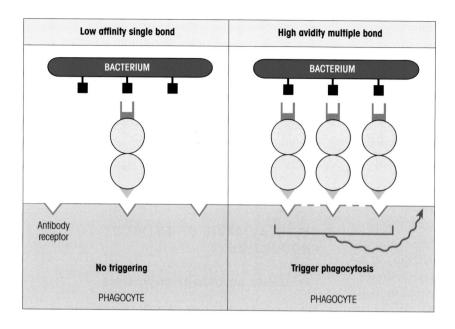

Figure 2.5. Binding of bacterium to phagocyte by multiple antibodies gives strong association forces and triggers phagocytosis by cross-linking the surface receptors for antibody.

**large granular lymphocytes** which includes the natural killer (NK) set referred to in Chapter 1.

The central role of the **small lymphocyte** in the production of antibody was established largely by the work of Gowans. He depleted rats of their lymphocytes by chronic drainage of lymph from the thoracic duct by an indwelling cannula, and showed that they had a grossly impaired ability to mount an antibody response to microbial challenge. The ability to form antibody could be restored by injecting thoracic duct lymphocytes obtained from another rat. The same effect could be obtained if, before injection, the thoracic duct cells were first incubated at 37°C for 24 hours under conditions which kill off large and medium sized cells and leave only the small lymphocytes. This shows that the small lymphocyte is necessary for the **antibody response**.

The small lymphocytes can be labeled if the donor rat is previously injected with tritiated thymidine; it then becomes possible to follow the fate of these lymphocytes when transferred to another rat of the same strain which is then injected with microorganisms to produce an antibody response (figure 2.8). It transpires that after contact with the injected microbes, some of the transferred labeled lymphocytes develop into **plasma cells** (figures 2.6g and 2.9) which can be shown to contain (figure 2.6h) and secrete antibody.

## Antigen selects the lymphocytes which make antibody

The molecules in the microorganisms which evoke and react with antibodies are called **antigens** (gener-

ates **anti**bodies). We now know that antibodies are formed before antigen is ever seen and that they are **selected** for by antigen.

It works in the following way. Each lymphocyte of a subset called the **B-lymphocytes**, because they differentiate in the *bone marrow*, is programmed to make one, and only one, antibody and it places this antibody on its outer surface to act as a receptor. This can be detected by using fluorescent probes and in figure 2.6f one can see the molecules of antibody on the surface of a human B-lymphocyte stained with a fluorescent rabbit antiserum raised against a preparation of human antibodies. Each lymphocyte has of the order of $10^5$ identical antibody molecules on its surface.

When an antigen enters the body, it is confronted by a dazzling array of lymphocytes all bearing different antibodies each with its own individual recognition site. The antigen will only bind to those receptors with which it makes a good fit. Lymphocytes whose receptors have bound antigen receive a triggering signal and develop into antibody-forming plasma cells and since the lymphocytes are programmed to make only one antibody, that secreted by the plasma cell will be identical with that originally acting as the lymphocyte receptor, i.e. it will bind well to the antigen. In this way, antigen selects for the antibodies which recognize it effectively (figure 2.10).

## The need for clonal expansion means humoral immunity must be acquired

Because we can make hundreds of thousands, maybe even millions, of different antibody molecules, it is

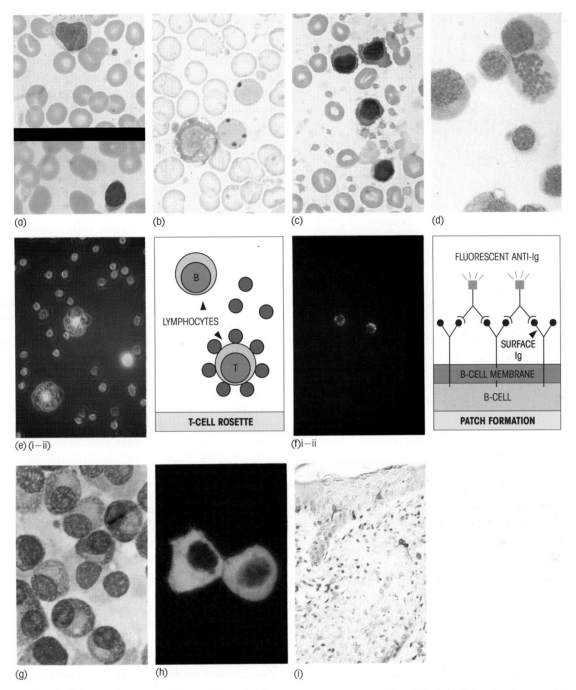

**Figure 2.6. Cells involved in the acquired immune response.** (a) Small lymphocytes. Condensed chromatin gives rise to heavy staining of the nucleus. The cell on the bottom is a typical resting agranular T-cell with a thin rim of cytoplasm. The upper nucleated cell is a large granular lymphocyte (LGL); it has more cytoplasm and azurophilic granules are evident. Isolated platelets are visible. B-lymphocytes range from small to intermediate in size and lack granules. (Giemsa stain.) (b) Small agranular T-cells stained with nonspecific esterase showing Gall bodies (each a cluster of primary lyso-somes associated with a lipid droplet) which appear as characteristic cyto-plasmic dot(s), stained for nonspecific esterase; compare with diffuse distribution in cytoplasm of monocyte at side. (c) T-lymphocytes from buffy coat stained with a monoclonal anti-T using the alkaline phosphatase immu-noenzymic method (cf. figure 6.10). Note the single unstained non-T lym-phocyte on the bottom. (d) Transformed lymphocytes (lymphoblasts) following stimulation of lymphocytes in culture with a polyclonal activator. The large lymphoblasts with their relatively high ratio of cytoplasm to nucleus may be compared in size with the isolated small lymphocyte. One cell is in mitosis. (May–Grünwald–Giemsa.) (e) Identification of lymphocytes by rosette formation with red cells visualized in UV light after staining with Acri-dine Orange which makes the lymphocyte nucleus fluorescent green. T-cell rosettes are formed by spontaneous binding of CD2 (cf. p. 152) to sheep erythrocytes. (f) Immunofluorescent staining of B-lymphocyte surface immunoglobulin using fluorescein-conjugated (■) anti-Ig. Provided the reaction is carried out in the cold to prevent pinocytosis, the labeled antibody cannot penetrate to the interior of the viable lymphocytes and reacts only with surface components. Patches of aggregated surface Ig are seen which are beginning to form a cap in the right-hand lymphocyte. During cap formation, submembranous myosin becomes redistributed in association with the surface Ig and induces locomotion of the previously sessile cell in a direction away from the cap. (g) Plasma cells. The nucleus is eccentric. The cytoplasm is strongly basophilic due to high RNA content. The juxtanuclear lightly stained zone corresponds with the Golgi region. (May–Grünwald–Giemsa.) (h) Plasma cells stained to show intracellular immunoglobulin using a fluo-rescein-labeled anti-IgG (green) and a rhodamine-conjugated anti-IgM (red). (i) Langerhans' cells in human epidermis in leprosy, increased in the subepi-dermal zone, possibly as a consequence of the disease process. Stained by the immunoperoxidase method with S-100 antibodies. (Material for (a), (b) and (c) was kindly supplied by Mr M. Watts of the Department of Haematol-ogy, Middlesex Hospital Medical School, (d), (e) and (f) by Dr P. Lydyard, (g) and (h) by Professor C. Grossi and (i) by Dr Marian Ridley.)

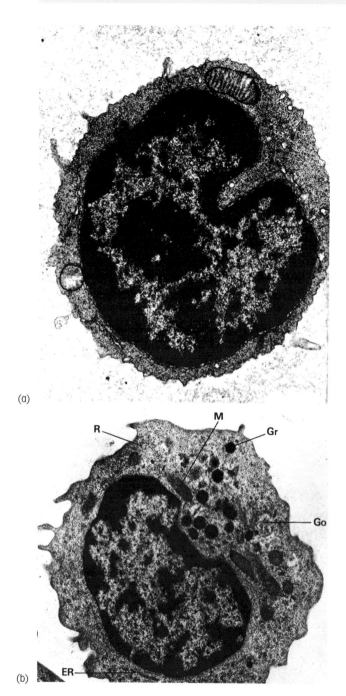

(a)

(b)

**Figure 2.7. Lymphocyte ultrastructure.** (a) Small agranular T-lymphocyte. Indented nucleus with condensed chromatin, sparse cytoplasm: single mitochondrion shown and many free ribosomes but otherwise few organelles (×13 000). B-lymphocytes are essentially similar with slightly more cytoplasm and occasional elements of rough-surfaced endoplasmic reticulum. (b) Large granular lymphocyte (LGL) (×7500). The more abundant cytoplasm contains several mitochondria (M), free ribosomes (R) with some minor elements of rough-surfaced endoplasmic reticulum (ER), prominent Golgi apparatus (Go) and characteristic membrane-bound electron-dense granules (Gr). The nuclear chromatin is less condensed than that of the agranular T-cell. (Courtesy of Drs A. Zicca and C.E. Grossi.)

not feasible for us to have too many lymphocytes producing each type of antibody; there just would not be enough room in the body to accommodate them. To compensate for this, lymphocytes which are triggered by contact with antigen undergo successive waves of proliferation (figure 2.6d) to build up a large clone of plasma cells which will be making antibody of the kind for which the parent lymphocyte was programmed. By this system of **clonal selection**, large enough concentrations of antibody can be produced to combat infection effectively (Milestone 2.1; figure 2.11).

The importance of proliferation for the development of a significant antibody response is highlighted by the ability of antimitotic drugs to abolish antibody production to a given antigen stimulus completely.

Because it takes time for the proliferating clone to build up its numbers sufficiently, it is usually several days before antibodies are detectable in the serum following primary contact with antigen. The newly formed antibodies are a consequence of antigen exposure and it is for this reason that we speak of the **acquired immune response**.

## ACQUIRED MEMORY

When we make an antibody response to a given infectious agent, by definition that microorganism must exist in our environment and we are likely to meet it again. It would make sense then for the immune mechanisms alerted by the first contact with antigen to leave behind some memory system which would enable the response to any subsequent exposure to be faster and greater in magnitude.

Our experience of many common infections tells us that this must be so. We rarely suffer twice from such diseases as measles, mumps, chickenpox, whooping cough and so forth. The first contact clearly imprints some information, imparts some **memory**, so that the body is effectively prepared to repel any later invasion by that organism and a state of immunity is established.

### Secondary antibody responses are better

By following the production of antibody on the first and second contacts with antigen we can see the basis for the development of immunity. For example, when we inject a bacterial product such as tetanus toxoid into a rabbit, for reasons already discussed, several days elapse before antibodies can be detected in the

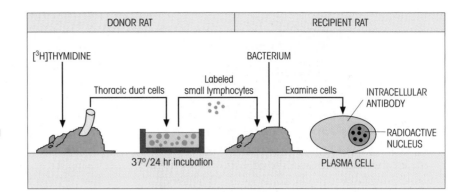

**Figure 2.8. Labeled small lymphocytes become antibody-forming plasma cells** when transferred to a recipient rat which is immunized with a bacterium. Transferred cell with radioactive nucleus shown by autoradiography. Intracellular antibody revealed by staining with fluorescent probes (cf. figure 2.6h).

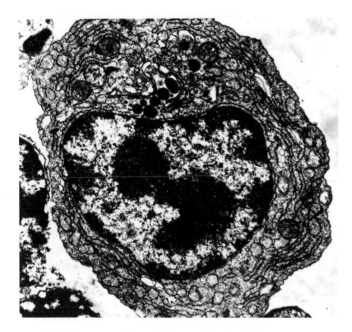

**Figure 2.9. Plasma cell** (× 10 000). Prominent rough-surfaced endoplasmic reticulum associated with the synthesis and secretion of Ig.

strated by **adoptive transfer** of lymphocytes to another animal, an experimental system frequently employed in immunology (cf. figure 2.8). In the present case, the immunologic potential of the transferred cells is expressed in a recipient treated with X-rays which destroy its own lymphocyte population; thus any immune response will be of donor not recipient origin. In the experiment described in figure 2.13, small lymphocytes are taken from an animal given a primary injection of tetanus toxoid and transferred to an irradiated host which is then boosted with the antigen; a rapid, intense production of antibody characteristic of a secondary response is seen. To exclude the possibility that the first antigen injection might exert a *nonspecific* stimulatory effect on the lympho-

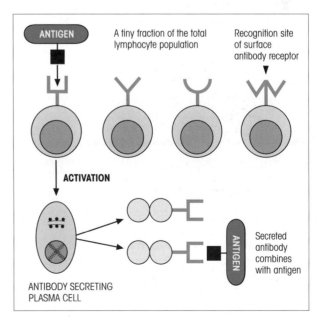

**Figure 2.10. Antigen activates those B-cells whose surface antibody receptors it can combine with firmly.**

blood; these reach a peak and then fall (figure 2.12). If we now allow the animal to rest and then give a second injection of toxoid, the course of events is dramatically altered. Within 2–3 days the antibody level in the blood rises steeply to reach much higher values than were observed in the **primary response**. This **secondary response** then is characterized by a more rapid and more abundant production of antibody resulting from the 'tuning up' or priming of the antibody-forming system.

With our knowledge of lymphocyte function, it is perhaps not surprising to realize that these are the cells which provide memory. This can be demon-

## Milestone 2.1—Clonal Selection Theory

### Antibody production according to Ehrlich

In 1894, well in advance of his time as usual, the remarkable Paul Ehrlich proposed the side-chain theory of antibody production. Each cell would make a large variety of surface receptors which bound foreign antigens by complementary shape 'lock and key' fit. Exposure to antigen would provoke over-production of receptors (antibodies) which would then be shed into the circulation (figure M2.1.1).

### Template theories

Ehrlich's hypothesis implied that antibodies were preformed prior to antigen exposure. However, this view

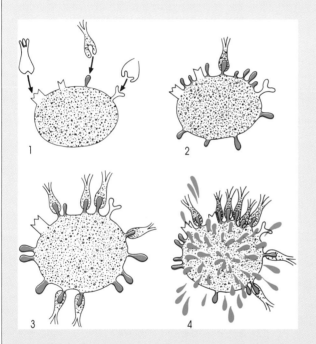

**Figure M2.1.1. Ehrlich's side-chain theory of Ab production.** (Reproduced from *Proceedings of the Royal Society B* (1900), **66**, 424.)

was difficult to accept when later work showed that antibodies could be formed to almost any organic structure synthesized in the chemist's laboratory (e.g. azobenzene arsonate; figure 5.1) despite the fact that such molecules would never be encountered in the natural environment. Thus was born the idea that antibodies were synthesized by using the antigen as a template. Twenty years passed before this idea was 'blown out of the water' by the observation that after an antibody molecule is unfolded by guanidinium salts in the absence of antigen, it spontaneously refolds to regenerate its original specificity. It became clear that each antibody has a different amino acid sequence which governs its final folded shape and hence its ability to recognize antigen.

### Selection theories

The wheel turns full circle and we once more live with the idea that since different antibodies must be encoded by separate genes, the information for making these antibodies must pre-exist in the host DNA. In 1955, Nils Jerne perceived that this could form the basis for a selective theory of antibody production. He suggested that the complete antibody repertoire is expressed at a low level and that when antigen enters the body, it selects its complementary antibody to form a complex which in some way provoked further synthesis of that particular antibody. But how?

Mac Burnet now brilliantly conceived of a cellular basis for this selection process. Let each lymphocyte be programmed to make its own singular antibody which is inserted like an Ehrlich 'side-chain' into its surface membrane. Antigen will now form the complex envisaged by Jerne, on the surface of the lymphocyte, and by triggering its activation and clonal proliferation, large amounts of the specific antibody will be synthesized (figure 2.11). Bow graciously to that soothsayer Ehrlich—he came so close in 1894!

---

cytes, the boosting injection includes influenza hemagglutinin as a control antigen. Furthermore, a 'criss-cross' control group primed with influenza hemagglutinin must also be included to ensure that this antigen is capable of giving a secondary booster response. I have explained the design of the experiment at some length to call attention to the need for careful selection of controls.

The higher response given by a primed lymphocyte population can be ascribed mainly to an expansion of the numbers of cells capable of being stimulated by

the antigen (figure 2.14), although we shall see later that there are some qualitative differences in these memory cells as well (pp. 196–198).

## ACQUIRED IMMUNITY HAS ANTIGEN SPECIFICITY

### Discrimination between different antigens

The establishment of memory or immunity by one organism does not confer protection against another

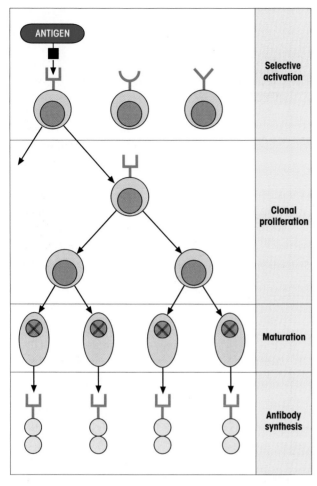

**Figure 2.11. Clonal selection.** The cell selected by antigen undergoes many divisions during the clonal proliferation and the progeny mature to give an expanded population of antibody-forming cells. The antibody response is particularly vulnerable to antimitotic agents at the proliferation stage.

unrelated organism. After an attack of measles we are immune to further infection but are susceptible to other agents such as the polio or mumps viruses. Acquired immunity then shows **specificity** and the immune system can differentiate specifically between the two organisms. A more formal experimental demonstration of this discriminatory power was seen in figure 2.13 where priming with tetanus toxoid evoked memory for that antigen but not for influenza and vice versa.

The basis for this lies of course in the ability of the recognition sites of the antibody molecules to distinguish between antigens; antibodies which react with

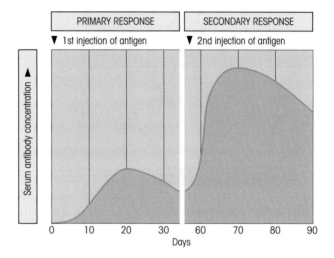

**Figure 2.12. Primary and secondary response.** A rabbit is injected on two separate occasions with tetanus toxoid. The antibody response on the second contact with antigen is more rapid and more intense.

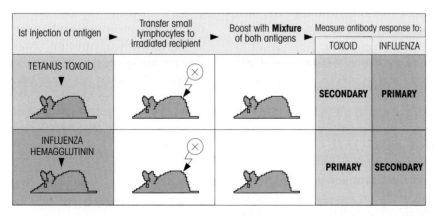

**Figure 2.13. Memory for a primary response can be transferred by small lymphocytes.** Recipients are treated with a dose of X-rays which directly kill lymphocytes (highly sensitive to radiation) but only affect other body cells when they divide; the recipient thus functions as a living 'test-tube' which permits the function of the donor cells to be followed. The reasons for the

design of the experiment are given in the text. In practice, because of the possibility of interference between the two antigens, it would be wiser to split each of the primary antigen-injected groups into two, giving a separate boosting antigen to each to avoid using a mixture.

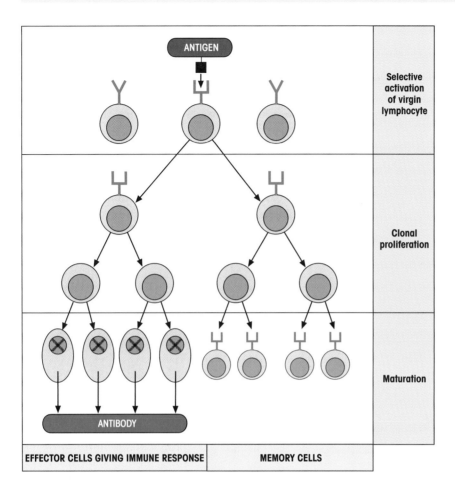

**Figure 2.14. The cellular basis for the generation of effector and memory cells after primary contact with antigen.** A fraction of the progeny of the original antigen-reactive lymphocytes become nondividing memory cells and others the effector cells of either humoral or, as we shall see subsequently, cell-mediated immunity. Memory cells require fewer cycles before they develop into effectors and this shortens the reaction time for the secondary response. The expanded clone of cells with memory for the original antigen provides the basis for the greater secondary relative to the primary immune response. Priming with low doses of antigen can often stimulate effective memory without producing very adequate antibody synthesis.

the toxoid do not bind to influenza and, *mutatis mutandis* as they say, anti-influenza is not particularly smitten with the toxoid.

### Discrimination between self and nonself

This ability to recognize one antigen and distinguish it from another goes even further. The individual must also recognize what is foreign, i.e. what is 'nonself'. The failure to discriminate between **self** and **nonself** could lead to the synthesis of antibodies directed against components of the subject's own body (**autoantibodies**), which in principle could prove to be highly embarrassing. On purely theoretical grounds it seemed to Burnet and Fenner that the body must develop some mechanism whereby 'self' and 'nonself' could be distinguished, and they postulated that those circulating body components which were able to reach the developing lymphoid system in the perinatal period could in some way be 'learnt' as 'self'. A permanent unresponsiveness or **tolerance** would then be created so that as immunologic maturity was reached there would normally be an inability

to respond to 'self' components. At this stage it is salutory to note that Burnet had the sagacity to realize that his clonal selection theory could readily provide the cellular basis for such a mechanism to operate. He argued that if each lymphocyte were preoccupied with making its own individual antibody, those cells programmed to express antibodies reacting with circulating self components could be rendered unresponsive without affecting those lymphocytes specific for foreign antigens. In other words, self-reacting lymphocytes could be selectively suppressed without undermining the ability of the host to respond immunologically to infectious agents. As we shall see in chapter 12, these predictions have been amply verified.

## VACCINATION DEPENDS ON ACQUIRED MEMORY

Nearly 200 years ago, Edward Jenner carried out the remarkable studies which mark the beginning of immunology as a systematic subject. Noting the pretty pox-free skin of the milkmaids, he reasoned that deliberate exposure to the pox virus of the cow, which is not virulent for the human, might confer protection against the related human smallpox organism. Accordingly, he inoculated a small boy with cowpox and was delighted—and I hope relieved—to observe that he was now protected against a subsequent exposure to smallpox (what would today's ethical committees have said about that?!). By injecting a harmless form of a disease organism, Jenner had utilized the specificity and memory of the acquired immune response to lay the foundations for modern **vaccination** (Latin *vacca*, cow).

The essential strategy is to prepare an innocuous form of the infectious organism or its toxins which still substantially retains the antigens responsible for establishing protective immunity. This has been done by using killed or live attenuated organisms, purified microbial components or chemically modified antigens (figure 2.15).

## CELL-MEDIATED IMMUNITY PROTECTS AGAINST INTRACELLULAR ORGANISMS

Many microorganisms live inside host cells where it is impossible for humoral antibody to reach them. Obligate intracellular parasites like viruses have to replicate inside cells; facultative intracellular parasites like *Mycobacteria* and *Leishmania* can replicate

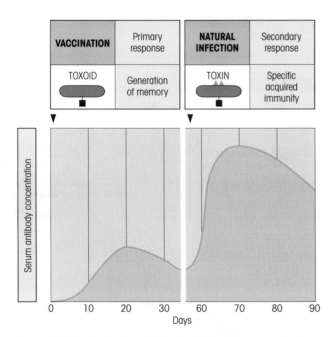

**Figure 2.15. The basis of vaccination** illustrated by the response to tetanus toxoid. Treatment of the bacterial toxin with formaldehyde destroys its toxicity (associated with ▲▲) but retains antigenicity. Exposure to toxin in a subsequent natural infection boosts the memory cells, producing high levels of neutralizing antibody which are protective.

within cells, particularly macrophages, but do not have to; they like the intracellular life because of the protection it affords. A totally separate acquired immunity system has evolved to deal with this situation based on a distinct lymphocyte subpopulation made up of **T-cells**, designated thus because, unlike the B-lymphocytes, they differentiate within the milieu of the **thymus gland**. Because they are specialized to operate against cells bearing intracellular organisms, T-cells only recognize antigen when it is on the surface of a body cell. Accordingly, the **T-cell surface receptors**, which are different from the antibody molecules used by B-lymphocytes, recognize antigen plus a surface marker which informs the T-lymphocyte that it is making contact with another cell. These cell markers belong to an important group of molecules known as the **major histocompatibility complex (MHC)**, identified originally through their ability to evoke powerful transplantation reactions in other members of the same species.

### Cytokine-producing T-cells help macrophages to kill intracellular parasites

These organisms only survive inside macrophages through their ability to subvert the innate killing mechanisms of these cells. Nonetheless, they cannot prevent the macrophage from processing small antigenic fragments (possibly of organisms which have spontaneously died) and placing them on the host cell surface. A subpopulation of T-lymphocytes called **T-helper cells**, if primed to that antigen, will recognize and bind to the combination of antigen with so-called class II MHC molecules on the macrophage surface and produce a variety of soluble factors termed **cytokines** which include the interleukins IL-2 etc. (p. 179). Different cytokines can be made by various cell types and generally act at a short range on neighboring cells. Some T-cell cytokines help B-cells to make antibodies while others such as γ-interferon (IFNγ) act as **macrophage activating factors** which switch on the previously subverted microbicidal mechanisms of the macrophage and bring about the death of the intracellular microorganisms (figure 2.16).

### Virally infected cells can be killed by cytotoxic T-cells and ADCC

We have already discussed the advantage to the host of killing virally infected cells before the virus begins to replicate and have seen that large granular lymphocytes with NK activity (p. 19) can subserve a cytotoxic

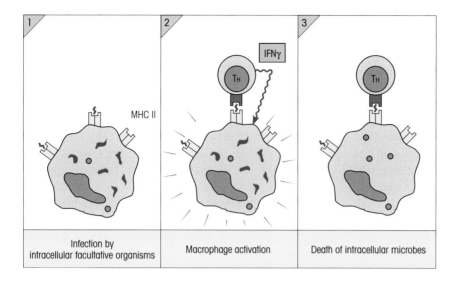

Figure 2.16. Intracellular killing of microorganisms by macrophages. (1) Surface antigen ($) derived from the intracellular microbes is complexed with class II MHC molecules (⊔). (2) The T-helper binds to this surface complex and is triggered to release the cytokine γ-interferon (IFNγ). This activates microbicidal mechanisms in the macrophage. (3) The infectious agent meets a timely death.

function. However, NK cells have a limited range of specificities and in order to improve their efficacy, this range needs to be expanded.

One way in which this can be achieved is by coating the target cell with antibodies specific for the virally coded surface antigens because NK cells have receptors for the constant part of the antibody molecule, rather like phagocytic cells. Thus antibodies will bring the NK cell very close to the target by forming a bridge, and the NK cell being activated by the complexed antibody molecules is able to kill the virally infected cell by its extracellular mechanisms (figure 2.17). This system, termed **antibody-dependent cell-mediated cytotoxicity (ADCC)**, is very impressive when studied *in vitro* but it has proved difficult to establish to what extent it operates within the body.

On the other hand, a subset of **cytotoxic T-cells** has evolved for which there is evidence of *in vivo* activity. Like the T-helpers, these cells have a very wide range of antigen specificities because they clonally express a large number of different surface receptors similar to, but not identical with, the surface antibody receptors on the B-lymphocytes. Again, each lymphocyte is programmed to make only one receptor and, again like the T-helper cell, recognizes antigen only in association with a cell marker, in this case the class I MHC molecule (figure 2.17). Through this recognition of surface antigen, the cytotoxic cell comes into intimate contact with its target and administers the 'kiss of apoptotic death'. It also releases **IFNγ** which would help to reduce the spread of virus to adjacent cells, particularly in cases where the virus itself may prove to be a weak inducer of IFNα or β.

In an entirely analogous fashion to the B-cell, T-cells are selected and activated by combination with antigen, expanded by clonal proliferation and mature to give T-helper and cytotoxic T-effectors, together with an enlarged population of memory cells. Thus both T- and B-cells provide **specific acquired immu-**

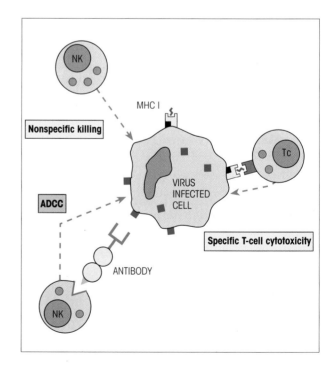

Figure 2.17. Killing virally infected cells. The nonspecific killing mechanism of the NK cell can be focused on the target by antibody to produce antibody-dependent cell-mediated cytotoxicity (ADCC). The cytotoxic T-cell homes onto its target specifically through receptor recognition of surface antigen in association with MHC class I molecules.

nity with a variety of mechanisms, which in most cases operate to extend the range of effectiveness of innate immunity and confer the valuable advantage that a first infection prepares us to withstand further contact with the same microorganism.

## IMMUNOPATHOLOGY

The immune system is clearly 'a good thing', but like mercenary armies, it can turn to bite the hand that feeds it, and cause damage to the host.

Thus where there is an especially heightened response or persistent exposure to exogenous antigens, tissue damaging or **hypersensitivity** reactions may result. Examples are allergy to grass pollens, blood dyscrasias associated with certain drugs, immune complex glomerulonephritis occurring after streptococcal infection, and chronic granulomas produced during tuberculosis or schistosomiasis.

In other cases, hypersensitivity to autoantigens may arise through a breakdown in the mechanisms which control self-tolerance, and a wide variety of **autoimmune diseases** such as thyrotoxicosis, myasthenia gravis and many of the rheumatologic disorders have now been recognized.

Another immunopathologic reaction of some consequence is **transplant rejection**, where the MHC antigens on the donor graft may well provoke a fierce reaction. Lastly, one should consider the by no means infrequent occurrence of inadequate functioning of the immune system — **immunodeficiency**. I would like to think that at this stage the reader would have no difficulty in predicting that the major problems in this condition relate to persistent infection, the type of infection being related to the elements of the immune system which are defective.

---

## SUMMARY

### Antibody—the specific adaptor

The antibody molecule evolved as a specific adaptor to attach to microorganisms which either fail to activate the alternative complement pathway or prevent activation of the phagocytic cells.

• The antibody fixes to the antigen by its specific recognition site and its constant structure regions activate complement through the classical pathway (binding C1 and generating a $\overline{C4b2b}$ convertase to split C3) and phagocytes through their antibody receptors.

• This supplementary route into the acute inflammatory reaction is enhanced by antibodies which sensitize mast cells and by immune complexes which stimulate mediator release from tissue macrophages (figure 2.18).

### Cellular basis of antibody production

• Antibodies are made by plasma cells derived from B-lymphocytes, each of which is programmed to make only one antibody which is placed on the cell surface as a receptor.

• Antigen binds to the cell with a complementary antibody, activates it and causes clonal proliferation and finally maturation to antibody-forming cells and memory cells. Thus the antigen brings about clonal selection of the cells making antibody to itself.

### Acquired memory and vaccination

• The increase in memory cells after priming means that the acquired secondary response is faster and greater, providing the basis for vaccination using a harmless form of the infective agent for the initial injection.

### Acquired immunity has antigen specificity

• Antibodies differentiate between antigens because recognition is based on molecular shape complementarity. Thus memory induced by one antigen will not extend to another unrelated antigen.

• The immune system differentiates self components from foreign antigens by making immature self-reacting lymphocytes unresponsive through contact with host molecules; lymphocytes reacting with foreign antigens are unaffected since they only make contact after reaching maturity.

### Cell-mediated immunity protects against intracellular organisms

• Another class of lymphocyte, the T-cell, is concerned with control of intracellular infections. Like the B-cell, each T-cell has its individual antigen receptor (although it differs structurally from antibody) which recognizes antigen and undergoes clonal expansion to form effector and memory cells providing specific acquired immunity.

(Continued on p. 36)

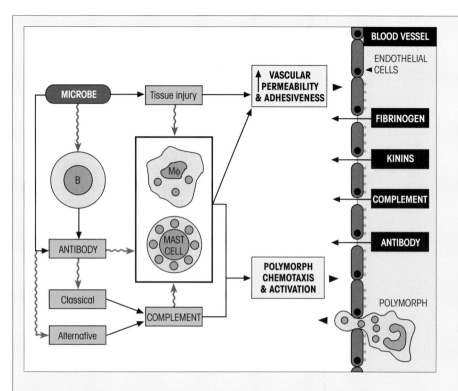

**Figure 2.18. Production of a protective acute inflammatory reaction by microbes** either (i) through tissue injury (e.g. bacterial toxin) or direct activation of the alternative complement pathway, or (ii) by antibody-dependent triggering of the classical complement pathway or mast cell degranulation (a special class of antibody, IgE, does this).

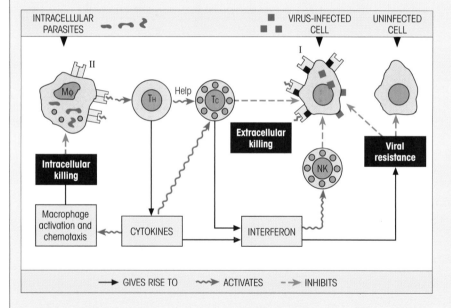

**Figure 2.19. T-cells link with the innate immune system to resist intracellular infection.** Class I (⊟) and class II (⊟) major histocompatibility molecules are important for T-cell recognition of surface antigen. The T-helper cells (TH) cooperate in the development of cytotoxic T-cells (Tc) from precursors. The macrophage (Mφ) microbicidal mechanisms are switched on by macrophage-activating lymphokines. Interferon inhibits viral replication and stimulates NK cells which together with Tc kill virus-infected cells.

• The T-cell recognizes cell surface antigens in association with molecules of the MHC.

• T-helper cells which see antigen with class II MHC on the surface of macrophages, release cytokines which in some cases can help B-cells to make antibody and in others, activate macrophages and enable them to kill intracellular parasites.

• Cytotoxic T-cells have the ability to recognize specific antigen plus class I MHC on the surface of virally infected cells which are killed before the virus replicates. They also release γ-interferon which can make surrounding cells resistant to viral spread (figure 2.19).

• NK cells have lectin-like 'non-specific' receptors for cells infected by viruses but do not have antigen-specific receptors; however, they can recognize antibody-coated virally infected cells through their Fcγ receptors and kill the target by antibody-dependent cell-mediated cytotoxicity (ADCC).

• Although the innate mechanisms do not improve with repeated exposure to infection as do the acquired, they

(Continued)

play a vital role since they are intimately linked to the acquired systems by **two different pathways** which all but **encapsulate the whole of immunology**. Antibody, complement and polymorphs give protection against most extracellular organisms, while T-cells, soluble cytokines, macrophages and NK cells deal with intracellular infections (figure 2.20).

## Immunopathology

• Immunopathologically mediated tissue damage to the host can occur as a result of:

inappropriate hypersensitivity reactions to exogenous antigens,

loss of tolerance to self-giving autoimmune disease,

reaction to foreign grafts.

• Immunodeficiency leaves the individual susceptible to infection.

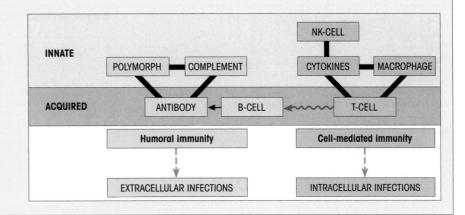

**Figure 2.20. The two pathways linking innate and acquired immunity** which provide the basis for humoral and cell-mediated immunity respectively.

# FURTHER READING

Alt F. & Marrack P. (eds) (1996) *Current Opinion in Immunology* **8**, Issue no. 1. (Articles on collectins, defensins, phagocytosis; see also Issue no. 1 of previous years.)

Cohen J.J., Sellins K.S. & Lamb C.A. (1996) Reviews of books on apoptosis. *Molecular Medicine* **2**, 230.

Ezekowitz R.A.B. & Hoffmann J.A. (eds) (1996) Innate immunity. *Current Opinion in Immunology* **8**, 82.

Gallin J., Goldstein I. & Snyderman R. (eds) (1987) *Inflammation: Basic Principles and Clinical Correlates.* Raven, New York.

Green D.R. (ed.) (1992) Apoptosis in the immune system. *Seminars in Immunology* **4**, 353.

Hofer E., Düchler M., Fuad S.A., Houchins J.P., Yabe T. & Bach F.H. (1992) Candidate natural killer cell receptors. *Immunology Today* **13**, 429.

Janeway C.A. (1995) Innate immunity acknowledged. *The Immunologist* **3**, 198.

Law S.K.A. & Reid K.B.M. (1988) In Male D.K. (ed.) *Complement.* (In Focus Series.) IRL, Oxford.

Levy O. (1996) Antibiotic proteins of polymorphonuclear leukocytes. *European Journal of Haematology* **56**, 263.

Morgan B.P. (1990) *Complement. Clinical Aspects and Relevance to Disease.* Academic Press, London.

Prince R.C. & Gunson D.E. (1993) *Trends in Biochemical Sciences* **18**, 35. (Rising interest in nitric oxide synthase.)

Reid K.B.M. (1995) The complement system — a major effector mechanism in humoral immunity. *The Immunologist* **3**, 206.

Segal A.W. & Abo A. (1993) *Trends in Biochemical Sciences* **18**, 43. (The biochemical basis of the NADPH oxidase of phagocytes.)

Shi L., Krant R.P., Aebersold R. & Greenberg A.H. (1992) An NK cell granule protein that induces DNA fragmentation and apoptosis (in perforin permeabilized cells). *Journal of Experimental Medicine* **175**, 553.

### General reading

Janeway C.A. Jr. & Travers P. (1996) *Immunobiology: The Immune System in Health and Disease*, 2nd edn. Current Biology Ltd, London. (In depth treatment of scientific basis of immunology.)

Kuby J. (1992) *Immunology.* W.H. Freeman & Co., New York. (In-depth single author book.)

Male D.K., Champion B., Cooke A. & Owen M.L. (1996) *Advanced Immunology*, 3rd edn. Gower Medical, London. (An excellent text for the advanced student.)

Playfair J.H.L. (1996) *Immunology at a Glance*, 6th edn. Blackwell Science Ltd, Oxford. (Very useful for revision.)

Roitt I.M., Brostoff J. & Male D.K. (eds) (1995) *Immunology*, 4th edn. Mosby Publishers, London. (An extensively and colorfully illustrated textbook.)

Stites D.P., Stobo J.D. & Wells J.V. (1997) *Basic and Clinical Immunology*, 9th edn. Lange Medical, California. (I find this of most use for reference purposes.)

### Reference work

Roitt I.M. & Delves P.J. (eds) (1992) *Encyclopedia of Immunology.* Academic Press, London. (Covers virtually all aspects of the subject and describes immune responses to most infections.)

## Historical

Clarke W.R. (1991) *The Experimental Foundations of Modern Immunology*, 4th edn. John Wiley & Sons, New York. (Important for those wishing to appreciate the experiments leading up to many of the major discoveries.)

Ehrlich P. (1890) On immunity with special reference to cell life. In Melchers F. *et al.* (eds) *Progress in Immunology* **VII**. Springer-Verlag, Berlin. (Translation of a lecture to the Royal Society (London) on the side-chain theory of antibody formation, showing this man's perceptive genius. A must!)

Landsteiner K. (1946) *The Specificity of Serological Reactions*. Harvard University Press (reprinted 1962 by Dover Publications, New York).

Mazumdar P.M.M. (ed.) (1989) *Immunology 1930–1980*. Wall & Thompson, Toronto.

Metchnikoff E. (1893) *Comparative Pathology of Inflammation*. Kegan Paul, Trench, Trubner, London (translated by F.A. & E.H. Starling).

Palmer R. (ed.) (1993) *Outstanding Papers in Biology*. Current Biology, London. (A delight to browse through some of the seminal papers which have shaped modern biology; wonderful material for teaching.)

Silverstein A.M. (1989) *A History of Immunology*. Academic, San Diego.

Tauber A.I. (1991) *Metchnikoff & The Origins of Immunology*. Oxford University Press, Oxford.

## In-depth series for the advanced reader

*Advances in Immunology* (Annual). Academic Press, London.

*Advances in Neuroimmunology* (edited by G.B. Stefano & E.M. Smith). Pergamon, Oxford.

*Annual Review of Immunology*. Ann Reviews Inc., California.

*Immunological Reviews* (edited by G. Moller). Munksgaard, Copenhagen. (Specialized, authoritative and thoughtful.)

*Progress in Allergy*. Karger, Basle.

*Seminars in Immunology*. Academic Press, Cambridge. (In-depth treatment of single subjects.)

## Current information

*Current Biology*. Current Biology, London. (What the complete biologist needs to know about significant current advances.)

*Current Opinion in Immunology*. Current Science, London. (Important personal opinions on focused highlights of the advances made in the previous year; most valuable for the serious immunologist.)

*Immunology Today*. Elsevier Science Publications, Amsterdam. (The immunologist's 'newspaper'. Excellent.)

*Molecular Medicine Today*. Elsevier Science Publications, Amsterdam. (Frequent articles of interest to immunologists with very good perspective.)

*The Immunologist*. Hogrefe & Huber Publishers, Seattle. (Official organ of the International Union of Immunological Societies — IUIS. Excellent, didactic and compact articles on current trends in immunology.)

## Multiple choice questions

Roitt I.M. & Delves P.J. (1995) *Essential Immunology Review*. Blackwell Science Ltd, Cambridge, Massachusetts. (400 MCQs each with 5 annotated learning responses.)

**Table 2.2.** The major immunological journals and their impact factors.

| GENERAL JOURNALS OF PARTICULAR INTEREST TO IMMUNOLOGISTS | *IMPACT FACTOR |
| --- | --- |
| Cell | 40.5 |
| EMBO J. | 13.5 |
| Lancet | 17.5 |
| Nature | 27.1 |
| Nature Medicine | N/A |
| New England Journal of Medicine | 22.4 |
| Proceedings of the National Academy of Science | 10.5 |
| Science | 21.9 |
| **IMMUNOLOGICAL JOURNALS** | ***IMPACT FACTOR** |
| Autoimmunity | 1.3 |
| Cancer Immunology | 1.7 |
| Cellular Immunology | 1.9 |
| Clinical and Experimental Allergy | 2.5 |
| Clinical and Experimental Immunology | 2.7 |
| European Journal of Immunology | 6.1 |
| Human Immunology | 2.7 |
| Immunity | 15.4 |
| Immunogenetics | 3.4 |
| Immunology | 2.8 |
| Clinical Immunology and Immunopathology | 2.1 |
| Immunopharmacology | 1.2 |
| Infection and Immunity | 3.7 |
| International Archives of Allergy and Applied Immunology | 1.3 |
| International Immunology | 4.3 |
| Journal of Allergy and Clinical Immunology | 3.5 |
| Journal of Autoimmunity | 2.0 |
| Journal of Clinical Immunology | 2.7 |
| Journal of Experimental Medicine | 15.1 |
| Journal of Immunology | 7.4 |
| Journal of Immunological Methods | 1.9 |
| Journal of Immunotherapy | 2.5 |
| Journal of Reproductive Immunology | 1.3 |
| Molecular Immunology | 2.3 |
| Parasite Immunology | 1.9 |
| Scandinavian Journal of Immunology | 1.8 |
| Therapeutic Immunology | N/A |
| Tissue Antigens | 3.3 |
| Transplantaion | 2.8 |
| Vaccine | 2.1 |

**\*IMPACT FACTOR** = relative frequency with which the journal's 'average article' has been cited in other publications

N/A, not available.

## Electronic publications (linked to 'Roitt's Essential Immunology')

Roitt I.M. & Delves P.J. (1995) *Immunology Textstack and Quizbank.* Keyboard Publishing, Blue Bell, Pennsylvania. (CD ROM Mac/Windows: Full text and illustrations of *Essential Immunology* with very rapid search facility. Cut and paste selected text. Transfer selected illustrations, amended as desired, to slide-making or overhead facility. Tutors can map out a 'theme' running through the book, insert updates at bookmarked points in the text, and network to other textbooks in the series, e.g. *Robbins' Pathologic Basis of Disease, Harrison's Principles of Internal Medicine,* the *Merck Manual,* etc. 400 multiple choice questions each with 5 annotated learning responses. 89 clinical immunology cases from Chapel H. & Haeney M.)

Roitt I.M. & Delves P.J. (1996) *Interactive Core Tutorials in Immunology.* Blackwell Science Ltd, Oxford. (CD ROM Mac/Windows: 110 fundamental immunological principles using animations accompanied by spoken explanations to clarify and guide. Reference to standard and advanced text in *Essential Immunology* and a selection of multiple choice questions.)

## Major journals

The major journals of interest and their impact factors are noted in table 2.2.

# THE RECOGNITION OF ANTIGEN

The reader now has a broad sense of the scope of immunological defense against infection. Constitutional mechanisms such as phagocytosis, which provide innate immunity and which are unaffected by repeated exposure to antigen, are enormously improved in efficiency by cooperation with acquired immune responses depending upon augmentation of antigen-specific effectors by antigen-driven expansion of individual T- and B-lymphocyte clones. This section of the book explores the processes involved in the recognition of foreign antigens by lymphocytes and their products. First, we characterize the molecules used for this purpose by the immune system. Chapter 3 describes the structural basis for the functions of **antibodies**, the soluble immunoglobulin secretion products of the B-lymphocyte. Provocation of clonal expansion requires the interaction of lymphocyte surface receptors with antigen, and in Chapter 4 we look at current views of the membrane-bound molecules concerned, namely **T- and B-cell antigen-specific receptors** and the **major histocompatibility complex (MHC)** which presents processed intracellular antigen to T-lymphocytes.

In Chapter 5 we are now ready to examine the mechanisms underlying the **primary recognition of antigen** by antibody, either in its soluble or B-cell membrane form, and by the T-cell receptor. Investigation of intracellular processing of protein antigen and the binding of the resulting peptides to the major histocompatibility molecular cleft for presentation to the T-cell receptor represents an area of truly prodigious scientific activity and breakneck advance.

# ANTIBODIES

## THE BASIC STRUCTURE IS A FOUR-PEPTIDE UNIT

The antibody molecule is made up of two identical heavy and two identical light chains held together by interchain disulfide bonds (figure M3.1.1). These chains can be separated by reduction of the S–S bonds and acidification. In the most abundant type of antibody, **immunoglobulin G**, the exposed hinge region is extended in structure due to the high proline content and is therefore vulnerable to proteolytic attack; thus the molecule is split by papain to yield two identical **Fab** fragments, each with a single combining site for antigen, and a third fragment, **Fc**, which lacks the ability to bind antigen. Pepsin strikes at a different point and cleaves the Fc from the remainder of the molecule to leave a large 5$S$ fragment which is formulated as F(ab′)$_2$ since it is still

divalent with respect to antigen binding just like the parent antibody (Milestone 3.1).

The location of the antigen combining sites was elegantly demonstrated by a study of purified antibodies to the dinitrophenyl (DNP) group mixed with the compound:

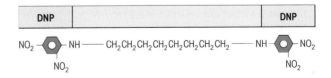

The two DNP groups are far enough apart not to interfere with each other's combination with antibody so that they can bring the antigen combining sites on two different antibodies together end to end. When viewed by negative staining in the electron

# Milestone 3.1—Four-peptide Structure of Immunoglobulin Monomers

Early studies showed the bulk of the antibody activity in serum to be in the slow electrophoretic fraction termed γ-globulin (subsequently immunoglobulin). The most abundant antibodies were divalent, i.e. had two combining sites for antigen and could thus form a precipitating complex (cf. figure 6.2).

To Rod Porter and Gerry Edelman must go the credit for unlocking the secrets of the basic structure of the immunoglobulin molecule. If the internal disulfide bonds are reduced, the component peptide chains still hang together by strong noncovalent attractions. However, if the reduced molecule is held under acid conditions, these attractive forces are lost as the chains become positively charged and can now be separated by gel filtration into larger so-called heavy chains and smaller light chains.

The clues to how the chains are assembled to form the antibody molecule came from selective cleavage using proteolytic enzymes. Papain destroyed the precipitating power of the intact molecule but produced two univalent Fab fragments still capable of binding to antigen (Fab = *fragment antigen binding*); the remaining fragment had no affinity for antigen and was termed Fc by Porter (*fragment crystallizable*). After digestion with pepsin, a smaller molecule, F(ab′)$_2$, was isolated; it still precipitated antigen and so retained both binding sites, but the Fc portion was further degraded. The structural basis for these observations is clearly evident from figure M3.1.1. In essence, with minor changes, all immunoglobulin molecules are constructed from one or more of the basic four-chain monomer units.

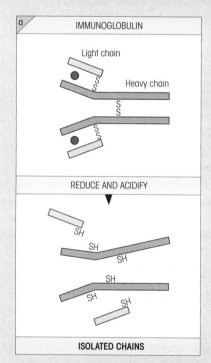 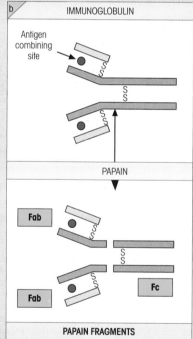 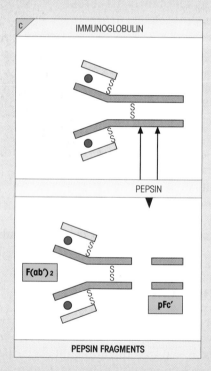

Figure M3.1.1. The antibody basic unit consisting of two identical heavy and two identical light chains held together by interchain disulfide bonds, can be broken down into its constituent peptide chains and to proteolytic fragments, the pepsin F(ab′)$_2$ retaining two binding sites for antigen and the papain Fab with one. After pepsin digestion the pFc′ fragment representing the C-terminal half of the Fc region is formed and is held together by noncovalent bonds. The portion of the heavy chain in the Fab fragment is given the symbol Fd. The N-terminal residue is on the left for each chain.

microscope, a series of geometric forms are observed which represent the different structures to be expected if a flexible Y-shaped hinged molecule with a combining site at the end of each of the two arms of the Y were to complex with this divalent antigen.

Triangular trimers, square tetramers and pentagonal pentamers may be readily discerned (figure 3.1). The way in which these polymeric forms arise is indicated in figure 3.2. The position of the Fc fragment and its lack of involvement in the combination with

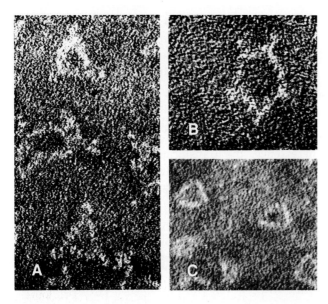

Figure 3.1. (A) and (B) Electron micrograph (× 1 000 000) of complexes formed on mixing the divalent DNP hapten with rabbit anti-DNP antibodies. The 'negative stain' phosphotungstic acid is an electron-dense solution which penetrates in the spaces between the protein molecules. Thus the protein stands out as a 'light' structure in the electron beam. The hapten links together the Y-shaped antibody molecules to form trimers (A), and pentamers (B) (cf. figure 3.2). The flexibility of the molecule at the hinge region is evident from the variation in angle of the arms of the 'Y'. (C) As in (A); trimers formed using the F(ab')$_2$ antibody fragment from which the Fc structures have been digested by pepsin (× 500 000). The trimers can be seen to lack the Fc projections at each corner evident in (A). (After Valentine R.C. & Green N.M. (1967) *Journal of Molecular Biology* **27**, 615; courtesy of Dr Green and with the permission of Academic Press, New York.)

antigen are apparent from the shape of the polymers formed using the pepsin F(ab')$_2$ fragment (figure 3.1C).

## AMINO ACID SEQUENCES REVEAL VARIATIONS IN IMMUNOGLOBULIN STRUCTURE

For good reasons, the antibody population in any given individual is just incredibly heterogeneous, and this has meant that determination of amino acid sequences was utterly useless until it proved possible to obtain the homogeneous product of a single clone. The opportunity to do this first came from the study of **myeloma proteins**.

In the human disease known as multiple myeloma, one cell making one particular individual immunoglobulin divides over and over again in the uncontrolled way a cancer cell does, without regard for the overall requirement of the host. The patient then possesses enormous numbers of identical cells derived as a clone from the original cell and they all synthesize the same immunoglobulin — the myeloma or M-protein — which appears in the serum, sometimes in

very high concentrations. By purification of the myeloma protein we can obtain a preparation of an immunoglobulin having a unique structure. **Monoclonal antibodies** can also be obtained by fusing individual antibody-forming cells with a B-cell tumor to produce a constantly dividing clone of cells dedicated to making the one antibody (cf. figures 2.11 and 6.20).

The sequencing of a number of such proteins has revealed that the N-terminal portions of both heavy and light chains show considerable variability, whereas the remaining parts of the chains are relatively constant, being grouped into a restricted number of structures. It is conventional to speak of variable and constant regions of both heavy and light chains (figure 3.3).

Certain sequences in the variable regions show quite remarkable diversity and systematic analysis localizes these hypervariable sequences to three segments on the light chain (figure 3.4) and three on the heavy chain.

## IMMUNOGLOBULIN GENES

### Immunoglobulins are encoded by multiple gene segments

Clusters of genes on three different chromosomes code for κ, λ and heavy chains respectively. Since a wide range of antibodies with differing amino acid sequences can be produced, there must be corre-

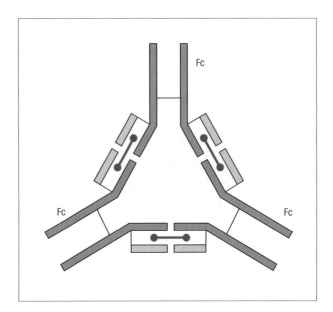

Figure 3.2. Three DNP antibody molecules held together as a trimer by the divalent antigen (●———●). Compare figure 3.1A. When the Fc fragments are first removed by pepsin, the corner pieces are no longer visible (figure 3.1C).

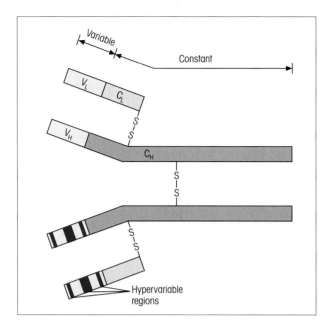

**Figure 3.3. Amino acid sequence variability in the antibody molecule.** The terms 'V region' and 'C region' are used to designate the variable and constant regions respectively, 'V_L' and 'C_L' are generic terms for these regions on the light chain and 'V_H' and 'C_H' specify variable and constant regions on the heavy chain. Certain segments of the variable region are hypervariable but adjacent framework regions are more conserved. As stressed previously, each pair of heavy chains is identical, as is each pair of light chains.

sponding nucleotide sequences to encode them. However, the complete gene encoding each heavy and light chain is not present as such in the germ-line DNA, but is created during early development of the B-cell by the joining together of minisegments of the gene. Take the human κ light chain for example; the variable region is made up of two gene segments, a large $V_\kappa$ and a small $J_\kappa$, while a single gene encodes the constant region (figure 3.5). There is a cluster of some 70 or more $V_\kappa$ genes and just five functional $J$ genes. In the immature B-cell, a translocation event leads to the joining of one of the $V_\kappa$ genes to one of the $J$ segments. Each $V$ segment has its own leader sequence and a number of upstream promoter sites including a characteristic octamer sequence, to which regulatory elements bind (figure 3.6). When the Ig gene is transcribed, splicing of the nuclear RNA brings the $V_\kappa J$ sequence into contiguity with the constant region $C_\kappa$ transcript, the whole being read off as a continuous κ chain peptide within the endoplasmic reticulum.

The same general principles apply to the arrangement of λ and heavy chain genes, although the latter constellation shows additional features: the subclass constant region genes form a single cluster and there

is a group of four highly variable $D$ segments inserted between the $V$ and $J$ regions (figure 3.7). The $D$ and $J$ segments together encode almost the entire third hypervariable region, the first two being contributed by the $V$ sequence.

## A special mechanism effects VDJ recombination

In essence, the translocation involves the mutual recognition of conserved heptamer–spacer–nonamer recombination signal sequences which flank each

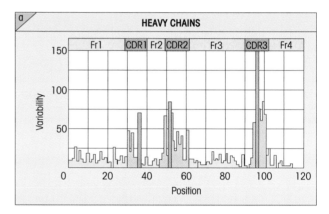

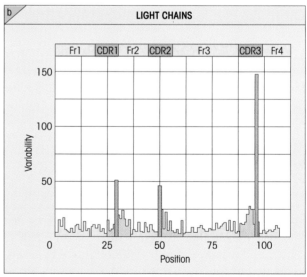

**Figure 3.4. Wu and Kabat plot of amino acid variability in the variable region of immunoglobulin heavy and light chains.** The sequences of chains from a large number of myeloma monoclonal proteins are compared and variability at each position is computed as the number of different amino acids found divided by the frequency of the most common amino acid. Obviously, the higher the number the greater the variability; for a residue at which all 20 amino acids occur randomly, the number will be 400 (20 ÷ 0.05) and at a completely invariant residue, the figure will be 1 (1 ÷ 1). The three hypervariable regions (darker blue) in the (a) heavy and (b) light chains, usually referred to as **Complementarity Determining Regions (CDR)**, are clearly defined. The intervening peptide sequences (grey) are termed framework regions (Fr1–4). (Courtesy of Professor E.A. Kabat.)

germ-line *V*, *D* and *J* segment (figure 3.8). Recombinase activation genes *RAG-1* and *RAG-2* catalyse the introduction of double-strand breaks between the elements to be joined and their respective flanking sequences. At this stage, nucleotides may either be deleted or inserted between the *VD*, *DJ* or *VJ* joining elements before they are ultimately ligated.

## STRUCTURAL VARIANTS OF THE BASIC IMMUNOGLOBULIN MOLECULE

### Isotypes

Based upon the structure of their heavy chain constant regions, immunoglobulins are classed into major groups termed **classes** which may be further subdivided into **subclasses**. In the human, for example, there are five classes: immunoglobulin G (IgG), IgA, IgM, IgD and IgE. They may be differentiated not only by their sequences but also by the antigenic structures to which these sequences give rise. Thus, by injecting a human IgG myeloma protein into a rabbit, it is possible to raise an antiserum which can be absorbed by mixtures of myelomas of other classes to remove cross-reacting antibodies and which will then be capable of reacting with IgG, but not IgA, IgM, IgD or IgE (figure 3.9).

Since all the heavy chain constant region ($C_H$) structures which give rise to classes and subclasses are expressed together in the serum of a normal subject, they are termed **isotypic variants** (table 3.1). Likewise, the light chain constant regions ($C_L$) exist in isotypic forms known as κ and λ which are associated with all heavy chain isotypes. Because the light chains in a given antibody are identical, immunoglobulins are either κ or λ but never mixed (unless specially engineered in the laboratory). Thus IgG exists as IgGκ or IgGλ, IgM as IgMκ or IgMλ, and so on.

### Allotypes

This type of variation depends upon the existence of allelic forms (encoded by alleles or alternative genes at a single locus) which therefore provide genetic

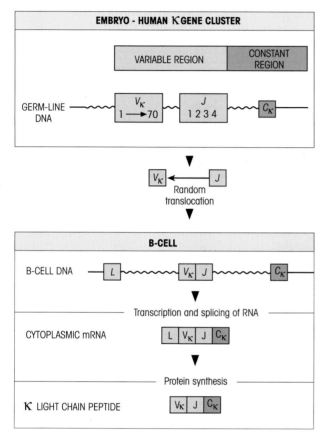

**Figure 3.5. Genetic basis for synthesis of human κ chains.** The $V_κ$ genes are arranged in a series of families or sets of a closely related sequence. Each $V_κ$ gene has its own leader sequence (*L*). As the cell becomes immunocompetent, the variable region is formed by the random combination of a $V_κ$ with a joining segment *J*, a translocation process facilitated by base sequences in the intron following the 3′ end of the $V_κ$-segment pairing up with sequences in the intron 5′ to *J*. The final joining occurs when the intervening intron sequence is spliced out of the RNA transcript. By convention, the genes are represented in italics and the antigens they encode in normal type.

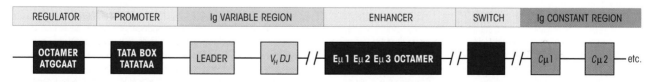

**Figure 3.6. Genes controlling immunoglobulin heavy chain transcription.** Each *VDJ* segment encoding the variable region is associated with a leader sequence. Closely upstream is the TATA box promoter which binds RNA polymerase II and the octamer motif which is one of a number of short sequences which bind transacting regulatory transcription factors. The *V*-region promoters are relatively inactive and only association with enhancers, which are also composites of short sequence motifs capable of binding nuclear proteins, will increase the transcription rate to levels typical of actively secreting B-cells. The enhancers are near to the regions which control switching from one Ig class constant region to another, e.g. IgM to IgG. Primary transcripts are initiated 20 nucleotides downstream of the TATA box and extend beyond the end of the constant region. These are spliced, cleaved at the 3′ end and polyadenylated to generate the translatable mRNA.

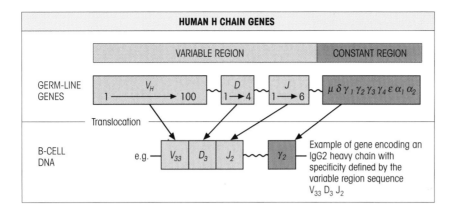

**Figure 3.7. Human *V*-region genes shuffled by translocation** to generate the single heavy chain specificity characteristic of each B-cell. Note the additional *D*-segment minigenes.

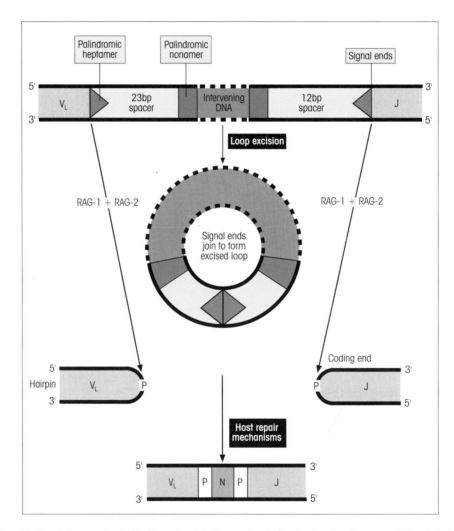

**Figure 3.8. The joining of *V*, *D* and *J* segments.** Joining is masterminded by the recombinase activation genes *RAG-1* and *RAG-2* which regulate expression of the recombinase, and it seems likely that they actually encode the recombinase itself. Supporting this view is the homology of RAG-1 to a yeast topoisomerase-like factor which is associated with site-specific recombination. RAG-1 and RAG-2 together produce several thousand times more efficient *VDJ* recombination than either alone. The introns adjoining the *V*, *D* and *J* gene segments contain specialized **recombination signal sequences (RSS)** which include palindromic heptamers and nonamers separated by spacers of either 12 or 23 base pairs. The two joining segments, in this example $V_L$ and $J_L$, are brought into proximity by interaction between their respective RSS and are cleaved by RAG-1 and RAG-2 which mediate the site-specific endonucleolytic cut at the border of the RSS. The excised signal sequences are joined in a loop containing the intervening DNA while the double strands of each coding segment form 'hairpin' ends with palindromic (P) insertions. These are spliced together by DNA repair mechanisms involving enzymes such as the catalytic component of the DNA-dependent protein kinase (mutation of which gives rise to mice with severe combined immunodeficiency (SCID)). Although the signal joint is precise, the joining of the coding ends is variable and can involve addition of base pairs resulting from the resolution of the hairpin loop (P nucleotides) or base pairs inserted by terminal deoxynucleotide transferase (N nucleotides). Since the coding elements are joined at random with respect to the reading frames, two out of three events have two coding elements out of frame. Although apparently wasteful, this is evolutionarily tolerated because it confers so much benefit in the form of important antigenic diversity. *VDJ* recombination products define the major antigen binding domains.

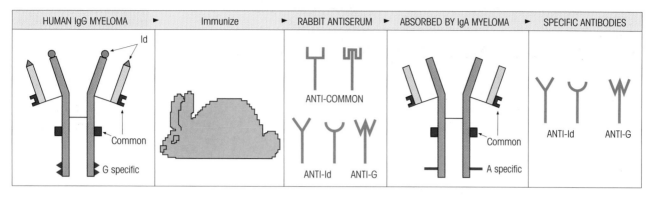

| HUMAN IgG MYELOMA | ▶ | Immunize | ▶ | RABBIT ANTISERUM | ▶ | ABSORBED BY IgA MYELOMA | ▶ | SPECIFIC ANTIBODIES |

**Figure 3.9. How to use monoclonal myeloma proteins to produce antibodies specific for different Ig structures.** The rabbit makes antibodies directed to different parts of the human IgG myeloma. Antibodies to those parts which are common to other Ig classes can be absorbed out with myelomas of those classes leaving other antibodies reacting with class-specific G and variable region-specific (idiotype = Id) structures on the original molecule. By the same token, further absorption with other IgG myelomas will remove the common IgG-specific antibodies leaving an antiserum directed to the idiotypic determinants alone. (In an attempt to simplify, I have ignored subclasses and allotypes, but the same principles can be extended to generating antisera specific for these variants.) The rabbit produces a mixture of polyclonal antibodies directed against each structural site on the antigen, i.e. they are produced by clones derived from a variety of antigen-specific parent cells which each react stereochemically in a slightly different way with the same structure (cf. p. 82).

markers (table 3.1). In somewhat the same way as the red cells in genetically different individuals can differ in terms of the blood group antigen system A, B, O, so the Ig heavy chains differ in the expression of their allotypic groups. Typical allotypes are the **Gm specificities** on IgG (Gm = *marker* on IgG). Allotypic differences at a given Gm locus usually involve one or two amino acids in the peptide chain. Take, for example, the G1m(a) locus on IgG1 (table 3.1). An individual with this allotype would have the peptide sequence: Asp . Glu . Leu . Thr . Lys on each of his IgG1 molecules. Another person whose IgG1 was a-negative would have the sequence Glu . Glu . Met . Thr . Lys, i.e. two amino acids different. To date, 25 Gm groups have been found on the γ-heavy chains and a further three (the Km—previously Inv groups) on the κ constant region.

As in other allelic systems, individuals may be homozygous or heterozygous for the genes encoding the markers; these are expressed codominantly and are inherited in simple Mendelian fashion. Take, for example, the b4, b5 allotypes on rabbit light chains: an animal of $b^4b^4$ genotype would express the b4 allotype, whereas a rabbit of $b^4b^5$ genotype derived from

**Table 3.1. Summary of immunoglobulin variants.**

| $V_H/V_L$ | | CONSTANT | |
|---|---|---|---|
| IDIOTYPE | ISOTYPE | | ISOTYPE |

Hypervariable (Ag combining site)    ALLOTYPE

| TYPE OF VARIATION | DISTRIBUTION | VARIANT | LOCATION | EXAMPLES |
|---|---|---|---|---|
| ISOTYPIC | All variants present in serum of a normal individual | Classes<br>Subclasses<br>Types<br>Subgroups<br>Subgroups | $C_H$<br>$C_H$<br>$C_L$<br>$C_L$<br>$V_H/V_L$ | IgM, IgE<br>IgA1, IgA2<br>κ, λ<br>$\lambda Oz^+$, $\lambda Oz^-$<br>$V_{\kappa I}$ $V_{\kappa II}$ $V_{\kappa III}$<br>$V_{HI}$ $V_{HII}$ $V_{HIII}$ |
| ALLOTYPIC | Alternative forms: genetically controlled so not present in all individuals | Allotypes | Mainly $C_H/C_L$ sometimes $V_H/V_L$ | Gm groups (human)<br>b4, b5, b6, b9 (rabbit light chains)<br>Igh-$1^a$, Igh-$1^b$ (mouse $\gamma_{2a}$ heavy chains) |
| IDIOTYPIC | Individually specific to each immunoglobulin molecule | Idiotypes | Variable regions | Probably one or more hypervariable regions forming the antigen-combining site |

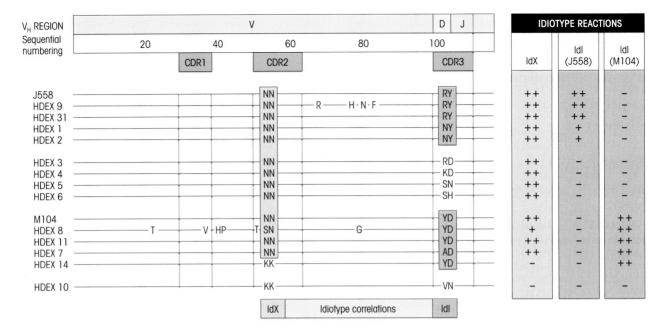

**Figure 3.10. Structural correlates of idiotopes (individual determinants on an idiotype) on antidextran antibodies.** Amino acid sequences of variable heavy chain regions of mouse monoclonal antidextran antibodies are shown. All antibodies have $\lambda_1$ L chains. Lines indicate identity to the sequence of the first protein, J558; letters (Dayhoff code) show differences or regions correlated with idiotopes (central boxed areas). The cross-reacting idiotope (IdX) is associated with the second complementarity determining region (CDR2) structures while the private idiotopes (IdI) are features of the CDR3 region in these antibodies. The presence of the idiotopes on each antibody molecule is assessed by reaction with antisera specific for IdX, J558 IdI, and M104 IdI (on the right). Cross-reacting idiotopes may also be associated with the CDR3 region in other systems. (Reproduced from Davie J.M. et al. (1986) Annual Review of Immunology **4**, 147 with permission. © by Annual Reviews Inc.)

$b^4b^4$ and $b^5b^5$ parents would express the b4 marker on one fraction and b5 on another fraction of its immunoglobulin molecules.

### Idiotypes

We have seen that it is possible to obtain antibodies that recognize isotypic and allotypic variants; one can also raise antiserums which are specific for individual antibody molecules and discriminate between one monoclonal antibody and another independently of isotypic or allotypic structures (figure 3.9). Such antiserums define the individual determinants characteristic of each antibody, collectively termed the **idiotype** (Kunkel & Oudin). Not surprisingly, it turns out that the idiotypic determinants are located in the variable part of the antibody associated with the hypervariable regions (figure 3.10).

Anti-idiotypes which react with one antibody and no other are said to recognize **private** idiotypes and provide further support for the idea that each antibody has a unique structure. Frequently, antibody molecules of closely similar amino acid structure may, in addition, share idiotypes (e.g. M104 and HDEX2 in figure 3.10) and we then speak of **public** or **cross-reacting** idiotypes.

Anti-idiotypic serums provide useful reagents for demonstrating the same V region on different heavy chains and on different cells, for identification of specific immune complexes in patients' serums, for recognition of $V_L$ type amyloid in subjects excreting Bence-Jones proteins, for detection of residual monoclonal protein after therapy and perhaps for selecting lymphocytes with certain surface receptors. The reader will (or should) be startled to learn that it is possible to raise autoanti-idiotypic sera since this means that individuals can make antibodies to their own idiotypes. This has quite momentous consequences, as will become apparent when we discuss the Jerne network theory in Chapter 11.

## IMMUNOGLOBULINS ARE FOLDED INTO GLOBULAR DOMAINS WHICH SUBSERVE DIFFERENT FUNCTIONS

### Immunoglobulin domains have a characteristic structure

In addition to the *interchain* disulfide bonds which bridge heavy and light chains, there are internal, *intrachain* disulfide links which form loops in the peptide chain. As Edelman predicted, the loops are compactly folded to form globular **domains** (figure 3.11) which have a characteristic β-pleated sheet protein structure.

Significantly, the hypervariable sequences appear at one end of the variable domain where they form parts of the β-turn loops and are clustered close to each other in space.

## The variable domain binds antigen

The clustering of the hypervariable loops at the tips of the variable regions where the antigen binding site is localized (figures 3.1 and 3.2) makes them the obvious candidates to subserve the function of antigen recognition (figures 3.11 and 3.12), and this has been confirmed by X-ray crystallographic analysis of complexes formed between the Fab fragments of monoclonal antibodies and their respective antigens. The issue has been put beyond doubt by the demonstration that the antigen specificity of a mouse monoclonal antibody could be conferred on a human immunoglobulin molecule by replacing the human hypervariable sequences with those of the mouse (cf. figure 6.21). The sequence heterogeneity of the three heavy and three light chain hypervariable loops ensures tremendous diversity in combining specificity for antigen through variation in the shape and nature of the surface they create. Thus each hypervariable region may be looked upon as an independent structure contributing to the complementarity of the binding site for antigen and one speaks of **complementarity determining regions (CDR)**.

That these variable regions of heavy and light chains both contribute to antibody specificity is suggested by experiments in which isolated chains were examined for their antigen combining power. In general, varying degrees of residual activity were associated with the heavy chains but relatively little with the light chains; on recombination, however, there was always a significant increase in antigen binding capacity.

Amino acids associated with the combining site can be identified by 'affinity labeling'. In this technique, a hapten (a well-defined chemical grouping to which antibodies can be formed, e.g. DNP in figure 3.1) is equipped with a chemically reactive side-chain which will form covalent links with adjacent amino acids after combination of the hapten with antibody, so labeling residues in the neighborhood of the combining site. A modification introduced by Porter and his colleagues utilizes a 'flick-knife' principle. The hapten with an azide side-chain combines with its antibody and is then illuminated with ultraviolet light; this converts the azide to the reactive nitrene radical which will covalently link to almost any organic group with which it comes in contact. The affinity label binds to both heavy and light chains in the hypervariable regions.

## Constant region domains determine secondary biological function

The classes of antibody differ from each other in many respects: in their half-life, their distribution throughout the body, their ability to fix complement and their binding to cell surface Fc receptors. Since the classes all have the same κ and λ light chains, and heavy and light variable region domains, these differences must lie in the heavy chain constant regions.

It has been possible to localize these biological activities to the various heavy chain domains by using myeloma proteins which have spontaneous domain deletions, or enzymic fragments produced by papain (Fc), pepsin (F(ab')$_2$ and pFc', the C-terminal portion of Fc) and plasmin (Facb from rabbit IgG lacks pFc' but retains the N-terminal half of Fc). Nowadays, of course, it can all be done by genetically engineered proteins.

A model of the IgG molecule is presented in figure 3.13 which indicates the spatial disposition and interaction of the domains in IgG and ascribes the various biological functions to the relevant structures. In principle, the V-region domains form the recognition unit (cf. figure 2.1) and constant-region domains mediate the secondary biological functions.

To enable the Fab arms to have the freedom to move and twist so they can align their hypervariable regions with the antigenic sites on large immobile carriers, and to permit the Fc structures to adjust spatially in order to trigger their effector functions, it is desirable for IgG to have a high degree of flexibility. And it has just that (figure 3.13b). Structural analysis shows that the Fab can 'elbow-bend' at its V–C junction and twist about the hinge, which itself can more properly be described as a *loose tether*, allowing the Fab and the Fc to drift relative to each other with remarkable suppleness (cf. figure 3.1). It could be said that movements like that make it a very sexy molecule!

## IMMUNOGLOBULIN CLASSES AND SUBCLASSES

The physical and biological characteristics of the five major immunoglobulin classes in the human are

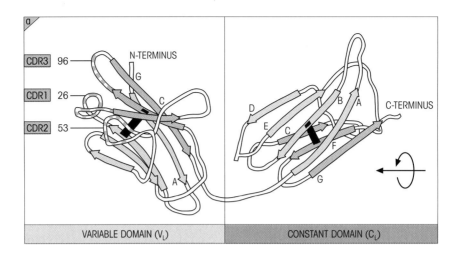

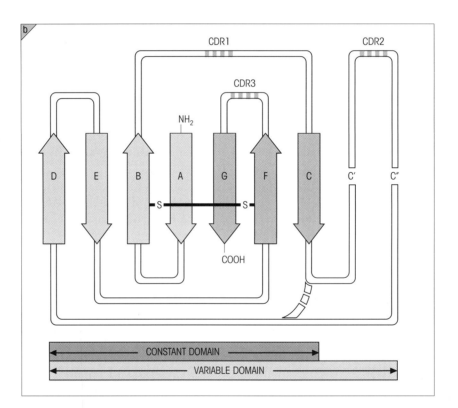

**Figure 3.11.  Ig domain structure.** (a) Structure of the globular domains of a light chain (from X-ray crystallographic studies of a Bence-Jones protein by Schiffler *et al.* (1973) *Biochemistry* **12**, 4620). One surface of each domain is composed essentially of four chains (light blue arrows) arranged in an antiparallel β-pleated structure stabilized by interchain H bonds between the amide CO· and NH· groups running along the peptide backbone, and the other surface of three such chains (darker blue arrows); the black bar represents the intrachain disulfide bond. This structure is characteristic of all immunoglobulin domains. Of particular interest is the location of the hypervariable regions ( ▪ ▪ ▪ ▪ ) in three separate loops which are closely disposed relative to each other and form the light chain contribution to the antigen binding site (cf. figure 3.12). One numbered residue from each complementarity determinant is identified. To generate a Fab fragment (cf. left side figure 3.13b), imagine a $V_H$–$C_H1$ segment just like the $V_L$–$C_L$ in the diagram, rotate it 180° around the axis of the arrow on the right of the figure and lay it on top of $V_L$–$C_L$ segment (Dr A. Feinstein). (b) Schematic view of folding pattern of constant and variable light-chain domains showing the β-strands (A–G) and the extra sequence C′C″ in the variable structure. Lettering and colors as in (a).

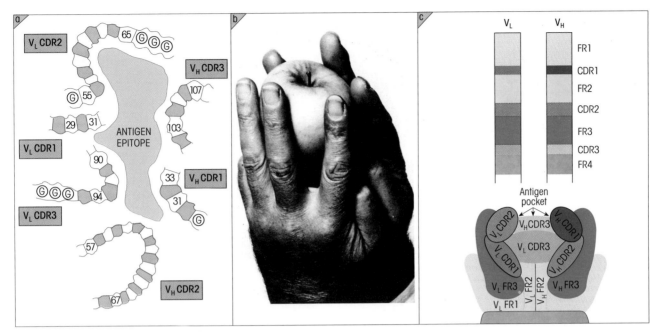

**Figure 3.12. The binding site.** (a) Idealized two-dimensional representation of an antigen binding site formed by spatial apposition of peptide loops containing the hypervariable regions (hot spots: ▪) on light and heavy chains. Numbers refer to amino acid residues. Glycine residues Ⓖ are invariably present at the positions indicated whatever the specificity or animal species of the immunoglobulin. They are of importance in allowing peptide chains to fold back and form β-pleated sheet structures which enable the hypervariable regions to lie close to each other (figure 3.9). Wu and Kabat have suggested that the flexibility of bond angle in this amino acid contributes to the effective formation of a binding site. On this basis the greater frequency of invariant glycines on the light chain might indicate that coarse specificity for antigen binding was provided by the heavy chain and 'fine tuning' by the light chain. By using different combinations of hypervariable regions and different residues within each of these regions, each antibody molecule can form a complex with a variety of antigenic determinants (with a comparable variety of affinities). (b) A simulated combining site for a hapten formed by apposing the three middle fingers of each hand, each finger representing a hypervariable loop. With protein epitopes the area of contact is usually greater and tends to involve more superficial residues (cf. figure 5.5). There appears to be a small repertoire of main chain conformations for at least five of the six CDRs, the particular configuration adopted being determined by a few key conserved residues (Chothia C. *et al.* (1989) *Nature* **342**, 877). (Photograph by B.N.A. Rice; inspired by A. Munro!) (c) An idealized space-filling model indicating the relative locations of the 6 CDR loops (taken from Silverman G.J. (1994) *The Immunologist* **2**, 52, with permission.)

## Immunoglobulin G has major but varied roles in extracellular defenses

Its relative abundance, its ability to develop high affinity binding for antigen and its wide spectrum of secondary biological properties, make IgG appear as the prime workhorse of the Ig stable. During the secondary response IgG is probably the major immunoglobulin to be synthesized. IgG diffuses more readily than the other immunoglobulins into the extravascular body spaces where, as the predominant species, it carries the major burden of neutralizing bacterial toxins and of binding to microorganisms to enhance their phagocytosis.

summarized in tables 3.2 and 3.3. The following comments are intended to supplement this information.

### Activation of the classical complement pathway

Complexes of bacteria with IgG antibody trigger the C1 complex when a minimum of two Fcγ regions in the complex bind C1q (figure 2.2, p. 23). As shown by site-specific mutagenesis of the Cγ2 domain, the common core motif for binding to C1q is Glu.318-X-Lys.320-X-Lys.322 where X, the residue separating these charged amino acids, can vary. In keeping with this analysis, it is comforting to note that synthetic peptides with this structure can block C1q binding to IgG. Activation of the next component C4 tends to produce attachment of C4b to the Cγ1 domain. Thereafter, one observes C3 convertase formation, covalent coupling of C3b to the bacteria and release of C3a and C5a leading to the chemotactic attraction of our friendly polymorphonuclear phagocytic cells (cf. p. 6). These adhere to the bacteria through surface

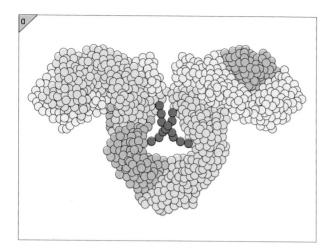

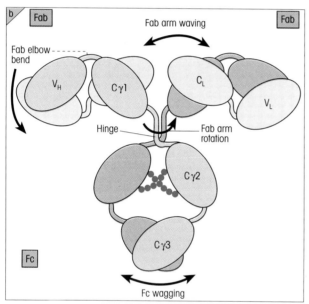

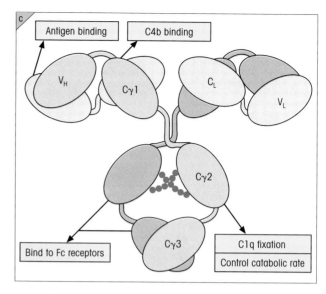

**Figure 3.13. The disposition, interaction and biological properties of the Ig domains in IgG.** (a) Computer-generated model of IgG. One heavy chain is depicted in light blue, the other in darker blue and the light chains in gray. Carbohydrate bound to and separating the Cγ2 domains is in red. The molecule analysed was a mutant with a truncated hinge region since the flexibility associated with the hinge (see (c) below) makes the X-ray pictures fuzzy and difficult to interpret. (The structure was determined by Silverton E.W., Navia M.A. & Davies J.R. (1977) *Proceedings of the National Academy of Science* **74**, 5140, and the figure generated by computer graphics using R.J. Feldmann's system (National Institute of Health).) (b) Diagram based on the model indicating IgG flexibility (cf. O.H. Brekke *et al.* (1995) *Immunology Today* **16**, 85) and showing apposing domains making contact through hydrophobic regions (after Dr A. Feinstein). The structures of these contact frameworks are highly conserved, an essential feature if different $V_H$ and $V_L$ domains are to associate in order to generate a wide variety of antibody specificities. These hydrophobic regions on the two complement fixing $CH_2$ (Cγ2) domains are partly masked by carbohydrate and remain independent, so allowing the formation of a hinge region which is extremely flexible both with respect to variation in the angle of the Fab fragments (waving) and their rotation about the hinge peptide chain. This flexibility enables combining sites in IgG to be readily adapted to spatial variations in the presentation of the antigenic epitopes; Fc 'wagging' permits optimal orientation to receptors on effector cells. (c) Location of biological function. The combined Cγ2 and Cγ3 domains bind to Fc receptors on phagocytic cells, NK cells and placental syncytiotrophoblast; also to staphylococcal protein A. (Note the IgG heavy chain is designated γ and the constant region domains Cγ1, Cγ2 and Cγ3.)

receptors for complement and the Fc portion of IgG (Fcγ) and then ingest the microorganisms through phagocytosis. In a similar way, the extracellular killing of target cells coated with IgG antibody is mediated largely through recognition of the surface Fcγ by NK cells bearing the appropriate receptors (cf. p. 18). The thesis that the **biological individuality of different immunoglobulin classes is dependent on the heavy chain constant regions, particularly the Fc,** is amply borne out in relationship to activities such as transplacental passage, complement fixation and binding to various cell types, where function has been shown to be mediated by the Fc part of the molecule.

## The diversity of Fcγ receptors

Since a wide variety of interactions between IgG complexes and different effector cells have been identified, we really should spend a little time looking at the membrane receptors for Fcγ which mediate these phenomena (figure 3.14). But first let me reiterate a point made earlier in figure 2.5 (p. 26). Simple occupancy of the receptor by its IgG ligand does *not* stimulate biological activity; that is only triggered when the receptors are cross-linked by immune complexes containing more than one IgG molecule.

All the receptors display immunoglobulin-like domains (p. 50) on the extracellular surface which

**Table 3.2. Physical properties of major human immunoglobulin classes.**

| DESIGNATION | IgG | IgA | IgM | IgD | IgE |
|---|---|---|---|---|---|
| Sedimentation coefficient | 7S | 7S,9S,11S* | 19S | 7S | 8S |
| Molecular weight | 150 000 | 160 000 and dimer | 900 000 | 185 000 | 200 000 |
| Number of basic four-peptide units | 1 | 1,2* | 5 | 1 | 1 |
| Heavy chains | $\gamma$ | $\alpha$ | $\mu$ | $\delta$ | $\varepsilon$ |
| Light chains $\kappa + \lambda$ | $\kappa + \lambda$ | $\kappa + \lambda$ | $\kappa + \lambda$ | $\kappa + \lambda$ | $\kappa + \lambda$ |
| Molecular formula† | $\gamma_2\kappa_2, \gamma_2\lambda_2$ | $(\alpha_2\kappa_2)_{1-2}$ $(\alpha_2\lambda_2)_{1-2}$ $(\alpha_2\kappa_2)_2S*$ $(\alpha_2\lambda_2)_2S*$ | $(\mu_2\kappa_2)_5$ $(\mu_2\lambda_2)_5$ | $\delta_2\kappa_2(\delta_2\lambda_2?)$ | $\varepsilon_2\kappa_2, \varepsilon_2\lambda_2$ |
| Valency for antigen binding | 2 | 2,4 | 5(10) | 2 | 2 |
| Concentration range in normal serum | 8-16 mg/ml | 1.4-4 mg/ml | 0.5-2 mg/ml | 0-0.4 mg/ml | 17-450 ng/ml‡ |
| % Total immunoglobin | 80 | 13 | 6 | 0-1 | 0.002 |
| % Carbohydrate content | 3 | 8 | 12 | 13 | 12 |

\* Dimer in external secretions carries secretory component—S
† IgA dimer and IgM contain J-chain
‡ ng $=10^{-9}$ g

**Table 3.3. Biological properties of major immunoglobulin classes in the human.**

| | IgG | IgA | IgM | IgD | IgE |
|---|---|---|---|---|---|
| Major characteristics | Most abundant Ig of internal body fluids particularly extravascular where it combats micro-organisms and their toxins | Major Ig in sero-mucous secretions where it defends external body surfaces | Very effective agglutinator; produced early in immune response – effective first-line defence vs. bacteremia | Most, if not all present on lymphocyte surface | Protection of external body surfaces. Recruits anti-microbial agents. Raised in parasitic infections. Responsible for symptoms of atopic allergy |
| Complement fixation | | | | | |
|   Classical | ++ | – | +++ | – | – |
|   Alternative | – | + | – | – | – |
| Cross placenta | ++ | – | – | – | – |
| Fix to homologous mast cells and basophils | – | – | – | – | +++ |
| Binding to macrophages and polymorphs | +++ | + | – | – | + |

they utilize for the binding of the Fc regions just as other molecules of related structure (the immunoglobulin 'superfamily' p. 247) are mutually attracted through domain interactions. Presumably the three domains of the high affinity Fcγ receptor I (**FcγRI**) provide a far more effective IgG binding site than the two-domain structures of the other receptors with their low affinity for monomeric IgG. FcγRI is present on monocytes and to a lesser extent on unstimulated macrophages. It is effective in mediating the extracellular killing of target cells coated with IgG antibody (ADCC; p. 337). Conceivably, it might be concerned with the overall regulation of IgG levels in the body, since the *catabolic rate* appears to depend directly upon the total IgG concentration and one might speculate that endocytosis of FcγRI, which is the only receptor to have a high affinity for monomeric IgG, could contribute significantly to this degradation. On the other hand, *synthesis* is largely governed by antigen stimulation, so that in germ-free animals, for example, IgG levels are extremely low but rise rapidly on transfer to a normal environment.

**FcγRII** is a low affinity receptor present on monocytes, neutrophils, eosinophils, platelets and B-cells. Binding of monomeric IgG is for all practical purposes insignificant. However, this lends itself to a cheeky play of outstanding simplicity for the uptake of immune complexes: because of the geometric increase in binding strength of polymeric vs monomeric ligands (cf. the 'bonus effect of multivalence' p. 88), complexes bind really well to these receptors and are selectively adsorbed to the cell surface in the face of competition from the dauntingly high concentrations of monomer IgG in the body fluids. Furthermore, because of their fixed spatial relationship within the immune complex, the bound IgG molecules bring about the cross-linking of Fc receptors mandatory for cellular activation. Thus the binding of IgG complexes triggers phagocytic cells and may provoke thrombosis through their reaction with platelets. On the other hand, occupation of B-cell Fc receptors leads to downregulation of cellular responsiveness, possibly being responsible for the negative feedback effect of IgG on antibody production (cf. p. 202). The B-cells have a different isoform of the receptor (FcγRIIB) from the other cell types (FcγRIIA) resulting from differential splicing of the message for a 13 amino acid region of the 47-residue cytoplasmic tail. Whereas the isoform in the phagocytic cells is associated with ligand internalization and delivery to lysosomes, that in the B-cell fails to internalize but concentrates instead on lymphocyte regulation.

Another low affinity receptor **FcγRIII** found on macrophages, polymorphs, eosinophils and NK cells would seem to be largely responsible for mediating ADCC by NK cells and clearance of immune complexes from the circulation by macrophages. For example, the clearance of IgG-coated erythrocytes from the blood of chimpanzees was essentially inhibited by the monovalent Fab fragment of a monoclonal anti-FcγIII (work out why the Fab fragment was used). The mad flurry of gene cloning and sequencing is revealing important similarities between proteins in different cells subserving comparable functions. In this connection, it is quite fascinating that the γ chain of human FcγRIII has close homology with the γ chain from the mast cell FcεRI and the ζ chain of the T-cell receptor complex, to be discussed later. Almost cer-

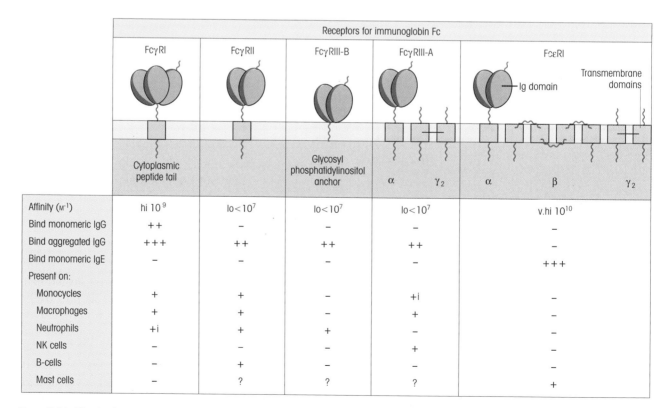

| | FcγRI | FcγRII | FcγRIII-B | FcγRIII-A | | FcεRI | | |
|---|---|---|---|---|---|---|---|---|
| | | | | α | γ₂ | α | β | γ₂ |
| | Cytoplasmic peptide tail | | Glycosyl phosphatidylinositol anchor | | | | | |
| Affinity (M⁻¹) | hi 10⁹ | lo<10⁷ | lo<10⁷ | lo<10⁷ | | v.hi 10¹⁰ | | |
| Bind monomeric IgG | ++ | – | – | – | | – | | |
| Bind aggregated IgG | +++ | ++ | ++ | ++ | | – | | |
| Bind monomeric IgE | – | – | – | – | | +++ | | |
| Present on: | | | | | | | | |
| Monocycles | + | + | – | +i | | – | | |
| Macrophages | + | + | – | + | | – | | |
| Neutrophils | +i | + | + | – | | – | | |
| NK cells | – | – | – | + | | – | | |
| B-cells | – | + | – | – | | – | | |
| Mast cells | – | ? | ? | ? | | + | | |

**Figure 3.14. The structures and characteristics of surface receptors for immunoglobulin Fc regions.** i = inducible; bars = disulfide bridge.

tainly, these represent a family of related proteins sharing a common role in a signal transducing pathway. Thus signals through the receptors are transmitted to initiate phagocytosis in macrophages, to bring out the killer in NK cells, and to trigger degranulation in mast cells.

Alone of the Ig classes, IgG possesses the crucially important ability to cross the human placenta so that it can provide a major line of defense for the first few weeks of a baby's life, and this may be further reinforced by the transfer of colostral IgG across the gut mucosa in the neonate. These transport processes involve translocation of IgG across the cell barrier by complexing to an Fcγ receptor. A recent study succeeded in cloning a **new FcγRn receptor** from the intestinal cells of the rat which transports IgG from mother's milk into the baby (figure 3.15). Note how the direction of transport is achieved by the differential binding of IgG to the receptor at the pH of the lumen versus that at the basal surface. Unlike

FcγRI, a member of the Ig superfamily (p. 247), FcγRn is an MHC class I molecule associated with $\beta_2$-microglobulin.

### Nonprecipitating 'univalent' antibodies

IgG has two combining sites for antigen and there has been a tendency to scoff at claims to have discovered 'univalent' antibodies. Sceptics must now accept that 5–15% of the IgG in all antiserums appears to consist of nonprecipitating asymmetric molecules with a single effective binding site. The other site is blocked stereochemically by a mannose-rich carbohydrate in the C1 domain. If one takes an antibody directed to a small molecule such as DNP (cf. p. 43), this spatial block by adjacent carbohydrate on binding of DNP linked to a larger carrier protein, can be overcome by distancing the DNP group from the bulky carrier with a spindly carbon chain spacer.

## Immunoglobulin A guards the mucosal surfaces

IgA appears selectively in the seromucous secretions such as saliva, tears, nasal fluids, sweat, colostrum, and secretions of the lung, genitourinary and gastrointestinal tracts, where it clearly has the job of defending the exposed external surfaces of the body against attack by microorganisms. This responsibility is clearly taken seriously since approximately 40 mg of secretory IgA/kg body weight is transported daily through the human intestinal crypt epithelium to the mucosal surface as compared with a *total* daily production of IgG of 30 mg/kg.

The IgA is synthesized locally by plasma cells and dimerized intracellularly together with a cysteine-rich polypeptide called J-chain of molecular weight 15 000. The dimeric molecule is effectively tetravalent and will have a much higher binding avidity for polymeric antigens than the monomeric form due to the bonus effect of multivalency (cf. p. 88). If dimerization occurred randomly *after* secretion, dimers of mixed specificity would be formed which would be no more effective in combining with antigen than the monomers. The dimeric IgA binds strongly through its J-chain to a receptor for polymeric Ig present in the membrane of mucosal epithelial cells. The complex is then actively endocytosed, transported across the cytoplasm and secreted into the external body fluids after cleavage of the poly Ig receptor peptide chain. The fragment of the receptor remaining bound to the IgA is termed secretory piece and the whole molecule, **secretory IgA** (figure 3.16). The reader is strongly recommended to turn to figure 8.10 (p. 161) for a

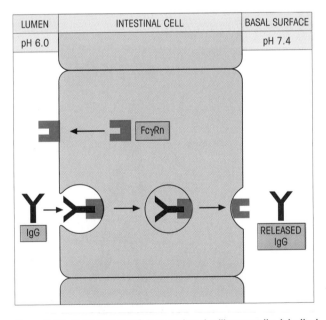

**Figure 3.15. Transport of IgG from maternal milk across the intestinal cells of the baby rat.** IgG binds to the receptor (FcγRn) at pH 6.0, is taken into the cell within a clathrin-coated vesicle and released at the pH of the basal surface. The directional movement of IgG is achieved by the asymmetric pH effect on Ig–receptor interaction. In the placenta, the receptor does not need to show differential binding because its function is to allow the fetal IgG concentration to rise to that in the maternal circulation. (Based on a diagram by Parham P. (1989) *Nature* **337**, 118.) FcγRn, somewhat surprisingly, contains $\beta_2$-microglobulin (cf. p.71) and knockout mice lacking this peptide are incapable of acquiring maternal Ig as neonates; furthermore, they have a grossly shortened IgG half-life suggesting that the FcγRn may be involved. The IgG half-life is unusually long compared with that of IgA and IgM and this enables the response to antigen to be sustained for many months following infection.

dramatic demonstration of secretory IgA held in the surface mucus of intestinal mucosal epithelial cells.

The function of the secretory piece may be to protect the IgA hinge from bacterial proteases. It would also be nice to think that it acted as a molecular Teflon to endow the IgA dimer with 'nonstick' potential, since IgA antibodies function by inhibiting the adherence of coated microorganisms to the surface of mucosal cells, thereby preventing entry into the body tissues. They will also combine with the myriad soluble antigens of dietary and microbial origin to block their access to the body. Aggregated IgA binds to polymorphs and can also activate the alternative (figure 2.3), as distinct from the classical, complement pathway, largely through its abundant carbohydrate groups. This may account for reports of a synergism between IgA, complement and lysozyme in the killing of certain coliform organisms where it is supposed that complement-induced disruption of the outer surface permits access of the enzyme to the peptidoglycan wall. Plasma IgA is predominantly monomeric and since this form is a relatively poor activator of secondary biological effects such as complement fixation which could lead to tissue damaging hypersensitivity reactions, it seems sensible for the body to use it for the neutralization of any antigens which breach the epithelial barrier to enter the circulation in appreciable quantities.

## Immunoglobulin M provides a defense against bacteremia

Often referred to as the macroglobulin antibodies because of their high molecular weight, IgM molecules are polymers of five four-peptide subunits each bearing an extra $C_H$ domain. As with IgA, a single J-chain is incorporated into the pentamer which has the structure shown in figure 3.17a. Under negative staining in the electron microscope, the free molecule in solution assumes a 'star' shape but when combined as an antibody with an antigenic surface membrane it can adopt a 'crab-like' configuration (figure 3.17b and c) in which multiple Fc regions are now accessible to C1q which is bound most firmly. It now seems that

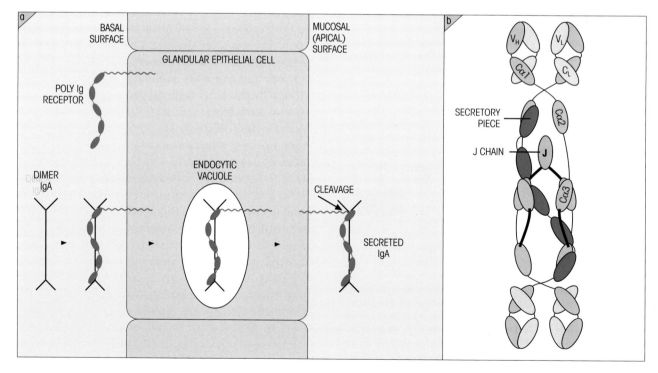

**Figure 3.16. Secretory IgA.** (a) The mechanism of IgA secretion at the mucosal surface. The mucosal cell synthesizes a receptor for polymeric Ig which is inserted into the basal membrane. Dimeric IgA binds to this receptor and is transported via an endocytic vacuole to the apical surface. Cleavage of the receptor releases secretory IgA still attached to part of the receptor termed secretory piece. Note how the receptor cleavage introduces an asymmetry which drives the transport of IgA dimers to the mucosal surface (in quite the opposite direction to the transcytosis of milk IgG in figure 3.15). (b) Schematic and still rather speculative view of the structure of secreted IgA. The J-chain which is an integral part of secreted polymeric Ig (IgA and IgM) is thought to form disulfide bonds with the penultimate cysteine residue(s) of the Cα3 domain and seems to be critical for the initial binding to the poly Ig receptor.

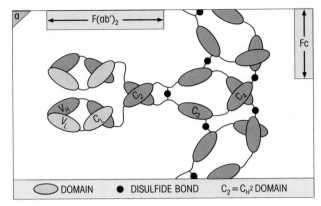
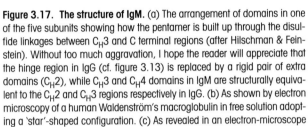
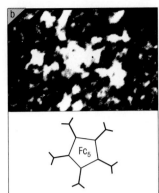
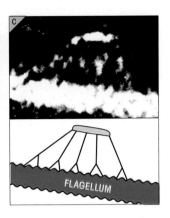

**Figure 3.17. The structure of IgM.** (a) The arrangement of domains in one of the five subunits showing how the pentamer is built up through the disulfide linkages between $C_H3$ and C terminal regions (after Hilschman & Feinstein). Without too much aggravation, I hope the reader will appreciate that the hinge region in IgG (cf. figure 3.13) is replaced by a rigid pair of extra domains ($C_H2$), while $C_H3$ and $C_H4$ domains in IgM are structurally equivalent to the $C_H2$ and $C_H3$ regions respectively in IgG. (b) As shown by electron microscopy of a human Waldenström's macroglobulin in free solution adopting a 'star'-shaped configuration. (c) As revealed in an electron-microscope preparation of specific sheep IgM antibody bound to *Salmonella paratyphi* flagellum where the immunoglobulin has assumed a 'crab-like' conformation in establishing its links with antigen. With the $F(ab')_2$ arms bent out of the plane of the central $Fc_5$ region, the $C_H3$ complement binding domains are now readily accessible to the first component of complement (cf. p. 23). The $Fc_5$ constellation obtained by papain cleavage can activate complement directly. (Electron micrographs are negatively stained preparations of magnification × 2 000 000, i.e. 1 mm represents 0.5 nm; kindly provided by Dr A. Feinstein and Dr E.A. Munn.)

IgM can also exist in a hexameric form and this is said to be 10–20 times more effective in activating complement-mediated lysis than the pentamer. The theoretical combining valency of the pentamer is of course 10 but this is only observed on interaction with small haptens; with larger antigens the effective valency falls to 5 and this must be attributed to some form of steric restriction due to lack of flexibility in the molecule. IgM antibodies tend to be of relatively low affinity as measured against single determinants (haptens) but, because of their high valency, they bind with quite respectable avidity to antigens with multiple epitopes (bonus effect of multivalency, p. 88). For the same reason, these antibodies are extremely efficient agglutinating and cytolytic agents and since they appear early in the response to infection and are largely confined to the bloodstream, it is likely that they play a role of particular importance in cases of bacteremia. The isohemagglutinins (anti-A, anti-B) and many of the 'natural' antibodies to microorganisms are usually IgM; antibodies to the typhoid 'O' antigen (endotoxin) and the 'WR' antibodies in syphilis are also found in this class. IgM would appear to precede IgG in the phylogeny of the immune response in vertebrates.

Monomeric IgM (i.e. a single four-peptide unit), with a hydrophobic sequence stitched into the C-terminal end of the heavy chain to anchor the molecule in the cell membrane, is the major antibody receptor used by B-lymphocytes to recognize antigen (cf. figure 2.10).

## Immunoglobulin D is a cell surface receptor

This class was recognized through the discovery of a myeloma protein which did not have the antigenic specificity of IgG, A or M, although it reacted with antibodies to immunoglobulin light chains and had the basic four-peptide structure. The hinge region is particularly extended and although protected to some degree by carbohydrate, it may be this feature which makes IgD, among the different immunoglobulin classes, uniquely susceptible to proteolytic degradation, and account for its short half-life in plasma (2.8 days). An exciting development has been the demonstration that nearly all the IgD is present, together with IgM, on the surface of a proportion of B-lymphocytes where it seems likely that they may operate as mutually interacting antigen receptors for the control of lymphocyte activation and suppression. The even greater susceptibility of IgD to proteolysis on combination with antigen could well be implicated in such a function.

## Immunoglobulin E triggers inflammatory reactions

Only very low concentrations of IgE are present in serum and only a very small proportion of the plasma cells in the body are synthesizing this immunoglobulin. It is not surprising, therefore, that so far only a handful of IgE myelomas have been recognized compared with tens of thousands of

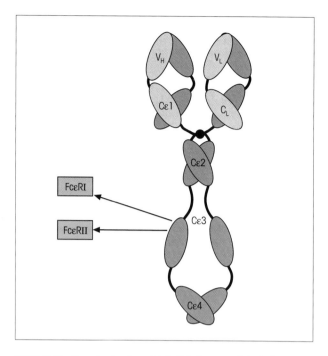

**Figure 3.18. Domain structure of IgE.** Note the general similarity in structure to the IgM basic unit in figure 3.17 with the IgG hinge replaced by the extra $C\varepsilon2$-coupled domains, but also the lack of association of the penultimate C-terminal domains (in this case $C\varepsilon3$) which is a consistent feature of all Ig classes. The $\alpha$-chain of the high affinity mast cell receptor for IgE ($Fc\varepsilon RI$) binds very avidly to a single site located in positions 301–304 of the $C\varepsilon2$ domain. The low affinity $Fc\varepsilon RII$ on inflammatory cells and B-lymphocytes requires the presence of both $C\varepsilon3$ domains for significant binding to IgE. 'Knockout' mice lacking the $Fc\varepsilon RI$ $\alpha$-chain do not express the receptor and cannot produce anaphylactic reactions; conclusion, the low affinity $Fc\varepsilon RII$ receptor which is expressed does not contribute significantly to IgE/mast cell mediated anaphylaxis.

IgG paraproteinemias. IgE antibodies (figure 3.18) remain firmly fixed for an extended period when injected into human skin where they are bound with high affinity to the $Fc\varepsilon RI$ receptor on mast cells (figure 3.14). Contact with antigen leads to degranulation of the mast cells with release of preformed vasoactive amines and cytokines, and the synthesis of a variety of inflammatory mediators derived from arachidonic acid (cf. figure 1.15). This process is responsible for the symptoms of hay fever and of extrinsic asthma when patients with atopic allergy come into contact with the allergen, e.g. grass pollen.

The main *physiological* role of IgE would appear to be protection of anatomical sites susceptible to trauma and pathogen entry, by local recruitment of plasma factors and effector cells through **triggering an acute inflammatory reaction**. Infectious agents penetrating the IgA defenses would combine with specific IgE on the mast cell surface and trigger the release of vasoactive agents and factors chemotactic for granulocytes, so leading to an influx of plasma IgG, complement, polymorphs and eosinophils (cf. p. 278). In such a context, the ability of eosinophils to damage IgG-coated helminths and the generous IgE response to such parasites would constitute an effective defense.

## Immunoglobulins are further subdivided into subclasses

Antigenic analysis of IgG myelomas revealed further variation and showed that they could be grouped into

| | IgG1 | IgG2 | IgG3 | IgG4 |
|---|---|---|---|---|
| % Total IgG in normal serum | 65 | 23 | 8 | 4 |
| Electrophoretic mobility | slow | slow | slow | slow |
| Spontaneous aggregation | – | – | +++ | – |
| Gm allotypes | a,z,f,x | n | b0,b1,b3 g,s,t,etc. | |
| Ga site reacting with rheumatoid factor* | +++ | +++ | – | +++ |
| Combination with staphylococcal A protein | +++ | +++ | – | +++ |
| Binding to staphylococcal protein G | +++ | +++ | +++ | +++ |
| Cross placenta | ++ | ± | ++ | ++ |
| Complement fixation (C1 pathway)** | +++ | ++ | ++++ | ± |
| Binding to monocytes | +++ | + | +++ | ± |
| Binding to heterologous skin | ++ | – | ++ | ++ |
| Blocking IgE binding | – | – | – | + |
| Antibody dominance | Anti-Rh | Anti-dextran Anti-levan | Anti-Rh | Anti-Factor VIII |

**Table 3.4.** Comparison of human IgG subclasses. *Other rheumatoid factors apparently react with Gm-specific sites. **The very poor complement-fixing ability of IgG4 cannot be ascribed to its rigid hinge region since substitution of serine 331 with proline (as in IgG1 and IgG3) endows the molecule with excellent C1q binding and C-mediated lytic capability. Intriguingly, substitution of proline 331 with serine in IgG1 maintains C1q binding but grossly diminishes lytic activity, a puzzle still to be resolved.

four isotypic **subclasses** now termed IgG1, IgG2, IgG3 and IgG4. The differences all lie in the heavy chains which have been labeled γ1, γ2, γ3 and γ4, respectively. These heavy chains show considerable homology and have certain structures in common with each other—the ones which react with specific anti-IgG antisera—but each has one or more additional structures characteristic of its own subclass arising from differences in primary amino acid composition and in interchain disulfide bridging. These

give rise to differences in biological behaviour which are summarized in table 3.4.

Two subclasses of IgA have also been found, of which IgA1 constitutes 80–90% of the total. The IgA2 subclass is unusual in that it lacks interchain disulfide bonds between heavy and light chains. Class and subclass variation is not restricted to human immunoglobulins but is a feature of all the mammals so far studied: monkey, sheep, rabbit, guinea-pig, rat and mouse.

## SUMMARY

### The basic structure is a four-peptide unit

- Immunoglobulins (Ig) have a basic four-peptide structure of two identical heavy and two identical light chains joined by interchain disulfide links.
- Papain splits the molecule at the exposed flexible hinge region to give two identical univalent antigen binding fragments (Fab) and a further fragment (Fc). Pepsin proteolysis gives a divalent antigen binding fragment F(ab')$_2$ lacking the Fc.

### Amino acid sequences reveal variations in immunoglobulin structure

- There are perhaps $10^8$ or more different Ig molecules in normal serum.
- Analysis of myeloma proteins which are homogeneous Ig produced by single clones of malignant plasma cells has shown the N-terminal region of heavy and light chains to have a variable amino acid structure and the remainder to be relatively constant in structure.

### Immunoglobulin genes

- Clusters of genes on three different chromosomes encode κ, λ and heavy Ig chains respectively. In each cluster there are approximately 100 or more variable region (*V*) genes and around five small *J* minisegments. Heavy chain clusters in addition contain of the order of four *D* minigenes. There is a single gene encoding each constant region.
- A special splicing mechanism involving mutual recognition of 5′ and 3′ flanking sequences, catalysed by recombinase enzymes, effects the *VD*, *VJ* and *DJ* translocations.

### Structural variants of the basic Ig molecule

- Isotypes are Ig variants based on different heavy chain constant structures, all of which are present in each individual; examples are the Ig classes IgG, IgA, etc.
- Allotypes are heavy chain variants encoded by allelic (alternative) genes at single loci and are therefore genetically distributed; examples are Gm groups.
- An idiotype is the collection of antigenic determinants on an antibody, usually associated with the hypervariable regions, recognized by other antigen-specific receptors either antibody (the anti-idiotype) or T-cell receptors.
- The variable region domains bind antigen, and three hypervariable loops on the heavy chain termed complementarity determining regions, and three on the light chain, form the antigen binding site.
- The constant region domains of the heavy chain (particularly the Fc) carry out a secondary biological function after the binding of antigen, e.g. complement fixation and macrophage binding.

### Immunoglobulin classes and subclasses

- In the human there are five major types of heavy chain giving five classes of Ig. IgG is the most abundant Ig particularly in the extravascular fluids where it neutralizes toxins and combats microorganisms by fixing complement via the C1 pathway, and facilitating the binding to phagocytic cells by receptors for C3b and Fcγ. It crosses the placenta in late pregnancy and the intestine in the neonate.
- Various Fcγ receptors are specialized for different functions such as phagocytosis, antibody-dependent cell-mediated cytotoxicity, placental transport and B-lymphocyte regulation.

*(Continued on p. 62)*

• IgA exists mainly as a monomer (basic four-peptide unit) in plasma, but in the seromucous secretions, where it is the major Ig concerned in the defense of the external body surfaces, it is present as a dimer linked to a secretory component.

• IgM is basically a pentameric molecule although a minor fraction may be hexameric. It is essentially intravascular and is produced early in the immune response. Because of its high valency it is a very effective bacterial agglutinator and mediator of complement-dependent cytolysis and is therefore a powerful first-line defense against bacteremia.

• IgD is largely present on the lymphocyte and probably functions as an antigen receptor.

• IgE binds firmly to mast cells and contact with antigen leads to local recruitment of antimicrobial agents through degranulation of the mast cells and release of inflammatory mediators. IgE is of importance in certain parasitic infections and is responsible for the symptoms of atopic allergy.

• Further diversity of function is possible through subdivision of classes into subclasses based on structural differences in heavy chains all present in each normal individual.

## FURTHER READING

Davie J.M. *et al.* (1986) Structural correlates of idiotopes. *Annual Review of Immunology* **4**, 147.

French M.A.H. (ed.) (1986) *Immunoglobulins in Health and Disease.* MTP, Lancaster, UK.

Harris L.J. *et al.* (1992) The 3-dimensional structure of an intact monoclonal antibody for canine lymphoma. *Nature* **360**, 369.

Metzger H. (1991) Fc receptors and membrane immunoglobulin. *Current Opinion in Immunology* **3**, 40.

Pascual V. & Capra J.D. (1991) Human immunoglobulin heavy chain variable region genes: organisation, polymorphism and expression. *Advances in Immunology* **49**, 1.

Ravetch J.V. & Kinet J.-P. (1991) Fc receptors. *Annual Review of Immunology* **9**, 457.

Roitt I.M. & Delves P.J. (eds) (1992) *Encyclopedia of Immunology.* Academic Press, London. (Articles on IgG, IgA, IgM, IgD and IgE and immunoglobulin function and domains.)

Sautes C. *et al.* (1992) Structures involved in the activities of murine low affinity Fcγ receptors. In Gergely J. *et al.* (eds) *Progress in Immunology.* VIII, p. 457. Springer-Verlag, Budapest.

Thompson C.B. (1995) New insights into *V(D)J* recombination and its role in the evolution of the immune system. *Immunity* **3**, 531.

# MEMBRANE RECEPTORS FOR ANTIGEN

## THE B-CELL SURFACE RECEPTOR FOR ANTIGEN

### The B-cell inserts a transmembrane immunoglobulin into its surface

In Chapter 2 we discussed the cunning system by which an antigen can be led inexorably to its doom by selecting the lymphocytes capable of making antibodies complementary in shape to itself through its ability to combine with a copy of the antibody molecule on the lymphocyte surface. It will be recalled that combination with the surface receptor can activate the cell to proliferate before maturing into a clone of plasma cells secreting antibody specific for the inciting antigen (cf. figure 2.11).

Immunofluorescent staining of live B-cells with labeled anti-Ig (e.g. figure 2.6f) reveals the earliest membrane Ig to be of the IgM class. The cell is committed to the production of just one antibody specificity and so transcribes its individual rearranged $VJC\kappa$ (or $\lambda$) and $VDJC\mu$ genes. The solution to the problem of secreting antibody with the same specificity as that present on the cell surface as a membrane Ig is found in a **differential splicing** mechanism. The initial nuclear μ-chain RNA transcript includes sequences coding for **hydrophobic transmembrane regions** which enable the IgM to sit in the membrane as a receptor, but if these are spliced out, the antibody molecules can be secreted in a soluble form (figure 4.1).

As the B-cell matures, it coexpresses surface IgD with the same specificity. This phenotype is abundant in the mantle zone lymphocytes of secondary lym-

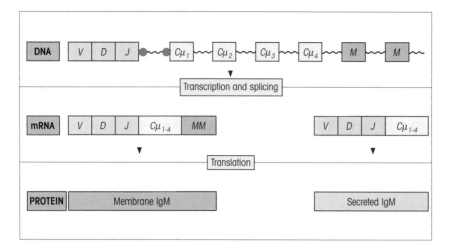

**Figure 4.1. Splicing mechanism for the switch from the membrane to the secreted form of IgM.** The hydrophobic sequence encoded by the exons *M–M* which anchors the receptor IgM to the membrane is spliced out in the secreted form. For simplicity, the leader sequence has been omitted. ⌇ = introns.

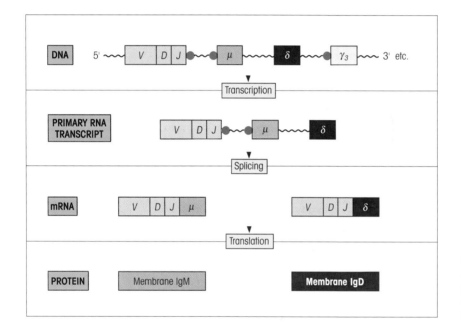

**Figure 4.2. Surface membrane IgM and IgD receptors** of identical specificity appear on the same cell through differential splicing of the composite primary RNA transcript (leader sequences again omitted for simplicity).

phoid follicles (cf. figure 8.7f) and is achieved by differential splicing of a single transcript containing *VDJ*, *Cμ* and *Cδ* segments producing either membrane IgM or IgD (figure 4.2). As the B-cell matures further, other isotypes such as IgG may be expressed (figure 4.3; cf. p. 240).

## The surface immunoglobulin is complexed with associated membrane proteins

The cytoplasmic tail of the surface IgM is a miserable three amino acids long. In no way could this accommodate the structural motifs required for interaction with intracellular protein tyrosine kinases or G proteins which mediate the activation of signal transduction cascades. However, the 25 amino acid

transmembrane-spanning region is the most conserved part of the μ chain, being identical in sequence between that old duo man and mouse and even showing 50% homology with the shark. It seems most likely that the surface Ig transduces signals through associated membrane proteins.

With some difficulty, it should be said, it has proved possible to isolate a disulfide-linked heterodimer which copurifies with the membrane Ig. This consists of two glycoprotein chains called Ig-α and Ig-β (figure 4.4). Interaction between Ig-α and μ chain is essential for transport of IgM to the cell surface. Both Ig-α and Ig-β fold extracellularly into immunoglobulin-like domains but have C-terminal cytoplasmic chains which become phosphorylated on cell activation by antibody-induced cross-linking of the membrane Ig

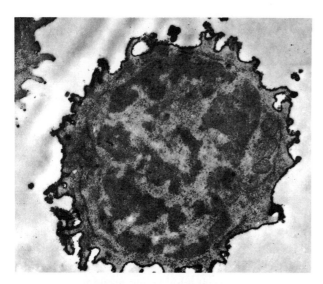

**Figure 4.3. Electron microscopic visualization of human IgG on the surface of a B-lymphocyte** by treatment of viable cell suspensions with peroxidase-coupled anti-IgG. Note the adjacent unstained lymphocyte. (Courtesy of Miss V. Petts.)

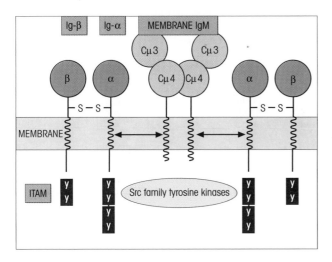

**Figure 4.4. Model of B-cell surface receptor complex.** The Ig-α/Ig-β heterodimer is encoded by the B-cell specific genes *mb-1* and *B29* respectively. Two of these heterodimers are shown with the Ig-α associating with a segment (sequence TAST) on the membrane-spanning region of the IgM μ chain. The Ig-like extracellular domains are colored blue. Each tyrosine (Y)-containing box possesses a recurrent sequence of general structure Tyr.$X_2$.Leu.$X_7$.Tyr.Ile (where X is not a conserved residue), referred to as the immunoreceptor tyrosine-based motif (ITAM). On activation of the B-cell, these ITAM sequences act as signal transducers through their ability to associate with and be phosphorylated by a series of tyrosine kinases.

or the Ig-α chain, an event also associated with rapid $Ca^{2+}$ mobilization.

A tyrosine-containing structural motif (ITAM) present in the cytoplasmic regions of the Ig-α/β heterodimer (figure 4.4) can associate with and undergo phosphorylation by tyrosine kinases. Homologous sequences have been identified in the C-

domains of the γ, δ and ζ chains of the T-cell receptor and β, γ chains of the high affinity IgE receptor, which must further strengthen the view that we are dealing with signal-transducing molecules.

## THE T-CELL SURFACE RECEPTOR FOR ANTIGEN

### The receptor for antigen is a transmembrane heterodimer

When it was eventually tracked down (Milestone 4.1), the antigen-specific **T-cell receptor** was identified as a membrane-bound molecule composed of two disulfide-linked chains, α and β. Each chain folds into two Ig-like domains, one having a relatively invariant structure, the other exhibiting a high degree of variability rather like an Ig Fab fragment. While it is safe to assume that the variable region has the job of binding to antigen, we do not yet have the X-ray diffraction data to define the structural basis of that recognition process.

Both α and β chains are required for antigen specificity as shown by transfection of the T-receptor genes from a cytotoxic T-cell clone specific for fluorescein to another clone of different specificity; when it expressed the new α and β genes, the transfected clone acquired the ability to lyse the fluoresceinated target cells. Another type of experiment utilized T-cell hybridomas formed by fusing single antigen-specific T-cells with T-cell tumors to achieve 'immortality'. One hybridoma recognizing chicken ovalbumin presented by a macrophage, gave rise spontaneously to two variants, one of which lost the chromosome encoding the α chain, and the other, the β chain. Neither variant recognized antigen but when they were physically fused together, each supplied the complementary receptor chain and reactivity with antigen was restored.

### There are two classes of T-cell receptors

Not long after the breakthrough in identifying the αβ T-cell receptor, came reports of the existence of a second type of receptor composed of γ and δ chains. Since it appears earlier in thymic ontogeny, the **γδ receptor** is termed **TCR1** and the αβ, **TCR2** (cf. p. 229).

In the human, γδ cells make up only 0.5–15% of the T-cells in peripheral blood but they show greater dominance in the intestinal epithelium and in skin. In contrast, between 30% and 80% of blood T-cells in ruminants are γδ, reflecting a somewhat different physiological life-style, but it does make the point

# Milestone 4.1—The T-cell Receptor

Since T-lymphocytes respond by activation and proliferation when they contact antigen presented by cells such as macrophages, it seemed reasonable to postulate that they did so by receptors on their surface. In any case, it would be difficult to fit T-cells into the clonal selection club if they lacked such receptors. Guided by Ockam's razor (the *Law of Parsimony*, which contends that it is the aim of science to present the facts of nature in the simplest and most economical conceptual formulations), most investigators plumped for the hypothesis that nature would not indulge in the extravagance of evolving two utterly separate molecular recognition species for B- and T-cells, and many fruitless years were spent looking for the Holy Grail of the T-cell receptor with anti-immunoglobulin serums or monoclonal antibodies (cf. p. 120). Success only came when a monoclonal directed to the idiotype of a T-cell was used to block the response to antigen. This was identified by its ability to block one individual T-cell clone out of a large number and it was correctly assumed

that the structure permitting this selectivity would be the combining site for antigen on the T-cell receptor. Immunoprecipitation with this monoclonal brought down a disulfide-linked heterodimer composed of 40–44 kDa subunits (figure M4.1.1).

The other approach went directly for the genes, arguing as follows. The T-cell receptor should be an integral membrane protein not present in B-cells. Hence, T-cell polysomal mRNA from the endoplasmic reticulum, which should provide an abundant source of the appropriate transcript, was used to prepare cDNA from which genes common to B- and T-cells were subtracted by hybridization to B-cell mRNA. The resulting T-specific clones were used to probe for a T-cell gene which is rearranged in all functionally mature T-cells but is in its germ-line configuration in all other cell types (figure M4.1.2.). In such a way were the genes encoding the β-subunit of the T-cell receptor uncovered.

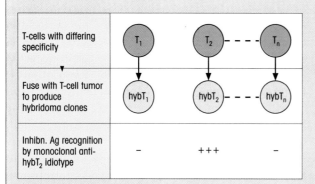

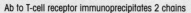
Ab to T-cell receptor immunoprecipitates 2 chains

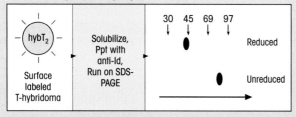

**Figure M4.1.1. Ab to T-cell receptor (anti-idiotype) blocks Ag recognition.** Based on Haskins K., Kubo R., White J., Pigeon M., Kappler J. & Marack P. (1983) *Journal of Experimental Medicine* **157**, 1149. (Simplified a little.)

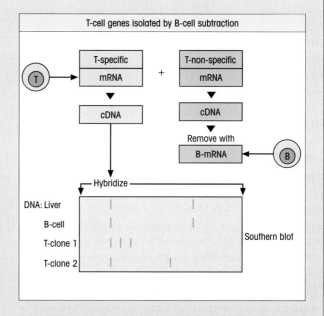

**Figure M4.1.2. Isolation of T-cell receptor genes.** Different size DNA fragments produced by a restriction enzyme are separated by electrophoresis and probed with the T-cell gene. The T-cells show rearrangement of one of the two germ line genes found in liver or B-cells. Based on Hendrick S.M., Cohen D.I., Nielsen E.A. & Davis M.M. (1984) *Nature* **308**, 149.

that these cells can play an important role in immune responses. In general, γδ T-cells seem to be strongly biased towards the recognition of mycobacterial antigens, particularly the highly conserved heat-shock protein hsp 65 which cross-reacts with self.

## The encoding of T-cell receptors is similar to that of immunoglobulins

The gene segments encoding the T-cell receptor *β* chains follow a similar arrangement of *V, D, J* and

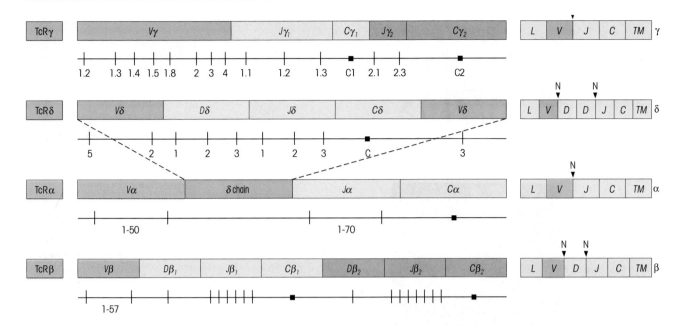

**Figure 4.5. Genes encoding γδ T-cell receptors (TCR1) and αβ receptors (TCR2).** Genes encoding the delta chains lie between the *V*α and *J*α clusters. Random nucleotide insertion (N) can occur at the positions arrowed on the right hand side which shows the recombined gene segments encoding the complete α, β, γ and δ peptide chains forming the T-cell receptors.

constant segments to that described for the immunoglobulins (figure 4.5). Similarly, as an immunocompetent T-cell is formed, rearrangement of *V*, *D* and *J* genes occurs to form a continuous *VDJ* sequence. The firmest evidence that B- and T-cells use similar recombination mechanisms comes from mice with severe combined immunodeficiency (SCID) which have a single autosomal recessive defect preventing successful linkage of *V*, *D* and *J* segments (cf. p. 48). Homozygous mutants fail to develop immunocompetent B- and T-cells and identical sequence defects in *VDJ* joint formation are seen in both pre-B- and pre-T-cell lines.

Looking first at the β-chain cluster, one of the large number of *V*β genes translocates to a preformed *D*β₁*J*β₁ or *D*β₂*J*β₂ segment. **Variability in junction formation** and the **random insertion of nucleotides** at the N region of *D* and *J* segment joins, parallels the same phenomenon seen with Ig gene rearrangements. Sequence analysis emphasizes the analogy with the antibody molecule; each *V* segment contains two hypervariable regions, while the *DJ* sequence provides a **very hypervariable** structure, making a total of six potential complementarity determining regions for antigen binding in each TCR (figure 4.6). As in the synthesis of antibody, the intron between *VDJ* and *C* is spliced out of the mRNA before translation with the restriction that *V*β*D*β₂*J*β₂ can only link to *C*β₂.

All the other chains are encoded by genes formed through similar translocations. The α-chain gene pool lacks *D* segments but more than makes up for it with a prodigious number of *J* segments. The number of *V*γ and *V*δ genes is very small in comparison with *V*α and *V*β. Like the α-chain pool, the γ chain cluster has no *D* segments. The awkward location of the locus within the gene cluster has been surprisingly informative with respect to the mechanism of translocation, since T-cells which have undergone *V*α–*J*α combination have no δ genes on the rearranged chromosome; in other words, the δ genes are completely excised.

## The CD3 complex is an integral part of the T-cell receptor

The T-cell antigen recognition complex and its B-cell counterpart, can be likened to specialized army platoons whose job is to send out a signal when the enemy has been sighted. When the TCR 'sights the enemy', i.e. ligates antigen, it relays a signal through an associated complex of transmembrane peptides (**CD3**) to the interior of the T-lymphocyte, instructing it to awaken from its slumbering G0 state and do something useful—like becoming an effector cell. In all immunocompetent T-cells, the antigen receptor is noncovalently but still intimately linked with CD3 in a complex which, as current wisdom has it, contains two heterodimeric TCRα/β or γδ recognition units closely apposed to the invariant CD3 peptide chains γ, δ, ε plus the disulfide-linked ζ–ζ dimer. The total complex has the structure TCR₂CD3γδε₂ζ₂ (figure 4.6, inset). The ITAM tyrosine motifs (cf. legend figure 4.4)

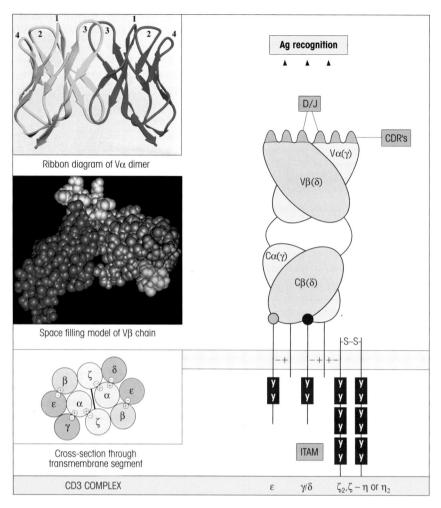

Ribbon diagram of Vα dimer

Space filling model of Vβ chain

Cross-section through
transmembrane segment

CD3 COMPLEX

**Figure 4.6. The T-cell receptor/CD3 complex.** The TCR resembles the immunoglobulin Fab antigen-binding fragment in structure. The variable and constant segments of the TCR2 α and β chains (VαCα/VβCβ) and of the corresponding TCR1 γ and δ chains belong structurally to the immunoglobulin domain family. The β-sheet strands of the Vα domains are shown in top inset with the numbered loops forming the complementarity-determining regions (CDR) clustering together. A fourth additional loop that could potentially interact with the peptide/MHC complex is shown. The Vα domains pack in the crystalline form analysed, as dimers. (Reproduced from Fields B.A. *et al.* (1995) *Science* **270**, 1821, with permission). The two-domain structure of the TCRβ chain and clustering of the CDRs is evident in the middle insert where the CDR1 is green, CDR2 violet (extreme right) and CDR3 yellow; Vβ is blue and Cβ red. (Reproduced from Bentley G. *et al.* (1995) *Science* **267**, 1984, with permission.) The TCRα and β CDR3 loops encoded by *D/J* genes are both short; the TCRγ CDR3 is also short with a narrow length distribution but the δ loop is long with a broad length distribution resembling the Ig light and heavy chain CDR3s respectively. The TCRs are probably expressed as dimeric structures linked to the CD3 complex (bottom inset). Negative charges on transmembrane segments of the 5 invariant chains of the CD3 complex contact the opposite charges on the TCR Cα and Cβ chains conceivably as depicted in the inset figure. The cytoplasmic domains of the CD3 peptide chains contain immunoreceptor tyrosine-based motifs (ITAM; cf. breakpoint cluster region (BCR), figure 4.4) which contact src protein tyrosine kinases (src is an oncogene). Try not to confuse the TCRγδ and the CD3γδ chains.

associate with src tyrosine kinases thereby transducing signals generated by ligand binding to the TCR.

Either or both of the ζ chains can be replaced by η. Both the ζ and η chains are encoded by the same gene locus and form heterodimers or homodimers. In the steady state, the ratio of ζ to η is around 50:1 but the proportions can probably vary and it is an attractive notion that dimers of different composition may mediate either positive or negative signals. The ζ chain can associate with the FcγRIII receptor in NK cells where it functions as part of the signal transduction mechanism in that context also.

## THE GENERATION OF DIVERSITY FOR ANTIGEN RECOGNITION

We know that the immune system has to be capable of recognizing virtually any pathogen that has arisen or might arise. The extravagant genetic solution to this problem of anticipating an unpredictable future involves the generation of millions of different specific antigen receptors, probably vastly more than the lifetime needs of the individual. Since this is likely to exceed the number of genes in the body, there must be some clever ways to generate all this diversity, particularly since the number of genes coding for antibodies and T-cell receptors is only of the order of 1000. Well, of course there are and we can now profitably examine the mechanisms which have evolved to generate tremendous diversity from such limited gene pools.

## Intrachain amplification of diversity

### Random VDJ combination increases diversity geometrically

Just as we can use a relatively small number of different building units in a child's construction set such as Lego to create a rich variety of architectural masterpieces, so the individual receptor gene segments can be viewed as building blocks to fashion a multiplicity of antigen-specific receptors for both B- and T-cells.

Take for example the immunoglobulin heavy-chain genes (table 4.1). There are 30 $D$ and 6 $J$ functional segments. If there were entirely random joining of any one $D$ to any one $J$ segment (compare figure 3.8), we would have the possibility of generating 180 $DJ$ combinations ($30 \times 6$). Let us go to the next stage. Since each of these 180 $DJ$ segments could join with any one of the 51 $V_H$ functional sequences, the net potential repertoire of $VDJ$ genes encoding the heavy-chain variable region would be $51 \times 180 = 9180$. In other words, just taking our $V$, $D$ and $J$ genes which add up

arithmetically to 87, we have produced a range of some 9000 different variable regions by **geometric recombination** of the basic elements. But that is only the beginning.

### Playing with the junctions

Another ploy to squeeze more variation out of the germ-line repertoire involves variable boundary recombinations of $V$, $D$ and $J$ to produce different junctional sequences (figure 4.7).

As discussed earlier, further diversity arises from the insertion of nucleotides at the N region of the $D$ and $J$ segments, a process associated with the expression of terminal deoxynucleotidyl transferase. This maneuver greatly increases the repertoire of T-receptor $\gamma$ and $\delta$ genes which are otherwise rather limited in number.

Just to make sure that we are really impressed, it transpires that even after a $V_H DJ_H$ rearrangement has occurred, an interchange with a quite different 5' $V_H$ gene can still take place; since the process is not precise, bases can be lost and/or added at the region joining the new $V_H$ to the N-terminal end of the $D$ sequence. This $V_H$ 'swapping' may prevent bias in the development of the heavy-chain $V$-region repertoire because the earliest differentiating B-cells utilize the $V_H$ segments most proximal to $D$ with high frequency to form their $V_H DJ_H$ rearrangements.

Yet additional mechanisms work on the $D$ regions: in some cases the $D$ segment can be read in three different reading frames and in others $DD$ combinations may be formed. Since the third complementarity determining regions (CDR3) in the various receptor

**Table 4.1. Calculations of human V gene diversity.** The minimum number of specificities generated by straightforward random combination of germ-line segments are calculated. These will be increased by the further mechanisms listed: *minimal assumption of approximately 10 variants for chains lacking D segments and 100 for chains with D segments. The calculation for

the T-cell receptor β-chain requires further explanation. The first of the two $D$ segments, $D\beta_1$ can combine with 57 $V$ genes and with all 13 $J_{\beta1}$ and $J_{\beta2}$ genes. $D_{\beta2}$ behaves similarly but can only combine with the seven downstream $J_{\beta2}$ genes.

| | TCR1 | | TCR2 | | Ig | | |
| | γ | δ | α | β | H | L κ | λ |
|---|---|---|---|---|---|---|---|
| V gene segments | 8 | 3 | 50 | 57 | 51 | ~70 | 25 |
| D gene segments | - | 3 | - | 1,1 | 30 | - | - |
| J gene segments | 3,2 | 3 | 70 | 6,7 | 6 | 5 | 8 |
| **Random Combinatorial joining** (without junctional diversity) | V x J  8 x 5 | V x D x J  3 x 3 x 3 | V x J  50 x 70 | V x D x J  57(13+7) | V x D x J  51 x 30 x 6 | V x J  70 x 5 | V x J  25 x 8 |
| Total | 40 | 27 | 3500 | 1140 | 9000 | 350 | 200 |
| **Combinatorial heterodimers** | 40 x 27 | | 3500 x 1140 | | 9000 x 350 | | 9000 x 200 |
| Total (rounded) | $10^3$ | | $4 \times 10^6$ | | $3.2 \times 10^6$ | | $1.8 \times 10^6$ |
| **Other mechanisms:** D's in 3 reading frames, junctional diversity, N region insertion;* x $10^3$ | $10^6$ | | $4 \times 10^9$ | | $3.2 \times 10^9$ | | $1.8 \times 10^9$ |
| **Somatic mutation** | - | | - | | +++ | | +++ |

chains are essentially composed of *(D)J* segments where junctional diversity mechanisms can introduce a very high degree of amino acid variability, one can see why it is that this hypervariable loop probably contributes the most flexibility in antigen-binding specificity within these molecules.

## Interchain amplification

The immune system took an ingenious step forward when two different types of chain were utilized for the recognition molecules because the combination produces not only a larger combining site with potentially greater affinity, but also new variability. Thus when one heavy chain is paired with different light chains the specificity of the final antibody is altered; for example, pairing of a heavy chain containing the T15 idiotype with three different light chains pro-

duced antibodies with different affinities for phosphorylcholine.

This random association between TCR1 γ and δ chains, TCR2 α and β chains, and Ig heavy and light chains yields a further geometric increase in diversity. From table 4.1 it can be seen that approximately 200 T-cell receptor and 200 Ig germ-line segments can give rise to 4 million and 5 million different combinations respectively, by straightforward associations *without* taking into account all of the fancy additional *D/J* mechanisms described above. Hats off to evolution!

## Somatic hypermutation

There is inescapable evidence that immunoglobulin *V*-region genes can undergo significant **somatic mutation**. Analysis of 18 murine λ myelomas revealed 12 with identical structure, four showing just one amino acid change, one with two changes and one with four changes, all within the hypervariable regions and indicative of somatic mutation of the single mouse λ germ-line gene. In another study, following immunization with pneumococcal antigen, a single germ-line T15 $V_H$ gene gave rise by mutation to several different $V_H$ genes all encoding phosphorylcholine antibodies (figure 4.8).

A number of features of this somatic diversification phenomenon deserve mention. The mutations are the result of single nucleotide substitutions, they are restricted to the variable as distinct from the constant region and occur in both framework and hypervariable regions. The mutation rate calculated by dividing the substitutions by the nucleotide bases sequenced is remarkably high, between 2 and 4% for $V_H$ genes as compared with a figure of less than 0.0001% for a non-immunological lymphocyte gene. In addition, the

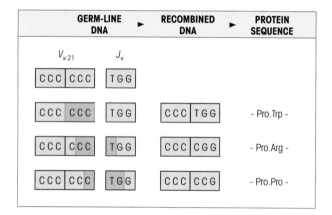

**Figure 4.7. Junctional diversity between two germ-line segments producing three variant protein sequences.** The nucleotide triplet which is spliced out is colored the darker blue.

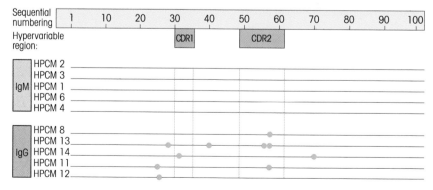

**Figure 4.8. Mutations in a germ-line gene.** The amino acid sequences of the $V_H$ regions of five IgM and five IgG monoclonal phosphorylcholine antibodies generated during an antipneumococcal response in a single mouse are compared with the primary structure of the T15 germ-line sequence. A line indicates identity with the T15 prototype and an orange circle a single amino acid difference. Mutations have only occurred in the IgG molecules and are seen in both hypervariable and framework segments. (After Gearhart P.J. (1982) *Immunology Today* **3**, 107.)

mutational mechanism is bound up in some way with class switch since mutations are more frequent in IgG and IgA than in IgM antibodies, affecting both heavy (figure 4.8) and light chains.

The view of the great and the good at the present time is that somatic mutation does not add to the repertoire available in the early phases of the primary response, but occurs during the generation of memory and is probably responsible for tuning the response towards higher affinity.

**T-cell receptor genes**, on the other hand, **do not appear to undergo serious somatic mutation**. Assuming this result is not biased by the selection of T-cell clones studied, it has been argued that this would be a useful safety measure since T-cells are so close fully to recognizing self, mutations could readily encourage the emergence of high affinity autoreactive receptors and autoimmunity.

One may ask how it is that this array of germ-line genes is protected from genetic drift. With a library of 400 or so *V* genes, selection would act only weakly on any single gene which had been functionally crippled by mutation and this implies that a major part of the library could be lost before evolutionary forces operated. One idea is that each subfamily of related *V* genes contains a prototype coding for an antibody indispensable for protection against some common pathogen so that mutation in this gene would put the host at a disadvantage and would therefore be selected against. If any of the other closely related genes in its set become defective through mutation, this indispensable gene could repair them by gene conversion, a mechanism in which it will be remembered that two genes interact in such a way that the nucleotide sequence of part or all of one becomes identical to that of the other. Although gene conversion has been invoked to account for the diversification of MHC genes, it can also act on other families of genes to maintain a degree of sequence homogeneity.

## THE MAJOR HISTOCOMPATIBILITY COMPLEX (MHC)

Molecules within this complex were originally defined by their ability to provoke vigorous rejection of grafts exchanged between different members of a species (Milestone 4.2). In Chapter 2, brief mention was made of the necessity for cell-surface antigens to be associated with class I or class II MHC molecules in order that they may be recognized by T-lymphocytes. The intention now is to give more insight into the nature of these molecules.

## Class I and class II molecules are membrane-bound heterodimers

### MHC class I

**Class I** molecules consist of a heavy peptide chain of 43 kDa noncovalently linked to a smaller 11 kDa peptide called $\beta_2$-**microglobulin**. The largest part of the heavy chain is organized into three globular domains ($\alpha_1$, $\alpha_2$ and $\alpha_3$; figure 4.9) which protrude from the cell surface; a hydrophobic section anchors the molecule in the membrane and a short hydrophilic sequence carries the C-terminus into the cytoplasm.

X-ray analysis of crystals of a human class I molecule has provided an exciting leap forwards in our understanding of MHC function. Both $\beta_2$-microglobulin and the $\alpha_3$ region resemble classic Ig domains in their folding pattern (cf. figure 4.9c). However, the $\alpha_1$ and $\alpha_2$ domains which are most distal to the membrane, form an utterly surprising structure composed of two extended $\alpha$-helices above a floor created by peptide strands held together in a $\beta$-pleated sheet, the whole forming an undeniable **cavity** (figure 4.9b and c). The appearance of these domains is so striking, I doubt whether the reader needs the help of gastronomic analogies such as 'two bananas on a plate' to prevent any class I structural amnesia. Another curious feature emerged. The cavity was occupied by a linear molecule, now known to be a peptide, which had cocrystallized with the class I protein. The significance of these unique findings for T-cell recognition of antigen will be revealed in the following chapter.

### MHC class II

**Class II MHC** molecules are also transmembrane glycoproteins, in this case consisting of $\alpha$ and $\beta$ polypeptide chains of molecular weight 34 kDa and 28 kDa respectively.

There is considerable sequence homology with class I and recent structural studies have shown that the $\alpha_2$ and $\beta_2$ domains, the ones nearest to the cell membrane, assume the characteristic Ig fold, while the $\alpha_1$ and $\beta_1$ domains mimic the class I $\alpha_1$ and $\alpha_2$ in forming a groove bounded by two $\alpha$-helices and a $\beta$-pleated sheet floor (figure 4.9a).

The organization of the genes encoding the $\alpha$-chain of the human class II molecule HLA-DR and the main regulatory sequences which control their transcription are shown in figure 4.10.

# Milestone 4.2—The Major Histocompatibility Complex

Peter Gorer raised rabbit antiserums to erythrocytes from pure strain mice (resulting from > 20 brother–sister matings), and by careful cross-absorption with red cells from different strains, he identified the strain-specific antigen II, now known as H-2 (table M4.2.1).

He next showed that the rejection of an albino (A) tumor by black (C57) mice was closely linked to the presence of the antigen II (table M4.2.2) and that tumor rejection was associated with the development of antibodies to this antigen.

Subsequently, George Snell introduced the term **histocompatibility (H)** antigen to describe antigens provoking graft rejection and demonstrated that of all the potential H antigens, differences at the H-2 (i.e. antigen II) locus provoked the strongest graft rejection seen between various mouse strains. *Poco a poco*, the painstaking studies gradually uncovered a remarkably complicated situation. Far from representing a single gene locus, H-2 proved to be a large complex of multiple genes, many of which were highly polymorphic, hence the term **major histocompatibility complex (MHC)**. The major components of the current genetic maps of the human HLA and mouse H-2 MHC are drawn in figure M4.2.1 to give the reader an overall grasp of the complex make-up of this important region (to immunologists I mean!—presumably all highly transcribed regions are important to the host in some way).

**Table M4.2.1. Identification of H-2 (antigen II).**

| Rabbit antiserum to: | Antigens detected on Albino red cells | | |
|---|---|---|---|
| | I | II | III |
| Albino (A) | +++ | +++ | ++ |
| Black (C57) | ++ | − | ++ |

**Table M4.2.2. Relationship of antigen II to tumor rejection.**

| Antigen II phenotype of recipient strain | Rejection of tumor inoculum (A strain) by: | | | |
|---|---|---|---|---|
| | *Pure strain | | **(A x C57) F1 backcross to C57 | |
| | − | + | − | + |
| Ag II +ve (A) | 39 | 0 | 17 (19.3) | 17 (19.5) |
| Ag II -ve (C57) | 0 | 45 | 0 | 44 (39) |

*A tumor inoculum derived from A strain bearing antigen II, is rejected by the C57 host. (+ = rejection; − = acceptance).

**Offspring of A × C57 mating were backcrossed to the C57 parent and the resulting progeny tested for Ag II and their ability to reject the tumor. The figures in brackets = number expected if tumor growth is influenced by two dominant genes, one of which determines the presence of Ag II.

| MAIN GENETIC REGIONS OF THE MAJOR HISTOCOMPATIBILITY COMPLEX | | | | | | | | | | | | |
|---|---|---|---|---|---|---|---|---|---|---|---|---|
| HUMAN | MHC CLASS | II | | | III | | | | I | | | | CHROMOSOME 6 |
| | HLA | DP | DQ | DR | C4 | C2 | FB | etc | B | C | A | G | |
| MOUSE | MHC CLASS | I | II | | III | | | | | I | | | CHROMOSOME 17 |
| | H-2 | K | A | E | C4 | C2 | FB | etc | | D | Q | T | |

Figure M4.2.1. Main genetic regions of the major histocompatibility complex.

## Complement genes contribute to the remaining class III region of the MHC

A variety of other genes which congregate within the MHC chromosome region are grouped under the heading of class III. Broadly, one could say that many are directly or indirectly related to immune defense functions. A notable cluster are the genes coding for two C4 isotypes and the two products, C2 and factor B, which each carry an active site for C3 convertase. Tumor necrosis factors (TNF) $\alpha$ and $\beta$ are encoded under the class III umbrella as are two members of the human 70 kDa heat-shock proteins. Although they are sited in the class II region (see below), the *LMP* and *TAP* genes concerned with the processing and transport of T-cell epitope peptides do not have the classical class II structure and should be classified more correctly in the class III cohort.

## Gene map of the MHC

An overall view of the main clusters of class I, II and III genes in the MHC of mouse and man may be gained from figure M4.2.1 in Milestone 4.2. More detailed maps of each region are provided in figures 4.11–4.13. A number of silent or pseudogenes have

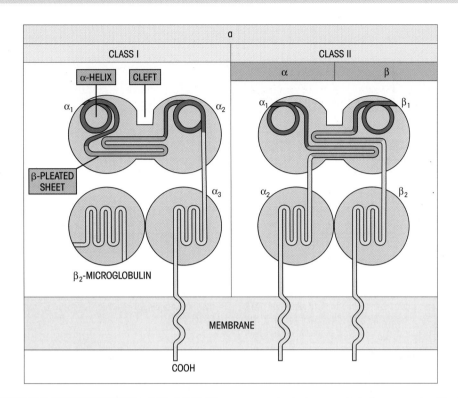

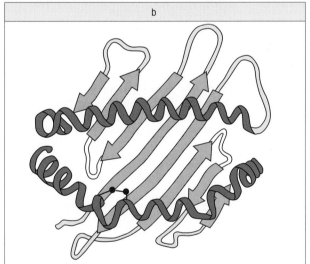

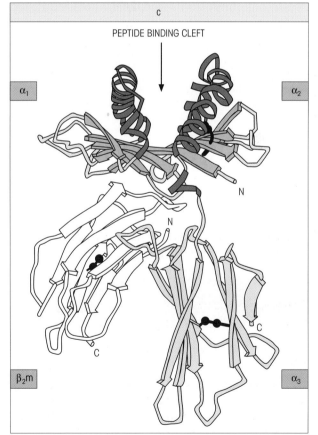

**Figure 4.9. Class I and class II MHC molecules.** (a) Diagram showing domains and transmembrane segments; the α-helices and β-sheets are viewed end on. (b) Schematic bird's eye representation of top surface of human class I molecule (HLA-A2) based on X-ray crystallographic structure. The strands making the β-pleated sheet are shown as thick gray arrows in the amino to carboxy direction, α-helices are represented as dark red helical ribbons. The inside-facing surfaces of the two helices and the upper surface of the β-sheet form a cleft. The two black spheres represent an intrachain disulfide bond. (c) Side view of the same molecule clearly showing the anatomy of the cleft and the typical Ig folding of the $\alpha_3$- and $\beta_2$-microglobulin domains (four antiparallel β-strands on one face and three on the other). (Reproduced from Bjorkman P.J. *et al.* (1987) *Nature* **329**, 506, with permission.)

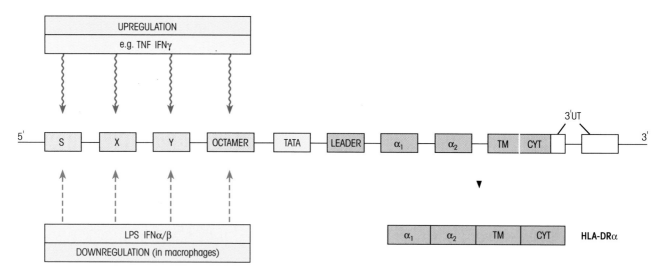

**Figure 4.10. Genes encoding human HLA-DRα chain (darker blue) and their controlling elements (regulatory sequences in light blue and TATA box promoter in yellow).** $\alpha_1/\alpha_2$ encode the two extracellular domains; TM and CYT encode the transmembrane and cytoplasmic segments respectively.

3' UT represents the 3' untranslated sequence. The octamer is identical with the corresponding 5' regulatory element controlling Ig chain transcription (cf. figure 3.6).

| HUMAN | HLA GENE | B | C | E | A | H | G | F |
|---|---|---|---|---|---|---|---|---|
| | GENE PRODUCT | HLA-B | HLA-C | HLA-E | HLA-A | HLA-H | HLA-G | HLA-F |

| MOUSE | H-2 GENE | K | D | L | Q | T | M |
|---|---|---|---|---|---|---|---|
| | GENE PRODUCT | H-2K | H-2D | H-2L | Qa | TI | H-2M3 |

**Figure 4.11. MHC class I gene map.** The 'classical' polymorphic class I genes highlighted with orange shading, encode peptide chains which together with $\beta_2$-microglobulin form the complete class I molecules originally identified as antigens by the antibodies they evoked on grafting into another member of the same species. The genes expressed most abundantly are *HLA-A* and *B* in the human and *H-2K* and *D* in the mouse. The other class I genes are termed 'non-classical' or 'class I-related' (now preferred to the older 'I-b'). They are oligo- rather than polymorphic or sometimes invariant, and many are silent or pseudogenes. *HLA-E* and *H-2M3* are closely related by their ability to bind mitochondrial and bacterial peptides possessing the *N*-terminal formyl group.

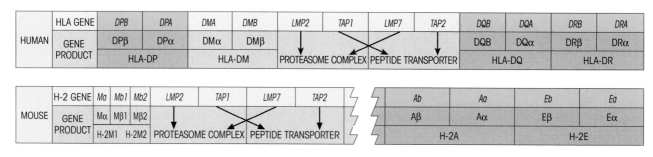

| HUMAN | HLA GENE | DPB | DPA | DMA | DMB | LMP2 | TAP1 | LMP7 | TAP2 | DQB | DQA | DRB | DRA |
|---|---|---|---|---|---|---|---|---|---|---|---|---|---|
| | GENE PRODUCT | DPβ | DPα | DMα | DMβ | | | | | DQB | DQα | DRβ | DRα |
| | | HLA-DP | | HLA-DM | | PROTEASOME COMPLEX | | PEPTIDE TRANSPORTER | | HLA-DQ | | HLA-DR | |

| MOUSE | H-2 GENE | Ma | Mb1 | Mb2 | LMP2 | TAP1 | LMP7 | TAP2 | Ab | Aa | Eb | Ea |
|---|---|---|---|---|---|---|---|---|---|---|---|---|
| | GENE PRODUCT | Mα | Mβ1 | Mβ2 | | | | | Aβ | Aα | Eβ | Eα |
| | | H-2M1 | H-2M2 | | PROTEASOME COMPLEX | | PEPTIDE TRANSPORTER | | H-2A | | H-2E | |

**Figure 4.12. MHC class II gene map** with 'classical' loci more heavily shaded. Both α and β chains of the class II heterodimer are transcribed from closely located genes. The *LMP2* and *7* genes encode part of a proteasome complex which cleaves cytosolic proteins into small peptides which are transported by the *TAP* gene products into the endoplasmic reticulum. Class II genes encoding the α and β chains of H-2O have been identified but no function has yet been assigned to the molecule; they are thought to be analogous to the *DNA* and *DOB* genes in the human. Two closely related molecules H-2M1 and H-2M2 sharing the same a chain have also surfaced recently.

been omitted from these gene maps in the interest of simplicity. The gap between class II and class I in the human can accommodate up to a 100 or so class III genes and new ones are constantly popping up.

The cell surface class I molecule based on a transmembrane chain with three extracellular domains associated with $\beta_2$-microglobulin has clearly proved to be an advantageous model for evolution to mould

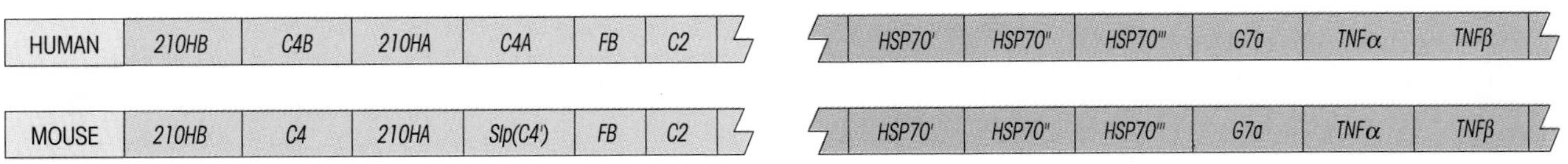

| HUMAN | 210HB | C4B | 210HA | C4A | FB | C2 |

| HSP70' | HSP70'' | HSP70''' | G7a | TNFα | TNFβ |

| MOUSE | 210HB | C4 | 210HA | Slp(C4') | FB | C2 |

| HSP70' | HSP70'' | HSP70''' | G7a | TNFα | TNFβ |

**Figure 4.13. MHC class III gene map.** The region is turning out to be something of a 'rag bag'. Aside from immunologically 'respectable' products like C2, C4, factor B, tumor necrosis factor (TNF) and possibly the 70 kDa heat-shock proteins (HSP), genes encoding tRNA synthetase (G7a), calmodulin, a member of the leucine zipper family of transcription factors, and tenascin, an extracellular matrix protein, have recently been winkled out and there are plenty more to come. Of course many genes may have drifted to this location during the long passage of evolutionary time without necessarily having to act in concert with their neighbors to subserve some integrated defensive function. The 21-hydroxylases (21OHA and B) are concerned with the hydroxylation of steroids such as cortisone and it would be curious if regulation of their expression were tied into a neuroimmunoendocrinological network. Slp (sex-limited protein) encodes a nonfunctional murine allele of C4, expressed under the influence of testosterone. No bright ideas concerning its function are making the rounds at the moment.

as evidenced by the variety of molecular species which utilize this structure (see Chapter 12). It is helpful to subdivide them, first into the **classical class I molecules**, HLA-A, B and C in the human and H-2K, D and L in the mouse. These were defined serologically by the antibodies arising in grafted individuals using methods developed from Gorer's pioneering studies (Milestone 4.2). Other loci, the human HLA-E, F, G and H and murine H-2Q, T and M, are far less polymorphic, often invariant, and many represent silent or pseudogenes. It is customary to refer to these as '**non-classical**' or '**class I-related**', the older term class Ib now being considered confusing because of the growing importance of **CD1**. This molecule incorporates the $\beta_2$-microglobulin subunit which is a *sine qua non* for membership of the class I club, although the relatively low homology with the classical archetypes is indicative of evolutionary divergence some ways back. Nevertheless CD1, like its true MHC counterparts, is involved in the presentation of antigens to T-cells, albeit in what for us seem to be quite novel ways. Two groups of loci have been delineated in the human: group I consisting of *CD1A*, B and C encodes cD1a, b and c transmembrane proteins and the group II genes *CD1D* and *E* give rise to CD1d and e. mCD1D 1 and 2 are the murine homologues of human CD1D.

## The genes of the MHC display remarkable polymorphism

Unlike the immunoglobulin system where, as we have seen, variability is achieved in each individual by a **multigenic** system, the MHC has evolved in terms of variability between individuals with a highly **polymorphic** (literally 'many shaped') system based on **multiple alleles** (i.e. alternative genes at each locus). Class I HLA-A and -B molecules are highly polymorphic, so are the class II peptides DQα, DQβ and DRβ, DPβ less so, while DRα and $\beta_2$-microglobulin are invariant in structure. The amino acid changes responsible for this polymorphism are restricted to the $\alpha_1$ and $\alpha_2$ domains of class I and to the $\alpha_1$ and $\beta_1$ domains of class II. It is of enormous significance that they occur essentially in the β-sheet floor and the inner surfaces of the α-helices which line the central cavity (figure 4.9a) and also on the upper surface of the helices.

The MHC region represents an outstanding hotspot with mutation rates two orders of magnitude higher than non-MHC loci. These multiple allelic forms can be generated by a variety of mechanisms: point mutations, recombination, homologous but unequal crossing over, and **gene conversion**.

The latter mechanism has been identified as an important contributory factor in the formation of a series of spontaneous mutations in the H-2K region of C57BL mice. Most of the mutations contain clusters of multiple amino acid substitutions and seem to arise by transfer of stretches of up to 95 nucleotides from class I *Q* genes to the $\alpha_1$ and $\alpha_2$ domains of H-2K. These intriguing findings have fostered the view that the large number of seemingly functionless *Q* genes may represent a stockpile of genetic information for the generation of polymorphic diversity in the 'working' class I molecules. Evidence for gene conversion has also been obtained for the class II genes.

Analysis of HLA polymorphism at the population level suggests that humans originated in Africa and then split into African and emigrating non-African groups. The latter subsequently divided into a Caucasoid grouping (Caucasian, East Asian, native American and Arctic) and the South-East Asian Pacific population.

## Nomenclature

Since much of the experimental work relating to the MHC is based on experiments in our little laboratory friend, the mouse, it may be helpful to explain the

| Strain | Haplotype | MHC Designation | I | II | | | | III | | I | |
|--------|-----------|-----------------|-----|------|------|------|------|------|--|-----|-----|
| C57BL | $b$ | $H\text{-}2^b$ | $K^b$ | $Ab^b$ | $Aa^b$ | $Eb^b$ | $Ea^b$ | $C4^b$ | | $D^b$ | etc |
| CBA | $k$ | $H\text{-}2^k$ | $K^k$ | $Ab^k$ | $Aa^k$ | $Eb^k$ | $Ea^k$ | $C4^k$ | | $D^k$ | etc |

**Figure 4.14. How the definition of H-2 haplotype works.** Pure strain mice homozygous for the whole H-2 region through prolonged brother–sister mating for at least 20 generations, are each arbitrarily assigned a **haplotype** designated by a superscript. Thus the particular set of alleles which happen to occur in the strain named C57BL is assigned the haplotype **H-2$^b$** and the particular nucleotide sequence of each allele in its MHC is labelled as **gene$^b$**, e.g. **H-2K$^b$** etc. It is obviously more convenient to describe a given allele by the haplotype than to trot out its whole nucleotide sequence and it is easier to follow the reactions of cells of known H-2 makeup by using the haplotype terminology—see for example the interpretation of the experiment in the following figure 4.15.

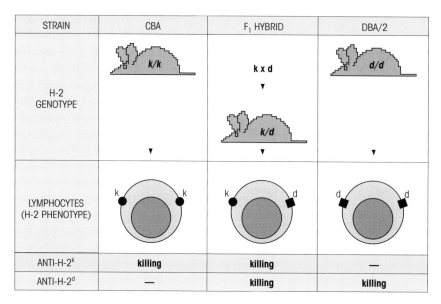

**Figure 4.15. Inheritance and codominant expression of MHC genes.** Each homozygous (pure) parental strain animal has two identical chromosomes bearing the H-2 haplotype, one paternal and the other maternal. Thus in the present example we designate a strain which is **H-2$^k$** as $k/k$. The first familial generation (F1) obtained by crossing the pure parental strains CBA (H-2$^k$) and DBA/2 (H-2$^d$) has the H-2 genotype $k/d$. Since 100% of F1 lymphocytes are killed in the presence of complement by antibodies to H-2$^k$ or to H-2$^d$ (raised by injecting H-2$^k$ lymphocytes into an H-2$^d$ animal and vice versa), the MHC molecules encoded by both parental genes must be expressed on every lymphocyte. The same holds true for other tissues in the body.

nomenclature used to describe the allelic genes and their products. If someone says to you in an obscure language 'we are having free elections', you fail to understand, not because the idea is complicated but because you do not comprehend the language. It is much the same with the shorthand used to describe the H-2 system which looks unnecessarily frightening to the uninitiated. In order to identify and compare allelic genes within the H-2 complex in different strains, it is usual to start with certain pure homozygous inbred strains, obtained by successive brother–sister matings, to provide the prototypes. The collection of genes in the H-2 complex is called the **haplotype** and the haplotype of each prototypic inbred strain will be allotted a given superscript. For example, the DBA strain haplotype is designated $H\text{-}2^d$ and the genes constituting the complex are therefore $H\text{-}2K^d$, $H\text{-}2Aa^d$, $H\text{-}2Ab^d$, $H\text{-}2D^d$ and so on; their products will be H-2K$^d$, H-2A$^d$ and H-2D$^d$ and so forth (figure 4.14). When new strains are derived from these by genetic recombination during breeding, they are assigned new haplotypes but the individual genes are designated by the haplotype of the prototype strain from which they were derived. Thus the A/J strain produced by genetic cross-over during interbreeding between ($H\text{-}2^k \times H\text{-}2^d$) F1 mice (cf. figure 4.15) is arbitrarily assigned the haplotype $H\text{-}2^d$, but table 4.2 shows that individual genes in the complex are identified by the haplotype symbol of the original parents.

If mixed haplotype heterodimers and interisotypic pairing (e.g. H-2A$\alpha^d$E$\beta^d$) could occur, this would increase the total range of MHC class II products dramatically, but the evidence for this is still controversial.

Table 4.2. The haplotypes of the H-2 complex of some commonly used mouse strains and recombinants derived from them. A/J was derived by interbreeding ($k \times d$) F1 mice, recombination occurring between E and S (class III) regions*.

| STRAIN | HAPLOTYPE | ORIGIN OF INDIVIDUAL REGIONS | | | | |
|--------|-----------|------|------|------|------|------|
| | | K | A | E | S | D |
| C57BL | b | b | b | b | b | b |
| CBA | k | k | k | k | k | k |
| DBA/2 | d | d | d | d | d | d |
| A/J | a | k | k | k* | d | d |
| B.10A(4R) | h4 | k | k | b | b | b |

## Inheritance of the MHC

Pure strain mice derived by prolonged brother–sister mating are homozygous for each pair of homologous chromosomes. Thus, in the present context, the haplotype of the MHC derived from the mother will be identical to that from the father; animals of the C57BL strain, for example, will each bear two chromosomes with the *H-2^d* haplotype (cf. table 4.2).

Let us see how the MHC behaves when we cross two pure strains of haplotypes *H-2^k* and *H-2^d* respectively. We find that the lymphocytes of the offspring (the F1 generation) all display *both* H-2^k and H-2^d molecules on their surface, i.e. there is **codominant expression** (figure 4.15). If we go further and breed F1s together, the progeny have the genotypes *k*, *k/d* and *d* in the proportions to be expected if the **haplotype segregates as a single Mendelian trait**. This happens because the H-2 complex spans 0.5 centimorgans, equivalent to a recombination frequency between the *K* and *D* ends of 0.5%, and the haplotype tends to be inherited *en bloc*. Only the relatively infrequent recombinations caused by meiotic cross-over events, as described for the A/J strain above, reveal the complexity of the system.

## The tissue distribution of MHC molecules

Essentially, all nucleated cells carry classical class I molecules. These are abundantly expressed on lymphoid cells, less so on liver, lung and kidney and only sparsely on brain and skeletal muscle. In the human, the surface of the villous trophoblast lacks HLA-A, B or C components; instead it bears HLA-G which does not appear on any other body cells in nonpregnant females. Human group I CD1 molecules are abundant on professional antigen-presenting cells (cf. p. 164) while molecules of group II and their murine counterpart mCD1d are expressed within intestinal epithelium. Class II molecules are also restricted, being especially associated with B-cells, antigen-presenting

cells and macrophages; however, when activated by agents such as γ-interferon, capillary endothelia and many epithelial cells can be stained for surface class II and increased expression of class I.

Under normal circumstances, a soluble form of HLA is present in serum; the level rises markedly during the course of a viral infection presumably due to an increase in HLA synthesis mediated by endogenous production of interferons and other cytokines.

## MHC functions

Although originally discovered through transplantation reactions, the MHC molecules are utilized for vital biological functions by the host. Their function as cell surface markers which enable infected cells to signal cytotoxic and helper T-cells will be explored in depth in subsequent chapters. There is no doubt that this role in immune responsiveness is immensely important, and in this respect the rich **polymorphism of the MHC** region would represent a species response to **maximize protection against diverse microorganisms**. An apparent example would be the malaria-driven selection at the HLA-B locus whereby resistance to severe malaria resulting from strains of *Plasmodium falciparum* in East Africa is associated with HLA-DRB1*0101 (cf. p. 363) whereas HLA-DRB1*1302 confers resistance to West African strains of the parasite. Aside from the potential role of *Q* genes in the generation of polymorphism, molecules encoded by the T complex are involved in differentiation events particularly in the embryo and possibly also in the placenta.

The MHC has been implicated in a variety of nonimmunological phenomena such as body weight in mice and egg production in chickens. The relationship between MHC and urinary odor profile is used by females to select partners of different haplotype, as evidenced by the much higher ratio of heterozygotes to homozygotes than would be expected by chance in wild populations of mice. In this way inbreeding is minimized and gene randomization maximized.

The social consequences of MHC perception are exploited yet further. House mice form communal nests and appear to nurse each other's pups indiscriminately. The communal nesting probably functions to reduce infanticide but makes females vulnerable to exploitation if nursing partners fail to provide their fair share of care. However, females prefer communal nesting partners that share MHC genes and this will minimize such exploitation. Expressed in more precious language, the MHC provides the basis for assortative preference during cooperative behavior but disassortative selection during mating. It may come as no surprise then to learn that $\beta_2$-microglobulin knockout mice in which the $\beta_2$-microglobulin gene is disrupted (cf. p. 144) have greatly reduced reproductive success even though otherwise hale and hearty, although failure to express the Fc$\gamma$Rn receptor which ferries immunoglobulin from mother's milk to the neonate (cf. p. 57) might also be a contributory factor.

Some of these phenomena may have a hormonal basis and the evidence that class I molecules also function as components of hormone receptors merits some consideration. For example, the Daudi tumor cell line which does not express surface class I because of a failure to synthesize $\beta_2$-microglobulin, lacks insulin receptors. If one strips class I, but not class II, from a cell surface by 'capping' with antibodies (see figure 2.6f), the binding of insulin is significantly diminished. Last, if a cell binds photoaffinity-labeled insulin, chemical links with H-2K but not H-2D may be seen. Associations with receptors for glucagon, epidermal growth factor and $\gamma$-endorphin have also

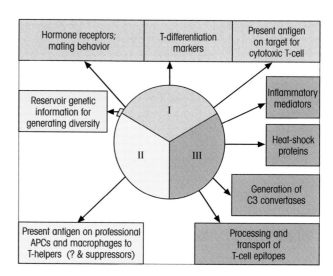

**Figure 4.16. The functions of MHC molecules.**

been described. Of course, one of the lessons to be learned is that we should never look at immunological events as phenomena isolated from the biology of the whole individual (figure 4.16).

## SUMMARY

### The B-cell surface receptor for antigen

• The B-cell inserts its Ig gene product containing a transmembrane segment into its surface where it acts as a specific receptor for antigen.
• The surface Ig is complexed with the membrane proteins IgM-$\alpha$ and Ig-$\beta$ which become phosphorylated on cell activation and presumably transduce signals received through the Ig antigen receptor.

### The T-cell surface receptor for antigen

• The receptor for antigen is a transmembrane dimer, each chain consisting of two Ig-like domains.
• The outer domains are variable in structure, the inner ones constant, rather like a membrane-bound Fab.
• Both chains are required for antigen recognition.
• Most T-cells express a receptor (TCR) with $\alpha$ and $\beta$ chains (TCR2). A separate lineage (TCR1) bearing $\gamma\delta$ receptors is transcribed strongly in early thymic ontogeny but is associated mainly with epithelial tissues in the adult.
• The encoding of the TCR is similar to that of immunoglobulins. The variable region coding sequence in the differentiating T-cell is formed by random translocation from clusters of $V$, $D$ (in most cases) and $J$ segments

to form a single recombinant $V(D)J$ sequence for each chain.
• Like the Ig chains, each variable region has three hypervariable sequences which are presumed to function in antigen recognition.
• The CD3 complex, composed of $\gamma$, $\delta$, $\varepsilon$ and either $\zeta_2$, $\zeta\eta$ or $\eta_2$ covalently linked dimers, forms an intimate part of the receptor and probably has a signal transducing role following ligand binding by the TCR.

### The generation of antibody diversity for antigen recognition

• Ig heavy and light chains and TCR$\alpha$ and $\beta$ chains generally are represented in the germ-line by between 25 and 70 variable region genes, between 1 and 30 $D$ segment minigenes (Ig heavy and TCR $\beta$ and $\delta$ only) and 3–70 short $J$ segments.
• TCR $\gamma$ and $\delta$ chains are encoded by far fewer genes.
• Random recombination of any single $V$, $D$ and $J$ from each gene cluster generates approximately $9 \times 10^3$ Ig heavy-chain $VDJ$ sequences, 500 light chains, $3 \times 10^3$ TCR$\alpha$, $1 \times 10^3$ TCR$\beta$, but only 40 TCR$\gamma$ and 27 TCR$\delta$.
• Random interchain combination produces roughly $5 \times 10^6$ Ig, $4 \times 10^6$ TCR2 and $10^3$ TCR1 receptors.
• Further diversity is introduced at the junctions

*(Continued)*

between *V, D* and *J* segments by variable combination as they are spliced together by recombinase enzymes and by the N-terminal insertion of random nontemplate nucleotide sequences. This mechanism may be particularly important in augmenting the number of specificities which can be squeezed out of the relatively small γδ pool.

• In addition, after a primary response, B-cells but not T-cells undergo high rate somatic mutation affecting the *V* regions.

## MHC

• Each vertebrate species has an MHC identified originally through its ability to evoke very powerful transplantation rejection.

• Each contains three classes of genes. Class I encodes 44 kDa transmembrane peptides associated at the cell surface with $β_2$-microglobulin. Class II molecules are transmembrane heterodimers. Class III products are heterogeneous but include complement components linked to the formation of C3 convertases, heat-shock proteins and tumor necrosis factors.

• The genes display remarkable polymorphism. A given MHC gene cluster is referred to as a 'haplotype' and is usually inherited *en bloc* as a single Mendelian trait, although its constituent genes have been revealed by cross-over recombination events.

• Classical class I molecules are present on virtually all cells in the body and signal cytotoxic T-cells. Structurally similar class I-related and CD1 molecules are probably also involved in antigen presentation to T-cells.

• Class II are particularly associated with B-cells and macrophages but can be induced on capillary endothelial cells and epithelial cells by γ-interferon. They signal T-helpers for B-cells and macrophages.

• Structural analysis indicates that the two domains distal to the cell membrane form a cavity bounded by two parallel α-helices sitting on a floor of β-sheet peptide strands; the walls and floor of the cavity and the upper surface of the helices are the sites of maximum polymorphic amino acid substitutions.

• Heterozygosity is encouraged by an effect on the mating behavior of female mice of MHC-controlled urinary odor profiles.

• Class I molecules may function as components of hormone receptors. Silent class I genes may increase polymorphism by gene conversion mechanisms.

# FURTHER READING

Alber G., Flaswinkel H., Kim K.-M., Weiser P. & Reth M. (1992) Structure and function of the B-cell antigen receptors. In Gergely J. *et al.* (eds) *Progress in Immunology* VIII, p. 27. Springer-Verlag, Berlin.

Brown J.H., Jardetzky T.S., Gorga J.C., Stern L.J., Urban R.G., Strominger J.L. & Wiley D.C. (1993) Three-dimensional structure of the human class II histocompatibility antigen HLA-DR1. *Nature* 364 (6432), 33.

Campbell R.D. & Trowsdale J. (1993) Map of the human MHC. *Immunology Today* 14, 349.

Campbell R.D. & Trowsdale J. (1997) Map of the human major histocompatibility complex. *Immunology Today* 18 (1), *pullout*.

Geraughty D.E. (1993) Structure of the HLA class I region and expression of its resident genes. *Current Opinion in Immunology* 5, 3.

Howard J.C. (1991) Disease and evolution. *Nature* 352, 565.

Imani F. & Soloski M.J. (1991) Heat shock proteins can regulate expression of the Tla region-encoded class I-b molecule Qa-1. *Proceedings of the National Academy of Science* 88, 10475.

Kara C. & Glimcher L.H. (1991) Regulation of MHC class II gene transcription. *Current Opinion in Immunology* 3, 16.

Kurlander R.J., Shawar S.M., Brown M. & Rich R.R. (1992) Specialized role for a murine class I-b MHC molecule in prokaryotic host defenses. *Science* 257, 678.

Mak T.W. (1992) T-cell receptor, αβ. In Roitt I.M. & Delves P.J. (eds) *Encyclopedia of Immunology*, p. 1425. (See also article by Hayday A. on the γδ TCR; *idem*, p. 1428.)

Moss P.A.H., Rosenberg W.M.C. & Bell J.I. (1992) The human T-cell receptor in health and disease. *Annual Review of Immunology* 10, 71.

# CHAPTER 5

# THE PRIMARY INTERACTION WITH ANTIGEN

## CONTENTS

## WHAT IS AN ANTIGEN?

A man cannot be a husband without a wife and a molecule cannot be an antigen without a corresponding antiserum or antibody or T-cell receptor. The term **antigen** is used in two senses, the first to describe a molecule which *gen*erates an immune response (also called an **immunogen**) and the second, a molecule which reacts with antibodies or primed T-cells irrespective of its ability to generate them. If this last situation sounds a trifle confusing, an example may help. A mouse injected with its own red cells, not too surprisingly, will not make any antibodies; if it is now given rat erythrocytes, antibodies are formed to both rat and *mouse* red cells and the latter bind to the animal's own cells *in vivo*, i.e. the mouse red cell acts

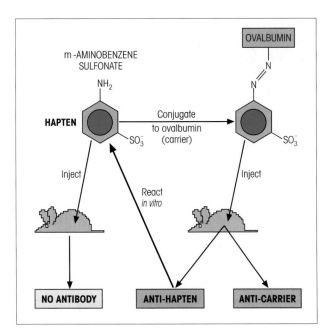

**Figure 5.1. A hapten on its own will not induce antibodies.** However, it will react *in vitro* with antibodies formed to a conjugate with an immunogenic carrier.

as antigen in binding antibodies even though unable to evoke their formation. Similarly, **haptens**, which are small well-defined chemical groupings such as dinitrophenyl (DNP; cf. p. 43) or *m*-aminobenzene sulfonate, are not immunogenic on their own but will react with preformed antibodies induced by injection of the hapten linked to a 'carrier' molecule which is itself an immunogen (figure 5.1).

The part of the hypervariable regions on the anti-body which contacts the antigen is termed the **paratope** and the part of the antigen which is in contact with the paratope is designated the **epitope**. To get some idea of size, if the antigen is a linear peptide or carbohydrate, the combining site can usually accommodate up to five or six amino acid residues or hexose units. With a globular protein as many as 16 or so amino acid side-chains may be in contact with an antibody (cf. figure 5.5).

## Of epitopes and antigen determinants

Antibodies formed in response to immunization with a native globular protein (as distinct from a fibrillar protein) do not tend to react well with denatured preparations and this is consistent with the view that the majority recognize topographic (surface) structures (i.e. epitopes) which depend upon the confor-mation of the native molecule. For this reason, antibodies to native proteins do not usually react as

strongly with peptides having the same primary sequence (figure 5.2). When individual epitopes are mapped using homogeneous monoclonal antibodies (cf. p. 120), they are frequently seen to involve amino acid residues far apart in the primary sequence, but brought together by the folding of the peptide chains in the native protein (figures 5.3 and 5.5). It seems rea-sonable to talk of **discontinuous** or assembled rather than **continuous** or sequential epitopes in these cases.

If one were to take each individual antibody within an antiserum raised to a protein antigen and plot the approximate center of the corresponding epitope on the antigen surface, one would almost certainly finish up with a 'contour map' of epitope density indicating regions on the antigen surface of **dominant epitope clusters** (figure 5.4a and b). Each of these clusters is as near as I can get to defining an antigen **determinant**. It is important to be aware that each antigen usually bears several determinants on its surface, which may well be structurally distinct from each other; thus a monoclonal antibody reacting with one determinant will usually not react with any other determinants on the same antigen unless the molecule has axes of symmetry (figure 5.4c).

## Identification of B-cell epitopes

This is a subject of particular interest to those wishing to make simple peptide substitutes for complex

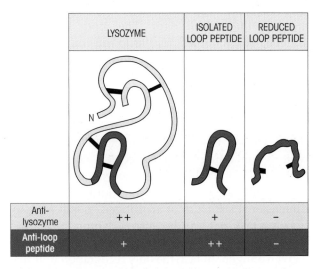

| | LYSOZYME | ISOLATED LOOP PEPTIDE | REDUCED LOOP PEPTIDE |
|---|---|---|---|
| Anti-lysozyme | ++ | + | – |
| Anti-loop peptide | + | ++ | – |

**Figure 5.2. Specificity and three-dimensional configuration in a globular protein, lysozyme.** Antibodies to the whole molecule and to the isolated loop peptide do not react with the peptide after reduction of its disulfide bond, showing that the linear reduced peptide has lost the antigenic configuration it had when held as a loop even though the amino acid sequence was unchanged. (From Maron E., Shiowa C., Arnon R. & Sela M. (1971) *Biochemistry* **10**, 763.)

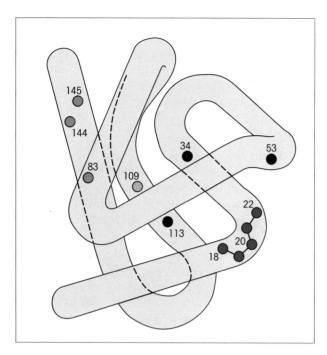

**Figure 5.3. Epitope residues on the folded peptide chain of sperm whale myoglobulin.** Amino acid residues 34, 53 and 113 (●) contribute to the epitope recognized by one homogeneous monoclonal antibody, 83, 144 and 145 (●) to another. These are clearly discontinuous epitopes. Amino acids 18–22 (●—●) are postulated to form part of a continuous epitope based on reactions with the isolated peptides. Much of the myoglobin chain is in the α-helical form. Residue 109 (○) is critical for T-cell recognition and so far no antibodies reacting with this site have been demonstrated. (Based on Benjamin D.C. *et al.* (1986) *Annual Review of Immunology* **2**, 67.)

mill scientist, being difficult, time-consuming and very 'high tech'. An alternative approach, applicable to protein antigens, is to carry out a series of mutations to locate the residues which provide the domi-

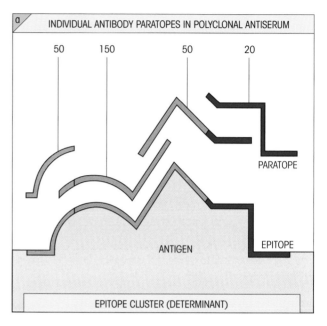

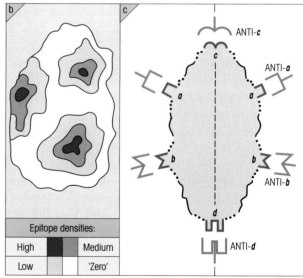

**Figure 5.4. A globular protein antigen usually bears a mosaic of determinants (dominant epitope clusters) on its surface,** defined by the heterogeneous population of antibody molecules in a given antiserum. (a) Highly idealized diagram illustrating the idea that individual antibodies in a polyclonal antiserum with different combining sites (paratopes) can react with overlapping epitopes forming a determinant on the surface of the antigen. The numbers refer to the imagined relative frequency of each antibody specificity. (b) Hypothetical 'contour' map of surface showing how determinants represent regions of clustering but overlapping epitopes, whose positions are plotted as the centre of the area making contact with antibody. The actual size of a single epitope may be gauged by looking at figure 5.5. (c) Cross-section of a theoretical antigen with an axis of symmetry displaying six determinants including two pairs which are identical. The clusters of overlapping antibodies to each determinant (one representative of each antibody cluster is shown) do not react with the other structurally unrelated determinants.

protein antigens. In general, large proteins, because they have more potential determinants, are better antigens than small ones. The more foreign an antigen, that is the less similar to self-configurations which induce tolerance, the more effective it is in provoking an immune response.

Parts of the peptide chains which protrude significantly from the globular surface tend to be sites of high epitope density. The least antigenic segments of the surface are associated with neighboring concave regions containing water molecules which may be more difficult to displace. However, prediction of B-cell epitopes, even when one knows the three-dimensional structure of an antigen, is still a pretty hopeless task, not least because each immunized host has its own way of recognizing the different regions of a given antigen. In fact, the only recognition unit that can be deployed to identify an epitope is that which defines it, namely the antibody bearing the complementary paratope.

The greatest precision is undoubtedly provided by X-ray crystallographic analysis of a complex of a monoclonal antibody (or fragment thereof) with the antigen (cf. figure 5.5), but this is not for the run of the nant binding to antibody—useful but not without its limitations. Attempts to mimic the epitope by building synthetic peptides will be described later (p. 297). To anticipate, this is good for linear epitopes and frustrating for those which are discontinuous.

## ANTIGENS AND ANTIBODIES INTERACT BY SPATIAL COMPLEMENTARITY NOT BY COVALENT BONDING

### Variation in hapten structure shows importance of shape

Once a method had been found for raising antibodies to small chemically defined haptens (figure 5.1), it then became possible to relate variations in the chemical structure of a hapten to its ability to bind to a given antibody. In one experiment, antibodies raised to *m*-aminobenzene sulfonate were tested for their ability to combine with *ortho*, *meta* and *para* isomers of the hapten and related molecules in which the sulfonate group was substituted by arsonate or carboxylate (table 5.1). The hapten with the sulfonate group in the *ortho* position combines somewhat less well with the antibody than the original *meta* isomer, but the *para*-substituted compound (chemically similar to the *ortho*) shows very poor reactivity. The substitution of arsonate for sulfonate leads to weaker combination with the antibody; both groups are negatively charged and have a tetrahedral structure but the arsonate group is larger in size and has an extra H atom. The aminobenzoates in which the sulfonate is substituted by the negatively charged but planar carboxylate group show even less affinity for the antibody. It would appear that the **overall** configuration of the hapten is even more important than its **chemical** nature, i.e. the hapten is recognized by the overall three-dimensional shape of its outer electron cloud as distinct from its chemical reactivity. The production of antibodies against such strange moieties as benzene sulfonate and arsonate becomes more comprehensible if they are thought to be directed against a particular electron-cloud shape rather than a specific chemical structure.

### Spatial complementarity of epitope and paratope can be demonstrated

It has proved possible, with not a little difficulty, to crystallize a complex of the Fab fragment of monoclonal antilysozyme with its antigen. X-ray analysis of these crystals was convincing; antigen and antibody fitted strongly together due to complementarity in shape over a wide area of contact (figure 5.5). Similar

**Table 5.1. Effect of variations in hapten structure on strength of binding to antibodies raised against m-aminobenzene sulfonate.** The reaction of the antibody with the original hapten against which it was raised is highlighted by the box. (From Landsteiner K. & van der Scheer J. (1936) *Journal of Experimental Medicine* **63**, 325.)

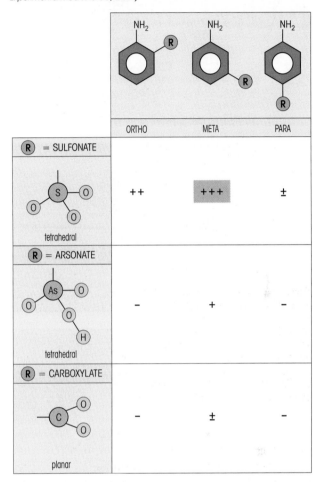

studies with three further monoclonal antibodies reacting with the same antigen confirmed the 'lock and key' type fit between paratope and epitope. It is important not to regard the 'lock and key' as inflexible entities like two pieces of rock, since this might make it very difficult for an animal to produce an antibody with such a unique complementary surface. In fact, three of these four studies revealed significant changes in the polypeptide backbone of up to 1.0 Å as the antibody complexed with its antigen (compare figure 5.6), and if one adds into the equation the possibility of rotational movement of the amino acid side-chains and alterations in the relative positions of the variable domains of light and heavy chains ($V_L/V_H$) in the Fab, it would seem more correct to think of antigen and antibody as surfaces which are to some extent mutually deformable — more like clouds than rocks as Lerner has so graphically expressed it. In this context, it is pertinent to draw attention to the associa-

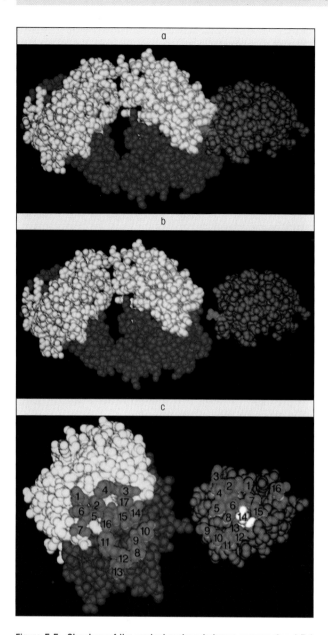

**Figure 5.5. Structure of the contact regions between a monoclonal Fab antilysozyme and lysozyme.** (a) Space-filling model showing Fab and lysozyme molecules fitting snugly together. Antibody heavy chain, blue; light chain, yellow; lysozyme, green with its glutamine 121 in red. (b) Fab and lysozyme models pulled apart to show how the protuberances and depressions of each are complementary to each other. (c) End-on views of antibody combining site (left) and the lysozyme epitope (right) obtained from (b) by rotating each molecule 90° about a vertical axis. Contact residues on both red, except Gln121 in light purple. The Gln121 fits into an antibody surface cavity surrounded by $V_L$ and $V_H$ residues 2, 5, 6, 7 and 16. The lysozyme epitope contact residues labeled 1–9 lie between residues 18–27 and labeled residues 10–16 are contributed by the peptide stretch from 117 to 128, i.e. this is clear evidence for a discontinuous epitope. All CDRs and two framework residues in the Fab make contact with the antigen. Most contacts are made by the heavy chain especially by the CDR3 region. All contacting residues may not contribute positively to the attractive forces between antigen and antibody; the striking influence of the Gln121 is revealed by the poor binding of lysozymes from other species in which the Gln121 is replaced by histidine. (Reproduced with permission from Amit A. *et al.* (1986) *Science* **233**, 747–753. Copyright 1986 by the AAAS.)

tion between those parts of a protein antigen which provide the dominant epitopes for antibody binding, and their peptide chain flexibility as measured by the temperature factors derived from X-ray crystallography. This mutual accommodation of structures on antigen and antibody obviously permits the maximum contact but there must be a price to pay, in that energy has to be expended in inducing these conformational changes. In general, though, this will be more than compensated by the intrinsic free energy change associated with the formation of the new binding sites (figure 5.7a and b). This input of energy to produce conformational change leading to strong binding appears to be the factor behind the frequent occurrence of normally 'buried' hydrophobic side-chains as contact residues for antibody.

With globular protein antigens, the area of contact between epitope and paratope is quite large, of the order of 75 $Å^2$, making it likely that residues on more than one peptide chain will be implicated; indeed, in each case the epitopes are discontinuous. It transpires that this contact area is within the range normally found for protein–protein interactions such as those between interacting C$\gamma$3 domains in the immunoglobulin Fc region. Nonetheless, as seen at a resolution of 2.8 Å, the atoms at the antigen–antibody interface are not as densely packed as at the $V_H/V_L$ boundary. Furthermore, only 60% of polar atoms are neutralized by salt bridges or hydrogen bonds, whereas, by contrast, around 90% of charged atoms are paired within the interior of a protein. Recently, however, more refined analysis at 1.8 Å resolution has revealed water molecules filling the voids not occupied by amino acid residues and these appear to neutralize most of the unpaired polar atoms at the interface. Tyrosines and tryptophans tend to occur with greater frequency in the combining site than they do in the remainder of the antibody molecule. Both can form H-bonds with solvent or antigen yet have large hydrophobic surfaces, undeniably useful characteristics for residues exposed to water when the antibody is free, but buried, i.e. excluded from solvent contact, when interacting closely with antigen.

## Antigen–antibody bonds are readily reversible

If the link between epitope and paratope is entirely dependent on spatial complementarity and does not involve the formation of covalent chemical bonds, it should not be too difficult to pull them apart. This can easily be put to the test. If one puts a mixture of the hapten with antibody inside a dialysis bag, the hapten

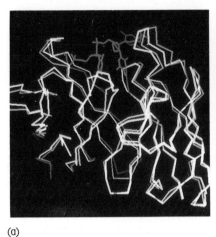

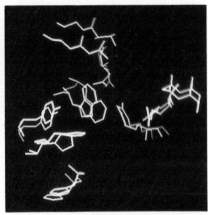

(a)               (b)

**Figure 5.6. Antibody structural flexibility on complexing with the antigen.** (a) Significant conformational changes (0.5–1.0 Å) occur in the Cα backbone of the complementarity determining regions (CDRs) of an autoantibody Fab specific for single-stranded DNA on complexing with a fragment of antigen (thymidine trimer). Only the Fv (V$_H$ + V$_L$) domains of the antibody are shown. The unliganded Fv is yellow and the ligand (antigen) red. In the complexed form, the V$_L$ is blue and the V$_H$ purple. (b) Movements in the contacting amino acid side-chains as a result of binding antigen. (Reproduced with permission from Herron J.N., He X.M., Ballard D.W., Blier P.R., Pace P.E., Bothwell A.L.M., Voss E.W. Jr. & Edmundson A.B. (1991) *Proteins* **11**, 150. Reprinted by permission of Wiley-Liss, a division of John Wiley and Sons, Inc.)

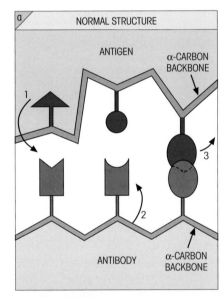

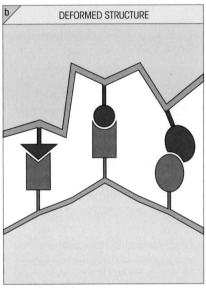

**Figure 5.7. Flexibility of antigen and antibody contributes to binding affinity.** In the illustration we show: (a) three types of energy-consuming reactions required to deform both molecules, thereby allowing (b) positive interaction between residues in the paratope and epitope—(1) bond rotation exposing a hydrophobic side-chain normally buried within the interior, (2) flexing of the α-carbon backbone to bring interacting residues close together, and (3) lateral displacement of a residue whose electron clouds would overlap with those of its opposite partner. Provided the total deformation energy is less than the energy of attraction of the deformed molecules, complex formation will be favored. Expressed mathematically:

$$\text{Free energy of deformation} = \left( \Delta G_1 + \Delta G_2 + \Delta G_3 \right) = \Delta G_{def}$$

where $\Delta G_1$ is the Gibbs free energy change of reaction 1 and so on.

Energy of association of deformed antigen and antibody = the sum of the individual binding energies = $\Delta G_{binding}$ (an attractive force gives a negative $\Delta G$).

Overall energy changes for complex formation

$$= \Delta G_{def} + \Delta G_{binding} = -RT \ln \mathbf{K_a}$$

Provided $-\Delta G_{binding} > \Delta G_{def}$, antigen and antibody will associate at equilibrium with a reasonable association affinity constant $\mathbf{K_a}$. (R, gas constant; T, absolute temperature; ln, natural logarithm.)

If the antigen were completely rigid, it would be unable to approach close enough to the antibody to generate significant binding energy.

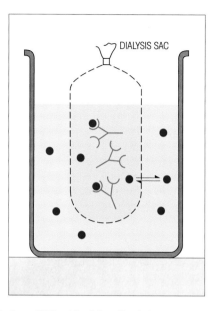

**Figure 5.8. Reversibility of the interaction between antibody ( ) and hapten ( ).** Within the dialysis sac the hapten is partly in the free form and partly bound to antibody according to the affinity of the antibody. Only hapten can diffuse through the dialysis membrane and the external concentration then will equal the concentration of unbound hapten within the sac. Measurement of total hapten in the dialysis sac then enables the amount bound to antibody to be calculated. Constant renewal of the external buffer will lead to total dissociation and loss of hapten from inside the dialysis sac showing the reversible nature of the antigen–antibody bond.

will be found to diffuse out into the surrounding fluid until an equilibrium is reached in which some hapten is bound to antibody and some is free; if this exterior fluid is continually renewed, all the hapten will be lost from the bag showing that it can be completely dissociated from the antibody (figure 5.8). With larger antigens, the complexes can be split by a change in pH which brings about alterations in protein conformation and destroys the complementarity of the two reactants. As will be seen subsequently (p. 127), this principle can be used for the purification of either antigens or antibodies by affinity chromatography.

## THE FORCES BINDING ANTIGEN TO ANTIBODY BECOME LARGE AS INTERMOLECULAR DISTANCES BECOME SMALL

It should be stressed immediately that the forces which hold antigen and antibody together are, in essence, no different from the so-called 'nonspecific' interactions which occur between any two unrelated proteins (or other macromolecules) as, for example, human serum albumin and human transferrin. These

intermolecular forces may be classified under four headings.

### 1 Electrostatic

These are due to the attraction between oppositely charged ionic groups on the two protein side-chains as, for example, an ionized amino group ($NH_3^+$) on a lysine of one protein and an ionized carboxyl group ($—COO^-$) of, say, glutamate on the other (figure 5.9a). The force of attraction ($F$) is inversely proportional to the square of the distance ($d$) between the charges, i.e.:

$$F \propto 1/k_D d^2$$

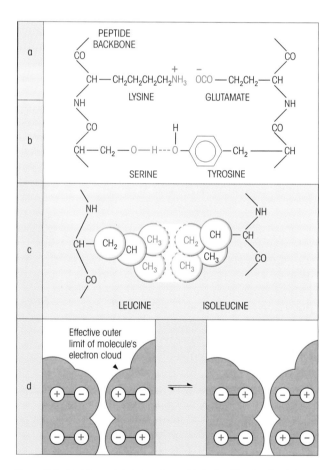

**Figure 5.9. Protein–protein interactions.** (a) Coulombic attraction between oppositely charged ionic groupings. (b) Hydrogen bonding between two proteins. (c) Hydrophobic bonding: the region in which the water molecules are in contact with the hydrophobic groups ( —— ) is considerably reduced when the hydrophobic groups on two proteins are in contact with each other ( – – – ) and the lower free energy of this system makes this a more probable state than separation of the hydrophobic groups. (d) Van der Waals force: the interaction between the electrons in the external orbitals of two different macromolecules may be envisaged (for simplicity!) as the attraction between induced oscillating dipoles in the two-electron clouds.

where $k_D$ is the dielectric constant. Thus as the charges come closer together, the attractive force increases considerably: if we halve the distance apart, we quadruple the attraction. Furthermore, since the dielectric constant of water is extremely high, the exclusion of water molecules through the contiguity of the interacting residues to which we have already drawn attention, would greatly increase $F$.

Dipoles on antigen and antibody can also attract each other. In addition, electrostatic forces may be generated by charge transfer reactions between antibody and antigen; for example, an electron-donating protein residue such as tryptophan could part with an electron to a group such as dinitrophenyl (DNP) which is electron accepting, thereby creating an effective +1 charge on the antibody and −1 on the antigen.

## 2  Hydrogen bonding

The formation of reversible hydrogen bridges between hydrophilic groups such as ·OH, ·NH$_2$ and ·COOH depends very much upon the close approach of the two molecules carrying these groups (figure 5.9b). Although H-bonds are relatively weak, because they are essentially electrostatic in nature, exclusion of water between the reacting side-chains would greatly enhance the binding energy through the gross reduction in dielectric constant.

## 3  Hydrophobic

In the same way that oil droplets in water merge to form a single large drop, so nonpolar, hydrophobic groups such as the side-chains of valine, leucine and phenylalanine tend to associate in an aqueous environment. The driving force for this hydrophobic bonding derives from the fact that water in contact with hydrophobic molecules, with which it cannot H-bond, will associate with other water molecules but the number of configurations which allow H-bonds to form will not be as great as that occurring when they are surrounded completely by other water molecules, i.e. the entropy is lower. The greater the area of contact between water and hydrophobic surfaces, the lower the entropy and the higher the energy state. Thus if hydrophobic groups on two proteins come together so as to exclude water molecules between them, the net surface in contact with water is reduced (figure 5.9c) and the proteins take up a lower energy state than when they are separated (in other words, there is a force of attraction between them). It has been estimated that hydrophobic forces may contribute up to 50% of the total strength of the antigen–antibody bond, although it must be appreciated that the relative contributions of these different types of molecular interaction will vary significantly from one complex to another.

## 4  Van der Waals

These are the forces between molecules which depend upon interaction between the external 'electron clouds'. The deviation of gaseous molecules of, say, nitrogen or hydrogen from 'ideal' behavior according to the kinetic theory is attributable to the Van der Waals attractions between them. The nature of this interaction is difficult to describe in nonmathematical terms but it has been likened to a temporary perturbation of electrons in one molecule effectively forming a dipole which induces a dipolar perturbation in the other molecule, the two dipoles then having a force of attraction between them; as the displaced electrons swing back through the equilibrium position and beyond, the dipoles oscillate (figure 5.9d). The force of attraction is inversely proportional to the seventh power of the distance, i.e.:

$$F \propto 1/d^7$$

and as a result this rises very rapidly as the interacting molecules come closer together.

This last point underlines one essential feature common to all four types of force—they depend upon the close approach of both molecules before the forces become of significant magnitude, the more so if water molecules are excluded. And this is at the heart of the combination of antigen and antibody. The **complementary** electron-cloud shapes on the combining site of the antibody and the surface determinant of the antigen enable the two molecules to fit snugly together (cf. figure 5.5) so that the **intermolecular distance becomes very small** and the 'nonspecific protein interaction forces' are considerably increased; the greater the areas of antigen and antibody which fit together, the greater the force of attraction, particularly if there is apposition of opposite charges and hydrophobic groupings.

By contrast, when the electron clouds of the two molecules effectively overlap, powerful repulsive forces are generated and energy must be expended in displacing the overlapping residues from their normal equilibrium positions.

## AFFINITY MEASURES STRENGTH OF BINDING OF ANTIGEN AND ANTIBODY

We saw from the electron microscope studies on the interaction between bifunctional DNP conjugates and antibody, that each DNP group fitted into one antibody combining site (figures 3.1 and 3.2). This means that small haptens by themselves are monovalent with respect to reaction with antibody. The experiment on mixing hapten with antibody in a dialysis bag (figure 5.8) showed that the combination with antibody was reversible and that the complex so formed could readily dissociate depending upon the strength of binding which we call **affinity**. This can be defined through the **equilibrium constant ($K_a$)** of the **association reaction:**

Ab + H ⇌ AbH

given by the mass action equation

$$K_a = \frac{[AbH]}{[Ab][H]}$$

where [Ab] is the concentration of free antibody combining sites and [H] the concentration of free hapten at equilibrium. If the antibody and hapten fit together very closely, the equilibrium will lie well over to the right; we refer to such antibodies which bind strongly to the hapten as **high affinity antibodies**. At a certain free hapten concentration [$H_c$] where half of the antibody sites are bound:

$$[AbH] = [Ab] \text{ and } K_a = 1/[H_c]$$

i.e. the affinity constant $K_a$ is equal to the reciprocal of the concentration of free hapten at the equilibrium point where half the antibody sites are in the bound form. In other words, when an antibody has a high affinity constant and binds hapten strongly, it only needs a low hapten concentration to half-saturate the antibody. It will be appreciated that an individual epitope on the surface of a complex antigen is also (by definition) monovalent and the strength of its combination with a univalent (Fab) antibody would also be defined by an affinity constant.

Affinity can equally well be formulated in terms of the **dissociation constant ($K_d$)** of the reaction:

AbH ⇌ Ab + H

Expressing concentrations in moles per liter:

$$K_d = \frac{[Ab \text{ moles/l}][H \text{ moles/l}]}{[AbH \text{ moles/l}]}$$

Clearly $K_d$ is the reciprocal of $K_a$, i.e. $1/K_a$, and has the units moles/l or M. Conversely, $K_a$ is expressed in the units l/mole or $M^{-1}$ and has the advantage that the stronger the binding, the higher the number.

The value of $K_a$ is determined by the difference in free energy ($\Delta G$) between the antigen and antibody in the free state on the one hand and in the complexed form on the other, according to the equation:

$$\Delta G = -RT \ln K_a$$

where $R$ is the universal gas constant, $T$ the absolute temperature and ln the natural logarithm.

One can study the interaction of hapten and antibody by the dialysis method described in figure 5.8 and use the data to calculate the affinity constant from the mass-action equation (figure 5.10). $K_a$ values may sometimes be as high as $10^{11}$ $M^{-1}$.

Analysis of the binding at different hapten concentrations generally shows a heterogeneity (figure 5.10) which indicates that most antiserums, even those raised against haptens with a simple structure, contain a variety of different antibodies with a range of binding affinities which depend upon the area of contact between the antibody and the hapten or epitope, the closeness of fit, conformation changes necessitated by electron-cloud overlap and the distribution of charged and hydrophobic groups.

### The avidity of antiserum for antigen— the bonus effect of multivalency

While the term affinity describes the binding of antibody to a monovalent hapten or single antigen determinant, in most practical circumstances we are concerned with the interaction of an antiserum (i.e. the serum from an immunized individual) with a multivalent antigen. The term employed to express this binding:

$$nAb + mAg \rightleftharpoons Ab_n Ag_m$$

(Ab = antibody; Ag = antigen) is **avidity** or **functional affinity**.

The factors which contribute to avidity are complicated, including as they do the heterogeneity of antibodies in a given serum which are directed against each determinant on the antigen, and the heterogeneity of the determinants themselves (figures 5.4 and 5.10). But yet a further factor must be considered. The multivalence of most antigens leads to an interesting **bonus** effect in which the binding of antigen to antibody by multiple links is always greater, usually many-fold greater, than the arithmetic sum of the individual antibody bonds. This is illustrated in

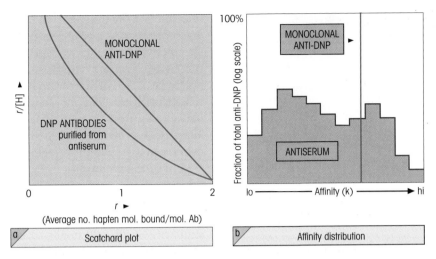

a | Scatchard plot

b | Affinity distribution

**Figure 5.10. Heterogeneity of IgG antihapten** (dinitrophenyl: DNP) antibodies from the serum of an immunized animal contrasting with the homogeneity of a monoclonal IgG anti-DNP. (a) A Scatchard plot of hapten binding to antibodies purified from the serum. If *r* represents the average number of DNP molecules bound to each antibody molecule, of affinity constant *k* and number of binding sites *n*, in the presence of a free hapten concentration [**H**], then from the mass-action equation of equilibrium relationships (p. 88) it can be shown that:

$$r/[\mathbf{H}] = nk - rk$$

Thus, a Scatchard plot of *r*/[**H**] against *r* for a single antibody species will be a straight line of slope −*k* as seen for the monoclonal antibody; the deviation from a straight line given by anti-DNP from the antiserum clearly indicates the existence of antibodies with different affinities, as may be confirmed by the binding of labeled DNP to many different bands after separation of the individual antibodies by isoelectric focusing of the serum. Extrapolation to *r*/[**H**] = 0 (at infinitely high concentration of antigen) gives the number of binding sites on each IgG molecule as two (cf. figure 3.2). For IgM antibodies the value would be 10. Because the slope of the Scatchard plot varies with *r*/**2** (the fractional occupancy of the antibody combining sites for a bivalent Ab), the affinity (which = −slope) will vary depending upon the range of values of *r* utilized in the experiments: thus affinity must be defined in terms of standard conditions of antibody dilution and concentration of hapten. (b) Histogram showing a typical distribution of antibody affinities in the anti-DNP serum. Measurable affinities tend to range between $10^4$ and $10^{10}$ or $10^{11}$ M$^{-1}$ and have skewed and not necessarily unimodal distributions. The monoclonal antibody of course gives a single affinity value since it is a homogeneous protein.

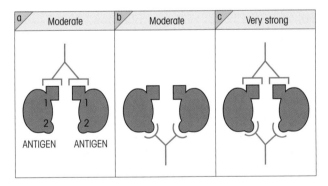

a | Moderate   b | Moderate   c | Very strong

ANTIGEN   ANTIGEN

**Figure 5.11. The 'bonus' effect of multivalent attachment on binding strength.** The force binding the two antigen molecules in (c) with two antibody bridges is many-fold greater than (a) + (b). If the affinity for determinant 1 is $k_1$ and for the second determinant $k_2$, the avidity of the mixture of antibodies for the antigen would be $K_{avid} = k_1 \times k_2$. To give a concrete example, if $k_1$ is $10^4$ and $k_2$ is $10^3$, $K_{avid}$ would be $10^7$ M$^{-1}$. Advanced readers should recognize that in practice, this bonus effect would be reduced by entropy losses resulting from any restriction of the flexibility of the antibody molecules required by adaptation to the spatial demands of the epitopes and from the restriction in translational movement of the individual components.

figure 5.11. The binding of the two antibodies to determinants 1 and 2 on the antigen can each be described by the individual change in free energy state on forming the epitope–paratope bond with its corresponding affinity constant, i.e.:

$$\Delta G_1 = -RT \ln k_1 \text{ and } \Delta G_2 = -RT \ln k_2$$

For both antibodies operating in conjunction, the *overall* free energy change giving the avidity ($K_{avid}$) would be:

$$\Delta G = \Delta G_1 + \Delta G_2 = -RT \ln k_1 - RT \ln k_2$$
$$= -RT(\ln k_1 + \ln k_2) = -RT(\ln k_1 \times k_2)$$

Since $\Delta G = -RT \ln K_{avid}$, $K_{avid} = k_1 \times k_2$.

The tremendous increase in equilibrium constant resulting from **multiplying the contributing affinities** (figure 5.11) is responsible for the bonus effect.

For those who prefer a more 'earthy' way of looking at molecular interactions, the mechanism of this effect may be interpreted by considering an analogy. Let us fabricate an unheard-of disease in which we cannot stop our hands opening and closing continuously. If we now try to hold an object in one hand, it will fall the moment we open that hand. However, if we use both hands to hold the object, provided we open and close our hands at different times, there is much less chance of the object falling. The reversible combination of antigen and antibody is like the opening and closing of the hand; the more valencies holding the

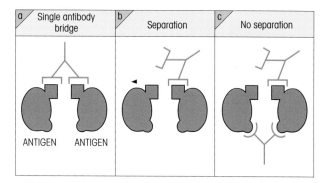

**Figure 5.12. The mechanism of the bonus effect.** Each antigen–antibody bond is reversible and with a single antibody bridge between two antigen molecules (a), dissociation of either bond could enable an antigen molecule to 'escape' as in (b). If there are two antibody bridges, even when one dissociates the other prevents the antigen molecule from escaping and holds it in position ready to reform the broken bond. In effect, the orientation of the broken bond greatly increases the effective combining concentration of antibody and thereby speeds up the velocity of the association reaction: $V_a = k_a [Ag][Ab\uparrow]$.

antigen the less likely it is to be lost when the complex dissociates at any one binding site (figure 5.12).

The same considerations apply to the binding of antibody to a polymeric antigen with repeating determinants such as ovalbumin substituted by several DNP groups, or most bacterial polysaccharides or red cells with repeating blood-group determinants. As one moves from a univalent Fab fragment to a divalent IgG to a pentameric IgM, the bonus effect of multivalency produces striking increases in the strength of antigen–antibody complex formation.

Avidity being a measure of the functional affinity of an antiserum for the whole antigen is of obvious relevance to the reaction with antigen in the body. High avidity is superior to low for a wide variety of functions *in vivo*, immune elimination of antigen, virus neutralization, protective role against bacteria and so on.

## THE SPECIFICITY OF ANTIGEN RECOGNITION BY ANTIBODY IS NOT ABSOLUTE

The ability of antibodies to discriminate between different antigens was well illustrated by the range of reactivity of an antihapten for a series of structurally related molecules as described in table 5.1. Since the strength of the reaction can be quantified by the affinity or avidity, we would relate the **specificity** of an antiserum to its relative avidity for the antigens which are being discriminated.

In so far as we recognize that an antiserum may have a relatively greater avidity for one antigen rather

than another, by the same token we are saying that the antiserum is displaying relative rather than absolute specificity; in practice we speak of degrees of **cross-reactivity**. An antiserum raised against a given antigen can cross-react with a partially related antigen which bears one or more identical or similar determinants. In figure 5.13 it can be seen that an antiserum to antigen$_1$ (Ag$_1$) will react less strongly with Ag$_2$ which bears just one identical determinant because only certain of the antibodies in the serum can bind. Ag$_3$, which possesses a similar but not identical determinant, will not fit as well with the antibody and the binding is even weaker. Ag$_4$, which has no structural similarity at all, will not react significantly with the antibody. Thus, based upon stereochemical considerations, we can see why the avidity of the antiserum for Ag$_2$ and Ag$_3$ is less than for the homologous antigen, while for the unrelated Ag$_4$ it is negligible. It would be customary to describe the antiserum as being highly specific for Ag$_1$ in relation to Ag$_4$ but cross-reacting with Ag$_2$ and Ag$_3$ to different extents.

By being directed towards single epitopes on the antigen, monoclonal antibodies frequently show high specificity in terms of their low cross-reactivity with other antigens. Occasionally, however, one sees quite unexpected binding to antigens which react poorly, if at all, with a specific antiserum. It is an instructive exercise to see how it is that a polyclonal antiserum containing a heterogeneous collection of antibodies can be more specific in discriminating between two antigens than a monoclonal antibody. The six hypervariable regions of an antibody encompass a relatively large molecular area composed of highly diverse amino acid side-chains and it is self-evident that a number of different epitopic structures could fit into different parts of this hypervariable 'terrain', albeit with a spectrum of combining affinities.

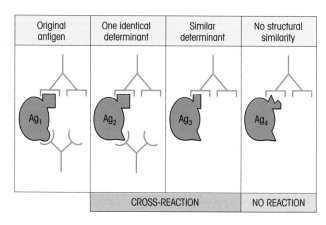

**Figure 5.13. Specificity and cross-reaction.** The avidity of the serum antibodies (⊣⊢ and ⟩—⟨) for Ag$_1$ > Ag$_2$ > Ag$_3$ >> Ag$_4$.

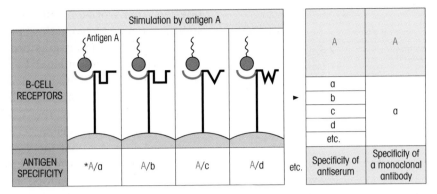

**Figure 5.14. The specificity of an antiserum derives from the reactivity common to the component antibodies.** Antigen A stimulates lymphocytes whose polyfunctional receptors bind A but could also bind other determinants as indicated (small letters). All antibodies in the resulting antiserum will have anti-A as a common specificity but the other specificities will be so diverse, none of them will reach appreciable concentrations to cross-react signifi- cantly with another antigen bearing a or b etc., i.e. the antiserum shows specificity for A. On the other hand, a monoclonal antibody cannot dilute out its alternative specificity so in the example shown with an asterisk there would be strong cross-reaction with an unrelated antigen a. (With acknowl- edgement to Talmage D.W. (1959) *Science* **129**, 1643.)

Thus, each antibody will react not only with the antigen which stimulated its production, but also with some possibly quite unrelated molecules. Figure 5.14 explains (I hope) how this may translate into a higher specificity for the polyclonal serum.

## WHAT THE T-CELL SEES

We have on several occasions alluded to the fact that the T-cell receptor sees antigen on the surface of cells associated with an MHC class I or II molecule. Now is the time for us to go into the nuts and bolts of this relationship.

### Haplotype restriction reveals the need for MHC participation

It has been established in tablets of stone that TCR2 T-cells bearing αβ receptors, with some exceptions (cf. p. 99), only respond when the antigen-presenting cells express the same MHC haplotype as the host from which the T-cells were derived (Milestone 5.1). This **haplotype restriction** on T-cell recognition tells us unequivocally that MHC molecules are intimately and necessarily involved in the interaction of the antigen-bearing cell with its corresponding antigen-specific T-lymphocyte. We also learn that cytotoxic T-cells recognize antigen in the context of class I MHC, and helper T-cells which interact with macrophages respond when the antigen is associated with class II molecules.

Accepting then the participation of MHC in T-cell recognition, what of the antigen? For some time it was perplexing that in so many systems antibodies raised to the native antigen failed to block cytotoxicity (cf.

Figure M5.1.1b), despite consistent success with anti-MHC class I sera. We now think we know why.

### T-cells recognize a linear peptide sequence from the antigen

In Milestone 5.1, we commented on experiments involving influenza nucleoprotein-specific T-cells which could kill cells infected with influenza virus. Killing occurs after the cytotoxic T-cell adheres strongly to its target through recognition of specific surface molecules. It is curious then that the nucleoprotein, which lacks a signal sequence or transmembrane region and so cannot be expressed on the cell surface, can nonetheless function as a target for cytotoxic T-cells, particularly since we have already noted that antibodies to native nucleoprotein have no influence on the killing reaction (figure M5.1.1b). Furthermore, uninfected cells do not become targets for the cytotoxic T-cells when whole nucleoprotein is added to the culture system. However, if instead, we add a series of short peptides with sequences derived from the primary structure of the nucleoprotein, the uninfected cells now become susceptible to cytolytic T-cell attack (figure 5.15).

Thus was the secret revealed! The startling reality is that T-cells recognize linear peptides derived from the antigen and that is why antibodies raised against nucleoprotein in its native three-dimensional conformation (cf. figure 5.2), do not inhibit killing. Note that only certain nucleoprotein peptides were recognized by the polyclonal T-cells in the donor population and these are to be regarded as T-cell epitopes. When clones of identical specificity are derived from these T-cells, each clone reacts with only one of the pep-

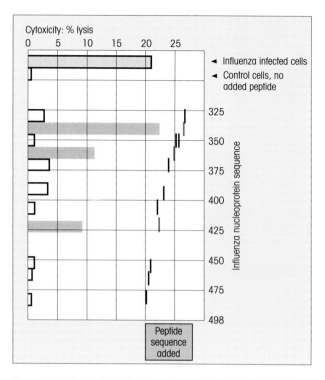

**Figure 5.15.** Cytotoxic T-cells, from a human donor, kill uninfected target cells in the presence of short influenza nucleoprotein peptides. The peptides indicated were added to $^{51}$Cr-labeled syngeneic (i.e. same as T-cell donor) mitogen-activated lymphoblasts and cytotoxicity assessed by $^{51}$Cr release with a killer : target ratio of 50 : 1. The three peptides indicated in red induced good killing. Blasts infected with influenza virus of a different strain served as a positive control. (Reproduced from Townsend A.R.M. et al. (1986) *Cell* **44**, 959, with permission. Copyright 1986 by Cell Press.)

tides; in other words, like B-cell clones, each clone is specific for one corresponding epitope.

Entirely analogous results are obtained when *T-helper* clones are stimulated by antigen-presenting cells to which certain peptides derived from the original antigen had been added. Again, by synthesizing a series of such peptides, the T-cell epitope can be mapped with some precision.

The conclusion is that the **T-cell recognizes both MHC and peptide** and we now know that the peptide which acts as a T-cell epitope lies along the groove formed by the α-helices and the β-sheet floor of the class I and class II outermost domains (figure 4.9). Just how does it get there?

## PROCESSING OF INTRACELLULAR ANTIGEN FOR PRESENTATION BY CLASS I MHC

Cytosolic proteins, including as an example the influenza nucleoprotein discussed above, are degraded to peptides via a ubiquitin-sensitive pathway, by an ATP-dependent complex of peptidases termed a **proteasome** (figure 5.16). This structure contains two MHC associated low molecular weight proteins, LMP2 and 7, which are polymorphic and may serve to optimize delivery of the peptides to the TAP1/TAP2 membrane-spanning transporter mechanism responsible for translocation of the peptides into the endoplasmic reticulum (ER) (figure 5.17). Now within the lumen of the ER, the peptides

## Milestone 5.1—MHC Restriction of T-cell Reactivity

The realization that the MHC, which had figured for so long as a dominant controlling element in tissue graft rejection, should come to occupy the center stage in T-cell reactions, has been a source of fascination and great pleasure to immunologists—almost as though a great universal plan had been slowly unfolding.

One of the seminal observations which helped to elevate the MHC to this lordly position was the dramatic Nobel prize-winning revelation by Doherty and Zinkernagel that cytotoxic T-cells taken from an individual recovering from a viral infection will only kill virally infected cells which share an MHC haplotype with the host. They found that cytotoxic T-cells from mice of the H-2$^d$ haplotype infected with lymphocytic choriomeningitis virus could kill virally infected cells derived from any H-2$^d$ strain but not cells of H-2$^k$ or other H-2 haplotype. The

reciprocal experiment with H-2$^k$ mice shows that this is not just a special property associated with H-2$^d$ (figure M5.1.1a). Studies with recombinant strains (cf. table 4.2) pin-pointed class I MHC as the restricting element and this was confirmed by showing that antibodies to class I MHC block the killing reaction.

The same phenomenon has been repeatedly observed in the human. HLA-A2 individuals recovering from influenza have cytolytic T-cells which kill HLA-A2 target cells infected with influenza virus but not cells of a different HLA-A tissue-type specificity (figure M5.1.1b). Note how cytotoxicity could be inhibited by antiserum specific for the donor HLA-A type but not by antisera to the allelic form HLA-A1 or the HLA-DR class II framework. Of striking significance is the inability of antibodies to the nucleoprotein to block T-cell recognition even though the

*(Continued)*

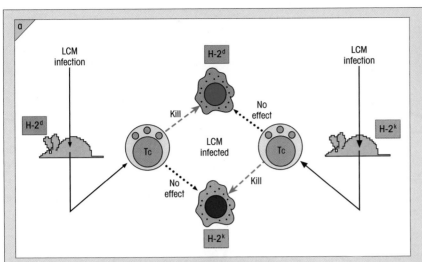

| b | | | |
|---|---|---|---|
| TARGET CELLS | | | % KILLING OF TARGET BY NP-SPECIFIC T-CELLS |
| Infected | Haplotype | Ab added | |
| − | HLA-A2 | − | |
| + | HLA-A2 | − | |
| + | HLA-A1 | − | |
| + | HLA-A2 | anti-HLA-A2 | |
| + | HLA-A2 | anti-HLA-A1 | |
| + | HLA-A2 | anti-HLA-DR | |
| + | HLA-A2 | anti-NP | |

**Figure M5.1.1. T-cell killing is restricted by the MHC haplotype of the virus-infected target cells.** (a) Haplotype restricted killing of lymphocytic choriomeningitis (LCM) virus-infected target cells by cytotoxic T-cells. Killer cells from H-2$^d$ hosts only killed H-2$^d$-infected targets, not those of H-2$^k$ haplotype and vice versa. (b) Killing of influenza-infected target cells by influenza nucleoprotein (NP)-specific T-cells from an HLA-A2 donor (cf. p. 362 for human MHC nomenclature). Killing was restricted to HLA-A2 targets and only inhibited by antibodies to A2, not to A1, nor to the class II HLA-DR framework or native NP antigen.

T-cell specificity in these studies was known to be directed towards this antigen. Since the antibodies react with nucleoprotein in its native form, the conformation of the antigen as presented to the T-cell must be quite different.

In parallel, an entirely comparable series of experiments has established the role of MHC class II molecules in antigen presentation to helper T-cells. Initially, it was shown by Schevach and Rosenthal that lymphocyte proliferation to antigen *in vitro*, could be blocked by antisera raised between two strains of guinea-pig which would have included antibodies to the MHC of the responding lymphocytes. More stringent evidence comes from the type of experiment in which a T-cell clone proliferating in response to ovalbumin on antigen-presenting cells with the H-2A$^b$ phenotype fails to respond if antigen is presented in the context of H-2A$^k$. However, if the H-2A$^k$ antigen-presenting cells are transfected with the genes encoding H-2A$^b$, they now communicate effectively with the T-cells (figure M5.1.2).

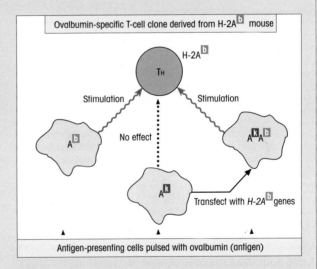

**Figure M5.1.2. The T-cell clone only responds by proliferation *in vitro* when the antigen-presenting cells (e.g. macrophages) pulsed with ovalbumin express the same class II MHC.**

complex with the membrane-bound class I MHC molecules thereby releasing them from their association with the TAP transporter. Thence, the complex traverses the Golgi stack, presumably picking up carbohydrate side-chains *en route*, and reaches the surface where it is a sitting target for the cytotoxic T-cell.

## PROCESSING OF ANTIGEN FOR CLASS II MHC PRESENTATION FOLLOWS A DIFFERENT PATHWAY

Class II MHC complexes with antigenic peptide are generated by a fundamentally different intracellular

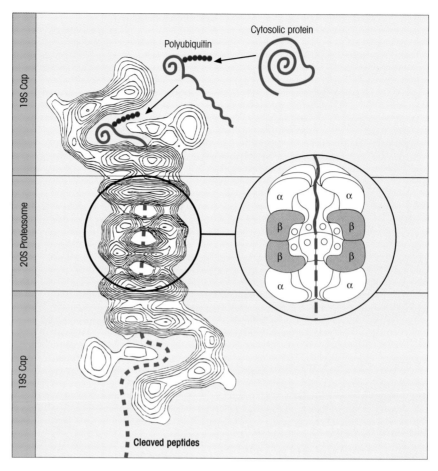

**Figure 5.16. Cleavage of cytosolic proteins by the proteasome.** The whole 26S protease complex consisting of the 20S proteasome with twin 19S caps is displayed as a contour plot derived from electron microscopy and image analysis. The cross-section of the proteasome reveals the sites of peptidase activity (o) within the inner core of the seven-membered rings of β-subunits. The ubiquitinated cytosolic protein binds to the ATPase-containing cap where

ATP drives the unfolded protein chain through the hydrophobic conducting channels of the α-subunits into the central hydrolytic chamber where it is exposed to a variety of proteolytic activities associated with the different β-subunits. (Based on Peters J.-M. *et al.* (1993) *Journal of Molecular Biology* **234**, 932 and Rubin D.M. & Finley D. (1995) *Current Biology* **5**, 854.)

mechanism, since the antigen-presenting cells which interact with T-helper cells need to sample the antigen from both the *extra*cellular and *intra*cellular compartments. In essence, a trans-Golgi vesicle containing class II has to intersect with a late endosome containing exogenous protein antigen taken into the cell by an endocytic mechanism.

First the class II molecules themselves. These are assembled from α- and β-chains in the endoplasmic reticulum in association with the transmembrane **invariant chain** (figure 5.18) which has several functions. It acts as a dedicated chaperone to ensure correct folding of the nascent class II molecule and it inhibits the precocious binding of peptides in the ER before the class II reaches the endocytic compartment containing antigen. Its combination with the αβ class II heterodimer inactivates a retention signal and allows transport to the Golgi. Finally, it uses its cyto-

plasmic tail to sort the class II-containing vesicle to the late endosomal compartment.

Meanwhile, exogenous protein is taken up by endocytosis and is subjected to partial degradation as the early endosome undergoes progressive acidification. The late endosome, having many of the characteristics of a lysosomal granule, now fuses with the vacuole containing the class II–invariant chain complex. Under the acidic conditions within this MHC class II-enriched compartment (MIIC), cathepsins B and D degrade the invariant chain but leave a constituent peptide, CLIP (class II-associated invariant chain peptide) lying within the MHC groove. Another MHC-related dimeric molecule, DM, now catalyzes the removal of CLIP and its replacement by other MIIC peptides (figure 5.19) after which the complexes are transported to the membrane for presentation to T-helper cells. The basis for the inhibition

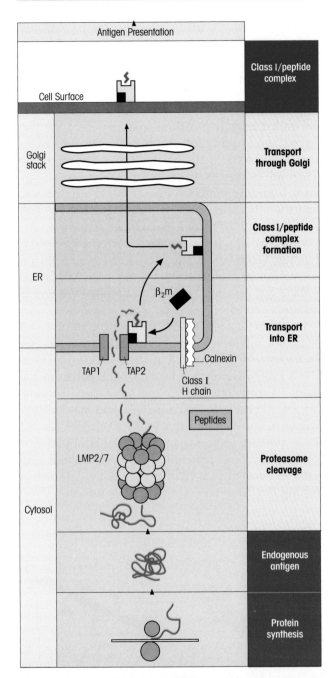

**Figure 5.17. Processing and presentation of endogenous antigen by class I MHC.** Cytosolic proteins are degraded by the proteasome complex into peptides which are transported into the endoplasmic reticulum (ER). There, they bind to membrane-bound class I MHC formed by $\beta_2$-microglobulin ($\beta_2$m)-induced dissociation of nascent class I heavy chains from its calnexin chaperone. The peptide/MHC complex is now released from its association with the TAP transporter, traverses the Golgi system, and appears on the cell surface ready for presentation to the T-cell receptor. Mutant cells deficient in TAP1/2 do not deliver peptides to class I and cannot function as cytotoxic T-cell targets. However, if they are transfected with a gene encoding the antigenic peptide linked to a cleavable signal sequence, the peptide is delivered to the ER without the need for TAP1/2 and the cells once again can become targets.

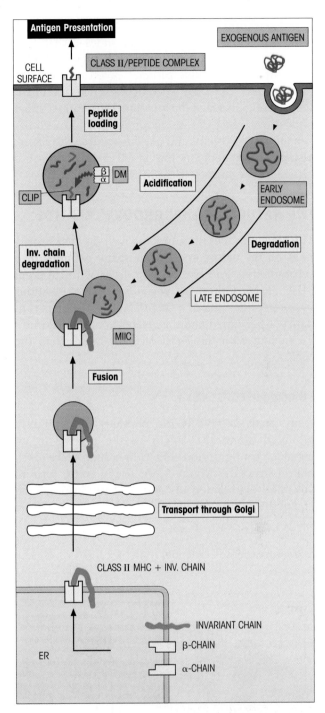

**Figure 5.18. Processing and presentation of exogenous antigen by class II MHC.** Class II molecules with invariant chain are assembled in the endoplasmic reticulum (ER) and transported through the Golgi to the trans-Golgi reticulum (actually as a nonamer consisting of three invariant, three $\alpha$- and three $\beta$-chains—not shown). There it is sorted to a late endosomal vesicle with lysosomal characteristics known as MIIC (meaning MHC class II enriched compartment) containing partially degraded protein derived from the endocytic uptake of exogenous antigen. Degradation of invariant chain leaves the CLIP (class II-associated invariant chain peptide) peptide lying in the groove but under the influence of the DM molecule, this is replaced by other peptides in the vesicle including those derived from exogenous antigen, and the complexes are transported to the cell surface for presentation to T-helper cells. This version of events is supported by the finding of high concentrations of invariant chain CLIP associated with class II in the MIIC vacuoles of DM-deficient mutant mice which are poor presenters of antigen to T-cells.

of antigen-processing by agents such as chloroquine which prevent acidification of lysosomes is clear.

Processing of antigens for class II presentation is not confined to soluble proteins taken up from the exterior but can also encompass microorganisms whose antigens reach the lysosomal structures, either after direct phagocytosis or prolonged intracellular cohabitation. Proteins and peptides within the ER are also potential clients for the class II groove and could also make the journey to the MIIC.

## THE NATURE OF THE 'GROOVY' PEPTIDE

The MHC grooves impose some well-defined restrictions on the nature and length of the peptides they accommodate and the pattern varies with different MHC alleles. Otherwise, at the majority of positions in the peptide ligand, a surprising degree of redundancy is permitted and this relates in part to residues interacting with the T-cell receptor rather than the MHC.

### Binding to MHC class I

X-ray analysis reveals the peptides to be tightly mounted along the length of the groove in an extended configuration with no breathing space for α-helical structures (figure 5.20). The N and C termini are tightly H-bonded to conserved residues at each end of the groove, independently of the MHC allele.

The naturally occurring peptides can be extracted from purified MHC class I and sequenced. They are predominantly octamers or nonamers; longer peptides bulge upwards out of the cleft. Analysis of the peptide pool sequences usually gives strong amino acid signals at certain key positions (table 5.2). These are called **anchor positions** and represent the preferred amino acid side-chains which fit into allele-specific pockets in the MHC groove (figure 5.21a). There are usually two such major anchor positions for class I binding peptides, one at the C-terminal end and the other frequently at position 2 (P2) but may also occur at P3, P5 or P7. Sometimes, a major anchor pocket may be replaced by two or three more weakly binding secondary binding pockets. Even with the constraints of 2 or 3 anchor motifs, each MHC class I allele can accommodate a considerable number of different peptides.

Except in the case of viral infection, the natural class I ligands will be self-peptides derived from proteins endogenously synthesized by the cell, histones, heat-shock proteins, enzymes, leader signal sequences and so on. It turns out that 75% or so of these peptides originate in the cytosol (figure 5.22) and most of them will be in low abundance, say 100–400 copies per cell. Thus proteins expressed with unusual abundance, such as oncofetal proteins in tumors and viral antigens in infected cells, should be readily detected by resting T-cells.

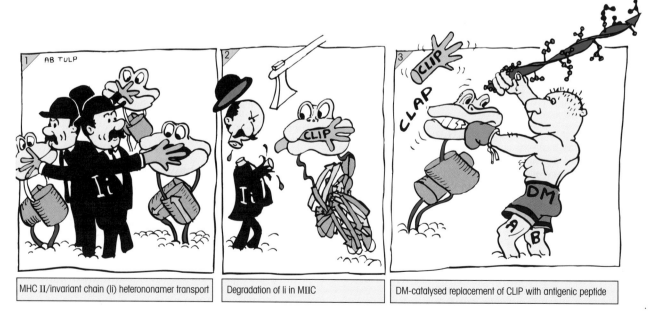

| MHC II/invariant chain (Ii) heterononamer transport | Degradation of Ii in MIIC | DM-catalysed replacement of CLIP with antigenic peptide |

**Figure 5.19. MHC class II transport and peptide loading** illustrated by Tulp's gently vulgar cartoon. (Reproduced from Benham A. *et al.* (1995) *Immunology Today* **16**, 361 with permission of the authors and Elsevier Science Ltd.)

**Table 5.2. Natural MHC class I peptide ligands contain two allele-specific anchor residues.** (Based on Rammensee H.-G., Falk K. & Rötzschke O. (1993) *Current Opinion in Immunology* **5**, 35.) Letters represent the Dayhoff code for amino acids; where more than one residue predominates at a given position, the alternative(s) is given; • = any residue.

| Class I allele | Amino acid position | | | | | | | | |
|---|---|---|---|---|---|---|---|---|---|
| | 1 | 2 | 3 | 4 | 5 | 6 | 7 | 8 | 9 |
| H-2K$^d$ | • | Y | • | • | • | • | • | • | L/I |
| H-2K$^b$ | • | • | • | • | F/Y | • | • | M/I/L | |
| H-2D$^b$ | • | • | • | • | N | • | • | • | I/L/M |
| HLA-A2 | • | L | • | • | • | • | • | • | V |
| HLA-B27 | • | R | • | • | • | • | • | • | R/K |

## Binding to MHC class II

Unlike class I where the allele-independent H-bonding to the peptide is focused at the N- and C-termini, the class II groove residues H-bond along the entire length of the peptide with links to the atoms forming the main chain. With respect to class II allele-specific binding pockets for peptide side-chains, motifs based on three major anchor residues seem to be the order of the day (figure 5.21b). Secondary binding pockets with less strict preference for individual side-chains can still modify the affinity of the peptide–MHC complex while 'non-pockets' may also influence preferences for particular peptide sequences especially if steric hindrance becomes a factor. Unfortunately we cannot establish these preferences for the individual residues within a given peptide because the open nature of the class II groove places no constraint on the length of the peptide which can dangle nonchalantly from each end of the groove quite unlike the strait-jacket of the class I ligand site (figures 5.20 and 5.21). Thus, as noted earlier, each class II molecule binds a collection of peptides with a spectrum of lengths ranging from 10 to 34mers and analysis of such a naturally occurring pool isolated from the MHC would not establish which amino acid side-chains were binding preferentially to the nine available sites within the groove. The modern approach is to study the binding of soluble class II molecules to very large libraries of random-sequence peptides expressed on the surface of bacteriophage (cf. the combinatorial phage libraries p. 125). The idea is emerging that each amino acid in a peptide contributes independently of the others to the total binding strength and it should be possible to compute each contribution quantitatively from this random binding data so that ultimately we could

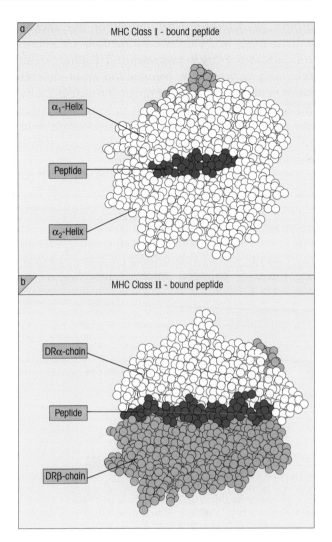

**Figure 5.20. Binding of peptides to the MHC cleft.** T-cell receptor 'view' looking down on the α-helices lining the cleft (cf. figure 4.9b) represented in space-filling models. (a) Peptide 309–317 from HIV-1 reverse transcriptase bound tightly within the class I HLA-A2 cleft. In general, 1 to 4 of the peptide side-chains are solvent exposed (17–27%) and thus are available to the T-cell receptor. (b) Influenza hemagglutinin 306–318 lying in the class II HLA-DR1 cleft. In contrast with class I, the peptide extends out of both ends of the binding groove and from 4 to 6 out of an average of 13 side-chains point towards the TCR increasing solvent accessibility to 35%. (Based on Vignali D.A.A. & Strominger J.L. (1994) *The Immunologist* **2**, 112, with permission of the authors and publisher.)

predict which sequences in a given protein antigen would bind to a given class II allele.

Because of the accessible nature of the groove, as the native molecule is unfolded and reduced, but before any degradation need occur, the high affinity epitopes could immediately bury themselves in the class II binding groove where they are protected from proteolysis. Trimming can take place afterwards leaving peptides 10–34 amino acids long. Several factors will influence the relative concentration of peptide–MHC complex formed: the affinity for the groove as determined by the fit of the anchors, enhancement or hindrance by flanking or internal residues, sensitivity to proteases and disulfide reduction, and downstream competition from determinants of higher affinity. The range of concentration of different peptide complexes which result will engender a hierarchy of epitopes with respect to their ability to interact with T-cells; the most effective will be **dominant**, the less so, **subdominant**.

Dominant, and presumably subdominant, **self** epitopes will generally induce tolerance during T-cell ontogeny in the thymus (see p. 231). Complexes with some self peptides which are of relatively low abundance will not tolerize their T-cell counterparts and these autoreactive T-cells constantly pose an underlying threat of potential autoimmunity. Sercarz has

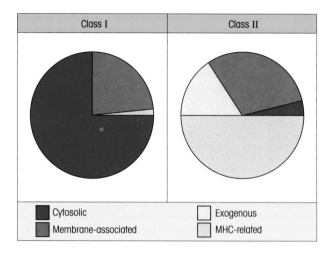

**Figure 5.22. The origins of class I- and class II-bound peptides.** Virtually all class I peptides are derived from endogenous proteins and even after viral infections, it is the intracellular antigens which are processed. Processing in the endosomal compartments ensures that proteins of endogenous origin and those derived from membranes constitute over 90% of the peptides bound to the class II grooves. (Diagram reproduced from Vignali D.A.A. & Strominger J.L. (1994) *The Immunologist* **2**, 112, with permission of the authors and publisher).

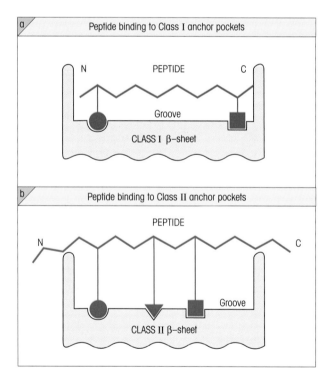

**Figure 5.21. Allele-specific pockets in the MHC binding grooves bind the major anchor residue motifs of the peptide ligands.** Cross-section through the longitudinal axis of the MHC groove. The two α-helices forming the lateral walls of the groove lie horizontally above and below the plane of the paper. (a) Tight interaction of peptide with the groove is critical for stable class I assembly and there is allele-independent strong H-bonding at the N- and C-termini of the peptide to tryptophan 167 and tyrosine 84 respectively at the ends of the class I closed groove. The anchor at the carboxy terminus is invariant but the second anchor very often at P2 may also be at P3, P5 or P7 depending on the MHC allele (cf. table 5.2). (b) The class II groove in contrast is open at both ends and does not constrain the length of the peptide. There are usually three major anchor pockets at P1, P4, P6, P7 or P9 with P1 being the most important.

labeled these **cryptic** epitopes and we will discuss their possible relationship to autoimmune disease in Chapter 19.

## THE αβ T-CELL RECEPTOR FORMS A TERNARY COMPLEX WITH MHC AND ANTIGENIC PEPTIDE

Soluble TCR preparations have been made in order to study the interaction with the MHC–peptide complex. One of the most cunning is derived from a TCR linked by a proteinase cleavage site to CD3 ζ chains. Insertion of the construct in a basophil cell line provides a direct biological readout for the retention of antigen recognition by the TCR construct. The soluble TCRs immobilized on a sensor chip can bind MHC–peptide complex specifically with rather low affinities ($K_a$) in the $10^4$ to $10^7$ $M^{-1}$ range. This low affinity and the relatively small number of links (40–1000) formed between the TCRs and their MHC/peptide ligands when T-cells contact their target cell, makes the contribution of TCR recognition to the binding energy of this cellular interaction fairly trivial. The brunt of the attraction rests on the antigen-independent major adhesion molecules such as ICAM1/2, LFA1/2 and CD2 but any subsequent triggering of the T-cell by MHC/peptide antigen must involve signalling through the T-cell receptor.

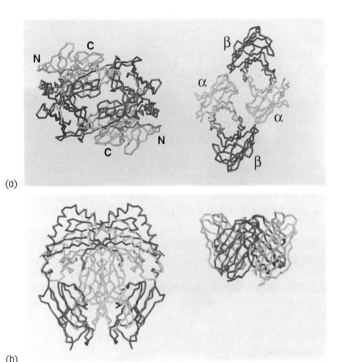

(a)

(b)

**Figure 5.23. Complementarity between MHC class II peptide and T-cell receptor.** The MHC class II exists as a dimer of αβ-heterodimers as is also probably the case with the TCR where X-ray analysis reveals the ability of Vα domains to pack closely together. (a) View from above the class II-peptide (red) complexes with the TCR (VαVβ)₂ tetramer pulled apart and rotated through 180°. The Vα and Vβ CDR3 loops are shown in red. If rotated back through 180° and placed above the MHC/peptide complex, the pair of CDR3 loops from each TCR are positioned to bind the two peptides as located within the class II tetramer with the Vα CDR3 contacting the N-terminus and the Vβ CDR3 the C-terminal end of the peptide in accord with most previous studies and by analogy, with the role of the CDRs in contact of antibody and antigen. The Vα CDR1 and CDR2 loops would bind to the class II β1 domain, the Vβ CDR1 and CDR2 to the class II α1 domain. (b) Side view of the complex pulled apart and rotated through 180°. The angle of the two bound peptides to each other and the essentially flat surface of the modelled TCR tetramer suggest that a conformational change in one or the other may be required for intimate contact between the two and could be one requirement for T-cell signalling. Mariuzza and colleagues suggest that a co-operative interaction involving the formation of stable TCR₂-MHC₂ signalling complexes from inherently weak individual TCR and class II dimers could provide a mechanism by which homogeneous peptide–MHC dimers could form on the surface of an antigen-presenting cell bearing a multiplicity of different peptide-MHC complexes. (Reproduced from Field B.A. *et al.* (1995) *Science* **270**, 1821 with permission.)

## Topology of the ternary complex

Of the three complementarity determinants assumed to be present in each TCR chain, CDR1 and CDR2 are much less variable than CDR3 which, like its immunoglobulin counterpart, has (D)J sequences which result from a multiplicity of combinatorial and nucleotide insertion mechanisms (cf. p. 69). Since the MHC elements in a given individual are fixed but great variability is expected in the antigenic peptide, a

logical model would have CDR1 and CDR2 of each TCR chain contacting the α-helices of the MHC, and the CDR3 concerned in binding to the peptide (figure 5.23). In accord with this view, several studies have shown that T-cells which recognize small variations in a peptide in the context of a given MHC restriction element, differ only in their CDR3 hypervariable regions. It now seems likely that complexes of two TCR molecules with two MHC/peptide moieties can form and may be linked to T-cell signalling (see figure 5.23 and legend).

## T-CELLS WITH A DIFFERENT OUTLOOK

### Non-classical class I molecules can also present antigen

#### MHC class I-like molecules

In addition to the highly polymorphic classical MHC class I molecules (HLA-A, B and C in the human and H-2K, D and L in the mouse) there are other loci encoding MHC molecules containing β₂-microglobulin with relatively non-polymorphic heavy chains. These are **H-2M, Q and T** in mice and **HLA-E, F and G** in *Homo sapiens*.

The best studied molecule encoded by the H-2M locus is **H-2M3** which is unusual in its ability to present bacterial *N*-formyl methionine peptides to T-cells. Expression of H-2M3 is limited by the availability of these peptides so that high levels are only seen during prokaryotic infections. The demonstration of H-2M3 restricted CD8 positive αβ T-cells specific for *Listeria monocytogenes* encourages the view that this class I-like molecule could underwrite a physiological function in infection. The role of HLA-G as a protector of human syncitiotrophoblast against natural killer (NK) cell attack will arise in Chapter 17 (p. 375).

#### The family of CD1 non-MHC class I-like molecules can present exotic antigens

After MHC class I and class II, the CD1 family represent a third lineage of antigen-presenting molecules recognized by T-lymphocytes. I know it's boring but it may be useful to record that there are 5 non-polymorphic *CD1* genes in the human (*CD1A* to *E* and 2 *CD1D* homologes in the mouse). Group I CD1 proteins (CD1a, -b, and -c) are abundant on 'professional' antigen-presenting cells, whereas group II CD1 proteins, e.g. CD1d, are strongly expressed on the intestinal epithelium. The CD1 peptide chains associate with β₂-microglobulin as becomes an honest class I-like moiety, but homology with classical class I molecules is negligible in the α1 domain and only rather tentative in the α2. Analysis of the α3 domain which has the characteristics of the Ig superfamily (cf. p. 247) suggests that CD1 evolved from an ancestral antigen-presenting molecule at about the same time as the MHC class I and II molecules diverged.

The exciting news is that human **CD1b** can act as a **restriction element** in the presentation of several **lipid and glycolipid mycobacterial antigens** to T-cells. There are also reports that cells belonging to a conserved CD1d-restricted subset bearing an invariant TCR and the NK1.1+ marker are amongst the first to produce interleukin (IL)-4 after antigen stimulation.

### γδ TCRs have some features of antibody

Unlike αβ T-cells, only a small fraction of the TCR1 subset bearing γδ receptors recognize allogeneic MHC molecules and when they do, neither the polymorphic residues associated with peptide binding nor the peptide itself are involved. Also, a γδ T-cell clone specific for the herpes simplex glycoprotein, can be stimulated by the intact protein, not in solution, but attached to plastic, suggesting that the cells are triggered by cross-linking of their receptors by the surface-bound antigen which they recognize in the intact native state just as antibodies do. There are structural arguments to give weight to this view. The CDR3 loops which are critical for foreign antigen recognition by T-cells and antibodies, are comparable in length and relatively constrained with respect to size in the α and β chains of the TCR1, presumably reflecting a relative constancy in the size of the MHC–peptide complexes which they bind to. CDR3 regions in the immunoglobulin light chains are short and similarly constrained in length but in the heavy chains they are longer on average and more variable in length, related perhaps to their need to recognize a wide range of epitopes. Quite strikingly, the γδ TCR1s resemble antibodies in that the γ chain CDR3 loops are short with a narrow length distribution, while in the δ chain they are long with a broad length distribution. Therefore m'Lud, as they say in court, the γδ **TCR resembles antibody** more than the αβ TCR and this could account for its ability to interact with intact rather than processed antigen.

More secrets are being teased out of the γδ T-cell sect. Heat-shock protein hsp-60 on autologous stressed keratinocytes, and mycobacteria are powerful activators of γδ cells. In the latter case, a distinct group of low molecular weight **phosphate-** containing **nonpeptides** such as isopentenyl pyrophosphate which occur in a range of microbial and mammalian cells, have been identified as potent stimulators, further extending the variety of non-peptide antigens which can be recognized by T-cells. These characteristics provide the γδ cells with a distinctive role complementary to that of the αβ population and enable them to function in the recognition of microbial pathogens and of damaged or stressed host cells.

## SUPERANTIGENS STIMULATE WHOLE FAMILIES OF LYMPHOCYTE RECEPTORS

### Bacterial toxins represent one major group of T-cell superantigens

Whereas an individual peptide complexed to MHC will react with antigen-specific T-cells which represent a relatively small percentage of the T-cell pool because of the requirement for specific binding to particular CDR3 regions, new classes of molecules have been identified, which stimulate that proportion of the total T-cell population which express the same TCR Vβ family structure irrespective of their antigen specificity. They have been described as **superantigens** by Kappler and Marrack.

*Staphylococcus aureus* enterotoxins (SEA, SEB and several others) are single-chain proteins which can cause food poisoning, vomiting and diarrhea. They are strongly mitogenic for T-cells with particular Vβ families in the presence of MHC class II accessory cells. SEA must be one of the most potent T-cell mitogens known, causing marked proliferation in the concentration range $10^{-13}$ to $10^{-16}$ M. It can cause the release of large amounts of cytokines and of mast cell leukotrienes which probably form the basis for its ability to produce toxic-shock syndrome.

Superantigens are not processed by the antigen-presenting cell but cross-link the class II and Vβ independently of direct interaction between MHC and TCR molecules (figure 5.24).

### Endogenous mouse mammary tumor viruses (MMTV) act as superantigens

Very many years ago, Festenstein made the curious observation that B-cells from certain mouse strains could produce powerful proliferative responses in roughly 20% of unprimed T-cells from another strain of identical MHC. The so-called Mls gene product responsible for inciting proliferation turns out to be encoded by the open reading frame (ORF) located in the 3' long terminal repeat of **MMTV**. They are type B

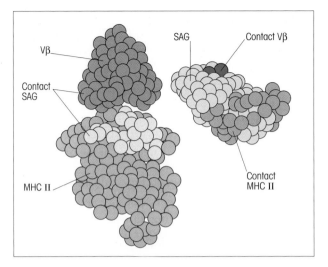

**Figure 5.24. Interaction of superantigen (SAG) with MHC and TCR.** Suggested model for cross-linking of MHC and TCR by SAG (in this case the *S. aureus* toxic-shock syndrome toxin-1). The interacting faces of both the MHC/TCR complex and the SAG are exposed by (opposed) 90° rotations of each about a vertical axis. The SAG contacts the α-helices of both class II α- and β-chains plus part of the peptide. The TCR region interacting with SAG is located in the DE loop (sometimes referred to as the HV4 loop) on the external β-sheet surface of the Vβ domain. (Based on Acharya R.A. *et al.* (1994) *Nature* **367**, 94). Another of the staphylococcal SAGs, *S. aureus* enterotoxin A (SEA), contacts the MHC differently, binding to the outer edge of the α-helix of the class II α-chain. The ability of SEA to enable class I restricted cytolytic T-cells expressing the correct Vβ family to kill target cells bearing MHC class II strongly supports a model in which the SAG cross-links the class II and TCR independently of their cognate interaction through peptide since the TCR will not recognize class II. It also tells us that the superantigen is not presented by class II in a processed form and also that CD4 is not involved.

retroviruses transmitted as infectious agents in milk and are specific for B-cells. They associate with class II MHC in the B-cell membrane and act as superantigens through their affinity for certain TCR Vβ families in a similar fashion to the bacterial toxins. No human counterparts of these retroviral superantigens have so far been uncovered.

## Microbes can also provide B-cell superantigens

Staphylococcal protein A reacts not only with the Fcγ region of IgG but also with 15–50% of polyclonal IgM, IgA and IgG F(ab')$_2$, all of which belong to the $V_H3$ family. The SAG is mitogenic for B-cells through its binding to positions 74–77 on framework 3 at a site distant from the conventional antigen binding pocket but similar to that on the TCR Vβ which is targetted by superantigen. The human immunodeficiency virus (HIV) glycoprotein gp120 and the polylactosamine elements in the I or i autoantigenic determinants react with framework structures of different $V_H$ families and are linked to superantigen-induced responses.

# THE RECOGNITION OF DIFFERENT FORMS OF ANTIGEN BY B- AND T-CELLS IS ADVANTAGEOUS TO THE HOST

It is my conviction that this section deals with a subject of the utmost importance which is at the epicenter of immunology.

Antibodies combat microbes and their products in the extracellular body fluids where they exist essentially in their native form (figure 5.25a). Clearly it is to the host's advantage for the B-cell receptor to recognize epitopes on the **native molecules**.

T-cells, be they cytotoxic or lymphokine producers, have quite a different job; they have to seek out and bind to infected cells and carry out their effector function face to face with the target. First, with respect to proteins produced by the intracellular infectious agent, the MHC molecules tell the effector T-lymphocyte that it is encountering a cell. Second, the T-cell does not want to attack an uninfected cell on whose surface a native microbial molecule is sitting adventitiously nor would it wish to have its antigenic target on the appropriate cell surface blocked by an excess of circulating antibody. Thus it is of benefit for the infected cell to express the microbial antigen on its surface in a form distinct from that of the native molecule. As will now be more than abundantly clear, the evolutionary solution was to make the T-cell recognize a processed peptide derived from the intra-

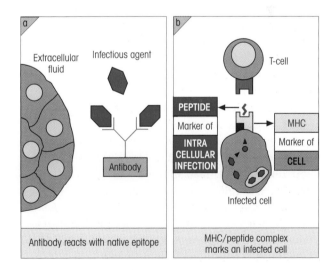

**Figure 5.25.** (a) **Antibodies are formed against the native, not denatured, form of infectious agents which are attacked in the extracellular fluids.** (b) Effector T-cells recognize infected cells by two surface markers: the MHC is a signal for cell, and the foreign peptide is there in the MHC groove since it is derived from the proteins of an intracellular infectious agent. Further microbial cell surface signals can be provided by undegraded antigens and low molecular weight phosphates (seen by γδ T-cells), and lipids and glycolipids presented by CD1 molecules.

cellular antigen and to hold it as a complex with the surface MHC molecules. The single T-cell receptor then recognizes both the **MHC cell marker** and the **peptide infection marker** in one operation (figure 5.25b).

A comparable situation arises when CD1 molecules substitute for MHC in antigen presentation to T-cells, in this case associating with processed microbial lipids and glycolipids. The physiological role of the $\gamma\delta$ cells has yet to be fully unravelled.

## SUMMARY

### The nature of antigens

• An antigen is defined by its antibody. The contact area with an antibody is called an **epitope** and the corresponding area on an antibody, a **paratope**.
• Antisera recognize a series of dominant epitope clusters on the surface of an antigen; each cluster is called a determinant.
• Most epitopes on globular proteins are **discontinuous** rather than **linear**, involving amino acids far apart in the primary sequence.
• The protruding regions and probably the 'flexible' segments of globular proteins tend to be associated with higher epitope densities.

### Antigens and antibodies interact by spatial complementarity, not by covalent binding

• The forces of interaction include electrostatic, hydrogen-bonding, hydrophobic and Van der Waals.
• The forces become large as separation of antigen and antibody diminishes, especially when water molecules are excluded.
• Antigen–antibody bonds are readily **reversible**.
• Antigens and antibodies are mutually deformable.

### Affinity

• The strength of binding to a single antibody combining site is measured by the **affinity**.
• The reaction of multivalent antigens with the heterogeneous mixture of antibodies in an antiserum is defined by **avidity (functional affinity)** and is usually much greater than affinity due to the 'bonus effect of multivalency'.
• **Specificity** of antibodies is not absolute and they may cross-react with other antigens to different extents measured by their relative avidities.

### T-cell recognition

• **Most T-cells see antigen in association with MHC molecules.**

• They are restricted to the haplotype of the cell which first primed the T-cell.
• Protein antigens are processed by antigen-presenting cells to form **small linear peptides** which associate with the MHC molecules, **binding to the central groove** formed by the $\alpha$-helices and the $\beta$-sheet floor.

### Processing of antigen for presentation by class I MHC

• Endogenous cytosolic antigens such as viral proteins are cleaved by **proteasomes** and the peptides so-formed **transported** to the ER by the TAP1/2 system.
• The peptide then cooperates with $\beta_2$-microglobulin to combine with newly synthesized class I MHC heavy chain to form a stable heterotrimer which dissociates from TAP1/2.
• This **peptide–MHC complex** is then transported to the surface for presentation to cytotoxic T-cells.

### Processing of antigen for presentation by class II MHC

• The $\alpha\beta$ **class II molecule** is synthesized in the ER and complexes with membrane-bound **invariant chain**.
• This facilitates transport of the vesicles containing class II across the Golgi and directs it to an acidified late endosome or lysosome containing exogenous protein taken into the cell by endocytosis or phagocytosis.
• Processing by cathepsins degrades the antigen to peptides which bind to class II now free of invariant chain.
• The **class II–peptide** complex now appears on the cell surface for presentation to T-helper cells.

### The nature of the peptide

• Class I peptides are held in extended conformation within the MHC groove.
• They are usually 9–11 residues in length and have two key **anchor** relatively invariant residues which bind to allele-specific pockets in the MHC.
• Class II peptides are between 12 and 25 residues long,

*(Continued)*

extend beyond the groove and usually have three anchor residues.

• The other amino acid residues are greatly variable and are recognized by the T-cell receptor (TCR).

### Complex between TCR, MHC and peptide

• The first and second hypervariable regions (CDR1 and CDR2) of each TCR chain contact the MHC α-helices while the CDR3s, having the greatest variability, interact with the antigenic peptide. Complexes of $TCR_2$ $(MHC/peptide)_2$ are probably formed.

### Some T-cells are independent of classical MHC molecules

• MHC class I-like molecules such as H-2M are relatively non-polymorphic and can present antigens such as bacterial $N$-formyl methionine peptides.

• The CD1 family of non-MHC class I-like molecules can present exotic antigens such as lipid and glycolipid mycobacterial antigens.

• γδ T-cells resemble antibodies in recognizing whole unprocessed molecules such as heat-shock proteins and low molecular weight phosphate containing non-peptides.

### Superantigens

• These are potent mitogens which stimulate whole T-cell subpopulations sharing the same TCR Vβ family independently of antigen specificity.

• *Staphylococcus aureus* enterotoxins are powerful human superantigens which cause food poisoning and toxic-shock syndrome.

• They are not processed but cross-link MHC class II and TCR Vβ independently of their direct interaction.

• Mouse mammary tumor viruses are B-cell retroviruses which are superantigens in the mouse.

### Recognition of different forms of antigen by B- and T-cells is an advantage

• B-cells recognize epitopes on the native antigen; this is important because antibodies react with native antigen in the extracellular fluid.

• T-cells must contact infected cells and to avoid confusion between the two systems, the infected cell signals itself to the T-cell by the combination of MHC and degraded antigen.

# FURTHER READING

Austyn J.M. (1989) Antigen-presenting cells. In Rickwood D. & Male D. (eds) *In Focus* series. IRL Press, Oxford.

Davies D.R. & Padlan E.A. (1992) Twisting into shape: evidence for induced fit in antibody–antigen interactions. *Current Biology* 2, 254.

Getzoff E.D., Tainer, J.A., Lerner R.A. & Geysen H.M. (1988) The chemistry and mechanism of antibody binding to protein antigens. *Advances in Immunology* 43, 1.

Groettrup M., Soza A., Kuckelkorn U. & Kloetzel P-M. (1996) Peptide antigen production by the proteasome: complexity provides efficiency. *Immunology Today* 17, 429.

Karush F. (1976) Multivalent binding and functional affinity. In Inman F.P. (ed.) *Contemporary Topics in Molecular Immunology*. Vol. 5, p. 217. Plenum Press, New York. (Bonus effect of multivalency.)

Lindahl K.F. & Rammensee H.-G. (eds) (1996) Antigen recognition. *Current Opinion in Immunology* 8, 1. (Series of articulate and coherent reviews with extensive citation of key supporting experimental work.)

MacCallum R.M., Martin A.C.R. & Thornton J.M. (1996) Antibody–antigen interactions: contact analysis and binding site topography. *Journal of Molecular Biology* 262, 732.

Nisonoff A. & Pressman D. (1957) Closeness of fit and forces involved in the reactions of antibody homologous to the *p*-(*p*′-N-azophenylazo)-benzoate ion group. *Journal of the American Chemistry Society* 79, 1616.

Novotny J., Bruccoleri R.E. & Saul F.A. (1989) On the attribution of binding energy in antigen–antibody complexes. *Biochemistry* 28, 4735. (View that only certain residues in epitope actively involved, others passive.)

Sekaly R.-P. (ed.) (1993) Bacterial superantigens. *Seminars in Immunology* 5, 1. (A very useful survey of current knowledge.)

Wong Y.W. *et al.* (1995) Modulation of antibody affinity by an engineered amino acid substitution. *Journal of Immunology* 154, 3351.

# PART 3

# TECHNOLOGY

The scientific method based on the creation of hypotheses and their test by experiment, has its own validity within the human quest for greater awareness and knowledge of the universe which surrounds us. So does **technology**, which embraces the application of science with its problem solving and establishment of new techniques. It seems reasonable, at this stage of the text, to mark time in the gradual build up of immunological concepts, and to focus on the most significant immunological techniques which have permitted the scientists to advance the subject so dramatically.

Chapter 6 gives an account of **immunochemical techniques** concerned essentially with the interaction of antibodies with individual molecules of antigen. It covers methods for the **measurement of antibodies**, the identification and **quantification of antigens**, the production of **antibodies to order** using genetic engineering and hybridoma technology, purification by **affinity chromatography** and the **functional interactions** with biologically active molecules.

Experimental techniques which apply to higher levels of organization, **the cell** and indeed **the whole organism**, are described in Chapter 7. We see how **lymphocyte subpopulations** can be isolated and individual clones produced. **Immunocytochemistry** enables us to probe the immunologically defined anatomy of the tissue and cell using both light and electron microscopy. **Flow cytofluorimetry** provides ever more parameters to define the **phenotype** of individual cells, and **tissue typing** for MHC and other alleles has fallen prey to the inevitable takeover by molecular biology. Another section is concerned with assessment of the **functional behavior** of white cells, their phagocytic activity, responsiveness to antigen, extracellular killing potential and so on. Last, the chapter reviews the expanding technologies concerning **manipulation of the genetic makeup** of cells and individuals and their exploitation to help delineate individual gene function within a physiological and pathological context.

# IMMUNOCHEMICAL TECHNIQUES

## ESTIMATION OF ANTIBODY

### Antigen–antibody interactions in solution

#### What does serum 'antibody content' mean?

If we have a solution of a monoclonal antibody, we can define its affinity and specificity with consider-able confidence and, if pure and in its native conformation, we will know that the concentration of antibody is the same as that of the measurable immunoglobulin in ng/ml or whatever. When it comes to measuring the antibody content of an antiserum, the problem is of a different order because the immunoglobulin fraction is composed of an almost infinite array of molecules of varying abundance and affinity. To illustrate the problem, I sometimes pose the following question: an adult individual's serum contains 10 mg/ml of IgG—what is the level of streptococcal M antibody? Given that the only numerical data given involves the number 10, the bright student guesses that the answer will be 0 or 10 and since the individual as an adult has almost certainly been exposed to infection, the answer 10 mg/ml is proffered, albeit with considerable diffidence. The answer is correct, but in terms of practical utility of course it is both useless and meaningless! It is important though to understand why.

The reason lies in the inadequacy of the question. As a consequence of weak intermolecular forces, all molecules have *some* attraction for each other when close, even if very small, and this can be expressed as an affinity value. Let us make a hypothetical plot of the abundance vs affinity for streptococcal M protein for the total IgG in the individual under discussion. One would probably expect a low concentration of high affinity antibody, a larger amount of antibody of moderate affinity, and then a gradual tailing off with more and more antibody species having a lower and lower affinity (figure 6.1a). No IgG would have a zero $K_a$ because, as we have stated, all molecules, even $N_2$, attract each other to some extent (for simplicity, I am ignoring gross effects such as those due to charged molecules for example). We can certainly obtain an **average** $K_a$ for the whole IgG by analysing the overall interaction with antigen as a Mass Action equation. But how can we define the **antibody content** of the IgG if all molecules interact with antigen? The answer is of course that we usually wish to describe antibody in practical functional terms: does a serum protect against a given infectious dose of virus, does it promote effective phagocytosis of bacteria (in this example streptococci), does it permit complement-mediated bacteriolysis, does it neutralize toxins, and so on? For such purposes, the very low affinity molecules would be useless because they form such inadequate amounts of complex with the antigen.

At the practical level in a diagnostic laboratory, the functional tests are labor intensive and therefore expensive, and we often compromise by using immunochemical assays which measure a composite of medium to high affinity antibodies and their abundance. The majority of such tests usually measure the total amount of antibody binding to a given amount of antigen; this could be a modest amount of high affinity antibody or much more antibody of lower affinity, or all combinations in between.

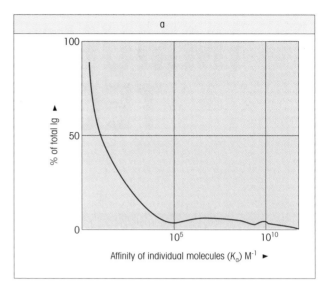

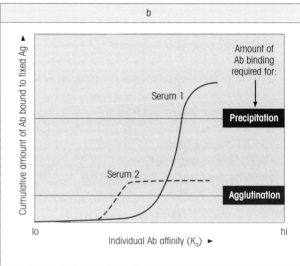

**Figure 6.1. Distribution of affinity and abundance of IgG molecules in an individual serum.** (a) Distribution of affinities of IgG molecules for a given antigen in the serum of a hypothetical individual. There is a great deal of low affinity antibody which would be incapable of binding to antigen effectively and much lower amounts of high affinity antibody whose skewed distribution is assumed to arise from exposure to infection. (b) Relationship of affinity distribution to positivity in tests for antigen binding. Rearranging the Mass Action equation, for all molecules of the same affinity $K_x$ and concentration of unbound antibody $[Ab_x]$:

the amount of complex formed $[AgAb] \propto K_x [Ab_x]$ for fixed $[Ag]$.

Starting with the lowest affinity molecules in the serum, we have charted the cumulative total of antibody bound for each antibody species up to and including the one being plotted. As might be expected, the very low affinity antibodies make no contribution to the tests. Serum 2 has more low affinity antibody and virtually no high affinity, but it can produce just enough complex to react in the sensitive agglutination test although unlike serum 1, it forms insufficient to give a positive precipitin. Because of its relatively high 'content' of antibody, serum 1 can be diluted to a much greater extent than serum 2 and yet still give positive agglutination, i.e. it has a higher titer. The precipitin test is less sensitive, requiring more complex formation, and serum 1 cannot be diluted much before this test becomes negative, i.e. the precipitin titer will be far lower than the agglutination titer for the same serum.

Sera are compared for high or low 'antibody content' either by seeing how much antibody binds to antigen at a fixed serum dilution, or testing a series of serum dilutions to see at which level a standard amount of antibody just sufficient to give a positive result is bound. This is the so-called **antibody titer**. To take an example, a serum might be diluted, say, 10 000 times and still just give a positive agglutination test (cf. figure 6.7). This titer of 1:10 000 enables comparison to be made with another much 'weaker' serum which has a titer of only, say, 1 : 100. Note that the titer of a given serum will vary with the sensitivity of the test, since much smaller amounts of antibody are needed to bind to antigen for a highly sensitive test such as agglutination, than a test of low sensitivity such as precipitation, which requires high concentrations of antibody–antigen product (figure 6.1b).

Let me summarize in case despair is setting in. We compare the '**effective antibody contents**' of different sera by seeing **how much antibody binds to the fixed amount of test antigen, or** we determine the titer, i.e. **how far the serum can be diluted before the test becomes negative.** This is a compromise between abundance and affinity and for practical purposes is used as an approximate indicator of biological effectiveness.

### The classical precipitin reaction

When an antigen solution is added progressively to a potent antiserum, antigen–antibody precipitates are formed (figures 6.2a and b). The cross-linking of antigen and antibody gives rise to three-dimensional lattice structures, as suggested by John Marrack, which coalesce, largely through Fc–Fc interaction, to form large precipitating aggregates. As more and more antigen is added, an optimum is reached (figure 6.2b) after which consistently less precipitate is formed. At this stage the supernatant can be shown to contain soluble complexes of antigen (Ag) and antibody (Ab), many of composition $Ag_4Ab_3$, $Ag_3Ab_2$ and $Ag_2Ab$ (figure 6.2c). In extreme antigen excess (figure 6.2c), ultracentrifugal analysis reveals the complexes to be mainly of the form $Ag_2Ab$, a result directly attributable to the two combining sites or divalence of the IgG antibody molecule (cf. EM study, figure 3.2, and Scatchard analysis, figure 5.10a).

Serums frequently contain up to 10% of nonprecipitating antibodies which are effectively univalent because of the asymmetric presence of a sugar on one Fd region which stereochemically blocks the adjacent

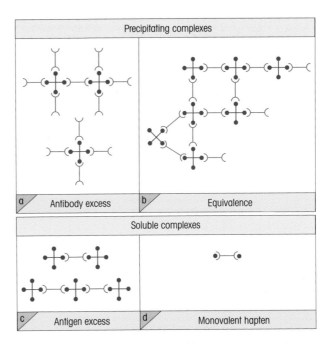

**Figure 6.2.** **Diagrammatic representation of complexes** formed between a hypothetical tetravalent antigen (•╬•) and bivalent antibody (◯——◯) mixed in different proportions. In practice, the antigen valencies are unlikely to lie in the same plane or to be formed by identical determinants as suggested in the figure. (a) In extreme antibody excess, the antigen valencies are saturated and the molar ratio Ab : Ag approximates to the valency of the antigen. (b) At equivalence, most of the antigen and antibody combines to form large lattices which aggregate to produce typical immune precipitates. This secondary aggregation, and hence precipitation, tends to be inhibited by high salt concentration. (c) In extreme antigen excess where the two valencies of each antibody molecule become rapidly saturated, the complex $Ag_2Ab$ tends to predominate. (d) A monovalent hapten binds but is unable to cross-link antibody molecules.

combining site. Also, frank precipitates are only observed when antigen, and particularly antibody, are present in fairly hefty concentrations. Thus, when complexes are formed which do not precipitate spontaneously, more devious methods must be applied to detect and estimate the antibody level.

### Nonprecipitating antibodies can be detected by nephelometry

The small aggregates formed when dilute solutions of antigen and antibody are mixed create a cloudiness or turbidity which can be measured by forward angle scattering of an incident light source (nephelometry). Greater sensitivity can be obtained by using monochromatic light from a laser and by adding polyethylene glycol to the solution so that aggregate size is increased. In practice, nephelometry is applied more to the detection of antigen than antibody and this will be dealt with in a later section.

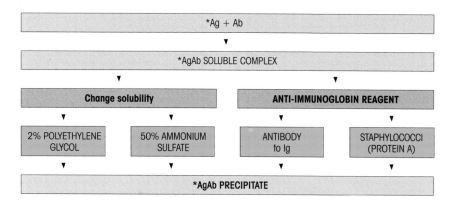

Figure 6.3. **Binding capacity of an antiserum for labeled antigen (*Ag) by precipitation of soluble complexes** either (i) by changing the solubility so that the complexes are precipitated while the uncombined Ag and Ab remain in solution, or (ii) by adding a precipitating anti-immunoglobulin antibody or staphylococcal organisms which bind immunoglobulin Fc to the protein A on their surface; the complex can then be spun down. The level of label (e.g. radioactivity) in the precipitate will be a measure of antigen-binding capacity.

### Complexes formed by nonprecipitating antibodies can be precipitated

The relative antigen-binding capacity of an antiserum which forms soluble complexes can be estimated using radiolabeled antigen. The complex can be brought out of solution either by changing its solubility or by adding an anti-immunoglobulin reagent as in figure 6.3.

### Enhancement of precipitation by countercurrent immunoelectrophoresis

This technique may be applied to antigens which migrate towards the positive pole on electrophoresis in agar (if necessary antigens can be substituted with negatively charged groups to achieve this end). Antigen and antiserum are placed in wells punched in the agar gel and a current applied (figure 6.4). The antigen migrates steadily into the antibody zone where it successively binds more and more antibody molecules, in essence artificially increasing the effective antibody concentration. The precipitin line which forms in the agar provides a fairly sensitive and rapid test that has been applied to the detection of antibodies (and by the same means, antigen) to hepatitis B antigen, DNA antibodies in systemic lupus erythematosus (SLE) (see p. 402), autoantibodies to soluble nuclear antigens in mixed connective tissue disease, and *Aspergillus* precipitins in cases with allergic bronchopulmonary aspergillosis.

### Measurement of antibody affinity

As discussed in earlier chapters (cf. p. 88), the binding strength of antibody for antigen is measured in terms of the association constant ($K_a$) or its reciprocal, the dissociation constant ($K_d$), governing the reversible

interaction between them and defined by the Mass Action equation at equilibrium:

$$K_a = \frac{[AgAb\ complex]}{[free\ Ag]\ [free\ Ab]}$$

With small haptens, the equilibrium dialysis method can be employed to measure $K_a$ (see p. 86), but usually one is dealing with larger antigens and other techniques must be used. In general, the approach is to add increasing amounts of radiolabeled antigen to a fixed amount of antibody, and then separate the free from bound antibody by precipitating the soluble complex as described above (e.g. by an anti-immunoglobulin). One can then plot, for example, the reciprocal of the bound, i.e. complexed, antibody concentration against the reciprocal of the free antigen concentration, so allowing the affinity constant to be calculated (figure 6.5a). For an antiserum this will give an affinity constant representing an average of the heterogeneous antibody compo-

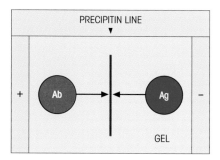

Figure 6.4. **Countercurrent immunoelectrophoresis.** Antibody moves towards the negative pole in the gel on electrophoresis due to endosmosis; an antigen which is negatively charged at the pH employed will move towards the positive pole and precipitate on contact with antibody.

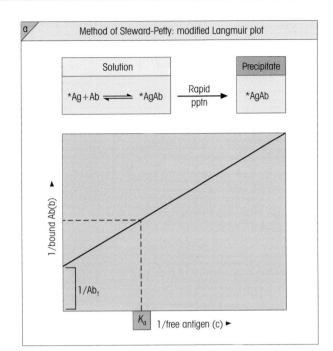

**Figure 6.5. Determination of affinity with large antigens.** The equilibria between Ab and Ag at different concentrations are determined as follows:

(a) For a polyclonal antiserum one can use the Steward–Petty modification of the Langmuir equation:

$$1/b = 1/(Ab_t \cdot c \cdot K_a) + 1/Ab_t$$

where $Ab_t$ = total Ab combining sites, $b$ = bound Ab concn, $c$ = free Ag concn and $K_a$ = average affinity constant. At infinite Ag concn, all Ab sites are bound and $1/b = 1/Ab_t$. When half the Ab sites are bound, $1/c = K_a$ (cf. p. 88).

(b) The method of Friguet *et al.* for monoclonal antibodies. First, a calibration curve for free antibody is established by estimating the proportion binding to solid phase antigen, bound antibody being measured by enzyme-labeled anti-Ig (ELISA: see text). Using the calibration curve, the amount of free Ab in equilibrium with Ag in solution is determined by seeing how much of the Ab binds to solid phase Ag (the amount of solid phase antigen is insufficient to affect the solution equilibrium materially). Combination of Klotz and Scatchard equations gives:

$$A_0/A_0 - A = 1 + k_d/a_0$$

where $A_0$ = ELISA optical density (OD) for Ab in absence of Ag, $A$ = OD in presence of Ag concn $a_0$ where $a_0$ is approximately $10 \times$ concn of Ab. The slope of the plot gives $K_d$. (Labeled molecules are marked with an asterisk.)

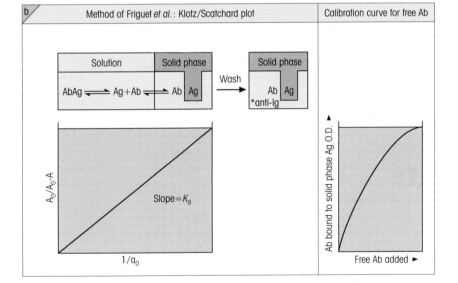

nents and a measure of the effective number of antigen binding sites operative at the highest levels of antigen used.

The number of studies on the affinity of monoclonal antibodies is burgeoning and the clear winner in the popularity stakes must surely be the indirect competitive system devised by Friguet and associates (figure 6.5b). A constant amount of antibody is incubated with a series of antigen concentrations and the free antibody at equilibrium assessed by secondary binding to solid phase antigen using the ELISA technique (see below). In this way, values for $K_a$ are not affected by any distortion of antigen by labeling. This again stresses the superiority of determining affinity by studying the **primary reaction** with antigen in the **soluble state** rather than conformationally altered through binding to a solid phase.

## Agglutination of antigen-coated particles

Whereas the cross-linking of multivalent protein antigens by antibody leads to precipitation, cross-linking of cells or large particles by antibody directed against surface antigens leads to agglutination. Since most cells are electrically charged, a reasonable number of antibody links between two cells is required before the mutual repulsion is overcome. Thus agglutination of cells bearing only a small number of determinants may be difficult to achieve unless special methods such as further treatment with an antiglobulin reagent are used. Similarly, the higher avidity of multivalent IgM antibody relative to IgG (cf. p. 90) makes the former more effective as an agglutinating agent, molecule for molecule (figure 6.6).

Agglutination reactions are used to identify bacteria and to type red cells; they have been observed with leukocytes and platelets, and even with spermatozoa in certain cases of male infertility due to sperm agglutinins. Because of its sensitivity and convenience, the test has been extended to the identification of antibodies to soluble antigens which have been artificially coated on to various types of particle. Red cells have been popular and they can be coated with proteins after first modifying their surface with tannic acid or chromium chloride, or by direct use of bifunctional cross-linking agents such as bisdiazobenzidine. The large, rapidly sedimenting red cells of the turkey are finding increasing favor for this purpose. The tests are usually carried out in the wells of plastic agglutination trays where the settling pattern of the cells on the bottom of the cup may be observed (figure 6.7); this provides a more sensitive indicator than macroscopic clumping. Inert particles such as bentonite and polystyrene latex have also been coated with antigens for agglutination reactions, particularly those used to detect the rheumatoid factors (figure 6.8). Latex particles have recently been improved by using a copolymer of glycidyl methacrylate and styrene which provides a mosaic of hydrophobic and hydrophilic domains. Nonspecific aggregation is said to be mini-

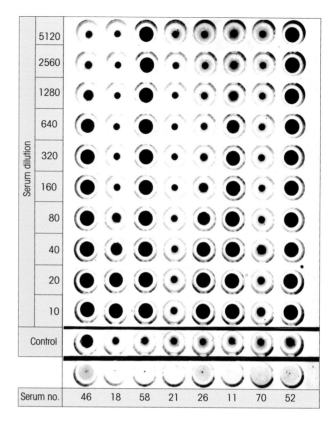

**Figure 6.7. Red cell hemagglutination test** for thyroglobulin autoantibodies. Thyroglobulin-coated cells were added to dilutions of patients' serums. Uncoated cells were added to a 1 : 10 dilution of serum as a control. In a positive reaction, the cells settle as a carpet over the bottom of the cup. Because of the 'V'-shaped cross-section of these cups, in negative reactions the cells fall into the base of the 'V', forming a small, easily recognizable button. The reciprocal of the highest serum dilution giving an unequivocally positive reaction is termed the titer. The titers reading from left to right are: 640, 20, >5120, neg, 40, 320, neg, > 5120. The control for serum no. 46 was slightly positive and this serum should be tested again after absorption with uncoated cells.

mized. Quantification of more subtle degrees of agglutination can be achieved by nephelometry or Coulter counting.

## Immunoassay for antibody using solid-phase antigen

### The principle

The antibody content of a serum can be assessed by the ability to bind to antigen which has been insolubilized by physical adsorption to a plastic tube or microagglutination tray with multiple wells; the bound immunoglobulin may then be estimated by addition of a labeled anti-Ig raised in another species (figure 6.9). Consider, for example, the determination of DNA autoantibodies in SLE (cf. p. 402). When a

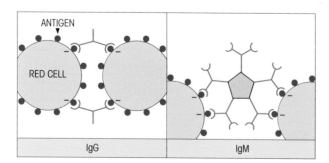

**Figure 6.6. Mechanism of agglutination of antigen-coated particles** by antibody cross-linking to form large macroscopic aggregates. If red cells are used, several cross-links are needed to overcome the electrical charge at the cell surface. IgM is superior to IgG as an agglutinator because of its multivalent binding and because the charged cells are further apart.

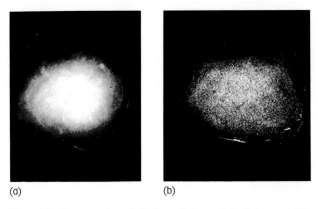

(a)                              (b)

**Figure 6.8. Macroscopic agglutination of latex** coated with human IgG by serum from a patient with rheumatoid arthritis. This contains rheumatoid factor, an autoantibody directed against determinants on IgG. (a) Normal serum. (b) Patient's serum.

patient's serum is added to a microwell coated with antigen (in this case DNA), the autoantibodies will bind to the plastic and remaining serum proteins can be readily washed away. Bound antibody can now be estimated by addition of $^{125}$I-labeled purified rabbit anti-human IgG; after rinsing out excess unbound reagent, the radioactivity of the tube will clearly be a measure of the autoantibody content of the patient's serum. The distribution of antibody in different classes can obviously be determined by using specific antisera. Take the radioallergosorbent test (RAST) for IgE antibodies in allergic patients. The allergen (e.g. pollen extract) is covalently coupled to an immunoabsorbent, in this case a paper disk, which is then treated with patient's serum. The amount of specific IgE bound to the paper can now be estimated by addition of labeled anti-IgE.

## A wide variety of labels is available

Because of health hazards and the deterioration of reagents through radiation damage, types of label for the antiglobulin reagent other than radioisotopes have been sought.

*ELISA (enzyme-linked immunosorbent assay).* Undoubtedly the most common alternative involves coupling to enzymes which give a colored soluble reaction product. Enzymes such as horseradish peroxidase and phosphatase which are readily available, stable and have a high turnover number, have been widely employed. One clever ploy for amplifying the phosphatase reaction is to use NADP as a substrate to generate NAD which now acts as a coenzyme for a second enzyme system (figure 6.10). Pyrophosphatase from *Escherichia coli* provides a good conjugate because the enzyme is not present in tissues, is stable and gives a good reaction color. Chemiluminescent systems based on enzymes such as luciferase can also be applied. A genetically engineered metapyrocatechase-protein A fusion molecule is a recent innovation for detection of IgG antibodies.

*Other labels.* Conjugation with the vitamin biotin is frequently used since this can readily be detected by its reaction with enzyme-linked avidin (or even better, streptavidin) to which it binds with ferocious specificity and affinity ($K = 10^{15}$ M$^{-1}$).

Acridinium luminescent molecules and new fluorescent labels have an important role to play in lowering the limits of detection of immunoassay methods and special mention should be made of time-resolved

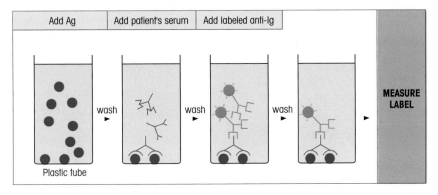

**Figure 6.9. Solid-phase immunoassay for antibody.** To reduce nonspecific binding of IgG to the solid phase after adsorption of the first reagent, it is usual to add an irrelevant protein such as gelatin, or more recently α$_1$-glycoprotein, to block any free sites on the plastic. Note that the conformation of a protein often alters on binding to plastic, e.g. a monoclonal antibody which distinguishes between the apo and holo forms of cytochrome c in solution combines equally well with both proteins on the solid phase. Covalent coupling to carboxy-derivatized plastic or capture of the antigen substrate by solid-phase antibody can sometimes improve this.

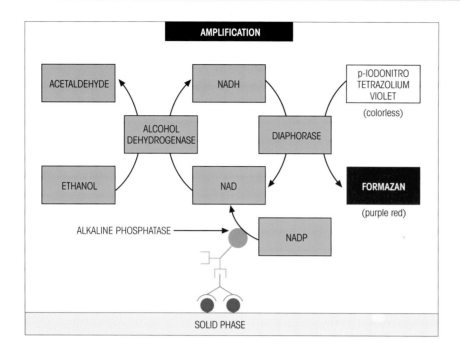

Figure 6.10. Coenzyme-geared amplification of the phosphatase reaction to reveal solid phase anti-immunoglobulin label.

fluorescence assay based upon chelates of rare earths such as europium 3+ (figure 6.11), although these have a more important role in antigen assays.

### Surface plasmon resonance

A sensor chip consisting of a monoclonal antibody coupled to dextran overlaying a gold film on a glass prism will totally internally reflect light at a given angle (figure 6.12a). Antigen present in a pulse of fluid will bind to the sensor chip and, by increasing its size, alter the angle of reflection. The system provides data on the kinetics of association and dissociation (and hence *K*) (figure 6.12b) and permits comparisons between monoclonal antibodies and also assessment of subtle effects of mutations.

## IDENTIFICATION AND MEASUREMENT OF ANTIGEN

### Precipitation reaction can be carried out in gels

### Characterization of antigens by electrophoresis and immunofixation

This technique is most often applied to the detection of an abnormal protein in serum or urine, usually a monoclonal paraprotein secreted by a B-cell tumor.

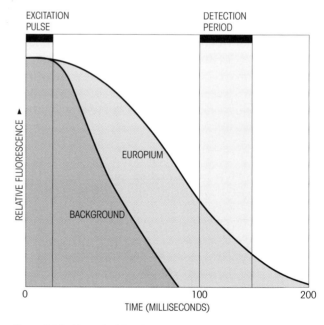

Figure 6.11. The principle of time-resolved fluorescence assay. The problem with conventional methods of detection of low fluorescent signals is interference from reflection of incident light and background instrument fluorescence. By using just a short excitation pulse and measuring the signal after background has fallen to zero but before the europium with its long fluorescence half-life has decayed completely, good discrimination between a weak signal and background becomes possible.

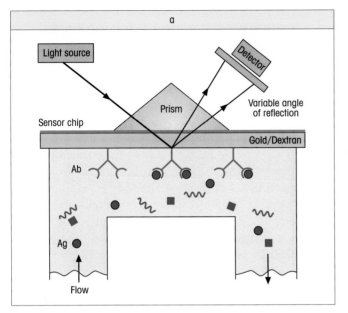

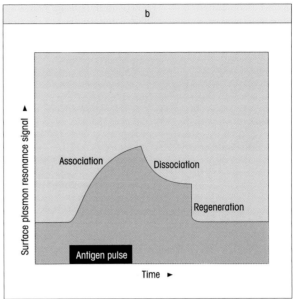

**Figure 6.12. Surface plasmon resonance.** (a) The principle: as antigen binds to the sensor chip it alters the angle of reflection. (b) This signals the rates of association during the antigen pulse and dissociation. The system can be applied to any other single ligand binding assay.

The paraprotein localizes as a dense compact 'M' band of defined electrophoretic mobility and its antigenic identity is then revealed by immunofixation with specific precipitating antiserums applied in paper strips overlying parallel lanes in the electrophoresis gel (figure 6.13).

### Quantification by single radial immunodiffusion (SRID)

When antigen diffuses from a well into agar containing suitably diluted antiserum, initially it is present in a relatively high concentration and forms soluble complexes; as the antigen diffuses further the concentration continuously falls until the point is reached at which the reactants are nearer optimal proportions and a ring of precipitate is formed. The higher the concentration of antigen, the greater the diameter of this ring (figure 6.14). By incorporating, say, three standards of known antigen concentration in the plate, a calibration curve can be obtained and used to determine the amount of antigen in the unknown samples tested (figure 6.15). The method was used routinely in clinical immunology, particularly for immunoglobulin determinations, and also for substances such as the third component of complement, transferrin, C-reactive protein (CRP) and the embry-

onic protein, α-fetoprotein, which is associated with certain liver tumors. More affluent laboratories now tend to use nephelometry (see below).

## The nephelometric assay for antigen

If antigen is added to a solution of excess antibody, the amount of complex which can be assessed by

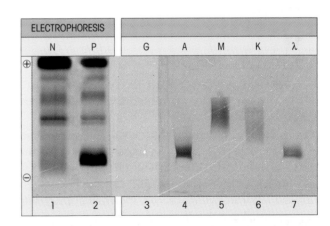

**Figure 6.13. Electrophoresis and immunofixation of a paraprotein in serum.** The sample is separated into its component bands by electrophoresis in agarose gel and these are visualized by direct staining after drying down the gel. The test sample is also run on a parallel gel which is then overlaid with strips of paper soaked in a specific antiserum. The antibodies diffuse into the gel and 'fix' the antigen by precipitation; after washing to remove the nonprecipitated soluble proteins, the gel is dried and stained to reveal the location of the paraprotein/antibody complex. N, normal serum; P, patient's serum showing compact paraprotein band; G, A, M, K and λ represent immunofixations with antiserum specific for each immunoglobulin chain. In the example chosen, the paraprotein is an IgGK. (Material kindly supplied by Mr. T. Heys).

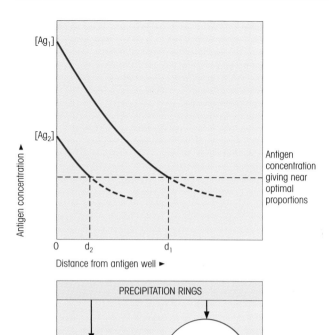

**Figure 6.14. Single radial immunodiffusion:** relation of antigen concentration to size of precipitation ring formed. Antigen at the higher concentration [Ag$_1$] diffuses further from the well before it falls to the level giving precipitation with antibody near optimal proportions.

## Sodium dodecyl sulfate–polyacrylamide gel electrophoresis (SDS–PAGE) for analysis of immunoprecipitates and immunoblotting

When proteins are denatured by SDS, the larger they are the more SDS they bind and the more negatively charged they become. Thus proteins of different size can be separated by electrophoresis in a gel such as polyacrylamide on the basis of their overall charge. If one or more antigens are radiolabeled and the complex with added antibody precipitated with an anti-Ig reagent such as staphylococci-bearing protein A, SDS–PAGE of the complex followed by autoradiography should define the **number** and **molecular weights of the antigens** concerned (figure 6.17).

After separation from a complex mixture by SDS–PAGE, antigens can be 'blotted' by transverse electrophoresis on to nitrocellulose sheets where they bind nonspecifically (**Western blots**) and can be identified by staining with appropriately labeled anti-

forward light scatter in a nephelometer (cf. p. 109) is linearly related to the concentration of antigen. With the ready availability of a wide range of monoclonal antibodies which facilitate the standardization of the method, nephelometry is replacing SRID for the estimation of immunoglobulins, C3, C4, haptoglobin, ceruloplasmin and CRP in those favored laboratories which can sport the appropriate equipment. Very small samples down in the range 1–10 μl can be analysed. Turbidity of the sample can be a problem; blanks lacking antibody can be deducted but a more satisfactory solution is to follow the **rate of formation** of complexes which is proportional to antigen concentration since this obviates the need for a separate blank (figure 6.16). Because soluble complexes begin to be formed in antigen excess, it is important to ensure that the value for antigen was obtained in antibody excess by running a further control in which additional antigen is included.

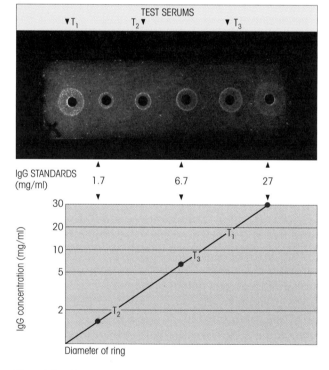

**Figure 6.15. Measurement of IgG concentration in serum by single radial immunodiffusion.** The diameter of the standards (●) enables a calibration curve to be drawn and the concentration of IgG in the serum under test can be read off:

T$_1$—serum from patient with IgG myeloma; 15 mg/ml

T$_2$—serum from patient with hypogammaglobulinemia; 2.6 mg/ml

T$_3$—normal serum; 9.6 mg/ml.

(Courtesy of Professor F.C. Hay.)

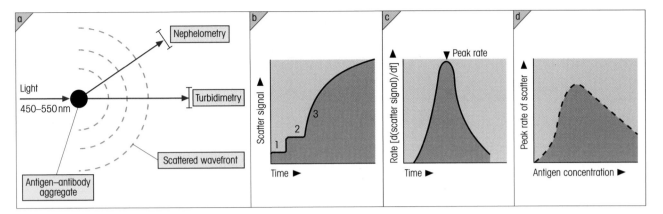

**Figure 6.16. Rate nephelometry.** (a) On addition of antiserum, small antigen–antibody aggregates form (cf. figure 6.2) which scatter incident light filtered to give a wavelength band of 450–550 nm. For nephelometry, the light scattered at a forward angle of 70° or so is measured. (b) After addition of the sample (1) and then the antibody (2), the rate at which the aggregates form (3) is determined from the scatter signal. (c) The software in the instrument then computes the maximum rate of light scatter which is related to the antigen concentration as shown in (d). (Copied from the operating manual for the 'Array' rate reaction automated immunonephelometer with permission from Beckman Instruments.)

bodies. This **immunoblotting** technique has been used widely, as for example in the identification of components of neurofilaments which have been separated by SDS–PAGE. Obviously, such a procedure will not work with antigens which are irreversibly denatured by this detergent and it is best to use polyclonal antisera for blotting to increase the chance of having antibodies to whichever epitopes do survive the denaturation procedure; a surprising number do (figure 6.18). Conversely, the spectrotype of an antiserum can be revealed by isoelectric focusing, blotting and then staining with labeled antigen.

### The immunoassay of antigens

The ability to measure the concentration of an analyte (i.e. a substance to be measured) through fractional occupancy of its specific binding reagent is a feature of any ligand-binding system (Milestone 6.1) but because antibodies can be raised to virtually any structure, its application is most versatile in immunoassay.

Large analytes, such as protein hormones, are usually estimated by a noncompetitive two-site assay in which the original ligand binder and the labeled detection reagent are both antibodies (figure M6.1.1). By using monoclonal antibodies directed to two different epitopes on the same analyte, the system has greater power to discriminate between two related analytes; if the fractional cross-reactivity of the first antibody for a related analyte is 0.1 and of the second also 0.1, the final readout for cross-reactivity will be as low as $0.1 \times 0.1$, i.e. 1%. Using chemiluminescent and time-resolved fluorescent probes, highly sensitive

assays are available for an astonishing range of analytes.

For small molecules like drugs or steroid hormones where two-site site binding is impractical, competitive assays (figure M6.1.1) are appropriate.

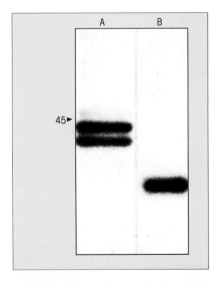

**Figure 6.17. Immunoprecipitation of membrane antigen.** Analysis of membrane-bound class I MHC antigens (cf. p. 71). The membranes from human cells pulsed with $^{35}$S-methionine were solubilized in a detergent, mixed with a monoclonal antibody to HLA-A and B molecules and immunoprecipitated with staphylococci. An autoradiograph (A) of the precipitate run in SDS–PAGE shows the HLA-A and B chains as a 43 000 molecular weight doublet (the position of a 45 000 marker is arrowed). If membrane vesicles were first digested with Proteinase K before solubilization, a labeled band of molecular weight 39 000 can be detected (B) consistent with a transmembrane orientation of the HLA chain: the 4000 hydrophilic C-terminal fragment extends into the cytoplasm and the major portion, recognized by the monoclonal antibody and by tissue typing reagents, is present on the cell surface (cf. figure 4.9). (From data and autoradiographs kindly supplied by Dr M.J. Owen.)

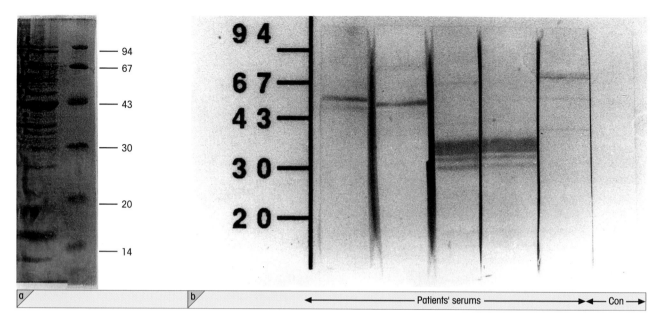

**Figure 6.18. Western blot analysis** of human polymorph primary granules with sera from patients with systemic vasculitis. Human polymorph postnuclear supernatant was run on SDS–PAGE. (a) Gel stained for protein with Coomassie Blue. Numbers refer to molecular weight markers (kDa). (b) Blots from gel stained with serums from five patients and one control (RHS) and visualized with alkaline phosphatase-conjugated goat anti-human IgG. Three different patterns of autoantibody reaction are evident. (Kindly supplied by Drs J. Cambridge & B. Leaker.) The antibodies used for immunoblotting are usually labeled with enzymes or biotin (followed by labeled avidin) but in many laboratories, colloidal gold conjugates are becoming the method of choice. Often IgG antibodies are picked up by labeled staphylococcal protein A, although this may well be superseded by streptococcal protein G which reacts with all IgG subclasses and with IgG from a wide variety of species. One method for relating the position of a peptide in a Western blot is to use colloidal gold for staining total protein red, and peroxidase labeled antibody to stain the immunoreactive band blue; the two colors can be differentiated by photography with appropriate filters.

## Immunoassay on multiple microspots

Paradoxically, minute spots of solid phase antibody are not completely saturated by analyte in the range of concentrations normally worked with in most immunoassays. Rather, analysis has shown that the fractional occupancies expected permit immunoassay technology, or any other ligand-specific binding system, to be practical options (Ekins), particularly with the advent of modern highly sensitive probes. Furthermore, when the amount of antibody on the microspot is very small, the fractional occupancy is independent of antibody level and also of analyte volume (**the ambient analyte principle**). Sensitivities compare very favorably with the best immunoassays and with such miniaturization, arrays of microspots which capture antibodies of different specificities can be placed on a single chip, opening the door to multiple analyte screening in a single test, with each analyte being identified by its grid coordinates in the array.

## Epitope mapping

### T-cell epitopes

Since T-cell epitopes are linear peptides, knowledge of the primary sequence of the whole protein makes identification of the epitopes relatively straightforward. Using multipin solid-phase synthesis, a series of overlapping peptides, 9-mers for cytotoxic T-cells and usually 12-mers for T-helpers, can be prepared (figure 6.19) and their ability to react with antigen-specific T-cell lines or clones deciphered to characterize the active epitopes.

Dissecting out T-cell epitopes where the antigen has not been characterized is a more daunting task. One would like to use T-cells to screen DNA libraries prepared from the antigen-bearing tissue. A possible approach might be to overlay the individual clones, each expressing whole or part of the antigen, with macrophages transfected with a reporter gene such as *lacZ* β-galactosidase linked to an interleukin-2 (IL-2) responsive element; addition of hyperstimulated T-cell lines should lead to IL-2 release at the site of the clone producing the epitope whereupon the upregulated β-galactosidase could be visualized by a color

# Milestone 6.1—Ligand-Binding Assays

The appreciation that a ligand could be measured by the fractional occupancy (F) of its specific binding agent heralded a new order of sensitive wide-ranging assays. Ligand-binding assays were first introduced for the measurement of thyroid hormone by thyroxine-binding protein (Ekins) and for the estimation of hormones by antibody (Berson & Yalow). These findings spawned the technology of radioimmunoassay, so called because the antigen had to be trace-labeled in some way and the most convenient candidates for this were radioisotopes.

The relationship between fractional occupancy and analyte concentration [An] is given by the equation:

$$F = 1 - \left(1/1 + K[\text{An}]\right)$$

where $K$ is the association constant of the ligand-binding reaction. $F$ can be measured by noncompetitive or competitive assays (figure M6.1.1) and related to a calibration curve constructed with standard amounts of analyte.

For competitive assays the maximum theoretical sensitivity is given by the term $\varepsilon/K$ where $\varepsilon$ is the experimental error (coefficient of variation). Suppose the error is 1% and $K$ is $10^{11}\,\text{M}^{-1}$, the maximum sensitivity will be $0.01 \times 10^{-11}\,\text{M} = 10^{-13}\,\text{M}$ or $6 \times 10^{7}$ molecules/ml. For noncompetitive assays, labels of very high specific activity could give sensitivities down to $10^{2}$–$10^{3}$ molecules/ml under ideal conditions. In practice, however, since the sensitivity represents the lowest analyte concentration which can be measured against a background containing zero analyte, the error of the measurement of background poses an ultimate constraint on sensitivity.

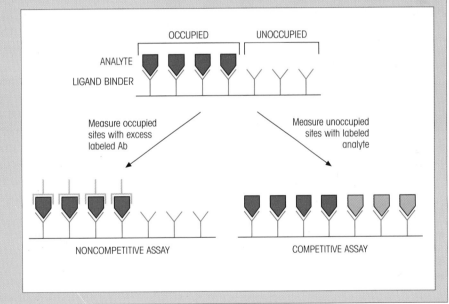

**Figure M6.1.1. The principle of ligand-binding assays.** The ligand-binding agent may be in the soluble phase or bound to a solid support as shown here, the advantage of the latter being the ease of separation of bound from free analyte. After exposure to analyte, the fractional occupancy of the ligand-binding sites can be determined by competitive or noncompetitive assays using labeled reagents (in orange) as shown.

reaction. Alternatively, the IL-2 enhancer—*lacZ* construct—can be introduced into the antigen-specific T-cells.

## B-cell epitopes

If they are linear protein epitopes formed directly from the primary amino acid sequence, then binding to individual overlapping peptides synthesized as described above will identify them. Unfortunately, most epitopes on globular proteins recognized by antibody are discontinuous and this makes the job rather demanding, since one cannot predict which residues are likely to be brought together in space to form the epitope. To the extent that small linear sequences may contribute to a discontinuous epitope, the overlapping peptide strategy may provide some clues. A potentially promising approach to this

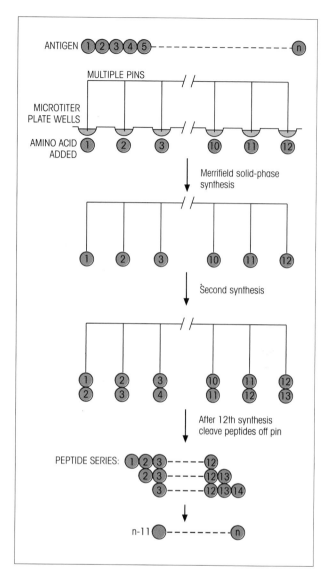

**Figure 6.19. Synthesis of overlapping peptide sequences for (PEPSCAN) epitope analysis.** A series of pins which sit individually in the wells of a 96-well microtiter plate each provide a site for solid phase synthesis of peptide. A sequence of such syntheses as shown in the figure provides the required nests of peptides. Incorporation of a readily cleavable linkage allows the soluble peptide to be released as the synthesis is terminated.

problem of mimicking the residues which constitute such epitopes (termed **mimotopes** by Geysen) is through the production of libraries of bacteriophages bearing all possible random hexapeptides. These are produced by ligating degenerate oligonucleotide inserts (coding for hexapeptides) to a bacteriophage coat protein in a suitable vector; appropriate expression in *E. coli* can provide up to $10^9$ different clones. The beauty of the system is that a bacteriophage expressing a given hexapeptide on its external coat protein, also bears the sequence encoding the hexapeptide in its genome (cf. p. 125). Accordingly, sequential rounds of selection in which the phages

react with a biotinylated monoclonal antibody and are then panned on a streptavidin plate should isolate those bearing the peptides which mimic the epitope recognized by the monoclonal; nucleotide sequencing will then give the peptide structure. Some encouraging progress is being made but the path is still rocky.

## DETECTION OF IMMUNE COMPLEX FORMATION

Many techniques for detecting circulating complexes have been described and because of variations in the size, complement-fixing ability and Ig class of different complexes, it is useful to apply more than one method. Two fairly robust methods for general use are:

**1** precipitation of complexed IgG from serum at concentrations of polyethylene glycol which do not bring down significant amounts of IgG monomer, followed by estimation of IgG in the precipitate by SRID or laser nephelometry, and

**2** binding of C3b-containing complexes to beads coated with bovine conglutinin (cf. p. 18) and estimation of the bound Ig with enzyme-labeled anti-Ig.

Other techniques include: (i) estimation of the binding of $^{125}$I-C1q to complexes by coprecipitation with polyethylene glycol, (ii) inhibition by complexes of rheumatoid factor-induced aggregation of IgG-coated particles, and (iii) detection with radiolabeled anti-Ig of serum complexes capable of binding to the C3b (and to a lesser extent the Fc) receptors on the Raji cell line. Sera from patients with immune complex disease often form a cryoprecipitate when allowed to stand at 4°C. Measurement of serum C3 and its conversion product C3c are sometimes useful.

Tissue-bound complexes are usually visualized by the immunofluorescent staining of biopsies with conjugated anti-immunoglobulins and anti-C3 (cf. figure 16.14).

## MAKING ANTIBODIES TO ORDER

### The monoclonal antibody revolution

*First in rodents*

A fantastic technological breakthrough was achieved by Milstein & Kohler who devised a technique for the production of 'immortal' clones of cells making single antibody specificities by fusing normal antibody-forming cells with an appropriate B-cell tumor line.

These so-called 'hybridomas' are selected out in a tissue culture medium which fails to support growth of the parental cell types, and by successive dilutions or by plating out, single clones can be established (figure 6.20). These clones can be grown up in the ascitic form in mice when quite prodigious titers of monoclonal antibody can be attained, but bearing in mind the imperative to avoid using animals wherever feasible, propagation in large-scale culture is to be preferred. Remember that even in a good antiserum, over 90% of the Ig molecules have little or no avidity for the antigen, and the 'specific antibodies' themselves represent a whole spectrum of molecules with different avidities directed against different determinants on the antigen. What a contrast is provided by the monoclonal antibodies, where all the molecules produced by a given hybridoma are identical: they have the same Ig class and allotype, the same variable region, structure, idiotype, affinity and specificity for a given epitope.

Whereas the large amount of nonspecific, relative to antigen-specific, Ig in an antiserum means that background binding to antigen in any given immunological test may be uncomfortably high, the problem is greatly reduced with a monoclonal antibody preparation, since all the Ig is antibody, thus giving a much superior 'signal:noise' ratio. By being directed towards single epitopes on the antigen, monoclonal antibodies frequently show high specificity in terms of their low cross-reactivity with other antigens. Occasionally, however, one sees quite unexpected binding to molecules which react poorly, if at all, with a specific antiserum directed to the original antigen. The reason for this has already been discussed (see p. 91). Suffice it to say here that the problem can be circumvented by using a group of overlapping monoclonals reacting with the same determinant or a combination of monoclonals to more than one determinant on the same antigen.

An outstanding advantage of the monoclonal antibody as a reagent is that it provides a single standard material for all laboratories throughout the world to use in an unending supply if the immortality and purity of the cell line is nurtured; antisera raised in different animals, on the other hand, may be as different from each other as chalk and cheese. The monoclonal approach again shows a clean pair of heels relative to conventional strategies in the production of antibodies specific for individual components in a complex mixture of antigens, which, for example, one may wish for in trying to identify which of a set of antigens on a given parasite can generate antibodies which are protective for the host. Whereas in the pre-hybridoma era we would have tried to purify individual antigens from the complex mixture and then raised antibodies to each component, now we would make a large number of hybridomas from the spleen of an animal immunized with the complete antigen mixture and separate the individual hybridomas by simple cloning. It must be clear that we now have in our hands a really powerful technique whose applications are truly legion. Some of these are touched upon in table 6.1 to give the reader an inkling of what is possible, but the potential defies the imagination: the separation of individual cell types with specific surface markers (lymphocyte subpopulations, neural cells, etc.), diagnosis of lymphoid and myeloid malignancies, tissue typing, radioimmunoassay, serotyping of microorganisms, elucidation of the fine structure of the antibody-combining site and the basis for variability, immunological intervention with passive antibody, anti-idiotype inhibition or 'magic bullet' therapy with cytotoxic agents coupled to antitumor-specific antibody — these and many other areas are being transformed by hybridoma technology.

### Catalytic antibodies

An especially interesting development with tremendous potential is the recognition that a monoclonal antibody to a stable analog of the transition state of a given reaction can act as an enzyme ('abzyme') in catalysing that reaction. The possibility of generating enzymes to order promises a very attractive future, and some exceedingly adroit chemical maneuvers have already extended the range of reactions which can be catalysed in this way. A recent demonstration of sequence-specific peptide cleavage with an antibody which incorporates a metal complex cofactor has raised the pulse rate of the *cognoscenti*, since this is an energetically difficult reaction which has an enormous range of applications. Another innovative approach is to immunize with an antigen which is so highly reactive that a chemical reaction occurs in the antibody combining site. This recruits antibodies which are not only complementary to the active chemical, but are also likely to have some enzymic catalytic power over the immunogen/substrate complex. Thus, using an organophosphorus diester as a hapten, it proved possible to recruit antibodies which catalysed the formation and cleavage of phosphorylated intermediates and subsequent ester hydrolysis.

Large combinatorial antibody libraries created by random association between pools of heavy and light chains and expressed on bacteriophage (see below)

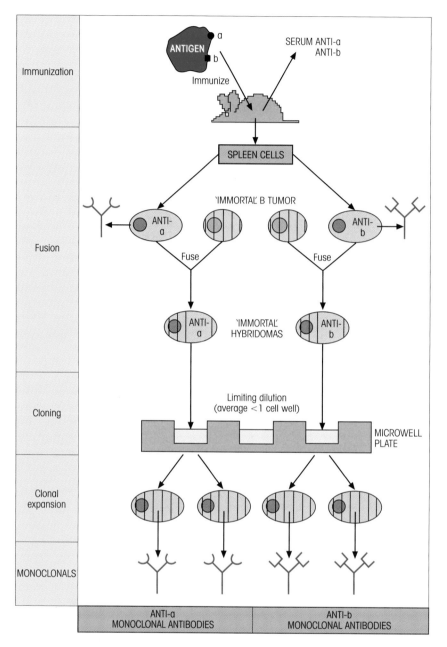

**Figure 6.20. Production of monoclonal antibodies.** Mice immunized with an antigen bearing (shall we say) two epitopes, a and b, develop spleen cells making anti-a and anti-b which appear as antibodies in the serum. The spleen is removed and the individual cells fused in polyethylene glycol with constantly dividing (i.e. 'immortal') B-tumor cells selected for a purine enzyme deficiency and often for their inability to secrete Ig. The resulting cells are distributed into micro-well plates in HAT (hypoxanthine, aminopterin, thymidine) medium which kills off the fusion partners, at such a dilution that *on average* each well will contain less than one hybridoma cell. Each hybridoma—the fusion product of a single antibody-forming cell and a tumor cell—will have the ability of the former to secrete a single species of antibody and the immortality of the latter enabling it to proliferate continuously. Thus, clonal progeny can provide an unending supply of antibody with a single specificity — the monoclonal antibody. In this example, we considered the production of hybridomas with specificity for just two epitopes, but the same technique enables monoclonal antibodies to be raised against complex mixtures of multiepitopic antigens. Fusions using rat cells instead of mouse may have certain advantages in giving a higher proportion of stable hybridomas, and monoclonals which are better at fixing human complement, a useful attribute in the context of therapeutic applications to humans involving cell depletion.

Naturally for use in the human, the ideal solution is the production of purely human monoclonals. Human myeloma fusion partners have not found wide acceptance since they tend to have low fusion efficiencies, poor growth and secretion of Ig which dilutes the desired monoclonal. A nonsecreting hetero-hybridoma obtained by fusing a mouse myeloma with human B-cells can be used as a productive fusion partner for antibody-producing human B-cells. Other groups have turned to the well-characterized murine fusion partners and the heterohybridomas so formed grow well, clone easily and are productive. There is some instability from chromosome loss and it appears that antibody production is maintained by translocation of human Ig genes to mouse chromosomes. Fusion frequency is even better if Epstein–Barr virus (EBV)-transformed lines are used instead of B-cells.

**Table 6.1. Some applications of monoclonal antibodies.**

| | |
|---|---|
| ENUMERATION OF HUMAN LYMPHOCYTE SUBPOPULATIONS | Anti-CD3 identifies all mature T-cells<br>Anti-CD4 identifies subset containing T-helpers<br>Anti-CD8 identifies cytotoxic-suppressor T-cells |
| CELL DEPLETION | Cocktail of anti-CD3 monoclonals + complement kills T-cells in human bone marrow to prevent graft-vs-host reaction (p. 356) |
| CELL ISOLATION | Enrichment of bone marrow stem cells by anti-CD34 in the FACS (p. 133) |
| IMMUNOSUPPRESSION | Anti-CD3 depresses T-cell function<br>Anti-CD4 induces tolerance |
| PASSIVE IMMUNIZATION | High titer antimicrobial human monoclonals can give passive protection |
| PROBING FUNCTION OF CELL SURFACE MOLECULES | Anti-CD8 inhibits killing by cytotoxic T-cells<br>Anti-class II MHC monoclonal inhibits T-cell response to macrophage-processed Ag |
| BLOOD GROUPING | Anti-A monoclonal provides more reliable standard reagent than conventional antisera |
| DIAGNOSIS IN CANCER | Monoclonal anti T-ALL allows differentiation from non T-ALL (cf. p. 387)<br>Follicle center cell lymphoma identified by peroxidase-labeled anticommon ALL in tissue sections |
| IMAGING | Radioactive anti-carcinoembryonic antigen (p. 397) used to localize colonic tumors or secondaries by scanning |
| NEPHELOMETRIC ASSAY | Routine estimation of individual soluble serum proteins e.g. IgG |
| SOLID-PHASE IMMUNOASSAY | Good discrimination for noncompetitive assay of antigen by monoclonals to more than one site (p. 119) |
| ANALYSIS OF COMPLEX ANTIGEN MIXTURES | Identification of the 'protective' antigen in parasite suitable for vaccine production<br>Identification of antigenic 'patch' on acetylcholine receptor involved in experimental myasthenia gravis (p. 425) |
| PURIFICATION OF ANTIGEN | Isolate from mixtures by monoclonal on affinity column |
| ANALYSIS OF EMBRYOLOGICAL RELATIONSHIPS | Separate monoclonals to neurons of neural tube and neural crest origin help to define embryological derivation of cells in nervous system |
| MONOCLONAL MUTANTS | Mutants lacking Fc structures used for *in vivo* neutralization of toxic drugs e.g. digoxin overdose, or for defining biological roles of Fc domains |
| GENETICALLY ENGINEERED ANTIBODIES | Transfer mouse CDRs to human Ig framework<br>Change Fc isotype to improve particular function |
| FUSED HYBRIDOMAS | Producing antibodies with dual specificity |
| ANALYSIS OF IMMUNE RESPONSE | Hybridomas made during an immune response give data on repertoire and on mutation events (the original reason for developing the hybridoma technology) |
| ARTIFICIAL ENZYMES (CATALYTIC ANTIBODIES) | Monoclonal antibodies which recognize the transitional state of the reactants in a reversible reaction can simulate an enzyme – early days but big potential |

can be screened for catalytic antibodies by using the substrate in a solid phase state. Cleavage by the catalytic antibody leaves a solid phase product which can now be identified by a double antibody system using antibodies specific for the *product* as distinct from the *substrate*.

Curiously, an autocatalytic antibody which catalyses the cleavage of vasoactive intestinal peptide (the neural mediator of nonadrenergic, noncholinergic relaxation of airway smooth muscle — no less) has been found in the serum IgG of around 16% of adult asthma patients and strenuously exercising healthy subjects. The autoantibody in nonasthmatics is bound to a small inhibitor and has a far lower affinity, but even so it does leave one wondering what else might be lurking in the murky depths of one's blood circulation.

### Human monoclonals can be made

Mouse monoclonals injected into human subjects for therapeutic purposes are frightfully immunogenic and the human anti-mouse antibodies (HAMA in the trade) so formed are a wretched nuisance, accelerating clearance of the monoclonal from the blood and possibly causing hypersensitivity reactions; they also prevent the mouse antibody from reaching its target and, in some cases, block its binding to antigen. In some circumstances it is conceivable that a mouse monoclonal taken up by a tumor cell could be processed and become the MHC-linked target of cytotoxic T-cells or help to boost the response to a weakly immunogenic antigen on the tumor cell surface. In general, however, logic points to removal of the xenogeneic (foreign) portions of the monoclonal antibody and their replacement by human Ig structures using recombinant DNA technology. Chimeric constructs, in which the $V_H$ and $V_L$ mouse domains are spliced onto human $C_H$ and $C_L$ genes (figure 6.21a), are far less immunogenic in humans.

Depend upon it, the restless human brain nags away at a problem to generate new solutions and such antibodies can now be produced in 'humanized' mice immunized by conventional antigens. One initiative involved the replacement of the mouse Cγ1 gene by its human counterpart in embryonic stem cells (cf. p. 144) using bacteriophage Cre-*loxP* site-specific recombination. The resulting mutant mice were crossed with animals expressing human in place of murine $C_\kappa$ chains; mice homozygous for both mutants produced humanized IgG1κ antibodies as effectively as the wild type synthesized mouse IgG1 in response to various thymus-dependent antigens (cf. p. 174).

There is still a snag in that such humanized rodent antibodies have a tendency to provoke anti-idiotype responses; these have to be circumvented by using chimeric antibodies bearing different idiotypes for subsequent injections.

Yet another approach is to graft the six complementarity determining regions (CDR) of a high affinity rodent monoclonal onto a completely human Ig framework without loss of specific reactivity (figure 6.21b). This is not a trivial exercise, however, and the objective of fusing human B-cells to make hybridomas is still appealing, taking into account not only the gross reduction in immunogenicity, but also the fact that within a species, antibodies can be made to subtle differences such as major histocompatibility complex (MHC) polymorphic molecules and tumor-associated antigens on other individuals, whereas xenogeneic responses are more directed to immunodominant structures common to most subjects. Notwithstanding the difficulties in finding good fusion partners, large numbers of human monoclonals have been established. A further restriction arises because the peripheral blood B-cells, which are the only B-cells readily available in the human, are not normally regarded as a good source of antibody-forming cells. If, as we are told, good primary responses with peripheral blood lymphocytes can be obtained *in vitro* by addition to the culture of the methyl *O*-ester of leucine which eliminates monocytes, NK cells and cytotoxic T-cells, then we have cause to hope that this approach will provide B-cells of wide specificities for human hybridomas. A radically different approach involves the production of immortalized Epstein–Barr virus transformed B-cell lines.

Many human monoclonals are awaiting the go-ahead for clinical use; one can cite IgG anti-RhD for the prevention of rhesus disease of the newborn (see p. 339), and highly potent monoclonals for protection against varicella zoster, cytomegalovirus, group B streptococci and lipopolysaccharide endotoxins of Gram-negative bacteria.

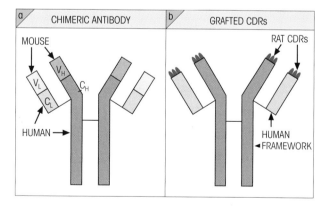

**Figure 6.21. Genetically engineering rodent antibody specificities into the human.** (a) Chimeric antibody with mouse variable regions fused to human Ig constant region. (b) 'Humanized' rat monoclonal in which gene segments coding for all six CDR are grafted onto a human Ig framework.

## Engineering antibodies

There are other ways around the problems associated with the production of human monoclonals which exploit the wiles of modern molecular biology. Reference has already been made to the 'humanizing' of rodent antibodies (figure 6.21) but an important new strategy based upon bacteriophage expression and **selection** has achieved a prominent position. In essence, mRNA from primed human B-cells is converted to cDNA and the antibody genes, or fragments therefrom, expanded by the polymerase chain reaction (PCR). Single constructs are then made in which the light- and heavy-chain genes are allowed to combine randomly in tandem with the bacteriophage pIII gene (figure 6.22). This **combinatorial library** containing most random pairings of heavy- and light-chain genes encodes a huge repertoire of antibodies (or their fragments) expressed as fusion proteins with the filamentous coat protein pIII on the bacteriophage surface. The extremely high number of phages produced by *E. coli* infection can now be panned on solid-phase antigen to select those bearing the highest affinity antibodies attached to their surface (figure 6.22). Because the genes which encode these highest affinity antibodies are already present within the selected phage, they can readily be cloned and the antibody expressed in bulk. It should be recognized that this **selection** procedure has an enormous advantage over techniques which employ **screening** because the number of phages which can be examined is several logs higher.

Combinatorial libraries have also been established using mRNA from **unimmunized** human donors. $V_H$, $V_\kappa$ and $V_\lambda$ genes are expanded by PCR and randomly recombined to form single-chain Fv (scFv) constructs (figure 6.23a) fused to phage pIII. Soluble fragments binding to a variety of antigens have been obtained. Of special interest are those which are autoantibodies to molecules with therapeutic potential such as CD4 and tumor necrosis factor (TNF)-$\alpha$; lymphocytes expressing such autoantibodies could not be obtained by normal immunization since they would probably be tolerized, but the random recombination of $V_H$ and $V_L$ can produce entirely new specificities under conditions *in vitro* where tolerance mechanisms do not operate.

Although a 'test-tube' operation, this approach to the generation of specific antibodies does resemble the affinity maturation of the immune response *in vivo* (see p. 195) in the sense that antigen is the

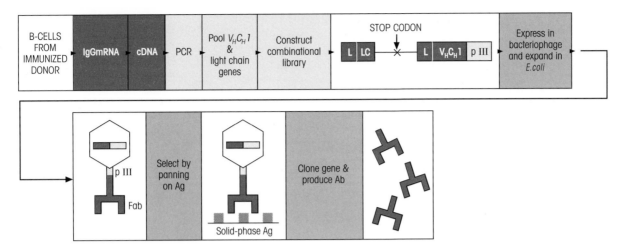

**Figure 6.22. Selection of antibody genes from a combinatorial library.** B-cells from an immunized donor (in one important experiment, human memory peripheral blood cells were boosted with tetanus toxoid antigen after transfer to SCID mice; Duchosal M.A. *et al.* (1992) *Nature* **355**, 258) are used for the extraction of IgG mRNA and the light-chain (*LC*) and $V_H C_H 1$ genes (encoding Fab) randomly combined in constructs fused to the bacte-riophage pIII coat protein gene as shown. These were incorporated into phagemids such as pHEN1 and expanded in *E. coli*. After infection with helper phage, the recombinant phages bearing the highest affinity were selected by rounds of panning on solid phase antigen so that the genes encoding the Fabs could be cloned. L = bacterial leader sequence.

determining factor in selecting out the highest affinity responders.

In order to increase the affinities of antibodies produced by these techniques, antigen can be used to select higher affinity mutants produced by random or site-directed mutagenesis (figure 6.23b), again mimicking the natural immune response which involves random mutation and antigen selection (see p. 192). Affinity has also been improved by gene 'shuffling' in which a $V_H$ gene encoding a reasonable affinity antibody is randomly combined with a pool of $V_L$ genes and subjected to antigen selection. The process can be further extended by mixing the $V_L$ from this combination with a pool of $V_H$ genes. It has also proved possible to shuffle individual CDR between variable regions of moderate affinity antibodies obtained by panning on antigen, thereby creating antibodies of high affinity from relatively small libraries.

Other novel antibodies have been created. In one construct, two scFv fragments associate to form an antibody with two different specificities (figure 6.23c). Another consists of a single heavy-chain variable region domain (DAB) whose affinity can be surprisingly high—of the order of 20 nM. If it were possible to overcome the 'stickiness' of these mini-antibodies, their small size could be exploited for tissue penetration and, as the authors aggressively state, for patent busting. Speaking of aggression, it must be the gang-

ster in me which is attracted to the design of potential 'magic bullets' for immunotherapy based on fusion of a toxin (e.g. ricin) to an antibody Fab (figure 6.23d).

### Fields of antibodies

Not only can the genes for a monoclonal antibody be expressed in bulk in the milk of lactating animals but plants can also be exploited for this purpose. So-called '**plantibodies**' have been expressed in bananas, potatoes and tobacco plants. One can imagine a high-tech farmer drawing the attention of a bemused visitor to one field growing anti-tetanus toxoid, another anti-meningococcal polysaccharide, and so on. Multifunctional plants might be quite profitable with, say, the root being harvested as a food crop and the leaves expressing some desirable gene product. At this rate there may not be much left for science fiction authors to write about!

### Drugs can be based on the CDRs of minibodies

Millions of **minibodies** composed of a segment of the $V_H$ region containing three β-strands and the H1 and H2 hypervariable loops (figure 6.24), were generated by randomization of the CDRs and expressed on the bacteriophage PIII protein (cf. figure 6.22). By panning the library on functionally important ligand-binding sites such as hormone receptors, useful lead

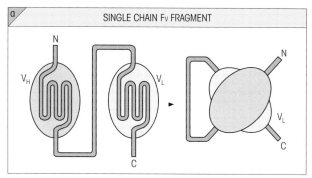

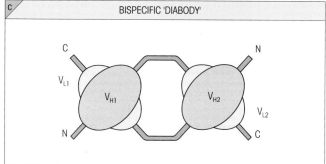

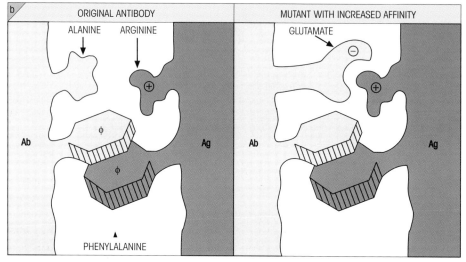

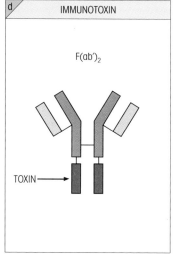

**Figure 6.23. Other engineered antibodies.** (a) A single gene encoding $V_H$ and $V_L$ joined by a sequence of suitable length gives rise to single chain Fv (scFv) antigen-binding fragment. (b) By site-specific mutagenesis of residues in or adjacent to the complementarity determining region (CDR), it is possible to increase the affinity of the antibody. (c) Two scFv constructs expressed simultaneously will associate to form a 'diabody' with two speci-ficities. These bispecific antibodies have a number of uses. Note that such a bispecific antibody directed to two different epitopes on the same antigen will have a much higher affinity due to the 'bonus effect' of cooperation between the two binding sites (cf. p. 89). (d) Potential 'magic bullets' can be constructed by fusing the gene for a toxin (e.g. ricin) to the Fab.

candidates for drug design programmes can be identified and their affinity improved by loop optimization, loop shuffling and further selection.

## PURIFICATION OF ANTIGENS AND ANTIBODIES BY AFFINITY CHROMATOGRAPHY

The principle is simple and *very* widely applied. Antigen or antibody is bound through its free amino groups to cyanogen bromide-activated Sepharose particles. Insolubilized antibody, for example, can be used to pull the corresponding antigen out of solution in which it is present as one component of a complex mixture, by absorption to its surface. The uninteresting garbage is washed away and the required ligand released from the affinity absorbent by disruption of

the antigen–antibody bonds by changing the pH or adding chaotropic ions such as thiocyanate (figure 6.25). Likewise, an antigen immunosorbent can be used to absorb out an antibody from a mixture whence it can be purified by elution. The potentially damaging effect of the eluting agent can be avoided by running the antiserum down an affinity column so prepared as to have relatively weak binding for the antibody being purified; under these circumstances, the antibody is retarded in flow rate rather than being firmly bound. If a protein mixture is separated by isoelectric focusing into discrete bands, an individual band can be used to affinity purify specific antibodies from a polyclonal antiserum; quite useful when supplies of antigen are painfully limited.

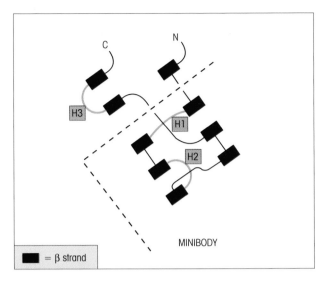

**Figure 6.24. The minibody** is a 61-residue protein composed of three β-strands from each of the two β-sheets of the $V_H$ domain of a murine Ab presenting the H1 and H2 hypervariable loop CDRs. The relationship to the whole $V_H$ is shown. Viewed along the axis of the β-strands. (From Sollazzo M. (1995) *The Immunologist* **3**, 5.)

# NEUTRALIZATION OF BIOLOGICAL ACTIVITY

## To detect antibody

A number of biological reactions can be inhibited by addition of specific antibody. Thus the agglutination of red cells by interaction of influenza virus with receptors on the erythrocyte surface can be blocked by antiviral antibodies and this forms the basis for their serological detection. Neutralization of the growth of hapten-conjugated bacteriophage provides an exquisitely sensitive assay for antihapten antibodies.

A test for antibodies to *Salmonella* H antigen present on the flagella depends upon their ability to inhibit the motility of the bacteria *in vitro*. Likewise, *Mycoplasma* antibodies can be demonstrated by their inhibitory effect on the metabolism of the organisms in culture.

## Using antibody as an inhibitor

The successful treatment of cases of drug overdose with the Fab fragment of specific antibodies has been described and may become a practical proposition if a range of hybridomas can be assembled. Conjugates of cocaine with keyhole limpet hemocyanin can provoke neutralizing antibodies. Antibodies to hormones such as insulin and thyroid-stimulating hormone (TSH), or to cytokines, can be used to probe the specificity of biological reactions *in vitro*. For example, the specificity of the insulin-like activity of a serum sample on rat epididymal fat pad can be checked by the neutralizing effect of an antiserum. Such antibodies can be effective *in vivo*, and anti-TNF has been injected into rheumatoid arthritis patients to reveal the role of this cytokine in the disease process. Likewise, as part of the worldwide effort to prevent disastrous overpopulation, attempts are in progress to immunize against chorionic gonadotropin using fragments of the β-chain coupled to appropriate carriers, since this hormone is needed to sustain the implanted ovum.

In a totally different context, antibodies raised against myelin-associated neurite growth inhibitory proteins revealed their importance in preventing nerve repair; treatment with these antibodies permitted regeneration of corticospinal axons after a spinal cord lesion had been induced in adult rats. This quite remarkable finding significantly advances our under-

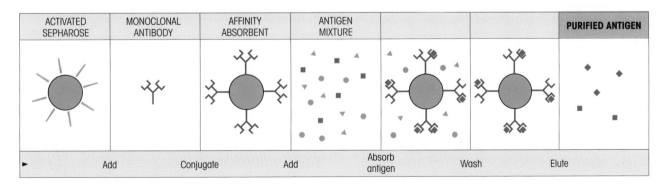

**Figure 6.25. Affinity chromatography.** A column is filled with Sepharose-linked antibody. The antigen mixture is poured down the column. Only the antigen binds and is released by change in pH, for example. An antigen-linked affinity column will purify antibody obviously.

standing of the processes involved in regeneration and gives ground for cautious optimism concerning the development of treatment for spinal cord resec-

tion, although for various reasons, this may not ultimately be based on antibody therapy.

## SUMMARY

### Estimation of antibody

• The antibody content of a polyclonal antiserum is defined entirely in operational terms by the nature of the assay employed.
• Antibody in solution can be assayed by the formation of frank precipitates which can be enhanced by counter-current electrophoresis in gels.
• Nonprecipitating antibodies can be measured by laser nephelometry or by salt or anti-Ig coprecipitation with radioactive antigen.
• Affinity is measured by a variety of methods which mostly determine the amount of antibody bound at various antigen concentrations.
• Antibodies can also be detected by macroscopic agglutination of antigen-coated particles, and by one of the most important methods, ELISA, a two-stage procedure in which antibody bound to solid phase antigen is detected by an enzyme-linked anti-Ig.
• The binding of antibody to solid phase antigen, and vice versa, can be followed physically by surface plasmon resonance which also give a measure of the on and off rates.

### Identification and measurement of antigen

• Antigens can be separated and their mobility in an electric field determined by electrophoresis and immunofixation.
• Antigens can be quantified by their reaction in gels with antibody using single radial immunodiffusion.
• Higher concentrations of antigens are frequently estimated by nephelometry.
• Exceedingly low concentrations of antigens can be measured by immunoassay techniques which depend upon the relationship between Ag concentration and fractional occupancy of the binding antibody. Occupied sites are measured with a high specific activity second antibody directed to a different epitope; alternatively, unoccupied sites can be estimated by labeled Ag. Multiple assays on arrays of antibody microspots are being developed.

• Overlapping nests of peptides derived from the linear sequence of a protein can map T-cell epitopes and the linear elements of B-cell epitopes. Bacteriophages encoding all possible hexapeptides on their surface have provided some limited success in identifying discontinuous B-cell determinants.

### Detection of immune complexes

• Serum complexes can be determined by precipitation with polyethylene glycol, reaction with C1q or bovine conglutinin, changes in C3 and C3c and binding to rheumatoid factors.

### Making antibodies to order

• Immortal hybridoma cell lines making monoclonal antibodies provide powerful new immunological reagents and insights into the immune response. Applications include enumeration of lymphocyte subpopulations, cell depletion, immunoassay, cancer diagnosis and imaging, purification of antigen from complex mixtures, and recently the use of monoclonals as artificial enzymes (abzymes).
• Genetically engineered human antibody fragments can be derived by expanding the $V_H$ and $V_L$ genes from unimmunized, but preferably immunized, donors and expressing them as completely randomized combinatorial libraries on the surface of bacteriophage. Phages bearing the highest affinity antibodies are selected by panning on antigens and the antibody genes can then be cloned from the isolated viruses.
• Single chain Fv (scFv) fragments encoded by linked $V_H$ and $V_L$ genes and even single heavy-chain domains can be created.
• Recombinant antibodies can be expressed on a large scale in plants.
• Combinatorial libraries of diabodies containing the H1 and H2 $V_H$ CDR may be used to develop new drugs.

### Affinity chromatography

• Insoluble immunoabsorbents prepared by coupling

*(Continued)*

antibody to Sepharose can be used to affinity-purify antigens from complex mixtures and reciprocally to purify antibodies.

## *Neutralization of biological activity*

• Antibodies can be detected by inhibition of biological

functions such as viral infectivity or bacterial growth.

• Inhibition of biological function by known antibodies helps to define the role of the antigen, be it a hormone or cytokine for example, in complex responses *in vivo* and *in vitro*.

## FURTHER READING

See end of Chapter 7.

# CHAPTER 7

# CELLULAR TECHNIQUES

## CONTENTS

## ISOLATION OF LEUKOCYTE SUBPOPULATIONS

### Bulk techniques

*Separation based on physical parameters*

Cells can be separated on the basis of their differential **sedimentation rate**, which is roughly correlated with **size**, by centrifugation through a density gradient whose purpose is to stabilize the liquid column. For very large volumes a centrifugal elutriator seems to help. Cells can be increased in mass by selectively binding particles such as red cells to their surface, the most notable example being the rosettes formed when sheep erythrocytes bind to the CD2 of human T-cells (cf. figure 2.6e).

**Buoyant density** is another useful parameter. Centrifugation of whole blood over isotonic Ficoll–Hypaque (sodium metrizoate) of density 1.077 leaves the mononuclear cells (lymphocytes, monocytes and natural killer (NK) cells) floating in a band at the interface, while the erythrocytes, being denser, keep on to the base of the tube. **Adherence** to plastic surfaces largely removes phagocytic cells, while passage down nylon-wool columns greatly enriches lymphocyte populations for T-cells at the expense of B-cells.

## Separation exploiting biological parameters

Actively phagocytic cells which take up small iron particles can be manipulated by a magnet deployed externally. Lymphocytes which divide in response to a polyclonal activator (see p. 168) or specific antigen, can be eliminated by allowing them to incorporate 5-bromodeoxyuridine (BUDR); this renders them susceptible to the lethal effect of UV irradiation.

## Selection by antibody coating

Several methods are available for the selection of cells which can be specifically coated on their surface with antibody (figure 7.1). Addition of complement or anti-Ig-toxin conjugates will eliminate such populations. Magnetic beads coated with anti-Ig will form clusters with the antibody-coated cells which can be readily separated from uncoated cells. High-grade positive selection of cells without loss of function can be achieved using super paramagnetic beads of less than 100 nm separated in high gradient magnetic fields. Another useful bulk selection technique is to pan the coated cells on anti-Ig adsorbed to a surface. One variation on this theme used to isolate bone marrow stem cells with anti-CD34 is to coat the cells with biotinylated antibody and select with an avidin-column or avidin magnetic beads.

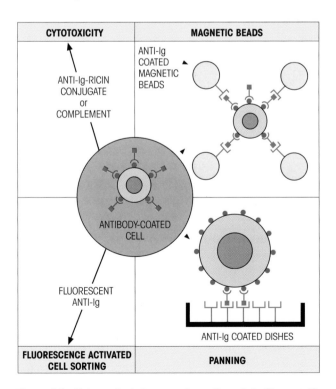

**Figure 7.1. Major methods for separating cells coated with a specific antibody.**

## Cell selection by the FACS

Smaller numbers of cells coated with fluorescent antibody can be separated in the fluorescence activated cell sorter (FACS) as described in Milestone 7.1 and figure 7.2. It should be appreciated that these instruments record quantitative data relating to the surface antigen content and physical nature of each individual cell, and that currently up to six different parameters per cell can be assessed giving very detailed phenotypic analysis on a single cell rather than a population average (see more in-depth discussion under 'Flow cytofluorimetry' p. 135).

## Enrichment of antigen-specific populations

Selective expansion of antigen-specific T-cells by repeated stimulation with antigen and presenting cells in culture, usually alternated with interleukin-2 (IL-2) treatment, leads to an enrichment of heterogeneous T-cells specific for different epitopes on the antigen. Such **T-cell lines** can be distributed in microtiter wells at a high enough dilution such that **on average** there is less than one cell per well; pushing the cells to proliferate with antigen or anti-CD3 produces single T-cell clones which can be maintained with much obsessional care and attention, but my goodness they can be a pain! Potentially immortal **T-cell hybridomas**, similar in principle to B-cell hybridomas, can be established by fusing cell lines with a T-tumor line and cloning. There should be considerable mileage in the use of *Herpes virus saimiri,* a lymphotropic agent of nonhuman primates, to **transform human T-cells and immortalize them** just as Epstein–Barr (EB) virus transforms and immortalizes B-cells. Growth is only IL-2 dependent. CD8 cells retain cytotoxicity and TH1 cells (cf. p. 184) continue to make γ-interferon (IFNγ) although TH2 cells tend to revert to TH0 or TH1 phenotype. These monoclonal immortalized T-cells have a range of potentially exciting applications: for biochemical studies of signalling pathways, as a source of T-cell receptors (TCR), for specificity analyses of T-cell clones, as a permissive system for lymphotropic viruses and even for immunotherapy and gene therapy.

Animals populated essentially by a single T-cell specificity can be produced by introducing the T-cell receptor α and β genes from a T-cell clone, as a transgene (see below); since the genes are already rearranged, their presence in every developing T-cell will switch off any other Vβ gene recombinations.

No one has succeeded in cloning B-cells except as hybridomas or EB virus-transformed cell lines,

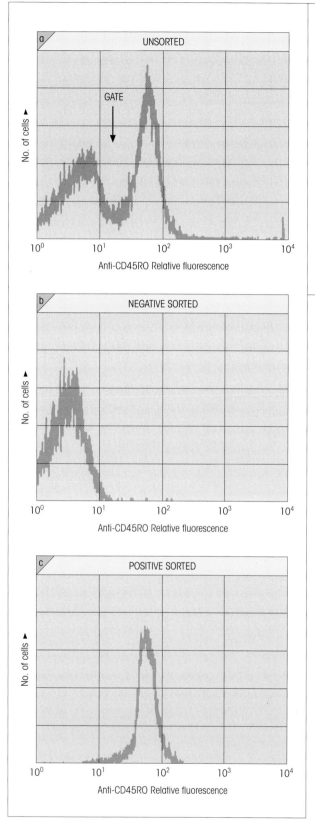

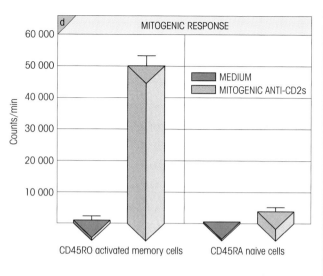

**Figure 7.2. Separation of activated peripheral blood memory T-cells (CD45RO positive) from naive T-cells** (CD45RO negative; but positive for the CD45RA isoform) in the FACS after staining the surface of the living cells in the cold with a fluorescent monoclonal antibody to the CD45RO (see p. 197). The unsorted cells showed two peaks (a) and cells with fluorescence intensity lower than the arbitrary gate are separated from those with higher intensity giving (b) negative (CD45RA) and (c) positive (CD45RO) populations which were each tested for their proliferative response to a mixture of two anti-CD2 monoclonals (OKT11 and GT2) in the presence of 10% antigen-presenting cells (d). 3H-Thymidine was added after 3 days and the cells counted after 15 h. Clearly the memory cell population proliferated whereas the naive population did not. (Data kindly provided by D. Wallace and R. Hicks.)

## Milestone 7.1 – The Fluorescence Activated Cell Sorter (FACS)

The FACS was developed by the Herzenbergs and their colleagues to quantify the surface molecules on individual white cells by their reaction with fluorochrome-labeled monoclonal antibodies and to use the signals so generated to separate cells of defined phenotype from a heterogeneous mixture.

In this elegant but complex machine, the fluorescent cells are made to flow obediently in a single stream past a laser beam. Quantitative measurement of the fluorescent signal in a suitably placed photomultiplier tube relays a signal to the cell as it emerges in a single droplet; the cell

becomes charged and can be separated in an electric field (figure M7.1.1). Extra sophistication can be introduced by using two lasers with four fluorochromes and both 90° and forward light scatter. This will be elaborated upon below in the section on flow cytofluorimetry describing how this technique can be used for quantitative multiparameter analysis of single-cell populations (cf. figure 7.8). Suffice to state that these latest FACS machines permit the isolation of cells with a complex phenotype from a heterogeneous population with a high degree of discrimination.

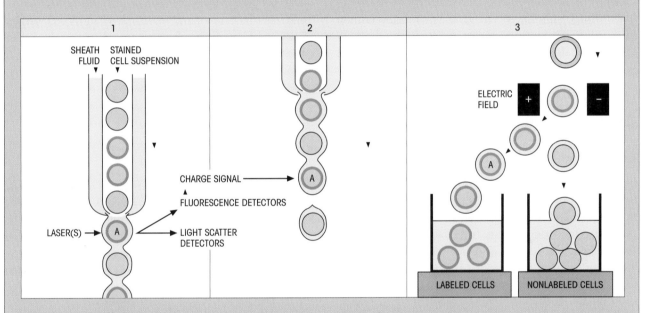

**Figure M7.1.1. The principle of the FACS**, designed by the Herzenbergs and colleagues, for flow cytofluorimetry of the fluorescence on stained cells (green rimmed circles) and physical separation from unstained cells (purple circles). The charge signal can be activated to separate cells of high from low fluorescence and, using light scatter, of large from small size and dead from living.

although as with T-cells, transgenic animals expressing the same antibody in all their B-cells have been generated.

## IMMUNOHISTOCHEMISTRY — LOCALIZATION OF ANTIGENS IN CELLS AND TISSUES

### Immunofluorescence techniques

Because fluorescent dyes such as fluorescein and rho-

damine can be coupled to antibodies without destroying their specificity, the conjugates can combine with antigen present in a tissue section and be visualized in the fluorescence microscope. In this way the distribution of antigen throughout a tissue and within cells can be demonstrated. Looked at another way, the method can also be used for the detection of antibodies directed against antigens already known to be present in a given tissue section or cell preparation. There are two general ways in which the test is carried out.

## Direct test with labeled antibody

The antibody to the tissue substrate is itself conjugated with the fluorochrome and applied directly (figure 7.3a). For example, suppose we wished to show the tissue distribution of a gastric autoantigen reacting with the autoantibodies present in the serum of a patient with pernicious anemia. We would isolate IgG from the patient's serum, conjugate it with fluorescein, and apply it to a section of human gastric mucosa on a slide. When viewed in the fluorescence microscope we would see that the cytoplasm of the parietal cells was brightly stained. By using antisera conjugated to dyes which emit fluorescence at different wavelengths, two different antigens can be identified simultaneously in the same preparation. In figure 2.6h, direct staining of fixed plasma cells with a mixture of rhodamine-labeled anti-IgG and fluorescein-conjugated anti-IgM craftily demonstrates that these two classes of antibody are produced by different cells. The technique of coupling biotin to the antiserum and then finally staining with fluorescent avidin is finding increasing favor.

## Indirect test for antibody

In this double-layer technique, the unlabeled antibody is applied directly to the tissue substrate and visualized by treatment with a fluorochrome-conjugated anti-immunoglobulin serum (figure 7.3b). In this case, in order to find out whether or not the serum of a patient has antibodies to gastric parietal cells, we would first treat a gastric section with the serum, wash well and then apply a fluorescein-labeled rabbit anti-human immunoglobulin; if antibodies were present, there would be staining of the parietal cells (figure 7.4a).

This technique has several advantages. In the first place the fluorescence is brighter than with the direct test since several fluorescent anti-immunoglobulins bind on to each of the antibody molecules present in the first layer (figure 7.3b). Second, since the conjugation process is lengthy, much time can be saved when many sera have to be screened for antibody because it is only necessary to prepare a single labeled reagent, viz. the anti-immunoglobulin. Furthermore, the method has great flexibility. For example, by using conjugates of antisera to individual immunoglobulin heavy chains, the distribution of antibodies among the various classes and subclasses can be assessed at least semiquantitatively. One can also test for complement fixation on the tissue section by adding a mixture of the first antibody plus a source of complement, followed by a fluorescent anticomplement reagent as the second layer. Even greater sensitivity can be attained by using a third layer. Thus, in the example quoted of antibodies to parietal cells, we could treat the stomach section sequentially with the following: patient's serum containing antibodies to parietal cells, then a rabbit anti-human IgG, and finally a fluorescein-conjugated goat anti-rabbit IgG. However, as with most immunological techniques as *sensitivity* is increased, *specificity* becomes progressively reduced and careful controls are essential.

Applications of the indirect test may also be seen in Chapter 19 (e.g. figure 19.1).

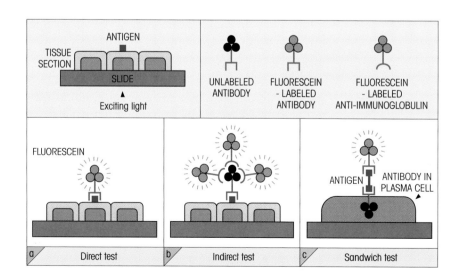

**Figure 7.3. The basis of fluorescence antibody tests for identification of tissue antigens or their antibodies.** ● = fluorescein labeled.

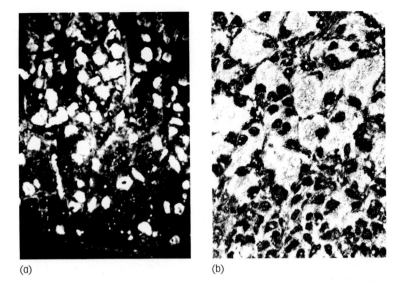

**Figure 7.4. Staining of gastric parietal cells by fluorescein (a) and peroxidase-linked antibody (b).** The sections were sequentially treated with human parietal cell autoantibodies and then with the conjugated rabbit anti-human IgG. The enzyme was visualized by the peroxidase reaction. (Courtesy of Miss V. Petts.)

(a)                                          (b)

### High resolution with the confocal microscope

Fluorescent images at high magnification are usually difficult to resolve because of the flare from slightly out of focus planes above and below that of the object. All that is now past, with the advent of commercially available **scanning confocal microscopes** which focus the image of the laser source in a fine plane within the cell and collect the fluorescence emission in a photomultiplier tube (PMT) with a confocal aperture (figure 7.5). Fluorescence from planes above and below the object plane fails to reach the PMT so the sharpness of the image is unaffected. An X–Y scanning unit enables the whole of the specimen plane to be interrogated *quantitatively* and with suitable optics, two different fluorophors can be used simultaneously. The instrument software can compute three-dimensional fluorescent images from an automatic series of such X–Y scans accumulated in the Z axis (figure 7.6) and rotate them at the whim of the operator.

### Flow cytofluorimetry

Surface antigens can be detected and localized by the use of labeled antibodies. Because antibodies cannot readily penetrate living cells except by endocytosis, treatment of cells with labeled antibody in the cold (to minimize endocytosis) leads to staining only of antigens on the surface (figure 7.2). Remember also a previous example of fluorescent staining of the surface of B-lymphocytes with anti-immunoglobulin (figure 2.6f).

It is now possible to stain single cells with up to four different fluorochromes (figure 7.7) and analyse the cells in individual droplets as they flow past the monitoring section of the FACS described above. Indeed

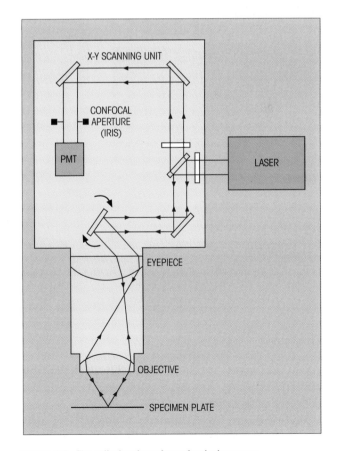

**Figure 7.5. The optical system of a confocal microscope.**

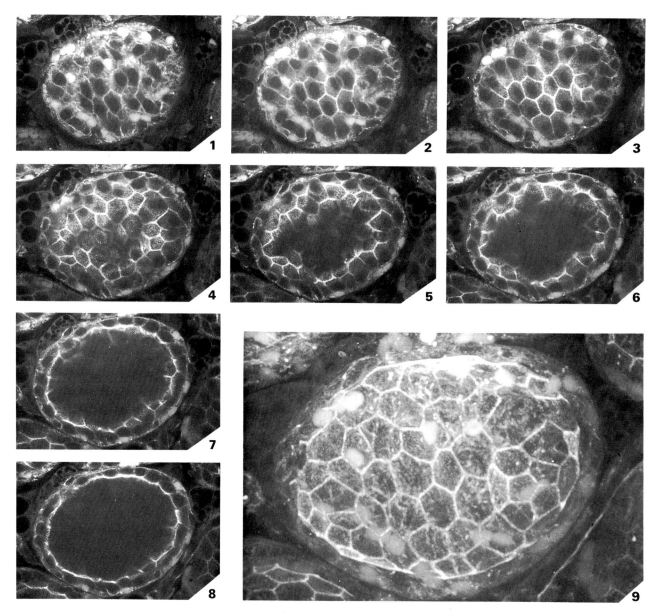

**Figure 7.6. Construction of a three-dimensional fluorescent image with the confocal microscope.** A spherical thyroid follicle in a thick razor-blade section of rat thyroid fixed in formalin, was stained with a rhodamine–phalloidin conjugate which binds F-actin (similar results obtained with antibody conjugates). Although the sample was very thick, the microscope was focused on successive planes at 1 μm intervals from the top of the follicle (image no. 1) to halfway through (image no. 8), the total of the images representing a hemisphere. Note how the fluorescence in one plane does not interfere with that in another and that the composite photograph (image no. 9) of images 1–8 shows all the fluorescent staining in focus throughout the depth of the hemisphere. Clearly the antibody is staining hexagonal structures close to the apical (inner) surface of the follicular epithelial cells. Erythrocytes are visible near the top of the follicle. (Negatives kindly supplied by Dr Anna Smallcombe were taken by Bio-Rad staff on a Bio-Rad MRC-600 confocal imaging system using material provided by Professor V. Herzog and Fr. Brix of Bonn University.)

there are many machines now which have this analytic capacity for **flow cytometry** without the cell-sorting facility of the FACS (figure 7.8).

With the impressive number of monoclonal antibodies to hand, highly detailed phenotypic analysis of single-cell populations is now a practical proposition. Of the ever-growing number of applications (see for example figure 7.9a), the contribution to diagnosis of leukemia (cf. p. 387) is quite notable.

We can also probe the cell *interior* in several ways. Permeabilization to allow penetration by fluorescent antibodies (preferably with small Fab or even single-chain Fv fragments) gives a readout of cytokines and other intracellular proteins. Cell cycle analysis and

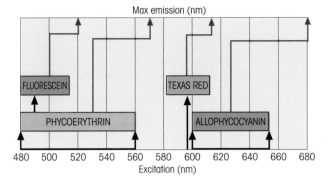

**Figure 7.7. Fluorescent labels used in flow cytofluorimetry.** The fluorescein longer wave emission overlaps with that of Texas Red and is corrected for in the software. The phycobiliproteins of red algae and cyanobacteria effect energy transfer of blue light to chlorophyll for photosynthesis; each molecule has many fluorescent groups (bilins) giving a broad excitation range, but fluorescence is emitted within a narrow wavelength band with such high quantum efficiency as to obviate the need for a second amplifying antibody.

enumeration of cells dying by apoptosis (figures 7.9b and c) can be achieved with DNA binding dyes such as propidium iodide. In addition, fluorescent probes for intracellular pH, thiol concentration, $Ca^{2+}$, $Mg^{2+}$ and $Na^+$ have been developed.

A powerful new string to the bow has been the introduction of methods for measuring the intracellular expression of the *LacZ* (*Escherichia coli* β-galactosidase) gene in mammalian cells by hydrolysis of the fluorogenic substrate fluorescein digalactoside. Depending on the construct introduced, the gene can be utilized as a marker for developmental and migration studies or as a reporter under the control of specified regulatory elements. By adapting this strategy, it was demonstrated that thiols, especially glutathione, control the cytokine-dependent activation of NFκB and hence the expression of HIV-1. Undoubtedly, the literature will be peppered with even more ingenious applications, but one further comment should be emphasized: unlike methods which average out results over a whole heterogeneous cell population, fluorocytometry provides data on individual cells each of which can be defined by a healthy number of parameters.

### The detection and isolation of rare cells

The limit of detection of rare cells by flow cytometry is 1 in $10^4$ allowing for autofluorescence and nonspecific staining plus difficulties in discrimination between

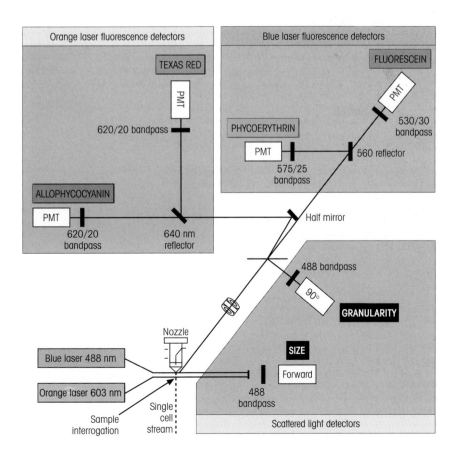

**Figure 7.8. Six-parameter flow cytometry optical system for multicolor immunofluorescence analysis.** Cell fluorescence excited by the blue laser is divided into green (fluorescein) and orange (phycoerythrin) signals, while fluorescence excited by the orange laser is reflected by a mirror and divided into near red (Texas Red) and far red (allophycocyanin) signals. Blue light scattered at small forward angles and at 90° is also measured in this system, providing information on cell size and internal granularity respectively. PMT, photomultiplier tube. (Based closely on Hardy R.R. (1992) In Roitt I.M. & Delves P.J. (eds) *Encyclopedia of Immunology*, p. 582. Academic Press, London.)

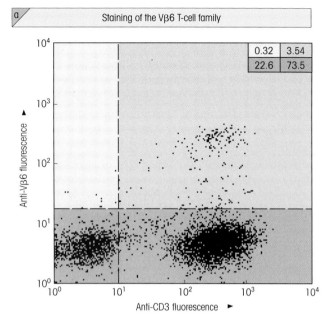

**Figure 7.9. Cytofluorimetric analysis of human peripheral blood lymphocytes.** (a) Cells stained with fluoresceinated anti-TCR Vβ6 and phycoerythrin conjugated anti-CD3. Each dot represents an individual lymphocyte and the numbers refer to the percentage of lymphocytes lying within the four quadrants formed by the two gating levels arbitrarily used to segregate positive from negative values. Virtually no lymphocytes bearing the T-cell receptors belonging to the Vβ6 family lack CD3, while 4.6% (3.5 out of 77.0) of the mature T-cells express Vβ6. (Data kindly provided by D. Morrison.) (b) Lymphocyte population stained for intracellular DNA with propidium iodide showing cells in apoptosis (purple) and in different stages of the mitotic cycle. (Data kindly supplied by R. Hicks.) (c) Amplification of the region showing apoptosis (cf. demonstration of apoptosis by nucleosome ladders, figure 1.18).

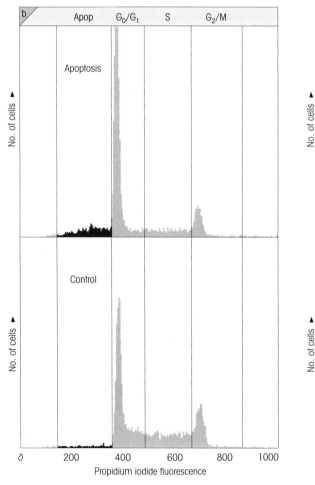

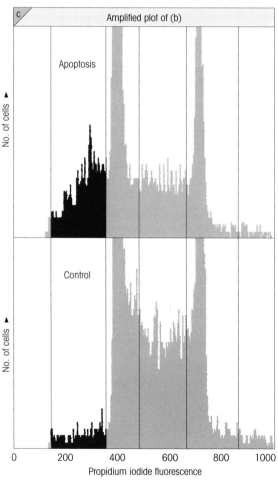

true staining and staining artefacts such as dead cells taking up stain non-specifically or aggregates of fluorescent conjugate. This background staining can be reduced dramatically by labeling the irrelevant cells with a mixture of antibodies tagged with a single fluorophor and then staining the rare cells using a specific antibody labeled with a second quite different fluorophor. At this stage it could even be scanned with a conventional fluorescence microscope!

## Other labeled antibody methods

In place of fluorescent markers, other workers have evolved methods in which enzymes such as alkaline phosphatase (cf. figure 18.6) or peroxidase are coupled to antibodies and these can be visualized by conventional histochemical methods at both light-microscope (figure 7.4b) and electron microscope (cf. figure 4.3) level.

Colloidal gold bound to antibody (figure 7.10) is being widely used as an electron-dense immunolabel by electron microscopists. At least three different antibodies can be applied to the same section by labeling them with gold particles of different size (cf. figure 9.10). A new ultra small probe consisting of Fab' fragments linked to undecagold clusters allows more accurate spatial localization of antigens and its small size enables it to mark sites which are inaccessible to the larger immunolabels. However, clear visualization requires a high-resolution scanning transmission electron microscope.

## Localization in tissues of a gene product

To get more feel for the way immunology interacts with other disciplines, it is instructive to follow the trail leading from the identification of a gene defect in Duchenne muscular dystrophy to the localization of the gene product within muscle tissue. The normal gene, which encodes the protein dystrophin, was sequenced and using either a peptide corresponding with part of this sequence, or a fusion protein produced when this gene was expressed in bacteria, rabbit antisera were raised and purified. Immunofluorescence showed binding of the antibodies to the surface membrane of intact human and mouse skeletal muscle. Excellent controls were provided by muscle from Duchenne patients and mdx mice (a model for Duchenne), neither of which express dystrophin. Electron microscopy (EM) studies with immunogold pinpointed the anatomical location of the antigen even more closely and showed convinc-

ingly that the major distribution of dystrophin was on the cytoplasmic face of the plasma membrane of muscle fibers (figure 7.10).

Note also that the multiple copies of mRNA produced by the cellular expression of a single gene can be localized by a labeled oligonucleotide probe which is complementary to the mRNA sequence and hybridizes with it *in situ*.

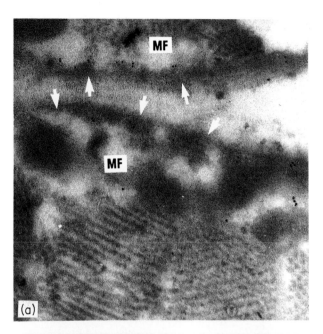

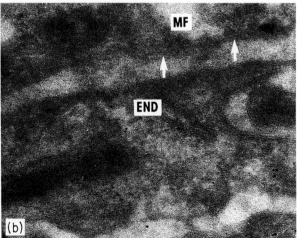

Figure 7.10. The immunolocalization of dystrophin in normal and mdx mouse skeletal muscle. mdx mice are a model for human Duchenne muscular dystrophy and both have a defective gene encoding dystrophin. Small dense round gold particles (5 nm) indicating the location of dystrophin immune complexes are seen along the plasma membrane (open arrows) of the normal mouse myofibers (a), but not the mdx plasma membrane (b). MF = myofiber; END = endothelial cell. (Reproduced with permission of the authors and the publishers from Watkins S.C., Hoffman E.P., Slayter H.S. & Kunkel L.M. (1988) *Nature* **333**, 863.)

## ASSESSMENT OF FUNCTIONAL ACTIVITY

### The activity of phagocytic cells

The major tests employed to assess polymorphonuclear neutrophil function are summarized in table 7.1.

### Lymphocyte responsiveness

When lymphocytes are stimulated by antigen or polyclonal activators *in vitro* they usually undergo mitosis (cf. figure 2.6d) and release soluble mediators termed cytokines. Mitosis is normally assessed by the incorporation of radiolabeled thymidine into the DNA of the dividing cells.

Cytokines released into the culture medium can be measured by a bioassay using a cell-line dependent on a particular cytokine for its growth and survival, or by immunoassay. Individual cells synthesizing cytokines can be enumerated in the flow cytometer by permeabilizing and staining intracellularly with labeled antibody: alternatively the 'Elispot' technique (see below) can be applied. As usual, molecular biology has a valuable, if more sophisticated, input since T-cells transfected with an IL-2 enhancer–*lacZ* construct will switch on *lacZ* β-galactosidase expression on activation of the IL-2 cytokine response (cf. p. 171) and this can be readily revealed with a fluorescent or chromogenic enzyme substrate.

The ability of cytotoxic T-cells to kill their cell targets extracellularly is usually evaluated by a chromium release assay. Target cells are labeled with $^{59}$Cr and the release of radioactive protein into the medium over and above that seen in the controls is the index of cytotoxicity. The test is repeated at different ratios of effector to target cells. A similar technique is used to measure extracellular killing of antibody-coated or uncoated targets by NK cells. Now a word of caution regarding the interpretation of *in vitro* assays. Since one can manipulate the culture conditions within wide limits, it is possible to achieve a result that might not be attainable *in vivo*. Let me illustrate this point by reference to cytotoxicity for murine cells infected with lymphocytic choriomeningitis virus (LCM) or vesicular stomatitis virus (VSV). The most sensitive *in vitro* technique proved to be chromium release from target cells after secondary stimulation of the lymphocytes. However, this needs five days during which time a relatively small number of memory CD8 cytotoxic T-cell precursors can replicate and surpass the threshold required to produce a measurable assay. Nonetheless, a weak cytotoxicity assay under these conditions was not reflected by any of the *in vivo* assessments of antiviral function implying that they had no biological relevance.

### Limiting dilution analysis

The magnitude of lymphocyte responses in culture is closely related to the number of antigen-specific lymphocytes capable of responding. Because of the clonality of the responses, it is possible to estimate the frequency of these antigen-specific precursors by **limiting dilution analysis**. In essence, the method depends upon the fact that if one takes several replicate aliquots of a given cell suspension which would be expected to contain *on average* one precursor per aliquot, then Poisson distribution analysis shows that 37% of the aliquots will contain *no* precursor cells (through the randomness of the sampling). Thus, if aliquots are made from a series of dilutions of a cell suspension and incubated under conditions which allow the precursors to mature and be recognized through some amplification scheme, the dilution at which 37% of the aliquots give negative responses will be known to contain an average of one precursor cell per aliquot and one can therefore calculate the precursor frequency in the original cell suspension. An example is shown in some detail in figure 7.11.

### Enumeration of antibody-forming cells

*The immunofluorescence sandwich test*

This is a double-layer procedure designed to visualize specific intracellular antibody. If, for example, we wished to see how many cells in a preparation of lymphoid tissue were synthesizing antibody to *Pneumococcus* polysaccharide, we would first fix the cells with

**Table 7.1.** Evaluation of neutrophil function.

| Function | Test |
|---|---|
| Phagocytosis | Measure uptake particles such as latex or bacteria by counting or by chemiluminescence |
| Respiratory burst | Measure reduction of nitroblue tetrazolium |
| Intracellular killing | Microbicidal test using viable *Staphylococcus aureus* |
| Directional migration | Movement through filters up concentration gradient of chemotactic agent such as formyl.Met.Leu.Phe |
| Surface LFA-1 and CR3 upregulation | Ascertained with monoclonal antibody staining |

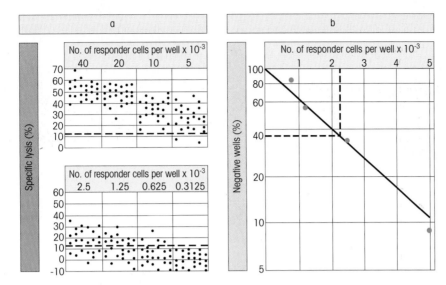

**Figure 7.11. Limiting dilution analysis of cytotoxic T-cell precursor frequency** in spleen cells from a BALB/c mouse stimulated with irradiated C57BL/6 spleen cells as antigen. BALB/c splenic responder cells were set up in 24 replicates at each concentration tested together with antigen and excess of T-helper factors. The generation of cytotoxicity in each well was looked for by adding $^{51}$Cr-labeled tumor cells (EL-4) of the C57BL/6 haplotype; cytotoxicity was then revealed by measuring the release of soluble $^{51}$Cr-labeled intracellular material into the medium. (a) The points show the percentage of specific lysis of individual wells. The dotted line indicates three standard deviations above the medium release control, and each point above that line is counted as positive for cytotoxicity. (b) The data replotted in terms of the percentage of negative wells at each concentration of responder cells over the range in which the data titrated ($5 \times 10^3$/well to $0.625 \times 10^3$/well). The dotted line is drawn at 37% negative wells and this intersects the regression line to give a precursor ($T_{cp}$) frequency of 1 in 2327 responder cells. The regression line has an $r^2$ value of 1.00 in this experiment. (Reproduced with permission from Simpson E. & Chandler P. (1986) In Weir D.M. (ed.) *Handbook of Experimental Immunology*, figure 68.2. Blackwell Scientific Publications, Oxford.)

ethanol to prevent the antibody being washed away during the test, and then treat with a solution of the polysaccharide antigen. After washing, a fluorescein-labeled antibody to the polysaccharide would then be added to locate those cells which had specifically bound the antigen.

The name of the test derives from the fact that antigen is sandwiched between the antibody present in the cell substrate and that added as the second layer (see figure 7.3c).

## Plaque techniques

Antibody-secreting cells can be counted by diluting them in an environment in which the antibody formed by each individual cell produces a readily observable effect. In one of the most widely used techniques, developed from the original method of Jerne and Nordin, the cells from an animal immunized with sheep erythrocytes are suspended together with an excess of sheep red cells and complement within a shallow chamber formed between two microscope sides. On incubation the antibody-forming cells release their immunoglobulin which coats the surrounding erythrocytes. The complement will then cause lysis of the coated cells and a **plaque** clear of red cells will be seen around each antibody-forming cell (figure 7.12). Direct plaques obtained in this way largely reveal IgM producers since this antibody has a high hemolytic efficiency. To demonstrate IgG-synthesizing cells it is necessary to increase the complement binding of the erythrocyte–IgG antibody complex by adding a rabbit anti-IgG serum; the 'indirect plaques' thus developed can be used to enumerate cells making antibodies in different immunoglobulin subclasses, provided the appropriate rabbit antisera are available. The method can be extended by coating an antigen such as *Pneumococcus* polysaccharide on to the red cell, or by coupling hapten groups to the erythrocyte surface.

In the '**Elispot**' modification, the antibody-forming cell suspension is incubated on a dish of immobilized antigen. The secreted antibody is captured locally and is visualized after removal of the cells, by treatment with peroxidase-labeled anti-Ig, and development of the color reaction by incorporating the substrate in a gel which is poured over the floor of the dish. Limited diffusion of the colored reaction product in the gel provides a series of macroscopic spots which can be readily enumerated (figure 7.13).

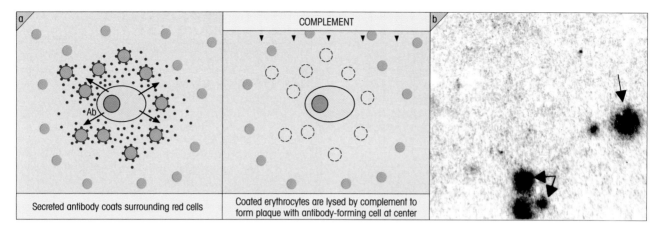

**Figure 7.12. Jerne plaque technique for enumerating antibody-forming cells (Cunningham modification).** (a) The *direct* technique for cells synthesizing IgM hemolysin is shown. The *indirect* technique for visualizing cells producing IgG hemolysins requires the addition of anti-IgG to the system. The difference between the plaques obtained by direct and indirect methods gives the number of 'IgG' plaques. The *reverse plaque* assay enumerates total Ig-producing cells by capturing secreted Ig on red cells coated with anti-Ig.

Multiple plaque assays can be carried out by a modification using microtiter plates. (b) Photograph of plaques which show as circular dark areas (some of which are arrowed) under dark-ground illumination. They vary in size depending upon the antibody affinity and the rate of secretion by the antibody-forming cell. (Courtesy of Mr C. Shapland, Ms P. Hutchings & Dr D. Male.)

## Analysis of functional activity by cellular reconstitution

### Radiation chimeras

The entire populations of lymphocytes and polymorphs can be inactivated by appropriate doses of X-irradiation. Such animals may be reconstituted by injection of bone marrow hemopoietic stem cells which provide the precursors of all the formed elements of the blood (cf. figure 12.1). These chimeras of host plus hemopoietic grafted cells can be manipulated in many ways to analyse cellular function such as the role of the thymus in the maturation of T-lymphocytes from bone marrow stem cells (figure 7.14).

### Mice with severe combined immunodeficiency (SCID)

Mice with defects in the genes encoding the IL-2 receptor γ-chain, or the nucleotide salvage pathway enzymes adenosine deaminase or purine nucleoside phosphorylase, develop SCID due to a failure of B- and T-cells to differentiate. These special animals can be reconstituted with various human lymphoid tissues and their functions and responses analysed. Coimplantation of contiguous fragments of human fetal liver (hematopoietic stem cells) and thymus allows T-lymphopoiesis, production of B-cells, and maintenance of colony-forming units of myeloid and erythroid lineages for 6–12 months. Adult peripheral blood cells injected into the peritoneal cavity of SCID mice treated with growth hormone can sustain production of human B-cells and antibodies and can be used to generate human hybridomas making defined monoclonal antibodies. Immunotherapeutic anti-tumor responses can also be played with in these animals.

### Cellular interactions in vitro

It is obvious that the methods outlined for depletion, enrichment and isolation of individual cell populations outlined at the beginning of the chapter, enable the investigator to study cellular interactions through judicious recombinations. These interactions are usually more effective when the cells are operating within some sort of stromal network resembling the set up of the tissues where their function is optimally expressed. For example, colonization of murine fetal thymus rudiments in culture with T-cell precursors enables one to follow the pattern of proliferation, maturation, TCR rearrangement and positive and negative selection normally seen *in vivo* (cf. p. 227). An even more refined system involves the addition of selected lymphoid populations to disaggregated stromal cells derived from fetal thymic lobes depleted of endogenous lymphoid cells with deoxyguanosine. The cells can be spun into a pellet and cocultured in

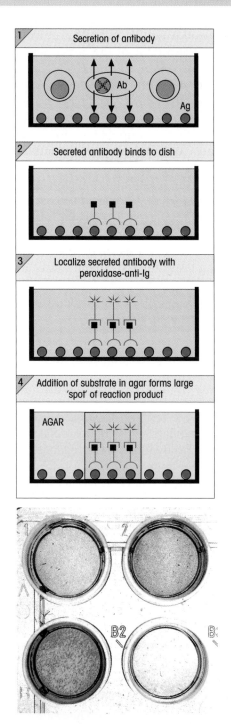

**1** Secretion of antibody

**2** Secreted antibody binds to dish

**3** Localize secreted antibody with peroxidase-anti-Ig

**4** Addition of substrate in agar forms large 'spot' of reaction product

**Figure 7.13.** **'Elispot' (from ELISA technique) system for enumerating antibody-forming cells.** The picture shows spots formed by hybridoma cells making autoantibodies to thyroglobulin revealed by alkaline phosphatase-linked anti-Ig (courtesy of P. Hutchings). Increasing numbers of hybridoma cells were added to the top two and bottom left-hand wells which show corresponding increases in the number of 'Elispots'. The bottom right-hand well is a control using a hybridoma of irrelevant specificity.

| | Operation | Irradiation | Restitution | Induction of cell-mediated immunity |
|---|---|---|---|---|
| 1 | Sham thymectomy | (X) | Bone marrow | ++ |
| 2 | Thymectomy | (X) | Bone marrow | – |
| 3 | Thymectomy | (X) | Bone marrow + adult lymphocytes | ++ |

**Figure 7.14.** **Maturation of bone marrow stem cells under the influence of the thymus** to become immunocompetent lymphocytes capable of cell-mediated immune reactions. X-irradiation (X) destroys the ability of host lymphocytes to mount a cellular immune response but the stem cells in injected bone marrow can become immunocompetent and restore the response (1) unless the thymus is removed (2), in which case only already immunocompetent lymphocytes are effective (3). Incidentally, the bone marrow stem cells also restore the levels of other formed elements of the blood (red cells, platelets, neutrophils, monocytes) which otherwise fall dramatically after X-irradiation, and such therapy is crucial in cases where accidental or therapeutic exposure to X-rays or other antimitotic agents seriously damages the hematopoietic cells.

## Probing function with antibodies

Antibodies can be used to confirm the importance of cross-linking cell surface components for a number of functions. An excellent example is the induction of histamine release from mast cells by divalent F(ab′)$_2$ anti-Fcε receptor I but not by the univalent fragment. Similarly, divalent anti-FcγR triggers phagocytosis in macrophages, while a bispecific antibody to CD3 and CD4 brings the two molecules together on the T-cell surface and induces activation.

I must tell you that antibodies can be made to cause spatially defined intracellular damage by chromophor-assisted laser inactivation. A neuronal growth cone in a living embryo, for example, can be permeabilized and loaded with anticalcineurin labeled with malachite green which absorbs light at 620 nm where most cellular constituents do not. A laser emitting light of this wavelength will irradiate the antibody–chromophor conjugate, so generating a pulse of highly reactive free radicals which cause inactivation in a small region of diameter around 15 Å. Figure 7.15 shows that the laser flash results in retraction of filopodial and lamellipodial membrane extensions. This in turn influences the direction of subsequent growth cone movement, so demonstrating the involvement of the calmodulin-dependent phosphatase, calcineurin in growth cone steering. By operating at different embryonic stages the investigator can knock out functions in a temporally as well as

hanging drops; on transfer to normal organ culture conditions after a few hours, reaggregation to intact lobes takes place quite magically and the various differentiation and maturation processes then unfold.

spatially restricted fashion. This should prove to be a discriminating cellular microsurgical tool of considerable utility and applicability.

## GENETIC ENGINEERING OF CELLS

### Insertion and modification of genes in mammalian cells

Because gene transfer into mammalian cells is inefficient, it is customary to use immortal cell lines for such **transfections** and to include a selectable marker such as neomycin resistance. Genes can be introduced into cells as calcium phosphate precipitates or by electroporation in which a brief electric pulse transiently creates holes in the cell membrane. Another approach is to incorporate the gene into liposomes which fuse with the cell membrane. Direct microinjection of DNA is also effective. Integration of the gene into the genome of a virus like vaccinia provides an easy ride into the cell, although more stable long-term transfections are obtained with modified retroviral vectors. The latest fad is transfection by biolistics, the buzz word for biological ballistics. DNA coated on to gold microparticles is literally fired from a high-pressure helium gun and penetrates the cells; even plant cells with their cellulose coats are easy meat for this technology. Skin and surgically exposed tissues can also be penetrated with ease.

Studying the effect of *adding* a gene then, does not offer too many technological problems. How does one assess the impact of *removing* a gene? One versatile strategy to delete endogenous gene function is to target the gene's mRNA as distinct from the gene itself. Nucleotide sequences of RNA or DNA complementary to the mRNA of the target gene are introduced into the cell in a form which allows them to replicate. The **antisense** molecules so produced base pair with the target mRNA and block translation into protein.

An important manipulation to achieve gene disruption is homologous recombination. A DNA sequence which disrupts the reading frame is inserted into the gene in question and microinjected directly into cells. In a small number of cells, the disrupted gene fragment replaces the resident normal gene by homologous recombination. These rare cells can be recovered by using a selectable marker or by a series of screening tests with the polymerase chain reaction (PCR) using oligonucleotide primers specific for the inserted DNA and upstream sequences on the adjacent normal gene (figure 7.16).

### Introducing new genes into animals

#### Establishing 'designer mice' bearing new genes

Female mice are induced to superovulate and then mated. The fertilized eggs are microinjected with the gene and surgically implanted in females. Between 5 and 40% of the implanted oocytes develop to term and of these, 10–25% have copies of the injected gene stably integrated into their chromosomes detectable by PCR. These 'founder' transgenic animals are mated with nontransgenic mice and pure transgenic lines eventually established (figure 7.17).

#### Transgenes introduced into embryonic stem cells

**Embryonic stem (ES) cells** can be obtained by culturing the inner cell mass of mouse blastocysts in the presence of a feeder layer of fibroblasts or leukemia inhibitory factor to prevent differentiation. After transfection with the appropriate gene, the transfected cells can be selected and reimplanted after injection into a new blastocyst. The resulting mice are chimeric, in that some cells carry the transgene and others do not. The same will be true of germ cells, and by breeding for germ-line transmission of the transgene, pure strains can be derived (figure 7.18).

The advantage over microinjection is that the cells can be selected after transfection, and this is especially important if homologous recombination with a disrupted gene is being used to develop '**knockout mice**' lacking the gene which has been targeted. This is a truly powerful technology with an awesome potential

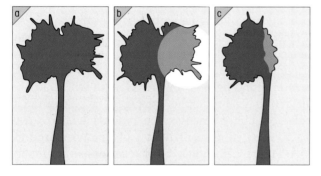

**Figure 7.15. Microsurgery of a neuronal growth cone loaded with a malachite green-labeled antibody to calcineurin.** The growth cone shows laser-induced retraction of membrane extensions: (a) before, (b) during and (c) after the laser flash. (Reproduced from a commentary by Muller B.K. and Bonhoeffer F. (1995) in *Current Biology* **11**, 1255 on experiments by Jay D.G. and colleagues (1995) *Nature* **376**, 686, with permission.)

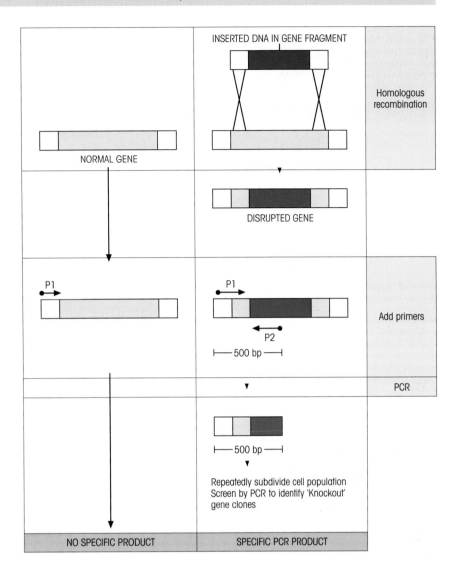

**Figure 7.16. Gene disruption by homologous recombination** with a DNA fragment containing a copy of the gene containing a 20-base pair insertion which interrupts the reading frame. Cells containing the disrupted gene can be recognized by looking for a specific PCR product using two primers, one annealing to the inserted sequence and the other to the natural DNA upstream of the fragment. After repeated rounds of subdivision and PCR testing, pure cell clones with the deleted gene can be recovered.

and the whole biological community has been suffused with boxing fever, knocking out genes right, left and center. Just a few examples of knockout mice of interest to immunologists, are listed in Table 7.2.

*Gene therapy in humans.* We seem to be catching up with science fiction and are in the early stages of civilized 'pseudo-Frankenstein' approaches to the correction of genetic misfortune by the introduction of 'good' genes. Effective gene delivery is still a major hurdle. Adenovirus vectors are good for delivering genes because they penetrate cells with high efficiency and enter the nucleus where they function in an epichromosomal manner to express the new gene. Needless to say, there are some disadvantages: slightly 'leaky' expression of adenovirus genes makes the cell a potential target for cytotoxic T-cells while

induction of humoral immunity can limit the efficacy of a second dose. In this respect, the production of IgA antibodies to the adenovirus vector thwarts attempts to administer gene therapy for cystic fibrosis via the airways more than once, although co-administration of IFNγ or IL-12 diminishes the formation of neutralizing antibody (cf. p. 184).

Liposomes (cf. p. 305) do not cause these problems but they are much less effective. They transfer genes to the target cell by fusion with the plasma membrane. Entry is relatively efficient but once inside, most of the liposomal DNA is shunted into lysosomal waste disposal systems and degraded. In the end, only 1 in 1000 plasmids reach the nucleus and are expressed. It reminds me of one of Nature's typically gruesome stories in which thousands of baby turtles hatch from their eggs on the beach but before they

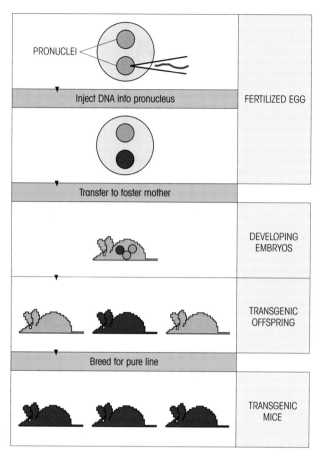

**Figure 7.17. Production of pure strain transgenic mice** by microinjection of fertilized egg, implantation into a foster mother and subsequent inbreeding.

**Table 7.2. Some gene 'knockouts' and their effects.**

| Knockout target | Phenotype of knockout mice |
|---|---|
| CD8 α-chain | Absence of cytotoxic T-cells |
| p59 $^{fynT}$ | Defective signalling in thymocytes but not peripheral T-cells |
| HOX 11 | No spleen |
| IgE | No defects observed! |
| FcεRI α-chain | Resistant to cutaneous and systemic anaphylaxis |
| IgM μ-chain membrane exon | Absence of B-cells |
| IL-6 | No bone loss when ovariectomized (implications for osteoporosis?) |
| MHC class II Aβ | Decreased CD4 T-cells; inflammatory bowel disease |
| Perforin | Impaired CTL and NK cell function |
| TAP1 | Lack CD8 cells |
| TNFR-1 | Resistant to endotoxic shock; susceptible to *Listeria* |
| Culled from Brandon (1995) *Current Biology* **5**, 625. | |

make the safety of the sea, nearly all get picked off by innumerable predators.

To return to our subject, genes can be selectively expressed in particular tissues by linking them to appropriate enhancer elements. To take an example, rats were made transgenic for human *bcl-2* linked to the regulatory sequences of a rat pyruvate kinase gene encoding a glycolytic enzyme expressed mainly in hepatocytes; the expression of *bcl-2* in liver, protected the animals from fulminating hepatic failure due to massive apoptosis induced by injection of antibodies to Fas. One could envisage a possible future therapy for the prevention of massive liver damage due to cytotoxic T-cells activated during viral hepatitis in humans.

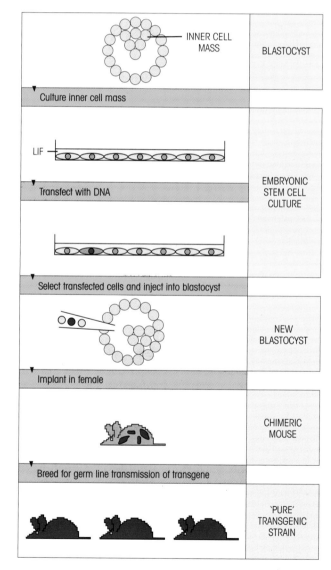

**Figure 7.18. Introduction of a transgene through transfection of embryonic stem cells.** The transfected cells can be selected, e.g. for homologous recombinant 'knockouts', before reimplantation. LIF, leukemia inhibiting factor.

# SUMMARY

## Isolation of leukocyte subpopulations

• Cells can be separated on the basis of physical characteristics such as size, buoyant density and adhesiveness.

• Phagocytic cells can be separated by a magnet after taking up iron particles and cells which divide in response to a specific stimulus, e.g. antigen, can be eliminated by ultraviolet light after incorporation of 5-bromodeoxyuridine.

• Antibody-coated cells can be eliminated by complement-mediated cytotoxicity or anti-Ig–ricin conjugates; they can be isolated by panning to solid-phase anti-Ig or by cluster formation with magnetic beads bearing anti-Ig on their surface.

• Smaller numbers of cells can be fractionated by coating with a fluorescent monoclonal antibody and separating them from nonfluorescent cells in the FACS.

• Antigen-specific T-cells can be enriched as lines or clones by driving them with antigen; fusion to appropriate T-cell tumor lines yields immortal antigen-specific T-cell hybridomas; antigen-specific immortalized T-cell clones can be obtained by transformation with the lymphotropic Herpes saimiri virus just as immortal B-cells can be derived by EB virus transformation.

## Immunohistochemical localization of antigens in cells and tissues

• Antigens can be localized if stained by fluorescent antibodies and viewed in an appropriate microscope. A new development, the confocal microscope, scans a very thin plane at high magnification and provides quantitative data on extremely sharp images of the antigen-containing structures which can also be examined in three dimensions.

• Antibodies can either be labeled directly or visualized by a second antibody, a labeled anti-Ig.

• Machines which employ the flow cytofluorimetric function of the FACS without the sorting facility are available. Single cells in individual droplets are interrogated by one or two lasers and quantitative data using up to four different fluorescent labels can be logged, giving a complex phenotypic analysis of each cell in a heterogeneous mixture. In addition, forward scatter of the laser light defines cell size and 90° scatter, cell granularity.

• Fluorescent antibodies or their fragments can also be used for staining intracellular antigens in permeabilized cells. Intracellular probes for pH, $Ca^{2+}$, $Mg^{2+}$, $Na^+$, thiols and the DNA of apoptotic cells are also available. Gene

regulatory elements linked to a reporter gene such as *lacZ* (galactosidase), which yields fluorescent enzyme products, can also now be studied at the single-cell level by flow cytometry.

• Antibodies can be labeled by enzymes for histochemical definition of antigens at the light microscope level, and with different-sized colloidal gold particles for ultrastructural visualization in the electron microscope.

• mRNA produced by a single gene can be localized by *in situ* hybridization using a complementary oligonucleotide probe.

## Assessment of functional activity

• Neutrophil polymorph chemotaxis, phagocytosis, NADH oxidase activity and microbicidal potency can all be studied, almost on a routine basis.

• Lymphocyte responses to antigen are monitored by proliferation and/or by cytokine release. Individual cells secreting cytokines can be identified by the 'Elispot' technique in which the secreted product is captured by a solid-phase antibody and then stained with a second labeled antibody.

• Extracellular killing by cytotoxic T-cells, and NK cells, can be measured by the release of radioactive chromium-59 from prelabeled target cells.

• The precursor frequency of effector T-cells can be measured by limiting dilution analysis.

• Antibody-forming cells can be enumerated, either by an immunofluorescence sandwich test or by plaque techniques in which the antibody secreted by the cells causes complement-mediated death of adjacent red cells, or is captured by solid-phase antigen in an 'Elispot' assay.

• Functional activity can be assessed by cellular reconstitution experiments in which leukocyte sets and selected lymphoid tissue can be transplanted into unresponsive hosts such as X-irradiated recipients or mice with severe combined immunodeficiency. Defined cell populations can also be separated and selectively recombined *in vitro*.

• Antibodies can be used to probe cellular function by cross-linking defined cell surface components or by selective destruction of particular intracellular sites by laser irradiation of chromophor-conjugated specific antibodies which localize to the target area by penetrating permeabilized cells.

## Genetic engineering of cells

• Genes can be inserted into mammalian cells by trans-

*(Continued on p. 148)*

fection using calcium phosphate precipitates, electroporation, liposomes and microinjection.

• Genes can also be taken into a cell after incorporation into vaccinia or retroviruses.

• Endogenous gene function can be inhibited by antisense RNA or by homologous recombination with a disrupted gene.

• Transgenic mice bearing an entirely new gene introduced into the fertilized egg by microinjection of DNA can be established as inbred lines.

• Genes can be introduced into embryonic stem cells with greater control by the operator; these modified stem cells are injected back into a blastocyst and can develop into founder mice from which pure transgenic animals can be bred. One very important application of this technique involves the disruption of a targeted gene in the embryonic stem cell by homologous recombination, producing so-called 'knockout' mice lacking a specific gene.

• Human gene therapy promises an exciting future. Delivery of genes by adenovirus vectors or liposomes is under intensive investigation but still poses problems.

## FURTHER READING

Ausubel F.M., Brent R., Kingston R.E., Moore D.D., Seidman J.G., Smith J.A. & Struhl K. (eds) (1987; continually updated) *Current Protocols in Molecular Biology, 1–2*. Greene Publishing Associates & Wiley-Interscience, New York.

Coligan J.E., Kruisbeek A.M., Margulies D.H., Shevach E.M. & Strober W. (eds) (1991; continually updated) *Current Protocols in Immunology, 1–2*. Greene Publishing Associates & Wiley-Interscience, New York.

Davis M.M. (ed.) (1996) Immunological techniques. *Current Opinion in Immunology* **8**, 255.

Fishwild D.M. *et al.* (1996) High-avidity human IgGκ monoclonal antibodies from a novel strain of minilocus transgenic mice. *Nature Biotechnology* **14**(7), 845.

Friguet B., Chafotte A.F., Djavadi-Ohaniance L. & Goldberg M.E.J. (1985) Measurements of the true affinity constant in solution of antigen–antibody complexes by enzyme-linked immunosorbent assay. *Immunological Methods* **77**, 305.

Gavrieli Y. *et al.* (1992) Identification of programmed cell death *in situ* via specific labelling of nuclear DNA fragmentation. *Journal of Cell Biology* **119**, 493. (Terminal deoxynucleotidyl transferase is used to add labeled nucleotides to the many free ends of the fragmented DNA seen in nuclear cells at the early stages of apoptosis.)

Malik V.S. & Lillehoj E.P. (1994) *Antibody Techniques*. Academic Press, London. (Laboratory manual of pertinent techniques for production and use of monoclonal antibodies for the non-immunologist.)

McGuinness B.T. *et al.* (1996) Phage diabody repertoires for selection of large numbers of bispecific antibody fragments. *Nature Biotechnology* **14**(9), 1149.

Mosier D.E. (ed.) (1996) Humanizing the mouse. *Seminars in Immunology* **8**, 185.

Ritter M.A. & Ladyman H.M. (1995) *Monoclonal Antibodies: Production, Engineering & Clinical Application*. Cambridge University Press, Cambridge. (An evaluation of different techniques available rather than a technical manual.)

Schauer U., Jung T., Krug N. & Frew A. (1996) Measurement of intracellular cytokines. *Immunology Today* **17**, 305.

Sikorski R.S. & Peters R. (1996) Antibodies on the web. *Nature Biotechnology* **14**(6), 775.

Staal F.J.T., Roederer M., Herzenberg L.A. & Herzenberg L.A. (1990) Intracellular thiols regulate NF-κB activation and HIV transcription. *Proceedings of the National Academy of Sciences* **87**, 9943. (Exploitation of *lacZ* (galactosidase) reporter gene technology using flow cytometry.)

Vaughan T.J. *et al.* (1996) Human antibodies with subnanomolar affinities isolated from a large nonimmunized phage display library. *Nature Biotechnology* **14**(3), 309.

Watson J.D., Gilman M., Witkowski J. & Zoller M. (1992) *Recombinant DNA*, 2nd edn. Scientific American Books, New York.

Weir D.M. *et al.* (eds) (1996) *Handbook of Experimental Immunology: Volume 4*, 5th edn. Blackwell Scientific Publications, Oxford.

Zola H. (1994) *Monoclonal Antibodies: the Second Generation*. Bios Scientific Publishers, Oxford. (New approaches including phage display combinatorial libraries.)

# THE ACQUIRED IMMUNE RESPONSE

Having looked in depth at the constituent parts of the immune system and the methods used to study them, the present section examines the interactions which lead to their integration in a coherent adaptive immune response.

Chapter 8 deals with the **anatomy of the immune response** and tries to explain just where it all happens within the body. The moment of truth for the slumbering lymphocyte when it is disturbed by its selective contact with antigen on a professional presenting cell complete with accessory costimulatory signals is described in Chapter 9 on **lymphocyte activation**. Next, in Chapter 10, we look at the factors which drive clonal proliferation of the activated lymphocytes and the subsequent **production of effectors** through differentiation into helper and cytotoxic T-cells, antibody-forming B-cells and the establishment of memory populations.

Since clonal proliferation is a potentially explosive event, there have to be effective **control mechanisms** — to take an analogy, if we are in the business of running nuclear power stations, we need to prevent them spontaneously becoming nuclear bombs. Chapter 11 describes the roles of both antigen and antibody as control elements and analyses the regulatory mechanisms based on T-cells and idiotype networks. Immune responses are strongly influenced by genetically linked factors and by neuro-endocrine interactions.

Finally, in Chapter 12, we identify the major events controlled by the microenvironment in the **ontogenic development** of lymphocyte progenitors to immunocompetent B- and T-cells with the concomitant silencing of self-reactions by **immunological tolerance**. A relatively brief account of **phylogenetic evolution** concludes the section.

# THE ANATOMY OF THE IMMUNE RESPONSE

## THE SURFACE MARKERS OF CELLS IN THE IMMUNE SYSTEM

In order to discuss the events which occur in the operation of the immune system as a whole, it is imperative to establish a nomenclature which identifies the surface markers on the cells involved since these are used for communication and are usually functional molecules reflecting the state of cellular differentiation. The nomenclature system is established as follows. Immunologists from the far corners of the world who have produced monoclonal antibodies directed to surface molecules on B- and T-cells, macrophages, neutrophils and natural killer (NK) cells and so on, get together every so often, to compare the specificities of their reagents in international workshops whose spirit of cooperation should be a lesson to most politicians. Where a cluster of monoclonals are found to react with the same polypeptide, they clearly represent a series of reagents

defining a given marker and we label it with a CD (**cluster of differentiation**) number. The number of CD specificities on leukocytes is well over the 100s(!) at the time of writing but I have selected just some of them in table 8.1 which are the ones most likely to be relevant to our discussions. This can be used for reference but I regret to have to tell the reader that familiarity with the numbers can be a great help. A more complete list of CD markers is given in Appendix 1.

## THE NEED FOR ORGANIZED LYMPHOID TISSUE

For an effective immune response an intricate series of cellular events must occur. Antigen must bind and if necessary be processed by antigen-presenting cells which must then make contact with and activate T- and B-cells; T-helpers must assist certain B-cells and cytotoxic T-cell precursors and there have to be mechanisms which amplify the numbers of potential

Table 8.1. Some of the major clusters of differentiation (CD) markers on human cells.

| CD | Main cellular association | Membrane component |
|---|---|---|
| CD2 | T | Receptor for LFA-3 and sheep rbc |
| CD2R | act. T | Ab's activate through these epitopes |
| CD3 | T | Transducing elements of T-cell receptor |
| CD4 | T-helper | MHC class II and HIV receptor |
| CD5 | T, B subset | Ab increases second messenger pool |
| CD8 | T-cytotoxic | MHC class I receptor |
| CD18 | Leukocytes | Integrin $\beta_2$-chain |
| CD19 | B | Pan B-cell marker associated with CD21 |
| CD21 | B subset | CR2, C3dg/EBV receptor |
| CD23 | B subset, act. M, Eo | FcεRII |
| CD25 | act. T, B, M | IL-2R $\beta$-chain |
| CD28 | T-cells | Receptor for B7 costimulator |
| CD29 | Leukocytes | VLA $\beta$, integrin $\beta_1$-chain |
| CD34 | Bone marrow | Stem cell marker |
| CD40 | B-cells | Receptor for CD40L costimulator |
| CD44 | Leukocytes | Homing receptor |
| CD45 | Leukocytes | Leukocyte common antigen |
| CD45 RA | T subset, B, G, M | Resting (naive?) T-cells |
| CD45 RO | T subset, B, G, M | Activated (memory?) T-cells |

M = macrophage; G = granulocyte; Eo = eosinophil. See Appendix 1 for more complete list.

effector cells by proliferation and then bring about differentiation to generate the mediators of humoral and cellular immunity. In addition, memory cells for secondary responses must be formed and the whole response controlled so that it is adequate but not excessive and is appropriate to the type of infection being dealt with. By working hard, we can isolate component cells of the immune system and persuade them to carry out a number of responses to antigen in the test tube, but compared with the efficacy of the overall development of immunity in the body, our efforts still leave much to be desired. *In vivo* the integration of the complex cellular interactions which form the basis of the immune response takes place within the organized architecture of peripheral, or secondary, lymphoid tissue which includes the lymph

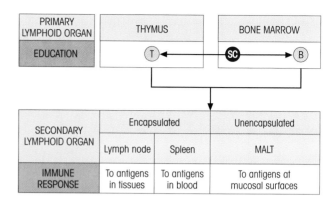

Figure 8.1. The functional organization of lymphoid tissue. Stem cells (SC) arising in the bone marrow differentiate into immunocompetent T- and B-cells in the primary lymphoid organs and then colonize the secondary lymphoid tissues where immune responses are organized. The mucosal-associated lymphoid tissue which produces the antibodies for mucosal secretions is often referred to as the MALT system.

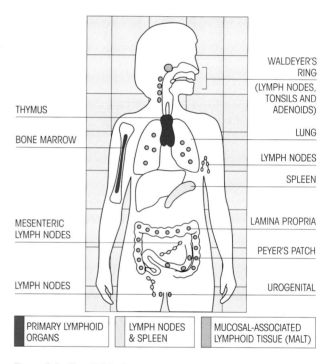

Figure 8.2. The distribution of major lymphoid organs and tissues throughout the body.

glands, spleen and unencapsulated tissue lining the respiratory, alimentary and genitourinary tracts.

These tissues become populated by cells of reticular origin and by macrophages and lymphocytes derived from bone marrow stem cells, the T-cells first differentiating into immunocompetent cells by a high pressure training period in the thymus, the B-cells undergoing their education in the bone marrow itself (figure 8.1). In essence, the lymph nodes filter off and, if necessary, respond to foreign material draining body tissues, the spleen monitors the blood and the

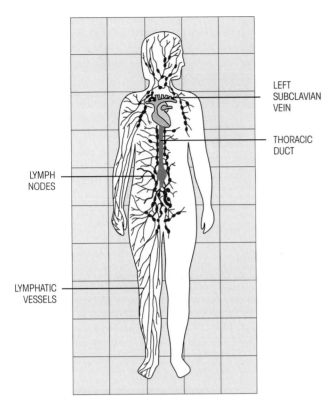

**Figure 8.3. The network of lymph nodes and lymphatics.** Lymph nodes occur at junctions of the draining lymphatics. The lymph finally collects in the thoracic duct and thence returns to the bloodstream via the left subclavian vein.

LEFT SUBCLAVIAN VEIN

THORACIC DUCT

LYMPH NODES

LYMPHATIC VESSELS

throughout the lymphoid system. Thus, antigen-reactive cells are depleted from the circulating pool of lymphocytes within 24 hours of antigen first localizing in the lymph nodes or spleen; several days later, after proliferation at the site of antigen localization, a peak of activated cells appears in the thoracic duct. When antigen reaches a node in a primed animal, there is a dramatic fall in the output of cells in the efferent lymphatics, a phenomenon described variously as 'cell shutdown' or 'lymphocyte trapping' and which probably results from the antigen-induced release of a T-cell soluble factor (cf. the lymphokines, p. 33); this is followed by an output of activated blast cells which peaks at around 80 hours.

## Lymphocytes home to their specific tissues

Naive lymphocytes enter a lymph node through the afferent lymphatics and by guided passage across the specialized **high-walled endothelium of the post-capillary venules (HEV)** (cf. figure 8.5). Comparable endothelial cells offer transit of cells concerned in mucosal immunity to Peyer's patches. In other cases involving migration into normal and inflamed tissues, the lymphocytes bind to and cross non-specialized flatter endothelia. Lymphoblasts and memory cell populations display tissue-restricted migration to extra lymphoid sites such as skin or mucosal epithelium, while lymphocytes, as well as neutrophils and monocytes, target and migrate into sites of inflammation in response to locally produced mediators.

This highly organized traffic is orchestrated by directing the relevant lymphocytes to different parts of the lymphoid system and the various other tissues by a series of **homing receptors** which recognize their complementary ligands, termed **vascular addressins**, on the surface of the appropriate endothelial cells of the blood vessels (figure 8.6). These act as selective gateways which allow lymphocytes access to the tissue in question.

## Transmigration occurs in three stages

### Step 1: Tethering and rolling

Lymphocytes normally travel in the fast lane down the centre of the blood vessels. However, blood flows slowly over the surface of the vessel wall and in order for the lymphocyte to become attached to the endothelial cell it has to overcome the shear forces that this creates. This is effected by a force of attraction between **selectins** and their ligands on the lym-

unencapsulated lymphoid tissue is strategically integrated into mucosal surfaces of the body as a forward defensive system based on IgA secretion.

The anatomical disposition of these lymphoid tissues is illustrated in figure 8.2. The lymphatics and associated lymph nodes form an impressive network, draining the viscera and the more superficial body structures before returning to the blood by way of the thoracic duct (figure 8.3).

Communication between these tissues and the rest of the body is maintained by a pool of recirculating lymphocytes which pass from the blood into the lymph nodes, spleen and other tissues and back to the blood by the major lymphatic channels such as the thoracic duct (figures 8.4 and 8.11).

## LYMPHOCYTES TRAFFIC BETWEEN LYMPHOID TISSUES

This traffic of lymphocytes between the tissues, the bloodstream and the lymph glands enables antigen-sensitive cells to seek the antigen and to be recruited to sites at which a response is occurring, while the dissemination of memory cells and their progeny enables a more widespread response to be organized

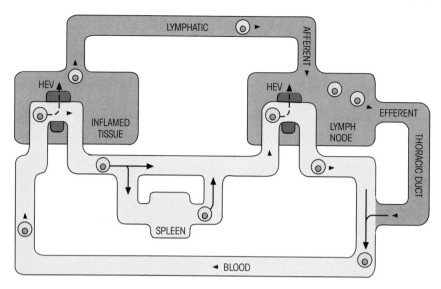

**Figure 8.4. Traffic and recirculation of lymphocytes through encapsulated lymphoid tissue and sites of inflammation.** Blood-borne lymphocytes enter the tissues and lymph nodes passing through the high-walled endothelium of the postcapillary venules (HEV) and leave via the draining lymphatics. The efferent lymphatics, finally emerging from the last node in each chain, join to form the thoracic duct which returns the lymphocytes to the bloodstream. In the spleen, lymphocytes enter the lymphoid area (white pulp) from the arterioles, pass to the sinusoids of the erythroid area (red pulp) and leave by the splenic vein. Traffic through the mucosal immune system is elaborated in figure 8.11.

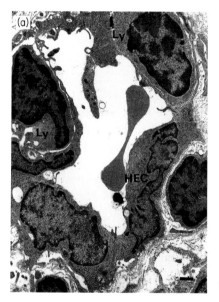

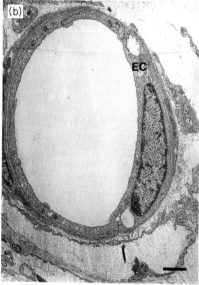

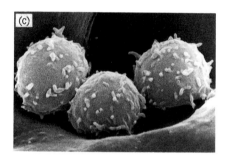

**Figure 8.5. Lymphocyte association with postcapillary venules.** (a) High-walled endothelial cells (HEC) of postcapillary venules in rat cervical lymph nodes showing intimate association with lymphocytes (Ly). (b) Flattened capillary endothelial cell (EC) for comparison. (c) Lymphocytes adhering to HEC (scanning electron micrograph). ((a) and (b) kindly provided by Dr Ann Ager and (c) by Dr W. van Ewijk.)

phocyte and vessel wall which operates through microvilli on the leucocyte surface (figure 8.6). After this tethering process, the lymphocyte rolls along the endothelial cell, partly through the selectin interactions but now increasingly through the binding of $\beta_1$ or $\beta_7$ integrins (table 8.2) to their respective ligands.

### Step 2: $\beta_2$ integrin activation and cell flattening

This process leads to activation and recruitment of members of $\beta_2$ integrin family (table 8.2) to the non-villous surface of the lymphocyte. In particular molecules such as LFA-1 bind very strongly to ICAM-1 and 2 on the endothelial cell, the intimate contact causing the lymphocyte to flatten.

### Step 3: Transmigration into the tissue (diapedesis)

The flattened lymphocyte now uses the LFA-1/ICAM interaction and PECAM-1 (CD31; see Appendix), an adhesion molecule of the immunoglobulin superfamily, to elbow its way between the endothelial cells and into the tissue.

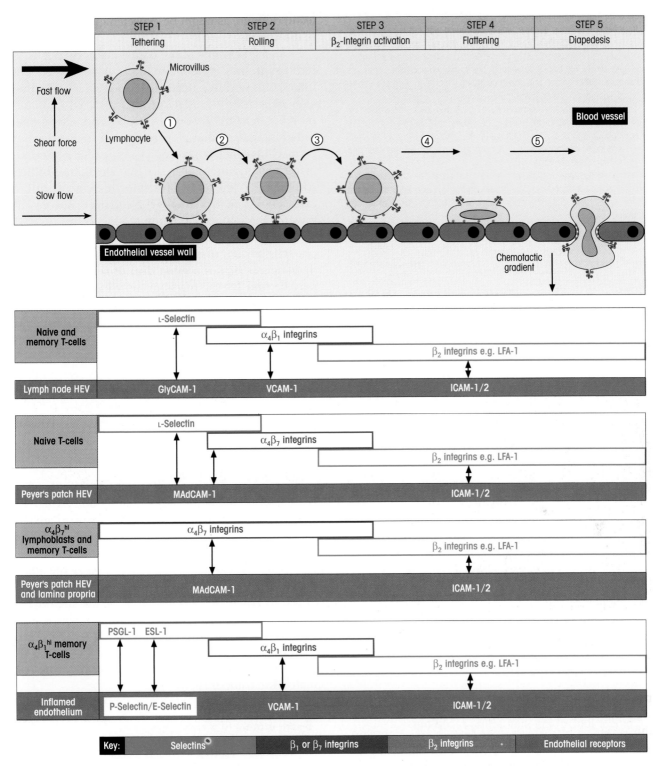

**Figure 8.6. Homing and transmigration of lymphocytes.** Fast-moving lymphocytes are tethered (Step 1) to the vessel walls of the tissue they are being guided to enter through an interaction between specific homing receptors and their ligands. After rolling along the surface of the endothelial cells making up the vessel wall, activation of β2 integrins (cf. table 8.2) occurs (Step 2) which leads to firm binding, cell flattening and (Step 3) migration of the lymphocyte between adjacent endothelial cells. Note that lymphoblasts and memory T-cells strongly positive for the α4β7 integrin can tether and roll

independently of selectins. Structures of some of the molecules concerned are given in figure 8.7.

LFA-1, lymphocyte function-associated molecule; ICAM-1/2, intercellular adhesion molecule 1 or 2; GlyCAM-1, glycosylation-dependent adhesion molecule; VCAM-1, vascular cell adhesion molecule; MAdCAM-1, mucosal addressin cell adhesion molecule-1; PSGL-1, P-selectin glycoprotein ligand; ESL-1, E-selectin ligand-1.

**Table 8.2. The integrin superfamily.**

In general, this group of molecules is concerned with tissue migration of cells during embryogenesis, tumor metastasis, wound healing, thrombosis and helper and cytotoxic T-cell functions. Some mediate intercellular adhesion and others adherence to extracellular matrix components. They are heterodimers with unique but related α-chains which can be grouped into subsets, each of which has a common β-chain.

The **VLA subfamily** took its name from VLA-1 and 2 which appeared as very late antigens (VLA) on T-cells, 2–4 weeks after *in vitro* activation. However, VLA-3, 4 and 5 belong to the same family but are not 'very late' and are found to different extents on lymphocytes, monocytes, platelets and probably hematopoietic progenitors.

A $Mg^{2+}$-dependent glutamate-containing structure (the so-called I domain) is present in many integrin subunits and seems to be the binding site for the Arg.Gly.Asp. (RGD) motif on many of the ligands essential for cell adhesion.

| Designation | Chain structure | β-chain phenotype | Cell type | Ligand |
|---|---|---|---|---|
| $β_1$ subfamily | | | | |
| VLA-1 | $α_1β_1$ | *CD29 | Widespread | LM, CO |
| VLA-2 | $α_2β_1$ | CD29 | Widespread | LM, CO |
| VLA-3 | $α_3β_1$ | CD29 | Widespread | FN, LM, CO |
| VLA-4 | $α_4β_1$ | CD29 | Leukocytes | FN, VCAM-1 |
| VLA-5 | $α_5β_1$ | CD29 | Widespread | FN |
| VLA-6 | $α_6β_1$ | CD29 | Widespread | LM |
| $β_2$ subfamily | | | | |
| LFA-1 | $α_Lβ_2$ | CD18 | Leukocytes | ICAM-1 |
| CR3 (Mac-1) | $α_Mβ_2$ | CD18 | Neutrophils Monocytes LGL | ICAM-1, C3bi |
| p150,95 | $α_Xβ_2$ | CD18 | Mononuclear phagocytes Neutrophils | FG |
| | $α_dβ_2$ | CD18 | Tissue macrophages | ICAM-3 |
| $β_3$ subfamily | | | | |
| VN receptor | $α_Vβ_3$ | CD61 | Widespread | VN |
| GPIIb/IIIa | $α_{IIb}β_3$ | CD61 | Megakaryocytes Platelets | FN,VN,FG,VWF |
| $β_7$ subfamily | | | | |
| | $α_4β_7$ | | Memory T lymphoblasts | MAdCAM-1 VCAM-1 FN |
| | $α_Eβ_7$ | | Intraepithelial T-cells | E-cadherin |

LM, laminin; CO, collagen; FN, fibronectin; LGL, large granular lymphocyte; VN, vitronectin; FG, fibrinogen; VWF, von Willebrand factor; *CD markers are explained on p. 151

## A closer look at the interacting receptors and their ligands

The structures of the major molecular families involved in the transmigration processes are outlined in figure 8.7.

The ligands for selectins tend to be mucinous molecules covered in dense patches of O-linked sugars. The selectins themselves appear to be the products of 'mongrel-like' evolution with motifs of quite diverse origin, but generally terminating in a lectin domain, as might be expected given the nature of the ligands.

P- and E-selectins allow $α_4β_1^{hi}$ memory T-cells to localize at sites of inflammation where subsequent interaction with the upregulated vascular cell adhesion molecule (VCAM-1) on the inflamed endothelium, and with various cytokine and chemokine inflammatory mediators presented on the surface of extracellular matrix proteoglycans, leads to lymphocyte transmigration. Secretion of heparanase by the stimulated T-cell could break down elements of the extracellular matrix thereby facilitating movement towards the sounds of inflammatory gunfire.

Homing previously activated and memory lymphocytes to sites of inflammation provoked by infectious agents makes a great deal of sense. The same may be said for the mechanisms which enable lymphocytes bearing receptors for mucosal-associated lymphoid tissue (MALT) to circulate within and between the collections of lymphoid tissue guarding the external body surfaces (figure 8.11). In this way, lymphocytes, such as those programmed to support the synthesis of IgA destined for secretion, will not waste time cooling their heels in encapsulated peripheral lymph nodes which play no role in mucosal protection.

## ENCAPSULATED LYMPH NODES

The encapsulated tissue of the lymph node contains a meshwork of reticular cells and their fibers organized into sinuses. These act as a filter for lymph draining the body tissues and possibly bearing foreign antigens which enters the subcapsular sinus by the afferent vessels and diffuses past the lymphocytes in the cortex to reach the macrophages of the medullary sinuses (figure 8.8) and thence the efferent lymphatics (figures 8.4 and 8.8). What is so striking about the organization of the lymph node is that the T- and B-lymphocytes are very largely separated into different anatomical compartments.

## B-cell areas

The follicular aggregations of B-lymphocytes are a prominent feature of the outer cortex. In the unstimulated node they are present as spherical collections of cells termed **primary nodules** (figure 8.8m), but after antigenic challenge they form **secondary follicles** (figure 8.8f) which consist of a corona or mantle of concentrically packed, resting small B-lymphocytes possessing both IgM and IgD on their surface surrounding a pale-staining **germinal center** (figure

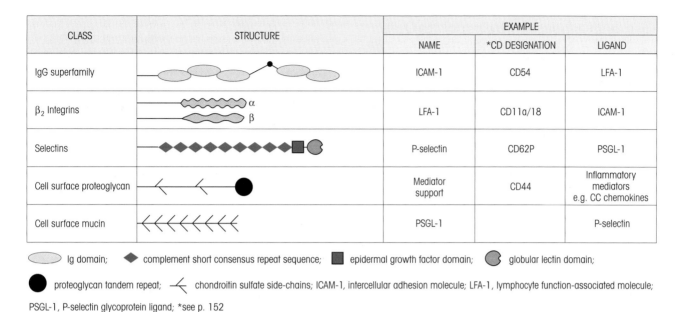

| CLASS | STRUCTURE | EXAMPLE | | |
|---|---|---|---|---|
| | | NAME | *CD DESIGNATION | LIGAND |
| IgG superfamily | | ICAM-1 | CD54 | LFA-1 |
| β₂ Integrins | α β | LFA-1 | CD11a/18 | ICAM-1 |
| Selectins | | P-selectin | CD62P | PSGL-1 |
| Cell surface proteoglycan | | Mediator support | CD44 | Inflammatory mediators e.g. CC chemokines |
| Cell surface mucin | | PSGL-1 | | P-selectin |

Ig domain;    ◆ complement short consensus repeat sequence;    ■ epidermal growth factor domain;    globular lectin domain;

● proteoglycan tandem repeat;    chondroitin sulfate side-chains; ICAM-1, intercellular adhesion molecule; LFA-1, lymphocyte function-associated molecule;

PSGL-1, P-selectin glycoprotein ligand; *see p. 152

**Figure 8.7. The structures of some leukocyte–endothelial cell adhesion molecules.**

8.8b). This contains large, usually proliferating, B-blasts, a minority of T-cells, scattered conventional reticular macrophages containing 'tingible bodies' of phagocytosed lymphocytes, and a tight network of specialized follicular dendritic cells with elongated cytoplasmic processes and few, if any, lysosomes. Germinal centers are greatly enlarged in secondary antibody responses and they are regarded as important sites of B-cell maturation and the generation of B-cell memory.

In the absence of antigen drive, the primary follicles are composed of a mesh of follicular dendritic cells (FDC; figure 8.8g) whose spaces are filled with recirculating but resting small B-lymphocytes. On priming with a single dose of a T-dependent antigen (i.e. antigen for which the B-cells require cooperation from T-helper cells; cf. p. 174), the FDC network can be colonized by as few as three primary B-blasts which undergo exponential growth, producing around 10⁴ so-called centroblasts (figure 8.8h) and displacing the original resting B-cells which now form the follicular mantle. These highly mitotic centroblasts with no surface IgD (sIgD) and very little sIgM, then differentiate into light zone centrocytes (figure 8.8i) which are noncycling and begin to upregulate their expression of sIg. At this stage there is very extensive apoptotic cell death, giving rise to DNA fragments which are visible as 'tingible bodies' within the macrophages which are the final resting place of the dead cells (figure 8.8j). The survivors undergo their final train-

ing in the apical light zone. A proportion of those which are shunted down the **memory** cell pathway take up residence in the mantle zone population, the remainder joining the recirculating B-cell pool. Other cells differentiate into plasmablasts with a well-defined endoplasmic reticulum, prominent Golgi apparatus and cytoplasmic Ig; these migrate to become plasma cells in the medullary cords of lymphoid cells which project between the medullary sinuses (figure 8.8d). This maturation of antibody-forming cells at a site distant from that at which antigen triggering has occurred is also seen in the spleen, where plasma cells are found predominantly in the marginal zone. One's guess is that this movement of cells acts to prevent the generation of high local concentrations of antibody within the germinal center, so avoiding neutralization of the antigen on the FDCs and premature shutting off of the immune response.

The remainder of the outer cortex is also essentially a B-cell area with scattered T-cells.

### T-cell areas

T-cells are mainly confined to a region referred to as the paracortical (or thymus-dependent) area (figure 8.8a); in nodes taken from children with selective T-cell deficiency (figure 15.5) or neonatally thymectomized mice (figure 8.8m), the paracortical region is seen to be virtually devoid of lymphocytes. Furthermore, when a T-cell-mediated response is elicited in a normal animal, say by a skin graft or by painting chemicals such as picryl chloride on the skin to

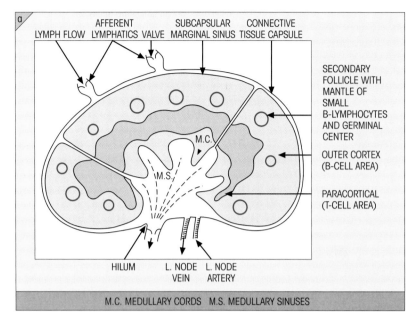

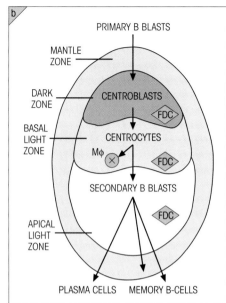

**Figure 8.8. Lymph node.** (a) Diagrammatic representation of section through a whole node. (b) Diagram showing differentiation of B-cells during passage through different regions of an active germinal center. FDC = follicular dendritic cell; Mφ = macrophage; × = apoptotic B-cell. *On facing page.* (c) Human lymph node, low-power view. (d) Medulla stained with methyl green (DNA)/pyronin (RNA) to show the basophilic (pink) cytoplasm of the plasma cells with their abundant ribosomes. (e) Medullary sinus of lymph node draining site of lithium carmine injection showing macrophages which have phagocytosed the colloidal dye (one is arrowed). (f) Secondary lymphoid follicle showing germinal center surrounded by a mantle of small B-lymphocytes stained by anti-human IgD labeled with horseradish peroxidase (brown color). There are few IgD-positive cells in the center but both areas contain IgM-positive B-lymphocytes. (g) The FDC network of a tonsil germinal center stained to show CD21 (CR2) expression using the immuno-alkaline phosphatase technique. The dense FDC network of the apical and basal light zones (LZ) contrasts with the finer FDC processes within the dark (DZ) and outer zones (OZ). (h) The germinal center dark zone showing closely packed centroblasts not separated by dendritic processes of FDC. Their variable size is typical of the dark zone. Occasional macrophages (Mφ) and mitoses (M) are seen. Giemsa stain. (i) The light zone of a human tonsil germinal center. The centrocytes are separated by the pale areas which are FDC and some macrophages. Apoptotic cells (A) exhibit condensed fragmented chromatin. Giemsa stain. (j) Germinal center from a reactive human lymph node stained with methyl green/pyronin. CC = centrocyte rich area; CB = centroblasts with abundant cytoplasmic RNA; A = apoptotic nuclei not obviously within macrophages; TBM = tingible body macrophages which have phagocytosed dead B-cells. (k) Node from mouse immunized with the thymus-independent antigen, pneumococcus polysaccharide SIII, revealing prominent stimulation of secondary follicles with germinal centers. (l) Methyl green/pyronin stain of lymph node draining site of skin painted with the contact sensitizer oxazolone, highlighting the generalized expansion and activation of the paracortical T-cells, the T-blasts being strongly basophilic. (m) The same study in a neonatally thymectomized mouse shows a lonely primary nodule (follicle) with complete lack of cellular response in the paracortical area.

SS = subcapsular sinus; PN = primary nodule; SF = secondary follicle; LM = lymphocyte mantle of SF; GC = germinal center; PA = paracortical area; MC = medullary cords; MS = medullary sinus; PC = plasma cell; SM = sinusoidal macrophage. ((c) Photographed by Professor PM. Lydyard; (d) and (f) photographed by Dr K.A. MacLennan; (e) courtesy of Anatomy Department, University College London Medical School; (g–j) kindly provided by Professor I.C.M. MacLennan; (k–m) courtesy of Dr M. de Sousa and Professor D.M.V. Parrott.)

induce contact hypersensitivity, there is a marked proliferation of cells in the thymus-dependent area and typical lymphoblasts are evident (figure 8.8l). In contrast, stimulation of antibody formation by the thymus-independent antigen, *Pneumococcus* polysaccharide SIII, leads to proliferation in the cortical lymphoid follicles with development of germinal centers, while the paracortical region remains inactive, reflecting the inability to develop cellular hypersensitivity to the polysaccharide (figure 8.8k). As expected, nodes taken from children with congenital hypogammaglobulinemia associated with failure of B-cell development conspicuously lack primary and secondary follicles.

## SPLEEN

On a fresh section of spleen, the lymphoid tissue forming the white pulp is seen as circular or elongated gray areas (figure 8.9b & c) within the erythrocyte-filled red pulp which consists of splenic cords lined with macrophages and venous sinusoids. As in the lymph node, T- and B-cell areas are segregated (figure 8.9a). The spleen is a very effective blood filter removing effete red and white cells and responding actively to blood-borne antigens, the more so if particulate. Plasmablasts and mature plasma cells are present in the marginal zone extending into the red pulp (figure 8.9c).

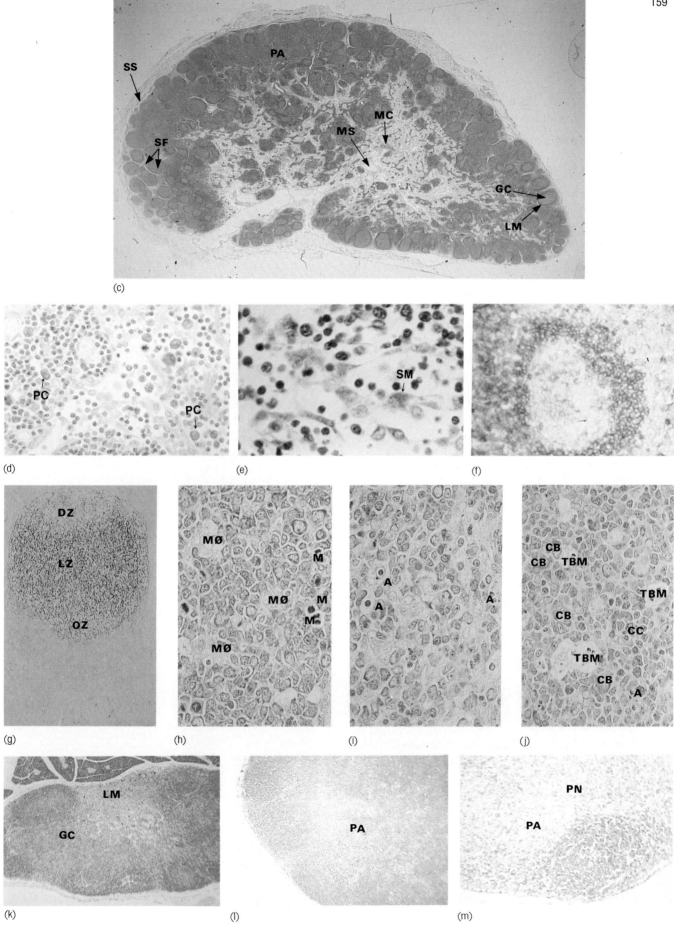

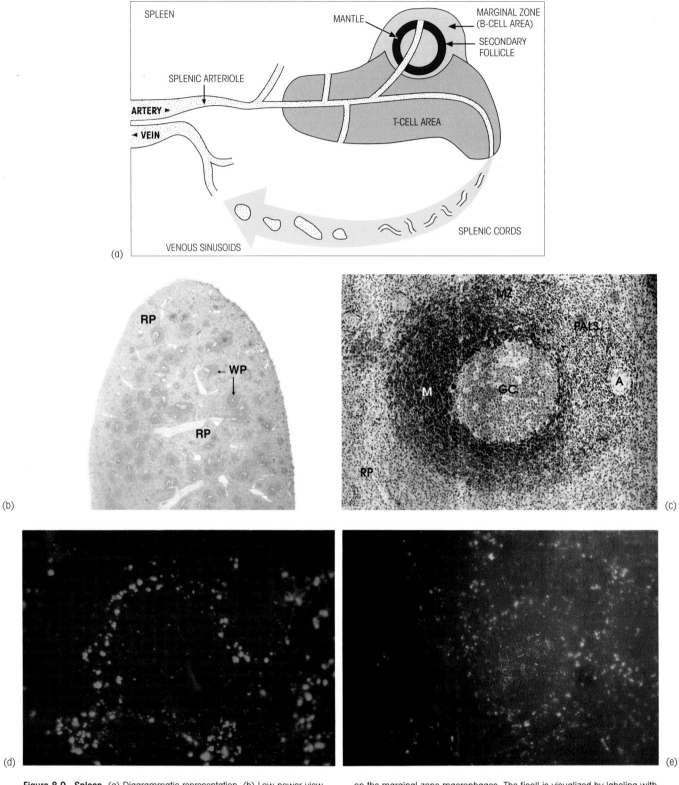

**Figure 8.9. Spleen.** (a) Diagrammatic representation. (b) Low-power view showing lymphoid white pulp (WP) and red pulp (RP). (c) High-power view of germinal center (GC) and lymphocyte mantle (M) surrounded by marginal zone (MZ) and red pulp (RP). Adjacent to the follicle, an arteriole (A) is surrounded by the periarteriolar lymphoid sheath (PALS) predominantly consisting of T-cells. Note that the marginal zone is only present above the secondary follicle. (d) Localization of the thymus-independent antigen, ficoll, on the marginal zone macrophages. The ficoll is visualized by labeling with the red fluorescent dye tetramethyl-rhodamine. (e) Preferential localization of a thymus-dependent antigen (conjugated to green fluorescein) on the follicular dendritic cells of a germinal center (ignore orange background fluorescence). ((b) Photographed by Professor P.M. Lydyard, (c) by Professor I.C.M. MacLennan; (d) and (e) kindly provided by Professor J.H. Humphrey.)

## MUCOSAL-ASSOCIATED LYMPHOID TISSUE (MALT)

The respiratory, alimentary and genitourinary tracts are guarded immunologically by subepithelial accumulations of lymphoid tissue which are not constrained by a connective tissue capsule (figure 8.10). These may occur as diffuse collections of lymphocytes, plasma cells and phagocytes throughout the lung and the lamina propria of the intestinal wall (figure 8.10a and b) or as more clearly organized tissue with well-formed follicles. In man, the latter includes the lingual, palatine and pharyngeal tonsils (figure 8.10c), the small intestinal Peyer's patches (figure 8.10d) and the appendix. It is generally agreed

that this MALT forms a separate interconnected secretory system within which cells committed to IgA or IgE synthesis may circulate.

In the gut, antigen enters the Peyer's patches (figure 8.10d) across specialized epithelial cells (cf. figure 8.15) and stimulates the antigen-sensitive lymphocytes. After activation these drain into the lymph and after a journey through the mesenteric lymph nodes and the thoracic duct, they pass from the bloodstream into the lamina propria (figure 8.11) where they become IgA-forming cells which, because they are now broadly distributed, protect a wide area of the bowel with protective antibody. The cells also appear in the lymphoid tissue of the lung and in other mucosal sites guided by the interactions of specific

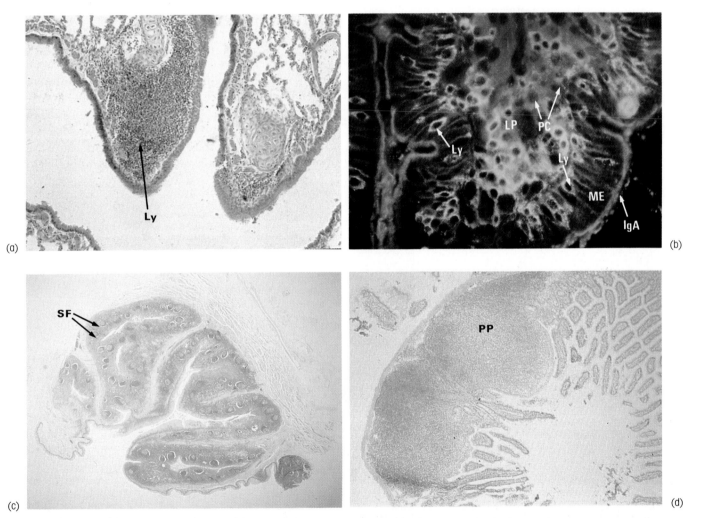

**Figure 8.10.  The IgA secretory immune system (MALT).** (a) Section of lung showing a diffuse accumulation of lymphocytes (Ly) in the bronchial wall. (b) Section of human jejunum showing lymphoid cells (Ly) stained green by a fluorescent anti-leukocyte monoclonal antibody, in the mucosal epithelium (ME) and in the lamina propria (LP). A red fluorescent anti-IgA conjugate stains the cytoplasm of plasma cells (PC) in the lamina propria and detects IgA in the surface mucus, altogether a super picture! (c) Low-power view of human tonsil showing the MALT with numerous secondary follicles (SF) containing germinal centers. (d) Peyer's patches (PP) in mouse ileum. The T-cell areas are stained brown by a peroxidase-labeled monoclonal antibody to Thy 1. ((a) Kindly provided by Professor P. Lydyard, (b) by Professor G. Janossy, (c) by Mr C. Symes and (d) by Dr E. Andrew.)

homing receptors with appropriate HEV addressins as discussed earlier.

### Intestinal lymphocytes

The intestinal **lamina propria** is home to a predominantly activated T-cell population rich in the $\alpha_4\beta_7$ integrin (cf. figure 8.6) and a phenotype roughly comparable to that of peripheral blood lymphocytes: viz. > 95% T-cell receptor (TCR) $\alpha\beta$ and a CD4:CD8 ratio of 7:3. There is also a generous sprinkling of activated B-blasts and plasma cells secreting IgA for transport by the poly-Ig receptor to the intestinal lumen (cf. p. 58).

**Intraepithelial lymphocytes** are quite a different kettle of fish. They are also mostly T-cells but 10–40% are TCR $\gamma\delta$ and 70% are CD8. They develop independently of the thymus and have a high degree of phenotypic heterogeneity including some novel T-cell subsets such as CD4+, 8+ TCR $\alpha\alpha$ and CD4−, 8+ TCR $\alpha\alpha$. The restriction element for antigen recognition tends to be the class I major histocompatibility complex (MHC)-unrelated CD1d molecule (cf. p. 99).

The relatively high proportion of TCR $\gamma\delta$ cells is also unusual. Since a number of cloned $\gamma\delta$-T-cells have been found to have specificity for heat-shock proteins, which are widely distributed in nature and usually highly immunogenic, it has been postulated that they act as a relatively primitive first line of defense at the outer surfaces of the body.

Reflect for a moment on the fact that roughly $10^{14}$ bacteria reside in the intestinal lumen of the normal adult human. That is a pretty impressive number of 'noughts' to swallow. Yet combined with the barrier of mucins produced by goblet cells and the protective zone of secreted IgA antibodies, these collections of intestinal lymphocytes represent a crucial line of defense. The development of various degrees of intestinal inflammation, for the most part restricted to the large bowel, which occurs in mice with disrupted genes for interleukin (IL)-2,10, TCR $\alpha/\beta$ or MHC class II must be telling us something.

## BONE MARROW CAN BE A MAJOR SITE OF ANTIBODY SYNTHESIS

A few days after a secondary response, activated memory B-cells can be shown to migrate to the bone marrow where they mature into plasma cells (figure 8.12). Bone marrow is a much neglected site of antibody synthesis which proves to be a major source of serum Ig, contributing up to 80% of the total Ig-secreting cells in the 100-week-old mouse. The peripheral lymphoid tissue responds rapidly to

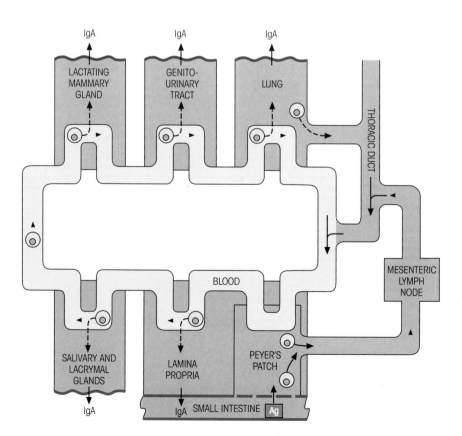

**Figure 8.11. Circulation of lymphocytes within the mucosal-associated lymphoid system.** Antigen-stimulated cells move from Peyer's patches (and probably lung and maybe all the mucosal member sites) to colonize the lamina propria and the other mucosal surfaces ( ∿∿∿ ).

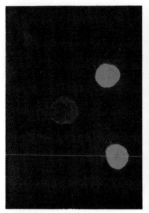 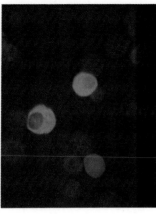

**Figure 8.12. Plasma cells in human bone marrow.** Cytospin preparation stained with rhodamine (orange) for IgA heavy chain and fluorescein (green) for lambda light chain. One cell is IgA.λ, another IgA.non-λ and the third is non-IgA.λ positive. (Photograph kindly supplied by Drs Benner, Hijmans and Haaijman.)

antigen, but only for a relatively short time, whereas bone marrow starts slowly and gives a long-lasting massive production of antibody to antigens which repeatedly challenge the host.

## THE ENJOYMENT OF PRIVILEGED SITES

Certain selected parts of the body, brain, anterior chamber of the eye and testis, have been designated **privileged immunological sites,** in the sense that antigens located within them do not provoke reactions against themselves. It has long been known for example that foreign corneal grafts can take up long-term residence, and a number of viruses have been expanded by repeated passage through animal brain.

Generally speaking, privileged sites are protected by rather strong blood–tissue barriers and low permeability to hydrophilic compounds and carrier-mediated transport systems. Functionally insignificant levels of complement reduce the threat of acute inflammatory reactions and unusually high concentrations of immunomodulators, such as transforming growth factor-β (TGFβ; cf. p. 181), endow macrophages with an immunosuppressive capacity. Lesley Brent put it rather well: 'It may be supposed that it is beneficial to the organism not to turn the anterior chamber or the cornea of the eye, or the brain, into an inflammatory battle-field, for the immunological response is sometimes more damaging than the antigen insult that provoked it.'

However, inflammatory reactions at the blood–tissue barrier can open the gates to invasion by immunological marauders — witness the inability of corneal grafts to take in the face of a local preexisting inflammation.

## THE HANDLING OF ANTIGEN

Where does antigen go when it enters the body? If it penetrates the tissues, it will tend to finish up in the draining lymph nodes. Antigens which are encountered in the upper respiratory tract or intestine are trapped by local mucosal-associated lymphoid tissue, whereas antigens in the blood provoke a reaction in the spleen. Macrophages in the liver will filter blood-borne antigens and degrade them without producing an immune response since they are not strategically placed with respect to lymphoid tissue.

### Macrophages are general antigen-presenting cells

'Classically', it has always been recognized that antigens draining into lymphoid tissue are taken up by macrophages. They are then partially, if not completely, broken down in the lysosomes; some may escape from the cell in a soluble form to be taken up by other antigen-presenting cells and a fraction may reappear at the surface, either as a large fragment or as a processed peptide associated with class II major histocompatibility molecules. Although resting, resident macrophages do not express MHC class II, antigens are usually encountered in the context of a microbial infectious agent which can induce the expression of class II by its adjuvant-like properties expressed through molecules such as bacterial lipopolysaccharide (LPS). There is general agreement that the antigen-presenting cell must bear antigen on its surface for effective activation of lymphocytes and we have ample evidence that antigen-pulsed macrophages can stimulate specific T- and B-cells both *in vitro* and when injected back *in vivo*. Some antigens, such as polymeric carbohydrates like ficoll, cannot be degraded because the macrophages lack the enzymes required; in these instances, specialized macrophages in the marginal zone of the spleen or the lymph node subcapsular sinus, trap and present the antigen to B-cells directly, apparently without any processing or intervention from T-cells (figure 8.9d).

## Interdigitating dendritic cells present antigen to T-lymphocytes

Notwithstanding this impressive account of the mighty macrophage in antigen presentation, there is one function where it is seemingly deficient, namely, the priming of naive lymphocytes. Animals which have been depleted of macrophages by selective uptake of liposomes containing the drug dichloromethylene diphosphonate, are as good as their controls with intact macrophages, in responding to T-dependent antigens. We must conclude that cells other than macrophages prime T-helper cells and it is now generally accepted that these belong to the group of dendritic cells which lack receptors for Ig and C3 but constitutively express high levels of the surface antigen-presenting heterodimers, MHC class I, II and CD1, are positive for the leukocyte common antigen (disclosing their bone marrow origin) and bear the β-integrin p150,95 and ICAM-3 adhesion molecules. Most importantly, they can display the surface costimulatory molecules B7-1/2 and CD40 (cf. pp. 169 and 177) and additionally secrete IL-2, IL-4 and γ-interferon (IFNγ), the significance of which for lymphocyte activation will I hope become blindingly clear in the following chapters. The dendritic cells have the awesome capacity to process four times their own volume of extracellular fluid in 1 hour thereby facilitating antigen capture and processing in their abundant intracellular MHC class II rich compartments (MIIC; cf. p. 94).

These are the crème de la crème of the antigen-presenting cells—the really gen-u-ine professionals—and if pulsed with soluble or allo-antigens or components of parasites, mycobacteria or tumors before injection into animals, usually produce stunning immune responses. In this connection, it is relevant to note that large numbers of these dendritic cells can be generated from peripheral blood by cultivation with granulocyte–macrophage colony-stimulating factor (GM-CSF) (cf. p. 181) to promote proliferation and IL-4 to suppress macrophage overgrowth; this means

that it is perfectly feasible to contemplate their use for immunotherapy, e.g. pulsing autologous dendritic cells with the patient's tumor antigens and then reinjecting them to evoke an immune response. There are hints of heterogeneity in the dendritic cell population. Some secrete IL-12 and would favor Th1 responses (cf. p. 184). It is also possible to derive MHC class I+II– lines which are potent stimulators of CD8 cytotoxic T-cells in the absence of CD4 helpers. It is worth noting that unlike macrophages which in a sense are 'brutal microbe crunchers', the dendritic cells are not strongly phagocytic (table 8.3) and they do need help from the macrophages in the preprocessing of particulate antigens, since these responses are completely abolished in macrophage-depleted animals.

The scenario for T-cell priming appears to be as follows. Peripheral immature dendritic cells such as the Langerhans' cells (cf. figure 2.6i), which bind to skin keratinocytes through surface expression of E-cadherin, can pick up and process antigen. As maturation proceeds, they lose their E-cadherin and travel as 'veiled' cells in the lymph (figure 8.13b) before settling down as interdigitating dendritic cells (IDC) in the paracortical T-cell zone of the draining lymph node (figure 8.13a). There, its maturation complete (figure 8.14), the IDC delivers the antigen with costimulatory signals for potent stimulation of naive specific T-cells which take advantage of the large surface area to bind to the MHC–peptide complex on the IDC membrane. Thus, dendritic cells from nodes draining the skin site of contact sensitization to picryl chloride can transfer sensitivity to a naive animal. It has also been shown that veiled cells isolated from gut lymphatics of appropriately infected rats were associated with *Salmonella* antigens. Sites of chronic T-cell inflammation seem to attract these cells, since abnormally high numbers are found closely adhering to activated T-lymphocytes in synovial tissue from patients with ongoing rheumatoid arthritis and in the glands of subjects with chronic autoimmune thyroiditis lesions.

There is a negative side to these dendritic cells.

**Table 8.3. Comparison of antigen handling by dendritic cells and macrophages.** (Based on Reis E., Sousa C., Austyn J.M. *et al.* (1992) *Seminars in Immunology* **4**, 230.)

| Function | Fresh Langerhans' cells | Cultured Langerhans' cells | Lymphoid interdigitating dendritic cells | Macrophages |
|---|---|---|---|---|
| Pinocytosis | +++ | + | ± | ++++ |
| Phagocytosis | + | – | – | ++++ |
| Antigen processing | +++ | – | – | ++ |
| T-cell priming | – | +++ | ++ | – |
| Ag presentation to activated cells | ++ | ++ | ++ | ++ |

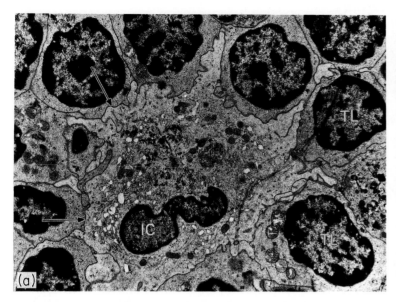
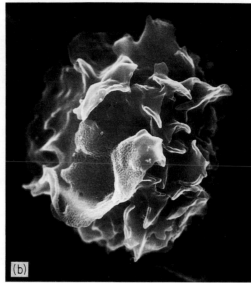

**Figure 8.13. Dendritic antigen-presenting cell.** (a) Interdigitating cell (IC) in the thymus-dependent area of the rat lymph node. This is thought to be an antigen-presenting cell derived from the Langerhans' cell in the skin and dendritic cells in other tissues, which travels to the node in the afferent lymph as a 'veiled' cell bearing antigen on its profuse surface processes. Intimate contacts are made with the surface membranes (arrows) of the surrounding T-lymphocytes (TL). The cytoplasm of the IC contains relatively few organelles and does not show Birbeck granules (racket-shaped cytoplasmic organelles, characteristic of the Langerhans' cell), but these granules appear after antigenic stimulation (× 2000). (b) Scanning electron micrograph of veiled cell. In contrast with these dendritic cells which present antigen to T-cells, the follicular dendritic cells in germinal centers stimulate B-cells. ((a) Reproduced with permission of the authors and publishers from Kamperdijk E.W.A., Hoefsmit E.Ch.H., Drexhage H.A. & Balfour B.H. (1980). In Van Furth R. (ed.) *Mononuclear Phagocytes*, 3rd edn. Rijhoff Publishers, The Hague. (b) Courtesy of Dr G.G. MacPherson.)

Nerve fibers containing calcitonin gene-related peptide, a neuropeptide vasodilator, impinge upon Langerhans' cells in the epidermis and inhibit antigen presentation. Do these then resemble ultraviolet irradiated dendritic cells in their ability to induce antigen-specific tolerance? Furthermore, there is every likelihood that dendritic cells within the thymus present self-peptides to developing autoreactive T-cells and trigger their apoptotic execution (known more gently as 'clonal abortion'; cf. p. 232).

Table 8.3 summarizes the properties of immature and mature dendritic cells in terms of their antigen handling, and compares them with macrophages. An important take-home message is that whereas dendritic cells at all stages of maturity and macrophages can present antigen to preactivated T-cells, only mature dendritic cells are capable of priming naive T-cells.

## Follicular dendritic cells stimulate B-cells in germinal centers

Secondary antibody responses can be boosted by quite small amounts of immunogen which complex with circulating antibody and fix C3 so that they localize very effectively on the surface of the follicular dendritic cells within the germinal centers of secondary follicles (figure 8.9e). These cells have very elongated processes which can make contact with numerous lymphocytes and their surface receptors for IgG Fc and iC3b enable them to trap the complexed antigen very efficiently and hold the antigen on their surface for extended periods, in keeping with the memory function of secondary follicles. Evidence for this notion may be derived from animals effectively depleted of complement by injection of cobra venom factor which contains the reptilian equivalent of C3b.

| BONE MARROW | BLOOD | THYMUS | | |
|---|---|---|---|---|
| | | | | Tolerance |
| | | NON-LYMPHOID TISSUE | LYMPH | LYMPH NODE |
| | | | BLOOD | SPLEEN |
| | | Ag processing | Migration | Immunostimulation |
| STEM CELLS | PRECURSORS | IMMATURE DC | MATURING DC | MATURE DC |

**Figure 8.14. Migration between tissues in relation to maturation of antigen-presenting capability of dendritic stem cells (DC).**

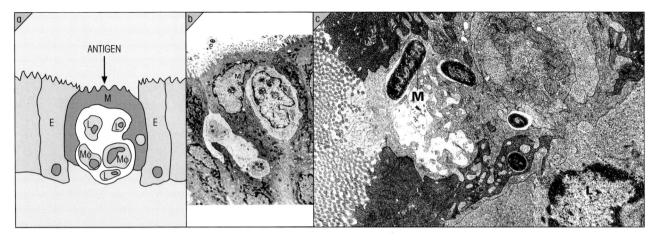

**Figure 8.15. M-cell within Peyer's patch epithelium.** (a) After uptake and transcellular transport by the M-cell, antigen is processed by macrophages and thence by dendritic cells which present antigen to T-cells in Peyer's patches and mesenteric lymph nodes. E = enterocyte; Mφ = macrophage; L = lymphocyte. (b) Electron photomicrograph of an M-cell (M in nucleus) with adjacent lymphocyte (L in nucleus). Note the flanking epithelial cells are both absorptive epithelial cells with a typical brush border. In some cases, proteases on the surface of the M-cells modify the pathogen so that it can adhere and be taken up by a sort of antigen sampling mechanism. Pathogenic *Salmonella* can invade and destroy M-cells, making a hole through which other bacteria can invade the underlying tissue. (Lead citrate and uranyl acetate, ×1600.) (c) An M-cell and an adjacent lymphocyte (L). A rod-shaped bacterium taken up from the intestinal lumen and packaged within an M-cell vesicle is indicated. (Lead citrate and uranyl acetate, ×4600.) ((a) Based on Sminia T. (1992) In Roitt I.M. & Delves P.J. (eds) *Encyclopedia of Immunology*, p. 107. Academic Press, London.)

This fires the alternative complement pathway by forming a complex with factor B but because of its insensitivity to the mammalian C3 inactivator, it persists long enough to discharge the feedback loop to exhaustion and deplete C3 completely. Such mice can neither localize antigen–antibody complexes on their follicular dendritic cells, nor generate B-memory cells in response to T-dependent antigens (see p. 174).

Classically, a secondary response would be initiated at the T-helper level by antigen, alone or as a complex, being taken up by dendritic cells and macrophages. However, the capture of immune complexes on the surface of **follicular dendritic cells** opens up an alternative pathway. One to three days after secondary challenge, the filamentous dendrites on the follicular cells to which the immune complexes are bound, form into beads which break off as 'immune-complex coated bodies'. These bind to and are processed by germinal center B-cells so that the antigen is now in a form in association with B-cell MHC class II, that can stimulate T-helper cells and kick off the secondary response. Cross-linking of B-cell surface receptors by the immune complexes may

also have an important function as we will see in chapter 9 (see figure 9.7).

## M-cells provide the gateway to the mucosal lymphoid system

As we have reflected already, the mucosal surface is in the front line facing a very unfriendly sea of microbes and, for the most part, antigens are excluded by the epithelium with its tight junctions and mucous layer. Gut lymphoid tissue, such as Peyer's patches, is separated from the lumen by a single layer of columnar epithelium interspersed with M-cells; these are specialized antigen-transporting cells with short, irregular microvillae, strong nonspecific esterase activity and no MHC class II. They overlay intraepithelial cells and macrophage-like dendritic cells (figure 8.15a and b). A diverse array of foreign material including bacteria is taken up by M-cells (figure 8.15c) and passed on to the underlying antigen-presenting cells which, in turn, migrate to the local lymphoid tissue to stir the appropriate lymphocytes into action.

## SUMMARY

### *The surface markers of cells in the immune system*

• Individual surface molecules are assigned a cluster of differentiation (CD) numbers defined by a cluster of monoclonal antibodies reacting with that molecule.

### *Organized lymphoid tissue*

• The complexity of immune responses is catered for by a sophisticated structure.
• Lymph nodes filter and screen lymph flowing from the

*(Continued)*

body tissues while spleen filters the blood.
- B- and T-cell areas are separated.
- B-cell structures appear in the lymph node cortex as primary nodules which become secondary follicles with germinal centers after antigen stimulation.
- Germinal centers with their meshwork of follicular dendritic cells expand B-cell blasts produced by secondary antigen challenge and direct their differentiation into memory cells and antibody forming plasma cells.

## Mucosal-associated lymphoid tissue

- Lymphoid tissue guarding the gastrointestinal tract is unencapsulated and somewhat structured (tonsils, Peyer's patches, appendix) or present as diffuse cellular collections in the lamina propria. Intraepithelial lymphocytes are mostly T-cells and include some novel subsets e.g. CD4$^-$8$^+$ TCR $\alpha\alpha$ which use CD1d as a restriction element for antigen presentation.
- Together with the subepithelial accumulations of cells lining the mucosal surfaces of the respiratory and genito-urinary tracts, this lymphoid tissue forms the 'secretory immune system' which bathes the surface with protective IgA antibodies.

## Other sites

- Bone marrow is a major site of antibody production.
- The brain, anterior chamber of the eye and testis are privileged sites in which antigens can be safely sequestered.

## Lymphocyte traffic

- Lymphocyte recirculation between the blood and lymphoid tissues is guided by specialized homing receptors on the surface of the high-walled endothelium of the postcapillary venules.
- Lymphocytes are tethered and then roll along the surface of the selected endothelial cells through interactions between selectins and integrins and their respective ligands. Flattening of the lymphocyte and transmigration across the endothelial cell follow LFA-1 activation.
- Entry of memory T-cells into sites of inflammation is facilitated by upregulation of integrin molecules ($\alpha_4\beta_1$ and LFA-1) on the lymphocyte and corresponding binding ligands on the vascular endothelium (VCAM-1 and ICAM-1/2 respectively).

## The handling of antigen

- Macrophages are general antigen-presenting cells for primed lymphocytes but cannot stimulate naive T-cells.
- This is effected by dendritic cells which process antigen, migrate to the draining lymph node and settle down as interdigitating dendritic cells which powerfully initiate primary T-cell responses.
- Follicular dendritic cells in germinal centers bind immune complexes to their surface through Ig and C3b receptors. The complexes are long-lived and provide a sustained source of antigenic stimulation for B-cells.
- Specialized antigen-transporting M-cells provide the gateway for antigens to the mucosal lymphoid tissue.

# FURTHER READING

Benner R., Hijmans W. & Haaijman J.J. (1981) The bone marrow: the major source of serum immunoglobulins, but still a neglected site of antibody formation. *Clinical and Experimental Immunology* **46**, 1–8.

Bradley L.M. & Watson S.R. (1996) Lymphocyte migration into tissue: the paradigm derived from CD4 subsets. *Current Opinion in Immunology* **8**, 312–320.

Caligaris-Cappio F. (1992) Germinal centres. In Roitt I.M. & Delves P.J. (eds) *Encyclopedia of Immunology*, p. 613. Academic Press, London.

Girard J-P. & Springer T.A. (1995) High endothelial (HEVs): specialized endothelium for lymphocyte migration. *Immunology Today* **16**, 449–457.

Hirsch E., Iglesias A. *et al.* (1996) Impaired migration but not differentiation of haematopoietic stem cells in the absence of $\beta_1$ integrins. *Nature* **380**(6570), 171–175.

Peters J.H., Gieseler R., Thiele B. & Steinbach F. (1996) Dendritic cells: from ontogenetic orphans to myelomonocytic descendants. *Immunology Today* **17**, 273–278.

Poussier P. & Julius M. (eds) (1995) T-cell development and selection in the intestinal epithelium. *Seminars in Immunology* **7**, 289–342.

Stingl G. (1995) Dendritic cells: a major story unfolds. *Immunology Today* **16**, 330–333.

Tew J.G. (ed.) (1992) Antigen trapping and presentation. *Seminars in Immunology* **4**, 203–274.

# C H A P T E R    9

# LYMPHOCYTE ACTIVATION

## IMMUNOCOMPETENT T- AND B-CELLS DIFFER IN MANY RESPECTS

These differences are sharply demarcated at the cell surface (table 9.1). The most clear-cut discrimination is established by reagents which recognize the antigen receptors, anti-CD3 for T-cells and anti-immunoglobulin for B-cells, and in laboratory practice these are the markers most often used to enumerate the two lymphocyte populations. The surface expression of receptors for Ig, C3b and certain viruses also distinguishes T- and B-cells, while the adventitious formation of rosettes through the binding of sheep erythrocytes to CD2 (figure 2.6e) is sometimes used for the detection and separation of T-cells.

Differences in the cluster of differentiation (CD) markers determined by monoclonal antibodies reflect disparate functional properties and in particular define specialized T-cell subsets. CD4 is a marker of T-helper cell populations which promote activation and maturation of B-cells and cytotoxic T-cells, and control antigen-specific chronic inflammatory reactions through stimulation of macrophages. CD4 molecules form subsidiary links with class II MHC on the cell presenting antigen. Similarly, the CD8 molecules on cytotoxic T-cells associate with major histocompatibility complex (MHC) class I (figure 9.1).

Attention should also be drawn to the so-called 'nonspecific mitogens' which activate populations and sometimes subpopulations of T- or B-cells in a way which is unrelated to the antigen specificity of the lymphocyte receptors because they react with constant, as distinct from highly variable, structures on the cell surface. For this reason, they are often termed polyclonal B- or T-cell activators (table 9.1). We have already drawn attention in Chapter 5 to the ability of superantigens such as staphylococcal

Table 9.1. Comparison of human T- and B-cells.

| | T | B |
|---|---|---|
| % in peripheral blood | 65–80 | 8–15 |
| **ANTIGEN RECEPTORS:** | | |
| Surface Ig | – | ++ |
| TCR/CD3 | ++ | – |
| **OTHER RECEPTORS:** | | |
| FcγRII | ± | ++ |
| C3b receptors (CR1, CR2) | ± | ++ |
| EBV receptors (=CR2) | – | ++ |
| Measles receptors | ++ | – |
| **OTHER MARKERS** | CD2 *4/5/*8/45 | CD *5/19/23/40/45 |
| MHC:  Class I | ++** | ++ |
|  Class II | ++** | ++ |
| POLYCLONAL ACTIVATION | anti-CD3 | anti-Ig |
| | phytohemagglutinin (PHA) | *Staph. aureus* (str. Cowan 1) |
| | pokeweed mitogen (PWM) | pokeweed mitogen (PWM) |
| | concanavalin A | |
| | *superantigen (e.g. enterotoxin) | EBV |

*subpopulation; **only activated cells; CD2 = receptor forming sheep cell rosettes; CR1/2 = complement receptors 1/2; EBV = Epstein–Barr virus.

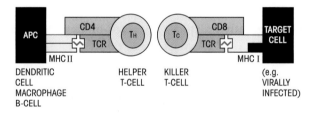

**Figure 9.1. Helper and killer T-cell subsets are restricted by MHC class.** CD4 on helpers contacts MHC class II; CD8 on killers associates with class I.

## T-LYMPHOCYTES AND ANTIGEN-PRESENTING CELLS INTERACT THROUGH SEVERAL PAIRS OF ACCESSORY MOLECULES

The affinity of an individual TCR for its specific MHC–antigen peptide complex is relatively low (figure 9.2) and a sufficiently stable association with the antigen-presenting cell (APC) can only be achieved by the interaction of complementary pairs of accessory molecules such as LFA-1/ICAM-1, CD2/LFA-3 and so on (figure 9.3). However, these molecular couplings are not necessarily concerned just with intercellular adhesion.

## THE ACTIVATION OF T-CELLS REQUIRES TWO SIGNALS

Antibodies to the TCR, either anti-idiotype or anti-CD3, when insolubilized by coupling to Sepharose, will not fully activate resting T-cells on their own. Addition of interleukin-1 (IL-1) now readily induces RNA and protein synthesis, the cell enlarges to a blast-like appearance, interleukin-2 (IL-2) synthesis begins and the cell moves from G0 into the G1 phase of the mitotic cycle. Thus, two signals are required for the activation of a resting T-cell (figure 9.3). Antigen in association with MHC class II on the surface of APCs is clearly capable of fulfilling these requirements. Complex formation between the TCR, antigen and MHC provides signal 1 through the receptor–CD3 complex and this is greatly enhanced by the coupling of CD4 with the MHC. The T-cell is now exposed to a costimulatory signal 2 from the APC. Although this could be IL-1, it would appear that the most potent costimulators are likely to be B7 on the APC binding

enterotoxins to act as polyclonal activators by stimulating all T-cells bearing certain T-cell receptor (TCR) Vβ families irrespective of their specificity for antigen.

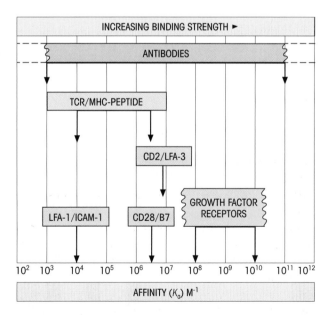

**Figure 9.2. The relative affinities of molecular pairs involved in interactions between T-lymphocytes and cells presenting antigen.** The range of affinities for growth factors and their receptors, and of antibodies, are shown for comparison. (Based on Davies M.M. & Chien Y.-H. (1993) *Current Opinion in Immunology* **5**, 45.)

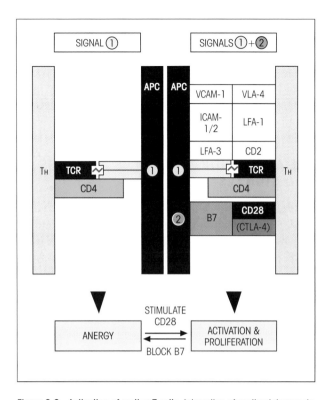

**Figure 9.3. Activation of resting T-cells.** Interaction of costimulatory molecules leads to activation of resting T-lymphocyte by antigen-presenting cell (APC) on engagement of the T-cell receptor (TCR) with its antigen–MHC complex. Engagement of the TCR signal 1 without accompanying costimulatory signal 2 leads to anergy. Note, a cytotoxic rather than a helper T-cell would, of course, involve coupling CD8 to MHC I. Engagement of CTLA-4 with B7 downregulates signal 1. LFA-1/2 = lymphocyte function associated molecule-1/2; ICAM-1/2 = intercellular adhesion molecule-1/2; VLA-4 = very late integrin antigen-4; VCAM-1 = vascular cell adhesion molecule-1. (Based on Liu Y. & Linsley P.S. (1992) *Current Opinion in Immunology* **4**, 265–270.)

to CD28. Thus activation of resting T-cells can be blocked by anti-B7; surprisingly, this renders the T-cell **anergic**, i.e. unresponsive to any further stimulation by antigen. As we shall see in later chapters, the principle that two signals activate but one may induce anergy in an antigen-specific cell, provides a potential for targeted immunosuppressive therapy. Unlike resting T-lymphocytes, **activated T-cells proliferate in response to a *single* signal**.

Adhesion molecules such as ICAM-1, VCAM-1 and LFA-3 are not themselves costimulatory but augment the effect of other signals; an important distinction.

## PROTEIN TYROSINE PHOSPHORYLATION IS AN EARLY EVENT IN T-CELL SIGNALING

The conversion of phosphorylase *b* to the active *a* form by phosphorylation originally drew attention to the importance of protein phosphorylation for the regulation of cellular processes and we now know that transforming proteins of certain oncogenic retroviruses and receptors for a number of growth factors or hormones have intrinsic protein tyrosine kinase (PTK) activity. If such a kinase phosphorylates and thereby activates a kinase precursor, which in turn switches on a second kinase precursor and so on, one has the basis for an enzymic phosphorylation cascade which could amplify an initial signal just as the proteolytic enzyme cascade amplifies the triggering event of the complement system (cf. p. 11).

The initial signal for T-cell activation through the TCR is greatly enhanced by cross-linking the TCR with CD4 which brings the CD4-associated PTK, p56lck, close to the ζ-chains of CD3. Immunostimulatory tyrosine-based activation motifs (ITAMs) on the ζ-chains become phosphorylated and bind to the SH2

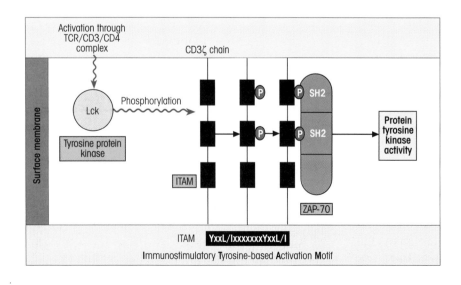

**Figure 9.4. Signals through the TCR/CD3/CD4/8 complex initiate a tyrosine protein kinase (TPK) cascade.** The TPK lck phosphorylates the tyrosine within the ITAM sequences of CD3 ζ-chains. These bind the ζ-associated protein (ZAP-70) through its SH2 groups and this in turn acquires TPK activity for downstream phosphorylation of later components in the chain. The other CD3 chains each bear a single ITAM.

domains of ZAP-70 which now becomes an active PTK (figure 9.4) capable of initiating a series of downstream biochemical events.

The CD4 lck may also be responsible for activating the p21 ras protein. The key role of these tyrosine kinases is underlined by the ability of the PTK inhibitor herbimycin-A to block proximal TCR-mediated signaling events such as phosphatidylinositol turnover as well as later manifestations like IL-2 production.

## DOWNSTREAM EVENTS FOLLOWING TCR SIGNALING

### The phosphatidylinositol pathway

Within 15 seconds of TCR stimulation, **phospholipase C$\gamma$1**, an enzyme which activates the phosphatidylinositol pathway, is phosphorylated and its catalytic activity increased. This early increase in phospholipase C activity accelerates the hydrolysis of phosphatidylinositol diphosphate to diacylglycerol and inositol triphosphate (figure 9.5). The triphosphate binds to specific receptors on specialized calcium storage vesicles and triggers the release of $Ca^{2+}$ into the cytosol; this is supplemented by an influx from the external milieu. The **raised $Ca^{2+}$** level has at least two consequences. First, it synergizes with diacylglycerol to activate **protein kinase C** (PKC); second, it increases the activity of a very important enzyme, **calcineurin**.

### p21 ras function

Following TCR signaling, there is an early increase in the level of active p21 ras–GTP complexes which regulate pivotal enzymes, *mitogen-activated protein kinases* (**MAPK** alias JNK or ERK, see legend figure 9.5) sequentially through Raf-1 and MAP kinase kinase. Thus, the phosphorylation amplifying cascade would make Raf-1 a MAP kinase kinase kinase or MAPKKK! MAP kinase may also be influenced by CD28 operating through phosphoinositide 3-kinase, and by protein kinase C and other factors as suggested in figure 9.5; it should be stressed, however, that these pathways are not yet inscribed in tablets of stone.

### Control of IL-2 gene transcription

Transcription of IL-2 is one of the key elements in preventing the signaled T-cell from lapsing into anergy and is controlled by multiple receptors for transcriptional factors in the promoter region (figure 9.5). The key enzyme MAP kinase phosphorylates the Jun protooncogene, which then binds as a binary complex with Fos to the **AP-1** site, deletion of which abrogates 90% of IL-2 enhancer activity.

Under the influence of calcineurin, the cytoplasmic component of the *nuclear factor of activated T-cells* (**NFAT$_C$**) becomes activated and translocates to the nucleus where it forms a binary complex with NFAT$_n$, its partner which is constitutively expressed in the nucleus. The NFAT complex binds to two different IL-2 regulatory sites (figure 9.5). Note here that the calcineurin effect is blocked by the anti-T-cell drugs cyclosporin and FK506 (see chapter 17). PKC brings about the liberation of another transcriptional factor NF$\kappa$B from its inhibitor I$\kappa$B. In addition, the ubiquitous transcriptional factor **Oct-1** interacts with specific octamer binding sequence motifs.

We have concentrated on IL-2 transcription as an early and central consequence of T-cell activation but finally, many genes become activated leading to T-cell proliferation and the synthesis of several other cytokines and their receptors (see chapter 10).

### Further thoughts on the control of T-cell triggering

*A serial TCR engagement model for T-cell activation*

I have already commented that the major docking forces which conjugate the APC and its T-lymphocyte counterpart must come from the complementary accessory molecules such as ICAM-1, LFA-1 and LFA-3/CD2, rather than through the relatively low affinity TCR–MHC/peptide links. Nonetheless, cognate antigen recognition by the TCR remains a *sine qua non* for T-cell activation. Fine, but how can as few as 100 MHC/peptide complexes on an APC, through their low affinity complexing with TCRs, effect the Herculean task of sustaining a raised intracellular calcium flux for the 60 minutes required for full cell activation? Any fall in calcium flux as may be occasioned by adding an antibody to the MHC, and NFAT$_c$ dutifully returns from the nucleus to its cytoplasmic location, so aborting the activation process.

Surprisingly, Valitutti and Lanzavecchia have shown that as few as 100 MHC/peptide complexes on an APC can downregulate 18 000 TCRs on its cognate T-lymphocyte partner. They suggest that each MHC/peptide complex can serially engage up to 200 TCRs. In their model, conjugation of an MHC/peptide dimer with two TCRs (cf. p. 99) activates signal transduction, phosphorylation of CD3 $\zeta$-

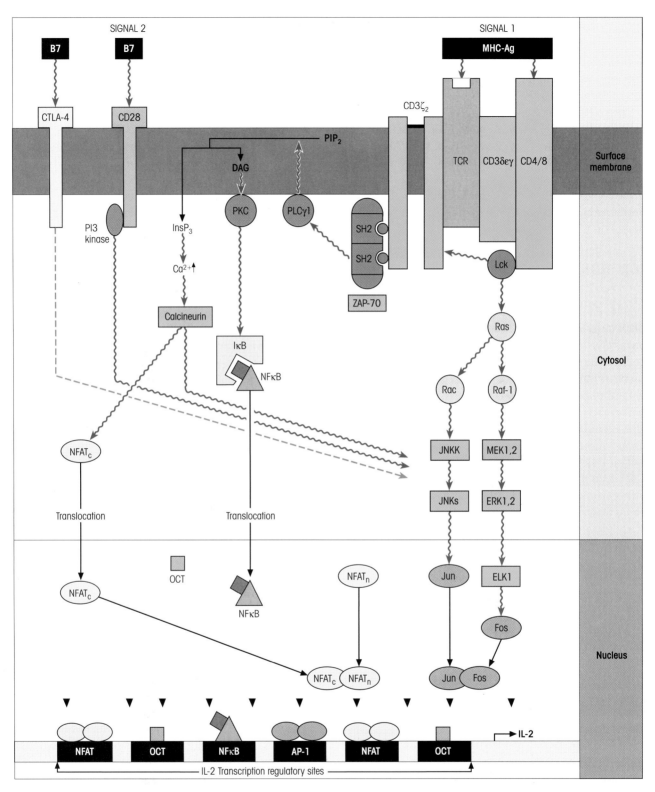

**Figure 9.5. T-cell signaling leads to activation.** The signals through the MHC–antigen complex and costimulator B7, initiate a protein kinase cascade and a rise in intracellular calcium; these activate transcription factors which control entry in the cell cycle from G0 and regulate the expression of IL-2 and many other cytokines (see text). Lck = *src*-related tyrosine protein kinase (TPK); ZAP-70 = $\zeta$ chain-associated protein kinase; PLC$\gamma$1 = phospholipase C; PIP$_2$ = phosphatidylinositol diphosphate; InsP$_3$ = inositol triphosphate; DAG = diacylglycerol; PKC = protein kinase C; PI3 kinase = phosphoinositide-3 kinase; Raf-1 = a kinase which activates a series of kinases through MEK1,2 and ERK1,2 (extracellular signal regulated kinase) and ELK1, and finally the transcription factor Fos; Rac phosphorylates JNKK,

the kinase which activates JNK (jun kinase) and finally the transcription factor jun which, complexed with fos binds to the AP-1 transcription site; NFAT$_c$ is the resting cytoplasmic component of the nuclear factor of activated T-cells which translocates to the nucleus when activated by calcineurin and complexes with the nuclear component NFAT$_n$ and then binds to the NFAT transcription sites. PKC and possibly calcineurin release NF$\kappa\beta$ (nuclear factor $\kappa\beta$) from its inhibitor I$\kappa\beta$ whence it translocates to the nucleus and binds to a specific regulatory site; ● = phosphate group; ■ = octamer 1,2 transcription factors (an Oct binding factor OBF-1 acts as a B-cell co-activator and is essential for adequate antibody responses and germinal center formation as shown by 'knockouts'). B7 incites a negative signal through CTLA-4.

chain with subsequent downstream events, and then downregulation of those TCRs. Intermediate affinity binding favors dissociation of the MHC/peptide, freeing it to engage and trigger another TCR, so sustaining the required intracellular activation events. The model for **agonist** action would also explain why peptides giving interactions of lower or higher affinity than the optimum could behave as **antagonists** (figure 9.6). The important phenomenon of modified peptides behaving as **partial agonists** with differential effects on the outcome of T-cell activation, is addressed in the legend to figure 9.6.

### Damping T-cell enthusiasm

I have frequently reiterated the premise that no self-respecting organism would permit the operation of an expanding enterprise such as a proliferating T-cell population without some sensible controlling mechanisms.

One such is the signal generated through B7–CTLA-4 coupling (figure 9.5), although the mecha-

nism is still unknown. Undoubtedly, phosphatases can undo the work of kinases and it is satisfying to note that the MAP kinase-mediated activation of gene transcription stimulates the production of a MAP kinase phosphatase with dual specificity for threonine and tyrosine phosphates which of course inactivates the MAP kinase itself.

Tempting though it might be, phosphatases should not automatically be equated with downregulation of a phosphorylation cascade. The observation that T-cell mutants lacking CD45 do not possess signal transduction capacity was at first sight deemed to be strange because CD45 has phosphatase activity and was thought thereby to downregulate signaling. However, the predominant form of the lck kinase in CD45-deficient cells is phosphorylated on tyrosine-505 which is a negative regulatory site for kinase activity; hence dephosphorylation by CD45 may activate the lck enzyme and the paradox is resolved.

## B-CELLS RESPOND TO THREE DIFFERENT TYPES OF ANTIGEN

### 1 Type 1 thymus-independent antigens

Certain antigens, such as bacterial lipopolysaccharides, at a high enough concentration, have the ability to activate a substantial proportion of the B-cell pool polyclonally, i.e. without reference to the antigen specificity of the surface receptor hypervariable regions. They do this through binding to a surface molecule which bypasses the early part of the biochemical pathway mediated by the specific antigen receptor. At concentrations which are too low to cause polyclonal activation through unaided binding to these mitogenic bypass molecules, the B-cell population with Ig receptors specific for these antigens will selectively and passively focus them on their surface where the resulting high local concentration will suffice to drive the activation process (figure 9.7a).

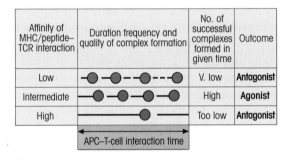

**Figure 9.6. Serial triggering model of TCR activation** (Valitutti S. & Lanzavecchia A. (1995) *The Immunologist* **3**, 122). Intermediate affinity complexes between MHC/peptide and TCR survive long enough for a successful activation signal to be transduced by the TCR and the MHC/peptide dissociates and fruitfully engages another TCR. A sustained high rate of formation of successful complexes is required for full T-cell activation. Low-affinity complexes have a short half-life which either has no effect on the TCR or produces inactivation, perhaps through partial phosphorylation of ζ-chains. (⬤= successful TCR activation; ⬤ = TCR inactivation;—= no effect: the length of the horizontal bar indicates the lifetime of that complex). Being of low affinity, they recycle rapidly and engage and inactivate a large number of TCRs. High-affinity complexes have such a long lifetime before dissociation that insufficient numbers of successful triggering events occur. Thus modified peptide ligands of either low or high affinity can act as antagonists by denying the agonist access to adequate numbers of vacant TCRs. Some modified peptides act as partial agonists in that they produce differential effects on the outcomes of T-cell activation. For example, a single residue change in a hemoglobin peptide reduced IL-4 secretion 10-fold but completely knocked out T-cell proliferation. The mechanism presumably involves incomplete or inadequately transduced phosphorylation events occurring through truncated half-life of TCR engagement, allosteric effects on the MHC/TCR partners, or orientational misalignment of the peptide within the complex. (Germain R.N., Levine E.H. & Madrenas J. (1995) *The Immunologist* **3**, 113.)

### 2 Type 2 thymus-independent antigens

Certain linear antigens which are not readily degraded in the body and which have an appropriately spaced, highly repeating determinant—*Pneumococcus* polysaccharide, ficoll, D-amino acid polymers and polyvinylpyrrolidone, for example — are also thymus independent in their ability to stimulate B-cells directly without the need for T-cell involvement. They persist for long periods on the surface of specialized macrophages located at the subcapsular sinus of the lymph nodes and the splenic marginal zone

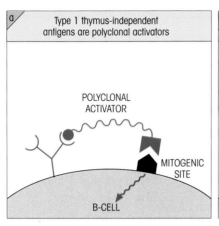

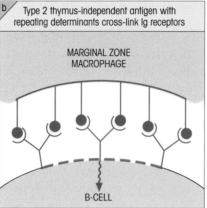

**Figure 9.7. B-cell recognition of (a) Type 1 and (b) Type 2 thymus-independent antigens.** The complex gives a sustained signal to the B-cell because of the long half-life of this type of molecule. ∿∿▶ = activation signal; ⌐⅄ = surface Ig receptor; ▬ ▬ ▬ = cross-linking of receptors.

(figure 8.9d), and can bind to antigen-specific B-cells with great avidity through their multivalent attachment to the complementary Ig receptors which they cross-link (figure 9.7b).

In general, the thymus-independent antigens give rise to predominantly low affinity IgM responses, some IgG3 in the mouse, and relatively poor, if any, memory. Neonatal B-cells do not respond well to type 2 antigens and this has important consequences for the efficacy of carbohydrate vaccines in young children.

## 3  Thymus-dependent antigens

### The need for collaboration with T-helper cells

Many antigens are thymus-dependent in that they provoke little or no antibody response in animals which have been thymectomized at birth and have few T-cells (Milestone 9.1). Such antigens cannot fulfil the molecular requirements for direct stimulation;

they may be univalent with respect to the specificity of each determinant; they may be readily degraded by phagocytic cells; and they may lack mitogenicity. If they bind to B-cell receptors, they will sit on the surface just like a hapten and do nothing to trigger the B-cell (figure 9.8). Cast your mind back to the definition of a hapten—a small molecule like dinitrophenyl (DNP) which binds to preformed antibody (e.g. the surface receptor of a specific B-cell) but fails to stimulate antibody production (i.e. stimulate the B-cell). Remember also that haptens become immunogenic when coupled to an appropriate carrier protein (see p. 81). Building on the knowledge that both T- and B-cells are necessary for antibody responses to thymus-dependent antigens (Milestone 9.1), we now know that the carrier functions to stimulate T-helper cells which cooperate with B-cells to enable them to respond to the hapten by providing accessory signals (figure 9.8). It should also be evident from figure 9.8 that while one determinant on a typical protein antigen is behaving as a hapten in binding to the B-cell, the other determinants subserve a carrier function in recruiting T-helper cells.

### Antigen processing by B-cells

The need for **physical linkage of hapten and carrier** strongly suggests that T-helpers must recognize the carrier determinants on the responding B-cell in order to provide the relevant accessory stimulatory signals. However, since T-cells only recognize processed membrane-bound antigen in association with MHC molecules, the T-helpers cannot recognize native antigen bound simply to the Ig-receptors of the B-cell as naively depicted in figure 9.8. All is not lost, however, since **primed B-cells can present antigen to T-helper cells** — in fact, they work at much lower antigen concentrations than conventional presenting

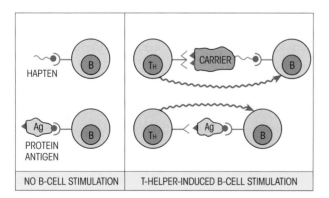

**Figure 9.8. T-helper cells cooperate through protein carrier determinants to help B-cells respond to hapten or equivalent determinants on antigens by providing accessory signals.** (For simplicity we are ignoring the MHC component and epitope processing in T-cell recognition, but we won't forget it.)

## Milestone 9.1 —T–B Collaboration for Antibody Production

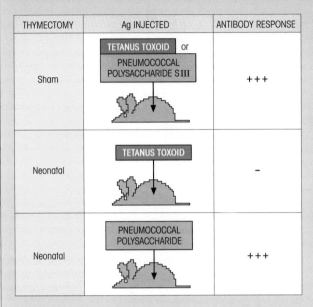

**Figure M9.1.1. The antibody response to some antigens is thymus-dependent and to others, thymus-independent.** The response to tetanus toxoid in the neonatally thymectomized animals could be restored by injection of thymocytes.

In the 1960s, as the mysteries of the thymus were slowly unravelled, our erstwhile colleagues pushing back the frontiers of knowledge discovered that neonatal thymectomy in the mouse abrogated not only the cellular rejection of skin grafts, but also the antibody response to some but not all antigens (figure M9.1.1). Subsequent investigations showed that both thymocytes and bone marrow cells were needed for optimal antibody responses to such **thymus-dependent antigens** (figure M9.1.2). By carrying out these transfers with cells from animals bearing a recognizable chromosome marker (T6), it became evident that the antibody forming cells were derived from the bone marrow inoculum, hence the nomenclature 'T' for **T**hymus-derived lymphocytes and 'B' for antibody-forming cell precursors originating in the **B**one marrow. This convenient nomenclature has stuck even though bone marrow contains embryonic T-cell precursors since the immunocompetent T- and B-cells differentiate in the thymus and bone marrow respectively (see Chapter 12).

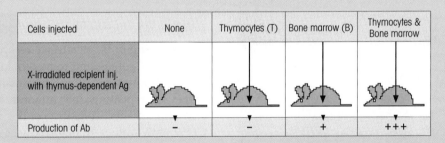

**Figure M9.1.2. The antibody response to a thymus-dependent antigen requires two different cell populations.** Different populations of cells from a normal mouse histocompatible with the recipient (i.e. of the same H-2 haplotype) were injected into recipients which had been X-irradiated to destroy their own lymphocyte responses. They were then primed with a thymus-dependent antigen such as sheep red blood cells (i.e. an antigen which fails to give a response in neonatally thymectomized mice; figure M9.1.1) and examined for the production of antibody after 2 weeks. The small amount of antibody synthesized by animals receiving bone marrow alone is due to the presence of thymocyte precursors in the cell inoculum which differentiate in the intact thymus gland of the recipient.

cells because they can focus antigen through their surface receptors. They must therefore be capable of 'processing' the antigen and the current view is that antigen bound to surface Ig is internalized in endosomes which then fuse with vesicles containing MHC class II molecules with their invariant chain. Processing of the protein antigen then occurs as described in Chapter 5 (see figure 5.17) and the resulting antigenic peptide is then recycled to the surface in association with the class II molecules where it is available for

recognition by specific T-helpers (figures 9.9 and 9.10). The need for the physical union of hapten and carrier is now revealed; the hapten leads the carrier to be processed into the cell which is programmed to make antihapten antibody and, following stimulus by the T-helper-recognizing processed carrier, it will carry out its program and ultimately produce antibodies which react with the hapten (is there no end to the wiliness of nature?!).

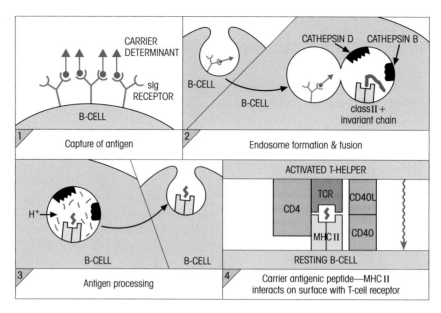

**Figure 9.9. B-cell handling of a thymus-dependent antigen.** Antigen captured by the surface Ig receptor is internalized within an endosome, processed and expressed on the surface with MHC class II (cf. figure 5.17). Costimulatory signals through the CD40–CD40L interaction are required for activation of the resting cell by the T-helper. sIg cross-linking by antigen on the surface of an antigen-presenting cell is likely during secondary responses within the germinal centers when complexes with C3b on follicular dendritic cells interact with B-lymphoblasts (cf. figure 8.9). ⟿ = activation signal; ⅄⅄⅄ = cross-linking of receptors.

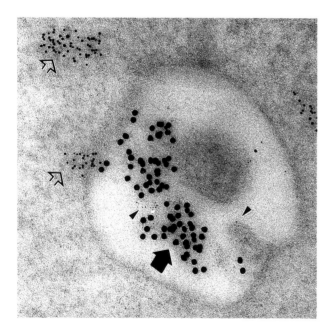

**Figure 9.10. Demonstration that endocytosed B-cell surface Ig receptors enter cytoplasmic vesicles geared for antigen processing.** Surface IgG was cross-linked with goat anti-human Ig and rabbit anti-goat Ig conjugated to 15-nm gold beads (large, dark arrow). After 2 minutes the cell sections were prepared and stained with anti-HLA-DR invariant chain (2-nm gold; arrowhead) and anti-cathepsin B (5-nm gold; clear arrow). Thus the internalized IgG is exposed to proteolysis in a vesicle containing class II molecules. The presence of invariant chain shows that the class II molecules derive from the endoplasmic reticulum and Golgi, not from the cell surface. Note the clever use of different-sized gold particles to distinguish the antibodies used for localizing the various intravesicular proteins, etc. (Photograph reproduced with permission from the authors and the publishers from Guagliardi L.E. *et al.* (1990) *Nature* **343**, 133. Copyright © 1990 Macmillan Magazines Ltd.)

## THE NATURE OF B-CELL ACTIVATION

### B-cells are stimulated by cross-linking surface Ig

Cross-linking of B-cell surface receptors, for example by anti-IgM conjugated to insoluble Sepharose particles or by polymeric type 2 thymus-independent antigens with repeating determinants, induces the early activation events. Coligation of the pan-B-cell marker CD19 with surface Ig (sIg) reduces the threshold for cell activation 100-fold. *In vivo* this could be brought about by bridging the Ig and CR2 complement receptors on the B-cell surface by antigen–C3b complexes bound to the surface of APC since CD19 and CR2 molecules enjoy mutual association. Current chit-chat likens CD19 to CD4, which is thought to deliver associated tyrosine kinase to the TCR. B-cells contain at least three src family kinases, fyn, lyn and blk, of which just the latter is specific for the B-lineage. Within 1 minute of surface Ig ligation, blk activity shoots up 5- to 8-fold and there is rapid phosphorylation of the sIg receptor chains Ig-$\alpha$ and Ig-$\beta$ and of phospholipase-C$\gamma$2, which kicks off the phosphatidylinositol 4,5-diphosphate pathway. Just as in the T-cell, this generates inositol triphosphate and diacylglycerol with a subsequent rise in intracellular calcium and activation of phosphokinase C (cf. figure 9.5). The $\kappa$-gene enhancer binding protein NF$\kappa$B, which exists as a dimer bound to an inhibitor in the cytoplasm, releases the inhibitor on activation of the protein kinase and moves into the nucleus where its appearance is associated with κ-gene transcription.

This cross-linking model seems appropriate for an understanding of stimulation by type 2 thymus-independent antigens, since their repeating determinants ensure strong binding to and cross-linking of multiple Ig receptors on the B-cell surface to form aggregates which persist owing to the long half-life of the antigen and sustain the high intracellular calcium needed for activation. On the other hand, type 1 T-independent antigens, like the T-cell polyclonal activators, probably bypass the specific receptor and act directly on downstream molecules such as diacylglycerol and protein kinase C since Ig-α and Ig-β are not phosphorylated.

## T-helper cells activate resting B-cells

T-dependent antigens pose a different problem, since they are usually univalent with respect to B-cell receptors, i.e. each epitope appears once on a monomeric protein, and as a result they cannot cross-link the surface Ig. However, we have discussed in some detail how antigen captured by a B-cell receptor can be internalized and processed for surface presentation as a peptide complexed with class II MHC (cf. figure 9.9). This can now be recognized by the TCR of a carrier-specific T-helper cell and with the assistance of costimulatory signals arising from the interaction of **CD40 with its ligand CD40L** (cf. figure 9.9), B-cell activation is ensured.

In effect, the B-lymphocyte is acting as an antigen-presenting cell and, as mentioned above, it is very efficient because of its ability to concentrate the antigen by focusing onto its surface Ig. Nonetheless, although a preactivated T-helper can mutually interact with and stimulate a resting B-cell, a *resting* T-cell can only be triggered by a B-cell that has acquired the B7 co-stimulator and this is only present on activated, not resting B-cells.

Presumably the immune complexes on follicular dendritic cells in germinal centers of secondary follicles can be taken up by the B-cells for presentation to T-helpers, but additionally, the complexes could cross-link the sIg of the B-cell blasts and drive their proliferation in a T-independent manner. This would be enhanced by the presence of C3 in the complexes since the B-cell complement receptor (CR2) is comitogenic.

## SUMMARY

*Immunocompetent T- and B-cells differ in many respects*

• Markers relating to the antigen-specific receptors TCR/CD3 on T-cells and surface Ig on B-cells provide clear discrimination.
• They differ in their receptors for C3b, IgG and certain viruses.
• There are distinct polyclonal activators of T-cells (concanavalin A, PHA, anti-CD3, superantigen) and of B-cells (anti-Ig, Epstein–Barr virus).

*T-lymphocytes and antigen-presenting cells interact through pairs of accessory molecules*

• The docking of T-cells and APCs depends upon strong mutual interactions between complementary molecular pairs on their surfaces: MHC II/CD4, MHC I/CD8, VCAM-1/VLA-4, ICAM-1/LFA-1, LFA-3/CD2, B7/CD28 (and CTLA-4) respectively.

*Activation of T-cells requires two signals*

• Two signals activate T-cells, but one alone produces unresponsiveness (anergy).
• One signal is provided by the low affinity cognate TCR/MHC–peptide interaction.
• The second costimulatory signal is mediated through ligation of CD28 by B7.

*Protein tyrosine phosphorylation is an early event in T-cell signaling*

• The TCR signal is transduced and amplified through a protein tyrosine kinase (PTK) enzymic cascade.
• CD4-TCR colocation leads to phosphorylation of tyrosine-based ITAM sequences on CD3 ζ-chains by the CD4-associated lck PTK. These bind and then activate the ZAP-70 kinase.

*(Continued on p. 178)*

## Downstream events following TCR

• Hydrolysis of phosphatidylinositol diphosphate by the phospholipase C$\gamma$1 produces inositol triphosphate (IP$_3$) and diacylglycerol (DAG).
• IP$_3$ mobilizes intracellular calcium.
• DAG and increased calcium activate protein kinase C.
• The raised calcium also stimulates calcineurin activity.
• Activation of ras sets off a kinase cascade operating through Raf-1, MAP kinase kinase (MEK) to the pivotal enzyme MAP kinase (also known as JNK or ERK). CD28 through PI-3 kinase and protein kinase C (PKC) perhaps through Vav, can also influence MAP kinase.
• The transcription factors, Fos, Jun, NFAT and NF$\kappa$B are activated by MAP kinase, calcineurin and PKC respectively and bind to regulatory sites in the IL-2 promoter region.
• A small number of MHC–peptide complexes can serially trigger a much larger number of TCRs thereby providing the sustained signal required for activation.
• B7 delivers a negative signal through CTLA-4. Gene activation mediated by MAP kinase generates a deactivating phosphatase. In contrast, the phosphatase domains on CD45 are required to remove phosphates at inhibitory sites on the kinases.

## B-cells respond to three different types of antigen

• Type 1 thymus-independent antigens are polyclonal activators focused onto the specific B-cells by sIg receptors.
• Type 2 thymus-independent antigens are polymeric molecules which cross-link many sIg receptors and, because of their long half-lives, provide a persistent signal to the B-cell.
• Thymus-dependent antigens require the cooperation of helper T-cells to stimulate antibody production by B-cells.
• Antigen captured by specific sIg receptors is taken into the B-cell, processed, and expressed on the surface as a peptide in association with MHC II.
• This complex is recognized by the T-helper cell which activates the resting B-cell.
• The ability of protein carriers to enable the antibody response to haptens is explained by T–B collaboration, with T-cells recognizing the carrier and B-cells the hapten.

## The nature of B-cell activation

• Cross-linking of surface Ig receptors (e.g. by type 2 thymus-independent antigens) activates B-cells.
• T-helper cells activate resting B-cells through TCR recognition of MHC II–carrier peptide complexes and costimulation through CD40L/CD40 interactions (analogous to the B7/CD28 second signal for T-cell activation).

## FURTHER READING

Garcia K.C., Scott C.A., Brunmark A. *et al.* (1996) CD8 enhances formation of stable T-cell receptor/MHC class I molecule complexes. *Nature* **384**, 577–581.
Sloan-Lancaster J., Steinberg T.H. & Allen P.M. (1996) Selective activation of the calcium signaling pathway by altered peptide ligands. *Journal of Experimental Medicine* **184**, 1525–1530.
Swain S.L. & Cambier J.C. (eds) (1996) Lymphocyte activation and effector functions. *Current Opinion in Immunology* **8**, 309–418.
Tew J.G. (ed.) (1992) Antigen trapping and presentation *in vivo*. *Seminars in Immunology* **4**, 203–283.
Valitutti S. *et al.* (1995) Serial triggering of many T-cell receptors by a few peptide-MHC complexes. *Nature* **375**, 148.
Ward S.G., June C.H. & Olive D. (1996) PI 3-kinase: a pivotal pathway in T-cell activation? *Immunology Today* **17**, 187.

# THE PRODUCTION OF EFFECTORS

## C O N T E N T S

## A SUCCESSION OF GENES ARE UPREGULATED BY T-CELL ACTIVATION

We have dwelt upon the early events in lymphocyte activation consequent upon the engagement of the T-cell receptor (TCR) and the provision of an appropriate costimulatory signal. A complex series of tyrosine and serine/threonine phosphorylation reactions produces the factors which push the cell into the mitotic cycle and drive clonal proliferation and their differentiation to effectors. Within the first half hour, nuclear transcription factors such as fos/jun and NFAT which regulate interleukin-2 (IL-2) expression and the cellular protooncogene c-*myc* are expressed, but the next few hours see the synthesis of a range of **soluble cytokines and their receptors** (figure 10.1). Much later we see molecules like the transferrin receptor related to cell division and very late antigens such as the adhesion molecule VLA-1.

## CYTOKINES ACT AS INTERCELLULAR MESSENGERS

In contrast with the initial activation of T-cells and T-

| ACTIVATION | 0 min | | |
|---|---|---|---|
| EARLY | 15 min | cfos/cjun | Nuclear binding transcription factor; binds to AP-1 |
| | | c-*myc* | Cellular oncogene; controls G0 → G1 |
| | | Nur77 | Function in TCR-mediated apoptosis in immature T-cells |
| | 30 min | NFAT | Nuclear transcription factor of activated-T; regulates IL-2 gene |
| | | NFκB | Nuclear binding protein; regulates expression of many genes |
| | | IκB-α | Inhibitor of NFκB |
| | | PAC-1 | Nuclear phosphatase which inactivates ERKs |
| MEDIUM TERM | Several hours | IL-2/3/4/5/6 | Cytokines and their receptors influencing growth and differentiation of myeloid and lymphoid cells, controlling viral growth and mediating chronic inflammatory processes |
| | | IL-9/10/13 | |
| | | GM-CSF | |
| | | IFNγ TGFβ | |
| LATE | 14h | Transferrin receptor | Related to cell division |
| | 16h | c-*myb* | Cellular oncogene |
| | 3-5 days | Class II MHC | Antigen presentation |
| | 7-14 days | VLA-1 | Very late 'antigen'; adhesion molecule |

Figure 10.1. Sequential gene activation on T-cell stimulation, appearance of mRNA.

dependent B-cells which involves intimate contact with the antigen-presenting cells (APCs), subsequent proliferation and maturation of the response is orchestrated by the T-cell cytokines which relay information between cells as soluble messengers. These T-cell products belong to a class of protein mediators generically termed cytokines which encompasses molecules previously called lymphokines, mono-kines, interleukins and interferons (IFN) (table 10.1).

## Cytokine action is transient and usually short range

These low molecular weight secreted proteins, usually 15–25 kDa, mediate cell growth, inflammation, immunity, differentiation and repair. Because they regulate the amplitude and duration of the immune–inflammatory responses, they must be produced in a transient manner tightly regulated by the presence of foreign material, and it is relevant that the AU-rich sequences in the 3'-untranslated regions of the mRNA of many cytokines are correlated directly with rapid degradation and therefore short half-life. Unlike endocrine hormones, the majority of cytokines normally act locally in a paracrine or even autocrine fashion. Thus lymphokines, the lymphoid cytokines, rarely persist in the circulation but nonlymphoid cells can be triggered by bacterial products to release cytokines which may be detected in the bloodstream, often to the detriment of the host. There is a growing suspicion that certain cytokines, perhaps IL-1 and tumour necrosis factor (TNF), may exist in membrane forms which could exert their stimulatory effects without becoming soluble.

## Cytokines act through cell surface receptors

Cytokines are highly potent, often acting at femtomolar ($10^{-15}$ M) concentrations, combining with small numbers of high affinity cell surface receptors to produce changes in the pattern of RNA and protein synthesis. A common feature in the triggering of the cytokine receptors is the ligand-induced association of receptor subunits which allows signal transduction through the interplay of their juxtaposed cytoplasmic domains.

There are at least three major cytokine receptor families, members of which each share a **common signal transducing component**.

**Table 10.1. Cytokines: their origin and function.**

| CYTOKINE | SOURCE | EFFECTOR FUNCTION |
|---|---|---|
| **INTERLEUKINS** | | |
| IL-1 | Mφ, fibroblasts | Proliferation activated B- & T-cells; induction PGE$_2$ & cytokines by Mφ; induction neutrophil & T-adhesion molecules on endothelial cells; induction IL-6, IFNβ1 & GM-CSF; induction fever, acute phase proteins, bone resorption by osteoclasts |
| IL-2 | T | Growth activated T- and B-cells; activation NK cells |
| IL-3 | T, MC | Growth & differentiation hematopoietic precursors Mast cell growth |
| IL-4 | CD4 T, MC, BM stroma | Proliferation activated B-, T-, mast & hematopoietic precursor; induction MHC class II and FcεR on B-cells, p75 IL-2R on T-cells; isotype switch to IgG1 & IgE; Mφ APC & cytotoxic function, Mφ fusion (migration inhibition) |
| IL-5 | CD4 T, MC | Proliferation activated B-cells; production IgM & IgA; proliferation eosinophils; expression p55 IL-2R |
| IL-6 | CD4 T, Mφ, MC, fibroblasts | Growth & differentiation B- and T-cell effectors, & hematopoietic precursors; induction acute phase proteins |
| IL-7 | BM stromal cells | Proliferation pre-B, CD4- CD8- T-cells & activated mature T-cells |
| IL-8 | Monocytes | Chemotaxis & activation neutrophils |
| IL-9 | T | Growth and proliferation T-cells |
| IL-10 | CD4 T, B, Mφ | Inhibits IFNγ secretion; inhibits mononuclear cell inflammation |
| IL-11 | BM stromal cells | Induction acute phase proteins |
| IL-12 | Monocytes, Mφ | Induction of TH1 cells |
| IL-13 | T | Inhibits mononuclear phagocyte inflammation; proliferation and differentiation B-cells |
| IL-16 | CD8 T, CD4 (not preformed) | Chemotaxis CD4 T-cells and eosinophils |
| **COLONY STIMULATING FACTORS** | | |
| GM-CSF | T, Mφ, fibroblasts MC, endothelium | Growth granulocyte & Mφ colonies Activates Mφ, neutrophils, eosinophils |
| G-CSF | Fibroblasts, endothelium | Growth mature granulocytes |
| M-CSF | Fibroblasts, endothelium, epithelium | Growth macrophage colonies |
| Steel factor | BM stromal cells | Stem cell division (c-kit ligand) |
| **TUMOR NECROSIS FACTORS** | | |
| TNFα TNFβ | Mφ, T } T } | Tumor cytotoxicity; cachexia; induction acute phase proteins; anti-viral & anti-parasitic activity; activation phagocytic cells; induction IFNγ, TNFα, IL-1, GM-CSF & IL-6; endotoxic shock |
| **INTERFERONS** | | |
| IFNα IFNβ | Leukocytes } Fibroblasts } | Anti-viral; expression MHC I |
| IFNγ | T | Anti-viral; Mφ activation; expression MHC class I & II on Mφ & other cells; differentiation of cytotoxic T; synthesis IgG2a by activated B; antagonism several IL-4 actions |
| **CHEMOKINES** | | |
| α e.g. IL-8, NAP-2 | Mφ, T | Chemotactic for neutrophils |
| β e.g. MCP, MIP, RANTES | Mφ } T } | Chemotactic for T-cells |
| **OTHERS** | | |
| TGFβ | T, B | Inhibition IL-2R upregulation and IL-2 dependent T- and B-cell proliferation Inhibition (by TGFβ1) of IL-3 + CSF induced hematopoiesis; isotype switch to IgA Wound repair (fibroblast chemotaxin) and angiogenesis Neoplastic transformation certain normal cells |
| LIF | T | Proliferation embryonic stem cells without affecting differentiation Chemoattraction & activation of eosinophils |

Mφ=macrophage; MC=mast cell; BM=bone marrow; IL=interleukin; GM-CSF=granulocyte–macrophage colony-stimulating factor; TGFβ=transforming growth factor-β; NAP=neutrophil activating peptide; MCP=membrane cofactor protein; MIP=membrane inhibitory peptide; LIF=leukemia inhibitory factor;chemokines are small basic heparin-binding polypeptides, mol.wt 8–14 kDa. IL-5 is chemotactic for eosinophils, IL-8 for neutrophils, and for eosinophils which have been primed with IL-5.

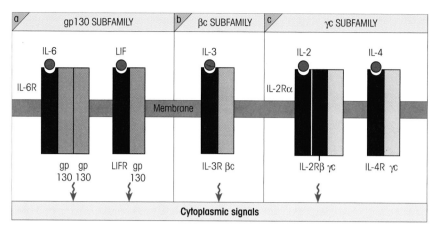

**Figure 10.2. The IL-6, GM-CSF and IL-2 subfamilies of cytokine receptors.** Each family operates through a common subunit which transduces the signal to the interior of the cell. In essence, binding of the cytokine to its receptor must initiate the signalling process by mediating hetero- or homo-dimer formation involving the common subunit. In some cases the cytokine is active when bound to the receptor either in soluble or membrane-bound form (e.g. IL-6). Soluble receptors such as TNFR, released from a cell following activation, can act as antagonists. The IL-2 receptor is interesting. It is composed of an α-chain (reacting with the CD25 Tac monoclonal) of low affinity, and a β-chain of intermediate affinity. IL-2 binds to and dissociates from the α-chain very rapidly but the same processes involving the β-chain occur at two or three orders of magnitude more slowly. When the α- and β-chains form a single receptor, the α-chain binds the IL-2 rapidly and facilitates its binding to a separate site on the β-chain from which it can only dissociate slowly. Since the final affinity ($K_d$) is based on the ratio of dissociation to association rate constants, then $K_d = 10^{-4}\,\text{s}^{-1}/10^7\,\text{M}^{-1}\,\text{s}^{-1} = 10^{-11}\,\text{M}$, which is a very high affinity.

## The gp130 subfamily

IL-6 and 11, leukemia inhibitory factor (LIF) and certain other cytokines all share the gp130 transmembrane molecule as a common signal transducing agent. For example, when IL-6 binds to its specific receptor it associates with gp130 and induces dimerization (figure 10.2a) thereby initiating a downstream signaling cascade.

## The βc and γc receptor subfamilies

Granulocyte–macrophage colony-stimulating factor (GM-CSF), IL-3 and 5 on binding to their respective receptors initiate heterodimerization with their common signal receptor component βc (figure 10.2b). The other subfamily which acts through the γc common chain includes IL-2, 4, 7 and 9 (figure 10.2c).

## Signal transduction through cytokine receptors

The ligand-induced dimerization of cytokine receptor subunits juxtaposes associated members of a novel class of protein tyrosine kinases, the **JAK family** (*j*ust *a*nother *k*inase?). Intermolecular phosphorylation of regulatory tyrosyl residues of associated JAK molecules is probably a crucial event in signal propagation. One of the most direct effects is the rapid tyrosine phosphorylation of a new group of transcription factors termed **STATs** (*s*ignal *t*ransducers and *a*ctivators of *t*ranscription), which dimerize and translocate to the nucleus where they play an important role in pushing the cell through the mitotic cycle (figure 10.3). JAKs may also act through src family kinases to generate other transcription factors through both the phosphoinositide-3 kinase/p70S6 kinase and the Ras/Raf/MEK/MAP kinase routes (figure 10.3).

## Cytokines often have multiple effects

In general, cytokines are **pleiotropic**, i.e. with multiple effects on growth and differentiation of a variety of cell types (table 10.1), and there is considerable overlapping and redundancy between them, partially accounted for by the induction of synthesis of common proteins.

Their roles in the generation of T- and B-cell effectors, and in the regulation of chronic inflammatory reactions (figure 10.4a and b) will be discussed at length later in this chapter. We should note here the important role of cytokines in the control of hematopoiesis (figure 10.4c). Thus we now realize that the differentiation of stem cells to become the formed elements of blood within the environment of the bone marrow is carefully nurtured through production of cytokines by the stromal cells. These include GM-CSF, G-CSF (granulocyte colony-stimulating factor), M-CSF (macrophage colony-stimulating factor), IL-6 and 7 and LIF (see table 10.1)

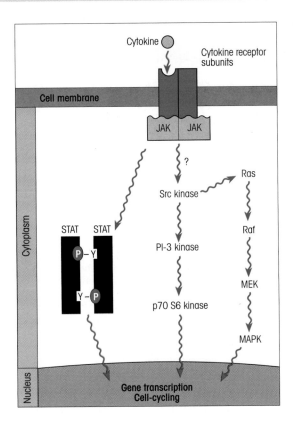

**Figure 10.3. Cytokinase receptor-mediated pathways for gene transcription.** Cytokine-induced receptor oligomerization activates the associated JAK kinases. These phosphorylate the STAT DNA-binding transcription factors which dimerize and translocate to the nucleus. JAK kinase may also activate src family kinases which could generate transcription factors via the two routes shown. IL-2 and IFNγ involve JAK/STAT but gp130 signaling may not. PI-3 kinase = phosphoinositide-3 kinase; MEK = kinase activator of MAPK; MAPK = mitogen-activated protein kinases (see figure 9.5).

and many of them are also derived from T-cells and macrophages. It is not surprising, therefore, that during a period of chronic inflammation, the cytokines that are produced recruit new precursors into the hematopoietic differentiation pathway — a useful exercise in the circumstances. One of the lymphokines, IL-3, should be highlighted for its exceptional ability to support the early cells in this pathway, particularly in synergy with IL-6 and G-CSF.

## Network interactions

The complex and integrated relationships between the different cytokines are mediated through cellular events. The genes for IL-3, 4 and 5 and GM-CSF are all tightly linked on chromosome 5 in a region containing genes for M-CSF and its receptor and several other growth factors and receptors. Interaction may occur through a cascade in which one cytokine induces the production of another, through transmodulation of

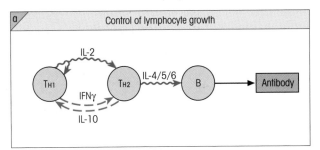

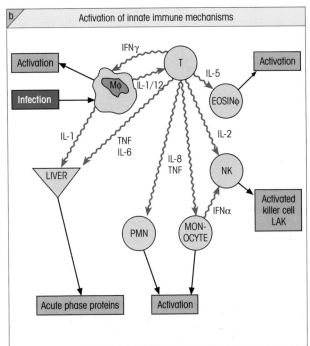

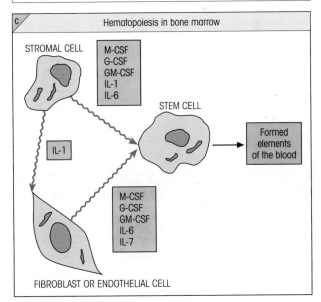

**Figure 10.4. Cytokine action.** A general but not entirely comprehensive guide to indicate the scope of cytokine interactions (e.g. for reasons of simplicity I have omitted the inhibitory effects of IL-10 on monocytes and the activation of NK cells by IL-12). Mφ = macrophage; PMN = polymorphonuclear neutrophil; NK = natural killer cell; LAK = lymphokine activated killer; eosinφ = eosinophil.

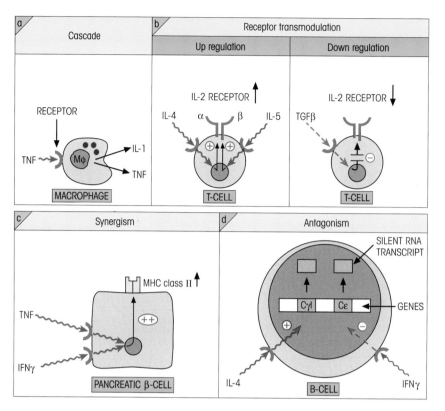

**Figure 10.5. Network interactions of cytokines.** (a) Cascade: in this example TNF induces secretion of IL-1 and of itself (autocrine) in the macrophage (note all diagrams in this figure are simplified in that the effects on the nucleus are due to messengers resulting from combination of cytokine with its surface receptor). (b) Receptor transmodulation showing upregula-tion of each chain forming the high-affinity IL-2 receptor in an activated T-cell by individual lymphokines and downregulation by TGFβ. (c) Synergy of TNF and IFNγ in upregulation of surface MHC class II molecules on cultured pancreatic insulin-secreting cells. (d) Antagonism of IL-4 and IFNγ on transcription of silent mRNA relating to isotype switch (cf. figure 10.16).

the receptor for another cytokine and through synergism or antagonism of two cytokines acting on the same cell (figure 10.5). Despite the widespread success in cloning and sequencing individual cytokines and their receptors, the means by which target cells integrate and interpret the complex patterns of stimuli induced by these multiple soluble factors is only slowly unfolding.

## DIFFERENT CD4 T-CELL SUBSETS CAN MAKE DIFFERENT CYTOKINE PATTERNS

### The bipolar TH1/TH2 concept

In the mouse, long-term TH clones can be divided into two types with distinct cytokine secretion phenotypes (table 10.2). This makes biological sense in that TH1 cells producing lymphokines like IFNγ would be especially effective against intracellular infections with viruses and organisms which grow in macrophages, whereas TH2 cells are very good helpers for B-cells and would seem to be adapted for defense against parasites which are vulnerable to IL-

4-switched IgE, IL-5-induced eosinophilia and IL-3/4-stimulated mast cell proliferation. The superiority of macrophages as antigen-presenting cells for TH1 clones and of B-cells for TH2 accords rather well with this hypothesis, as do studies on the infection of mice with the pathogenic protozoan *Leishmania major*. Intravenous or intraperitoneal injection of killed promastigotes leads to protection against challenge with live parasites associated with high expression of IFNγ mRNA and low levels of IL-4 mRNA; the reciprocal finding of low IFNγ and high IL-4 expression was made after subcutaneous immunization which failed to provide protection. Furthermore, nonvaccinated mice infected with live organisms could be saved by injection of IFNγ and anti-IL-4. These results are consistent with preferential expansion of a population of protective IFNγ-secreting TH1 cells by intraperitoneal or intravenous immunization, and of nonprotective TH2 cells producing IL-4 in the subcutaneously injected animals. The ability of IFNγ, the characteristic TH1 lymphokine, to inhibit proliferation of TH2 clones, and of TH2-derived IL-4 and 10 to block both proliferation and cytokine release by TH1 cells, would

**Table 10.2. Cytokine patterns of mouse T-cell clones** (from Mosmann *et al.* (1989) In Melchers F. *et al.* (eds) *Progress in Immunology* **7**, 611. Springer-Verlag, Berlin).

| CYTOKINE PATTERNS OF MOUSE T-CELL CLONES | | | |
|---|---|---|---|
|  | TH1 | TH2 | Tc |
| IFN-γ | ++ |  | ++ |
| IL-2 | ++ |  |  |
| TNFβ | ++ |  |  |
| TNFα | ++ |  |  |
| GM-CSF | ++ | ++ |  |
| IL-3 | ++ | ++ |  |
| Met. enkephalin | ++ | ++ |  |
| IL-4 |  | ++ |  |
| IL-5 |  | ++ |  |
| IL-6 |  | ++ |  |
| IL-10 |  | ++ |  |

██ ++     ▒▒ +     ☐ Negative

TH1/2 = T-helper-1/2; Tc = cytotoxic T-cell

seem to put the issue beyond reasonable doubt (figure 10.6).

And yet, having said all that, no such clear-cut patterns of secreted lymphokines were originally demonstrable in human or rat T-cell clones, or even in murine cells early after immunization. We should recall that the original Mosmann–Coffman classification into TH1 and TH2 subsets was predicted on data obtained with clones which had been maintained in culture for long periods and might have been artefacts of conditions *in vitro*. Perhaps the most sensible view to take at this juncture is to look upon T-cells as producing the whole spectrum of cytokine profiles (TH0, figure 10.6) with possible skewing of the responses towards the extreme TH1 and TH2 patterns depending on the nature of the antigen stimulus.

## Interactions with cells of the innate immune system may bias the TH1/TH2 response

Invasion of phagocytic cells by intracellular pathogens induces copious secretion of IL-12, which in turn stimulates IFNγ production by NK cells. These two cytokines selectively drive differentiation of TH1 development and inhibit TH2 responses (figure 10.6).

On the other side of the coin, a source of IL-4 would favor TH2 development and it just so happens that a novel subset of T-cells bearing the murine NK1+ marker rapidly release an IL-4 dominated pattern of cytokines on stimulation. This subset has many

unusual features. They may be CD4⁻8⁻ or CD4⁺8⁻ and they express low levels of T-cell αβ receptors with an invariant α chain and very restricted β which recognize MHC class 1b CD1. Their morphology and

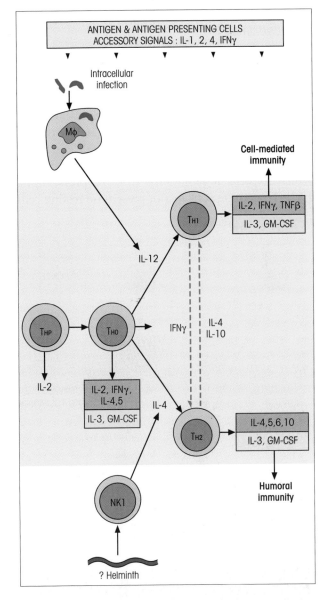

**Figure 10.6. The generation of TH1 and TH2 CD4 subsets.** It is envisaged that following initial stimulation of T-cells, a range of cells producing a spectrum of cytokine patterns emerges. Under different conditions, the resulting population can be biased towards two extremes. IL-12, possibly produced through an 'innate' type effect of an intracellular infection on macrophages, encourages the development of TH1 cells which produce the cytokines characteristic of *cell-mediated immunity*. IL-4, possibly produced by interaction of micro-organisms with the lectin-like NK1.1+ receptor on a specialized population of murine low density TCRαβ cells, skews the development to production of TH2 cells whose cytokines assist the progression of B-cells to antibody secretion and the provision of *humoral immunity*. Cytokines produced by polarized TH1 and TH2 subpopulations are mutually inhibitory. THP = T-helper precursor; TH0 = early helper cell producing a spectrum of cytokines; other abbreviations as in Table 10.1.

granule content are intermediate between T-cells and NK cells. Although they express TCRαβ, there is an inclination to classify them on the fringe of the 'innate' immune system having regard to their primitive characteristics and possession of several NK markers including NK1 which is lectin-like and could be stimulated by NK1 recognition of microbial carbohydrates.

## ACTIVATED T-CELLS PROLIFERATE IN RESPONSE TO CYTOKINES

In so far as T-cells are concerned, amplification following activation is critically dependent upon IL-2 (figure 10.7). This lymphokine is a single peptide of molecular weight 15.5 kDa which acts only on cells which express high affinity IL-2 receptors (figure 10.2). These receptors are not present on resting cells,

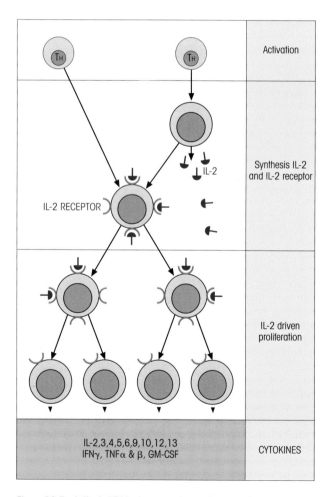

**Figure 10.7. Activated T-blasts expressing surface receptors for IL-2 proliferate in response to IL-2** produced by itself or by another T-cell subset. Expansion is controlled through downregulation of the IL-2 receptor by IL-2 itself. The expanded population secretes a wide variety of biologically active lymphokines of which IL-4 also enhances T-cell proliferation.

but are synthesized within a few hours after activation (figure 10.1).

Separation of an activated T-cell population into those with high and low affinity IL-2 receptors showed clearly that an adequate number of high affinity receptors were mandatory for the mitogenic action of IL-2. It is the skewed cellular distribution of these high affinity receptors which is responsible for the asynchronous division of activated T-cells on addition of IL-2. The numbers of these receptors on the cell increase under the action of antigen and of IL-2, and as antigen is cleared, so the receptor numbers decline and, with that, the responsiveness to IL-2. It should be appreciated that although IL-2 is an immunologically nonspecific T-cell growth factor, it only functions appropriately in specific responses because unstimulated T-cells do not express IL-2 receptors.

The T-cell blasts also produce an impressive array of other cytokines and the proliferative effect of IL-2 is reinforced by the action of IL-4 and, to some extent, IL-6, which react with corresponding receptors on the dividing T-cells. We must not lose sight of the importance of control mechanisms, and obvious candidates to subsume this role are transforming growth factor-β (TGFβ), which blocks IL-2-induced proliferation (figure 10.3b) and production of TNFα and β, and the cytokines IFNγ, IL-4 and IL-10 which mediate the mutual antagonism of TH1 and TH2 subsets.

## T-CELL EFFECTORS IN CELL-MEDIATED IMMUNITY

### Cytokines mediate chronic inflammatory responses

In addition to their role in the adaptive response, the T-cell lymphokines are responsible for generating antigen-specific chronic inflammatory reactions which deal with intracellular parasites (figure 10.4b and 10.8), although there is a different emphasis on the pattern of factors involved (cf. p. 278).

*Early events*

The initiating event is probably a local inflammatory response to tissue injury caused by the infectious agent which would upregulate the synthesis of adhesion molecules such as VCAM-1 and ICAM-1 on adjacent vascular endothelial cells. These would permit entry of memory T-cells to the infected site

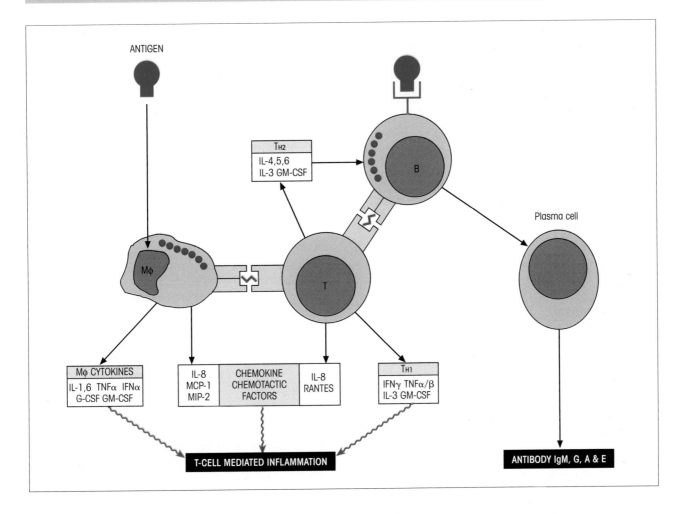

**Figure 10.8. Cytokines controlling the antibody and T-cell-mediated inflammatory responses.** Abbreviations as in table 10.1.

through their VLA-4 and LFA-1 homing receptors (cf. p. 155). Contact with processed antigen derived from the intracellular parasite will activate the specific T-cell and induce the release of secreted cytokines. TNF will further enhance the expression of endothelial accessory molecules and increase the chances of other memory cells in the circulation homing in to meet the antigen provoking inflammation.

*Chemotaxis*

The recruitment of T-cells and macrophages to the inflammatory site is greatly enhanced by the action of chemotactic cytokines termed **chemokines** (*chemo*attractant cyto*kine*). These are divided into two families based on sequence homology and the disposition of the first two of four canonical cysteine residues (cf table 13.1). In essence, the CXC or α-chemokines, of which IL-8 is an example, attract neutrophils but not monocytes. The reverse is true for the CC or β-

chemokines which include MCP, MIP and RANTES (see figure 10.8), but additionally may attract T-cells and NK cells.

*Macrophage activation*

Macrophages with intracellular organisms are activated by agents such as IFNγ, GM-CSF, IL-2 and TNF and should become endowed with microbicidal powers. During this process, some macrophages may die (helped along by cytotoxic T-cells?) and release living parasites, but these will be dealt with by fresh macrophages brought to the site by chemotaxis and newly activated by local cytokines so that they have passed the stage of differentiation at which the intracellular parasites can subvert their killing mechanisms (cf. p. 267).

*Combating viral infection*

Virally infected cells require a different strategy and one strand of that strategy exploits the innate interferon mechanism to deny the virus access to the cell's

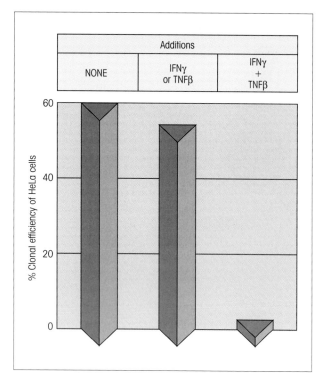

**Figure 10.9. Synergism of γ-interferon (IFNγ) and tumour necrosis factor-β (TNFβ) in the growth inhibition of the HeLa tumor cell line.** (Data from Stone-Wolff D.S. *et al.* (1984) *Journal of Experimental Medicine* **159**, 828.)

replicative machinery. IFNγ of course does this but note that TNFα and β both induce 2'–5'(A) synthetase, a protein also switched on by IFN and which is involved in viral protection. TNF has another string to its bow in its ability to kill certain cells, since death of an infected cell before viral replication has occurred is obviously beneficial to the host. Its cytotoxic potential was first recognized using tumor cells as targets (hence the name), and recent work with cloned products reveals a synergism between IFNγ and TNFβ (figure 10.9) in which IFNγ sets up the cell for destruction by inducing the formation of TNF receptors (see also figure 10.5c). It is interesting to note also that IFNγ can affect the growth of intracellular parasites in cells other than macrophages; for example, it inhibits the growth of *Rickettsia prowazekii* in mouse fibroblast cultures.

## Killer T-cells

### The generation of cytotoxic T-cells

Cytotoxic T-cells (Tc) represent the other major arm of the cell-mediated immune response and are generally thought to be of strategic importance in the killing of virally infected cells and possibly in contributing to

the postulated surveillance mechanisms against cancer cells.

The cytotoxic cell precursors recognize antigen on the surface of cells in association with class I major histocompatibility complex (MHC), and like B-cells they require help from T-cells. The mechanism by which help is proffered may, however, be quite different. As explained earlier (see p. 174), effective T–B collaboration is usually 'cognate' in that the collaborating cells recognize two epitopes which are physically linked (usually on the same molecule). If I may remind the reader without causing offence, the reason for this is that the surface Ig receptors on the B-cell capture native antigen, process it internally and present it to the Th as a peptide in association with MHC class II. Although it has been shown that linked epitopes on the antigen are also necessary for cooperation between Th and cytotoxic T-cell precursor (Tcp), the nature of T-cell recognition prevents native antigen being focused onto the Tcp by its receptor for subsequent processing, even if that cell were to express MHC II, which in its resting state it does not. It seems most likely that Th and Tcp bind to the same APC which has processed viral antigen and displays processed viral peptides in association with both class II (for the Th cell) and class I (for the Tcp) on its surface; one cannot exclude the possibility that the APC could be the virally infected cell itself. Cytokines from the triggered Th will be released in close proximity to the Tcp which is engaging the antigen–MHC signal and will be stimulated to proliferate and differentiate into a Tc under the influence of IL-2 and 6. The possibility of a Th-independent mechanism by which the virally infected cell triggers the antigen-specific Tcp through the CD2 molecule has also been mooted, but this requires greater clarification.

### The lethal process

Cytotoxic T-cells (Tc) are generally of the CD8 subset and their binding to the target cell through T-receptor recognition of antigen plus class I MHC is assisted by association between CD8 and class I and by other accessory molecules such as LFA-1 and CD2 (see figure 9.3). MHC recognition is important for this binding but it does not seem to be involved in the signals leading to cell death, since B-cell hybridomas making anti-CD3 or antibodies to the T-receptor idiotype are killed by Tc independently of their MHC haplotype; what does appear to be vital is an intimate signaling to the T-receptor or the CD3 transducer.

Tc are **unusual secretory cells** which use a modified lysosome to secrete their lytic proteins. Following delivery of the TCR/CD3 signal, the **lytic granules** are driven at a rare old speed (up to 1.2 μm sec$^{-1}$) along the microtubule system and delivered to the point of contact between the Tc and its target (figure 10.10). This guarantees the specificity of killing dictated by TCR recognition of the target and limits any damage to bystander cells. As argued earlier when we discussed cytotoxicity by NK cells which have comparable granules (cf. p. 19), there is evidence for exocytosis of the granule contents including perforins, granzymes and TNF which cause lesions in the target cell membrane and death by inducing apoptosis. Tc are endowed with a second killing mechanism involving fas and its ligand (cf. p. 19) but the inability of perforin knockout mice to clear viruses effectively,

suggests that the secretory granules provide the dominant attack on virally infected cells. Perhaps the fas pathway is more concerned in control of the immune system.

Videomicroscopy shows that Tc are serial killers. After the 'kiss of death', the T-cell can disengage and seek a further victim, there being rapid synthesis of new granules.

One should also not lose sight of the fact that CD8 cells synthesize other cytokines such as IFNγ which also have antiviral potential.

### Inflammation must be regulated

Once the inflammatory process has cleared the inciting agent, the body needs to switch it off. IL-10 has profound anti-inflammatory and immunoregulatory effects, acting on macrophages and TH1 cells to inhibit release of factors such as IL-1 and TNFα. It induces the release of soluble TNF receptors which are endogenous inhibitors of TNF, and downregulates surface TNF receptor. Soluble IL-1 receptors released during inflammation can act to 'decoy' IL-1 itself. IL-4 not only acts to constrain TH1 cells but also upregulates production of the natural inhibitor of IL-1, the IL-1 receptor antagonist (IL-1Ra). The role of TGFβ is more difficult to tease out because it has some pro- and other anti-inflammatory effects, although it undoubtedly promotes tissue repair after resolution of the inflammation.

### PROLIFERATION AND MATURATION OF B-CELL RESPONSES ARE MEDIATED BY CYTOKINES

The activation of B-cells by TH through the TCR recognition of MHC-linked antigenic peptide plus the costimulatory **CD40L/CD40 interaction**, leads to upregulation of the surface receptor for IL-4. Copious local release of this cytokine from the TH then drives powerful clonal proliferation and expansion of the activated B-cell population. IL-2 and IL-13 also contribute to this process (figure 10.11).

Under the influence of IL-4 alone, the expanded clones can differentiate and mature into IgE synthesizing cells. TGFβ encourages cells to switch their Ig class to IgA and IL-5 can then stimulate them to become IgA producers. IgM plasma cells emerge under the tutelage of IL-4 plus 5, and IgG producers result from the combined influence of IL-4, 5 and 6 with a probable contribution from IFNγ (figure 10.11).

Type 2 thymus-independent antigens can activate

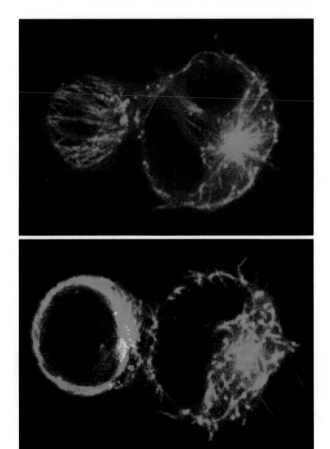

**Figure 10.10. Conjugation of a cytotoxic T-cell (on left) to its target,** here a mouse mastocytoma, showing polarization of the granules towards the target at the point of contact. The cytoskeletons of both cells are revealed by immunofluorescent staining with an antibody to tubulin (green) and the lytic granules with an antibody to granzyme A (red). Twenty minutes after conjugation the target cell cytoskeleton may still be intact (above), but this rapidly becomes disrupted (below). (Photographs kindly provided by Dr. Gillian Griffiths.)

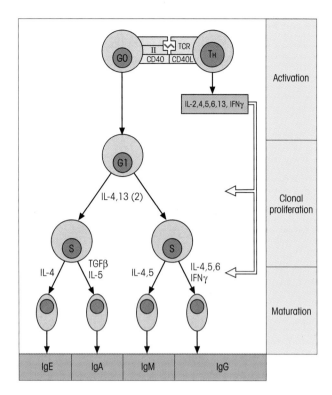

**Figure 10.11. B-cell response to thymus-dependent antigen: clonal expansion and maturation of activated B-cells under the influence of T-cell-derived soluble factors.** Costimulation through the CD40L/CD40 interaction is essential for primary and secondary immune responses to TD antigens and for the formation of germinal centers and memory. c-*myc* expression, which is maximal 2 hours after antigen or anti-μ stimulation, parallels sensitivity to growth factors; transfection with c-*myc* substitutes for anti-μ.

B-cells directly (cf. p. 173) but nonetheless still need cytokines for efficient proliferation and Ig production. These may come from accessory cells such as NK and NK1+ T-cells which bear lectin-like receptors.

## WHAT IS GOING ON IN THE GERMINAL CENTER?

The secondary follicle with its corona or mantle of small lymphocytes surrounding the pale germinal center is a striking and unique cellular structure, often picked out proudly by immunologists with a rather untutored histological background (like myself) to bolster their otherwise shaky morphological prowess. Nonetheless, until recently, the nature of the events occurring within it were shrouded in mystery, as if it were yet another 'black box'. First, let us recall the overall events described in Chapter 8.

Secondary challenge with antigen or immune complexes induces enlargement of germinal centers, formation of new ones, appearance of B-memory cells and development of Ig-producing cells of higher affinity. B-cells entering the germinal center become

**centroblasts** which divide with a very short cycle time of 6 hours, and then become nondividing **centrocytes** in the basal light zone, many of which die from apoptosis (figure 10.12). As the surviving centrocytes mature, they differentiate either into **immunoblast plasma cell precursors** which secrete Ig in the absence of antigen or **memory B-cells**.

What then is the underlying scenario? Following secondary antigen challenge, primed B-cells may be activated by paracortical TH cells in association with interdigitating dendritic cells or macrophages, and migrate to the germinal center. There they divide in response to powerful stimuli from complexes on follicular dendritic cells (cf. p. 165), cleaved CD23 derived from the surface of the dendritic cells and stimulated B-cells, and T-cell lymphokines released in response to antigen-presenting B-cells. During this particularly frenetic bout of cell division, it is now established that **somatic mutation** of B-cell Ig genes occurs with high frequency. The cells also undergo **Ig class-switching**. Thereafter, as they transform to centrocytes, they are vulnerable and die readily whence they are taken up as the 'tingible bodies' by macrophages, unless rescued by association with antigen on a follicular dendritic cell. This could result from cross-linking of surface Ig receptors and is accompanied by expression of bcl-2, a molecule known to protect against death by apoptosis. Signaling through CD40 by presentation of antigen to TH cells, would also prolong the life of the centrocyte. In either case, the interactions will only occur if the mutated surface Ig receptor still binds antigen and, as the concentration of antigen gradually falls, only if the receptor is of high affinity. In other words, the system can deliver high-affinity antibody by a Darwinian process of high-frequency mutation of the Ig genes and selection by antigen of the cells bearing the antibody which binds most strongly (figure 10.13). This increase of affinity as the antibody level falls late in the response is of obvious benefit, since a small amount of high-affinity antibody can do the job of a large amount of low affinity (as in boxing, a small 'goodun' will generally be a match for a mediocre 'bigun').

Further differentiation now occurs. The cells either migrate to the sites of plasma cell activity (e.g. lymph node medulla) or go to expand the memory B-cell pool depending upon the signals received. Soluble CD23 and IL-1α, presumably derived from follicular dendritic cells, stimulate the formation of antibody forming cells, whereas CD40, signalled through a T-cell, guides the cell into the memory compartment.

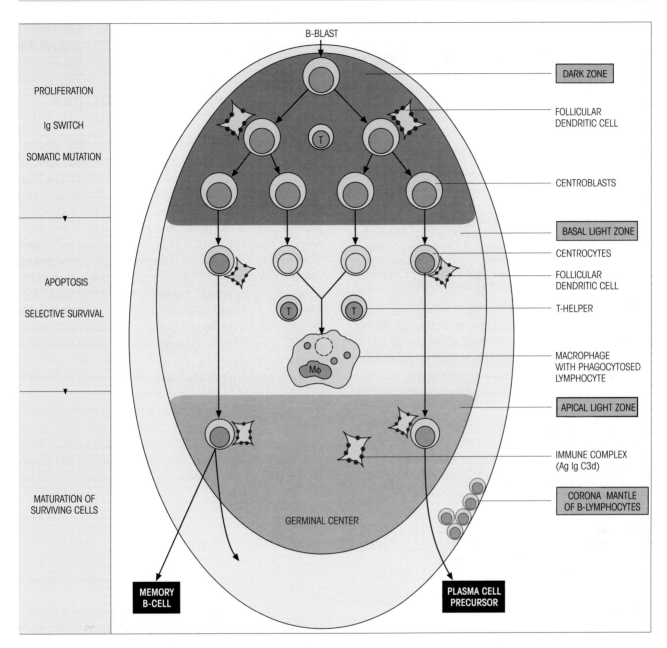

**Figure 10.12. The events occurring in lymphoid germinal centers.** Germinal center B-cells can be enriched through their affinity for the peanut agglutinin lectin. They show numerous mutations in the antibody genes. Expression of LFA-1 and ICAM-1 on B-cells and follicular dendritic cells (FDC) in the germinal center makes them 'sticky'. Centroblasts at the base of the follicle are strongly CD77 positive. The TH cells bear the unusual CD57 marker. The FDC all express CD21 and CD54; those in the apical light zone are strongly CD23 positive, those in the basal light zone express little CD23. Through their surface receptors, FDC bind immune complexes containing antigen and C3 which, in turn, are very effective B-cell stimulators since coligation of the surface receptors for antigen and C3 (CR2) lowers their threshold for activation. The costimulatory molecules CD40 and B7 play pivotal roles. Antibodies to CD40 prevent formation of germinal centers and anti-CD40L can disrupt established germinal centers within 12 hours. Anti-B7-2 given early in the immune response prevents germinal center formation and when given at the onset of hypermutation, suppresses that process.

## THE SYNTHESIS OF ANTIBODY

The sequential processes by which secreted Ig arises by translation of mRNA are illustrated in figure 10.14. In the normal antibody-forming cell there is a rapid turnover of light chains which are present in slight excess. Defective control occurs in many myeloma cells and one may see excessive production of light chains or complete suppression of heavy-chain synthesis.

Using 'pulse and chase' techniques with radioactive amino acids, it was found that the build-up of both light and heavy chains proceeds continuously starting from the N-terminal end. Furthermore, isola-

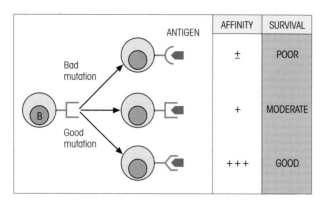

| | AFFINITY | SURVIVAL |
|---|---|---|
| Bad mutation | ± | POOR |
| | + | MODERATE |
| Good mutation | +++ | GOOD |

**Figure 10.13. Darwinian selection by antigen of B-cells with antibody mutants of high affinity** protects against cell death in the germinal center, either through cross-linking of sIg by antigen on follicular dendritic cells, or through TH cell recognition of processed antigen and signaling through CD40. In both cases, capture of antigen, particularly as the concentration falls, will be critically affected by the affinity of the surface receptor.

tion of the mRNA for each type of chain has shown them to be of appropriate size to allow synthesis of the complete peptides. The evidence therefore confirms the present view that the messenger regions for variable and constant regions are spliced together before leaving the nucleus.

Differential splicing mechanisms also provide a rational explanation for the co-expression of surface IgM and IgD with identical V regions on a single cell, and for the switch from production of membrane-bound IgM receptor to secretory IgM in the antibody-forming cell as discussed previously (cf. figures 4.1 and 4.2).

## IMMUNOGLOBULIN CLASS SWITCHING OCCURS IN INDIVIDUAL B-CELLS

The synthesis of antibodies belonging to the various immunoglobulin classes proceeds at different rates. Usually there is an early IgM response which tends to fall off rapidly. IgG antibody synthesis builds up to its maximum over a longer time period. On secondary challenge with antigen, the time-course of the IgM response resembles that seen in the primary. By contrast, the synthesis of IgG antibodies rapidly accelerates to a much higher titer and there is a relatively slow fall-off in serum antibody levels (figure 10.15). The same probably holds for IgA, and in a sense both these immunoglobulin classes provide the main immediate defense against future penetration by foreign antigens.

There is evidence that individual cells can switch over from IgM to IgG production. Several days after immunization with *Salmonella* flagella, isolated cells taken into micro-drop cultures were shown to produce both IgM and IgG immobilizing antibodies. In another study it was shown that antigen challenge of irradiated recipients receiving relatively small

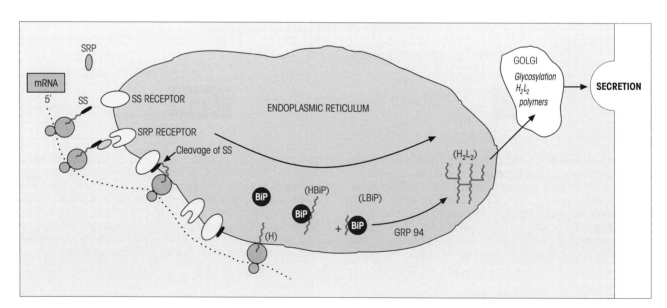

**Figure 10.14. Synthesis of immunoglobulin.** As mRNA is translated on the ribosome, the N-terminal signal sequence (SS) is bound by a complex signal recognition particle (SRP) which docks onto a receptor on the outer membrane of the endoplasmic reticulum (ER) and facilitates entry of the nascent Ig chain into the ER lumen. The SS associates with a specific membrane receptor and is cleaved; the remainder of the chain, as it elongates, complexes with the chaperonin BiP (heavy chain binding protein) which catalyses protein folding. BiP binds to the heavy chain $C_H1$ and $V_L$ domains to control protein folding. Another chaperone GRP94 now associates with the unassembled chains which oxidize and dissociate as the full $H_2L_2$ Ig molecule. The assembled $H_2L_2$ molecules can now leave the ER for terminal glycosylation in the Golgi and final secretion. Surface receptor Ig would be inserted by its hydrophobic sequences into the membrane of the endoplasmic reticulum as it was synthesized.

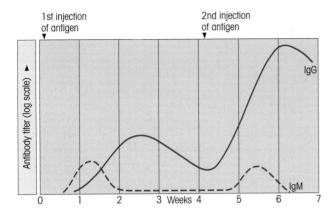

**Figure 10.15.** Synthesis of IgM and IgG antibody classes in the primary and secondary responses to antigen.

numbers of lymphoid cells, produced splenic foci of cells, each synthesizing antibodies of different heavy-chain class bearing a single idiotype; the common idiotype suggests that each focus is derived from a single precursor cell whose progeny can form antibodies of different class.

Antibody synthesis in most classes shows considerable dependence upon T-cooperation in that the responses in T-deprived animals are strikingly deficient; such is true of mouse IgG1, IgG2a, IgA, IgE and part of the IgM antibody responses. T-independent antigens such as the polyclonal activator, lipopolysaccharide (LPS) endotoxin, induce synthesis of IgM with some IgG2b and IgG3. Immunopotentiation by complete Freund's adjuvant, a water-in-oil emulsion containing antigen in the aqueous phase and a suspension of killed tubercle bacilli in the oily phase (see p. 304), seems to occur, at least in part, through the activation of Th cells which stimulate antibody production in T-dependent classes. The prediction from this that the response to T-independent antigens (e.g. *Pneumococcus* polysaccharide, p. 173) should not be potentiated by Freund's adjuvant is borne out in practice; furthermore, as mentioned previously, these antigens evoke primarily IgM antibodies and poorly defined immunological memory, as do T-dependent antigens injected into T-cell-deficient, neonatally thymectomized hosts.

Thus, in rodents at least, the switch from IgM to IgG and other classes appears to be largely under T-cell control critically mediated by CD40 and presumably also by cytokines as described earlier (see p. 189), although it is often difficult to establish whether a given agent is itself causing the switch or is a particularly good growth promoter for the Ig class resulting from the switch. Let us take another look at the stimulation of small surface IgM-positive B-cells by LPS; as

we noted, on its own the nonspecific mitogen evokes the synthesis of IgM, IgG3 and some IgG2b. Following addition of IL-4 to the system, there is heightened production of IgE and IgG1, whereas IFNγ stimulates IgG2a secretion at concentrations that inhibit the effects of IL-4. IL-5 promotes maturation without affecting Ig class. The notion that IL-4 was a switch factor for IgA stemmed largely from results with a given lymphoma but with no confirmatory data using normal B-cells. Rather more convincing was the 5–10-fold increase in IgA production when TGFβ was introduced into the LPS system and the demonstration of a switch from surface IgA-negative to -positive in Peyer's patch cells so treated. Significantly, TGFβ induced the formation of sterile transcripts consisting of a 5′ exon derived from germ-line sequences upstream of the α-switch region (cf. figure 10.16) spliced to the IgA class $C_\alpha$ gene. The 5′ exons contain stop codons in the open-reading frame of the $C_\alpha$ gene and so cannot encode large proteins. This is now seen to be one instance of a more general phenomenon in which sterile transcripts of a $C_H$ gene are associated with a switch to that class (figure 10.16). Perhaps the transcripts facilitate the action of the recombinase in some way. Under the influence of the recombinase, a given *VDJ* gene segment is transferred from μδ to an alternative constant region gene by utilizing the specialized switch region sequences (figure 10.16), so yielding antibodies of the same specificity but of different class.

## Class-switched B-cells are subject to high mutation rates after the initial response

The reader will no doubt recollect that this idea was raised in Chapter 4 when discussing the generation of diversity and that the germinal center has been identified as the site of intense mutagenesis. The normal V region mutation rate is of the order of $10^{-5}$/base pair/cell division, but this rises to $10^{-3}$/base pair/generation in B-cells as a result of antigenic stimulation. This process is illustrated well in figure 10.17 which charts the accumulation of somatic mutations in the immunodominant $V_H/V_K$ antibody structure during the immune response to phenyloxazolone. With time and successive boosting the mutation rate is seen to rise dramatically, and in the context of the present discussion it is clear that the strategically targeted hypermutations occurring within or adjacent to the complementarity determining hypervariable loops can give rise to cells which secrete antibodies having a different combining affinity to that of the original parent cell. Randomly, some mutated daughter cells

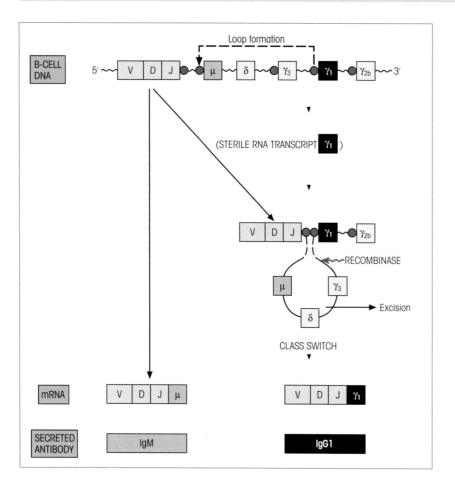

Figure 10.16. Class-switching to produce antibodies of identical specificity but different immunoglobulin isotype (in this example from IgM to IgG1) is achieved by a recombinase process which utilizes the specialized switch sequences (●) and leads to a loss of the intervening DNA loop (μ, δ and γ3). The $C_H$ transcript which always accompanies the phenomenon somehow helps formation of the junction between the *VDJ* segment and the appropriate $C_H$ gene. Rare examples of mutant clones expressing an isotypic gene 5′ of the parent heavy chain gene suggest that switching to constant region genes on the sister chromatid may sometimes occur.

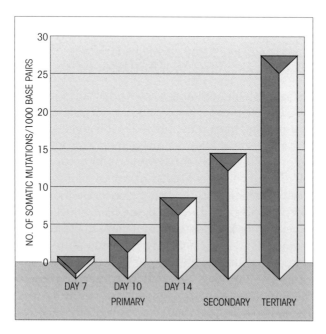

Figure 10.17. Increasing somatic mutations in the immunodominant germ-line antibody observed in hybridomas isolated following repeated immunization with phenyloxazolone. (Data from Berek C. & Apel M. (1989) In Melchers F. *et al.* (eds) *Progress in Immunology* **7**, 99. Springer-Verlag, Berlin.)

will have higher affinity for antigen, some the same or lower and others perhaps none at all (cf. figure 10.13). Similarly, mutations in the framework regions may be 'silent' or, if they perturb the ability of the molecule to fold properly, give rise to nonfunctional molecules. Pertinently, the proportions of germinal center B-cells with 'silent' mutations is high early in the immune response but falls dramatically with time, suggesting that early diversification is followed by preferential expansion of clones expressing mutations which improve their chances of reacting with and being stimulated by antigen.

## FACTORS AFFECTING ANTIBODY AFFINITY IN THE IMMUNE RESPONSE

### The effect of antigen dose

Other things being equal, the binding strength of an antigen for the surface antibody receptor of a B-cell will be determined by the usual affinity constant of the reaction:

$$Ag + (surface)Ab \rightleftharpoons Ag\,Ab$$

and the reactants will behave according to the Law of Mass Action (cf. p. 88).

It may be supposed that when a sufficient number of antigen molecules are bound to the antibody receptors on the cell surface and processed for presentation to T-cells, the lymphocyte will be stimulated to develop into an antibody-producing clone. When only small amounts of antigen are present, only those lymphocytes with high-affinity antibody receptors will be able to bind sufficient antigen for stimulation to occur and their daughter cells will, of course, also produce high-affinity antibody. Consideration of the antigen–antibody equilibrium equation will show that, as the concentration of antigen is increased, even antibodies with relatively low affinity will bind more antigen; therefore at high doses of antigen the lymphocytes with lower affinity antibody receptors will also be stimulated and, as may be seen from figure 10.18, these are more abundant than those with receptors of high affinity. Furthermore, there is a strong possibility that cells with the highest affinity will bind so much antigen as to become tolerized (cf. p. 241). Thus, in summary, low amounts of antigen produce high affinity antibodies, whereas high antigen concentrations give rise to an antiserum with low to moderate affinity.

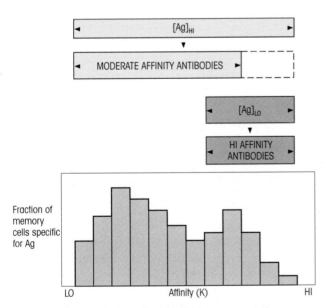

**Figure 10.18. Relationship of antigen concentration to affinity of antibodies produced.** Low concentrations of antigen ($[Ag]_{LO}$) bind to and permit stimulation of a range of high affinity memory cells and the resulting antibodies are of high affinity. High doses of antigen ($[Ag]_{HI}$) are able to bind sufficiently to the low affinity cells and thereby allow their stimulation, whilst the highest affinity cells may bind an excess of antigen and be tolerized (dashed line); the resulting antiserum will have a population of low to moderate affinity antibodies.

## Maturation of affinity

In addition to being brisker and fatter, secondary responses tend to be of higher affinity, which from our point of view is a particularly felicitous state of affairs. There are probably two main reasons for this maturation of affinity after primary stimulation. First, once the primary response gets under way and the antigen concentration declines to low levels, only successively higher affinity cells will bind sufficient antigen to maintain proliferation. Second, at this stage the cells are mutating madly in the germinal centers and any mutants with an adventitiously higher affinity will bind well to antigen on follicular dendritic cells and be positively selected for by its persistent clonal expansion. The increase in somatic mutation which occurs *pari passu* with the maturation of affinity accords well with this analysis and argues against the view that high affinity clones largely arise without mutation from very small numbers of precursors in the preimmune population. Modification of antibody specificity by point mutations allows gradual diversification on which positive selection for affinity can act during clonal expansion; on the other hand, other mechanisms, such as gene conversion, which produce gross changes, are more likely to destroy the antigen binding structure.

It is worth noting that responses to thymus-independent antigens which have poorly developed memory with very rare mutations do not show this phenomenon of affinity maturation. Overall, the ability of $T_H$ to facilitate responses to nonpolymeric, nonpolyclonally activating antigens, to induce expansive clonal proliferation, to effect class-switching and, lastly, to fine-tune responses to higher affinity has provided us with bigger, better and more flexible immune responses.

## MEMORY CELLS

Antibodies encoded by unmutated germ-line genes represent a form of evolutionary memory, in the sense that they tend to include specificities for commonly encountered pathogens which appear in the so-called 'natural antibody' fraction of serum. Memory acquired during the adaptive immune response requires contact with antigen and expansion of antigen-specific memory cells, as seen for example in the 20-fold increase in cytotoxic T-cell precursors after immunization of females with the male H-Y antigen.

Memory of early infections such as measles is long-lived and the question arises as to whether the

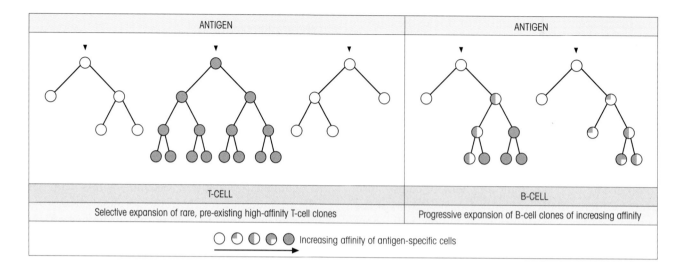

Figure 10.19. Antigen selects high-affinity memory T- and B-cells by different mechanisms.

memory cells are long-lived or are subject to repeated antigen stimulation from persisting antigen or subclinical reinfection. Fanum in 1847 described a measles epidemic on the Faroe Islands in the previous year in which almost the entire population suffered from infection except for a few old people who had been infected 65 years earlier. While this evidence favors the long half-life hypothesis, recent studies show that the memory function of B-cells transferred to an irradiated syngeneic recipient is lost within a month unless antigen is given or the donor is transgenic for the *bcl*-2 gene (remember that signals in the germinal center which prevent apoptosis of centrocytic B-cells also upregulate *bcl*-2 expression). It is envisaged that B-cell memory is a dynamic state in which survival of the memory cells is maintained by recurrent signals from follicular dendritic cells in the germinal centers, the only long-term repository of antigen. Curiously, nerve growth factor is an autocrine survival factor for memory B-cells.

T-cell memory, too, is probably dependent upon repeated stimulation by antigen, and if we accept the proposition that antigen usually only persists as complexes on follicular dendritic cells, one must further assume that they are driven by germinal center memory B-cells which capture and process this complexed antigen before presenting it to the T-cells. However, it seems not unlikely that memory T-cells may be perpetuated to some extent through 'bystander' stimulation by IFNα and β released as a result of local infections.

## The memory population is not simply an expansion of corresponding naive cells

There are studies based on the abundance of the murine surface heat-stable antigen (HSA) which indicate that the precursors of primary B-cell responses represent a different lineage to precursors capable of giving rise to secondary responses. Whether these subsets diverged from a common lineage before any contact with antigen or whether the majority of naive cells undergo preliminary differentiation before conventional antigen challenge through mild encounter with cross-reacting antigen or natural anti-idiotype, is still a debatable issue.

In general, memory cells are more readily stimulated by a given dose of antigen because they have a higher affinity. In the case of B-cells we have been satisfied by the evidence linking mutation and antigen selection to the creation of high-affinity memory cells within the germinal center of secondary lymph node follicles. The receptors for antigen on memory T-cells also have higher affinity but since they do not undergo significant somatic mutation during the priming response, it would seem that pre-existing receptors of relatively higher affinity in the population of naive cells proliferate selectively through preferential binding to the antigen (figure 10.19).

Intuitively one would not expect to improve on affinity to the same extent that somatic mutation can achieve for the B-cells, but nonetheless memory T-cells augment their binding avidity for the antigen-presenting cell through increased expression of accessory adhesion molecules, CD2, LFA-1, LFA-3 and ICAM-1 (table 10.3). Since several of these molecules also function to enhance signal transduction, the

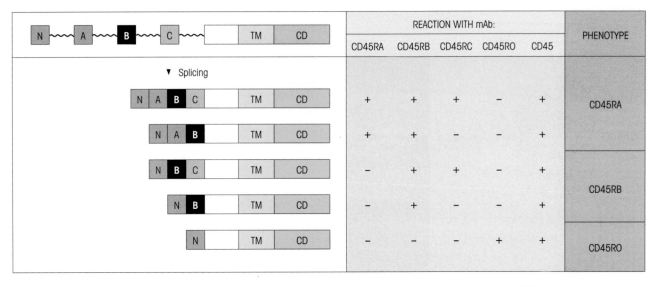

**Figure 10.20. The isoforms of human CD45** generated by alternative splicing of the N-terminal exons (boxed) and identified by different monoclonal antibodies (mAb). N = N-terminal segment; TM = transmembrane segment; CD = cytoplasmic domain; wavy lines = introns.

memory T-cell is more readily triggered than its naive cell counterpart.

An important phenotypic change in the isoform of the leukocyte common antigen CD45R, derived by differential splicing (figure 10.20), allows a useful distinction to be made between naive and memory cells. Monoclonal antibodies to CD45RA molecules, which express exon A, define naive T-cells and monoclonals which only react with the lower molecular weight form CD45RO, identify the memory cells capable of responding to recall antigens (table 10.3).

The realization that most, if not all, memory cells are subject to repeated bombardment from antigen makes it likely that most of the features associated with the CD45RO subset are in fact manifestations of **activated cells**. The expression of homing receptors for the endothelium of inflamed sites gives them a better chance of meeting an antigenic infectious agent than random searching through the entire tract of extravascular tissue. However there is growing evidence that CD45RO cells can revert to the RA phenotype, and the inclination is that memory cells, perhaps in the absence of antigenic stimulation, may lose their activated status and join a resting pool (figure 10.21).

Virgin B-cells lose their surface IgM and IgD and switch receptor isotype on becoming memory cells, and the differential expression of these surface markers has greatly facilitated the separation of B- and T-cells into naive and memory populations for the use of further study. The costimulatory molecules B7.1 and B7.2 are rapidly upregulated on memory B-cells and their potent antigen-presenting capacity for T-cells could well account for the brisk and robust nature of secondary responses.

| Phenotype | CD45RA Naive T-cells | CD45RA Memory T-cells |
|---|---|---|
| CD45RA | +++ | ±/- |
| CD45RO | ±/- | +++ |
| VLA-β (CD29) | ++ | +++ |
| CD2 | ++ | +++ |
| IL-2R (CD25) | ±/- | + |
| CD44 | ++ | +++ |
| LFA-1 | ++ | +++ |
| ICAM-1 | ±/- | ++ |
| LFA-3 | + | ++ |
| MHC class I | ++ | +++ |
| MHC class II | ±/- | ++ |
| **Function** | | |
| Intermitotic life-span | Long | Short |
| Response to recall antigens | ±/- | +++ |
| Response to alloantigens | +++ | +++ |
| Response to anti-CD2 | ±/- | +++ |
| Response to anti-CD3 | ++ | +++ |
| Secretion of IL-2 | ++ | ++ |
| Secretion of other cytokines | ±/- | ++ |

■ +++    ▨ ++    ▢ +    □ ±/-

**Table 10.3. The phenotype and function of naive and memory human T-cell subsets** defined by the presence of the CD45RA and CD45RO isoforms. (Based on Beverley P.C.L. (1992) *Seminars in Immunology* **4**, 35.)

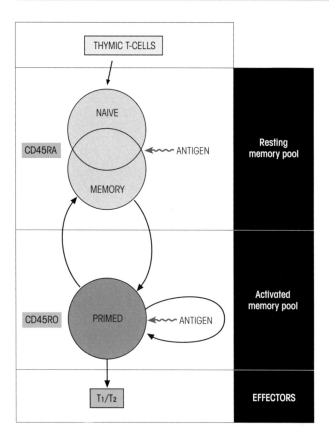

**Figure 10.21. Memory T-cells and CD45 isoforms.** Naive CD45RA T-cells transform to CD45RO-activated primed cells when stimulated by antigen. Continued stimulation by the original or by cross-reacting antigens maintains an activated memory pool but some cells exit, either to join a CD45RA resting memory pool or to become T1 or T2 effectors. (Note there is an increasing tendency to consider that both CD4 and CD8 cells have functionally distinct T1/T2 subsets and thus to talk generally of T1 and T2 cells.)

## SUMMARY

### *A succession of genes are upregulated by T-cell activation*

• Within 15–30 minutes genes for transcription factors concerned in the progression G0 to G1 and control of IL-2 are expressed.

• Up to 14 hours cytokines and their receptors are expressed.

• Later, a variety of genes related to cell division and adhesion are upregulated.

### *Cytokines act as intercellular messengers*

• Cytokines act transiently and usually at short range, although circulating IL-1 and IL-6 can mediate release of acute-phase proteins from the liver.

• They act through surface receptors belonging to three subfamilies, each with a common chain.

• Cytokine-induced dimerization of receptor subunits activates protein tyrosine kinases, including the JAK family, and leads to phosphorylation and activation of STAT transcription factors.

• Cytokines are pleiotropic, i.e. have multiple effects in

the general areas of (i) control of lymphocyte growth, (ii) activation of innate immune mechanisms (including inflammation), and (iii) control of bone marrow hematopoiesis (cf. figure 10.2).

• Cytokines may act sequentially, through one cytokine inducing production of another or by transmodulation of the receptor for another cytokine; they can also act synergistically or antagonistically.

• Their roles *in vivo* can be assessed by gene 'knockout', transfection or inhibition by specific antibodies.

### *Different CD4 T-cell subsets can make different cytokines*

• As immunization proceeds, TH tend to develop into two subsets: TH1 cells concerned in inflammatory processes, macrophage activation and delayed sensitivity make IL-2 and 3, IFNγ, TNFβ and GM-CSF; TH2 cells help B-cells to synthesize antibody and secrete IL-3, 4, 5, 6 and 10, TNFα and GM-CSF.

• Early interaction of antigen with macrophages producing IL-12 or with an NK1+ T-cell subset secreting IL-4 will skew the responses to TH1 or TH2 respectively.

### Activated T-cells proliferate in response to cytokines

• IL-2 acts as an autocrine growth factor for TH1 and paracrine for TH2 cells which have upregulated their IL-2 receptors.
• Cytokines act on cells which express receptors.

### T-cell effectors in cell-mediated immunity

• Cytokines mediate chronic inflammatory responses and induce the expression of MHC class II on endothelial cells, a variety of epithelial cells and many tumor cell lines, so facilitating interactions between T-cells and non-lymphoid cells.
• α-Chemokines are cytokines which chemoattract neutrophils and β-chemokines attract T-cells and macrophages.
• TNF synergizes with IFNγ in killing cells.
• Cytotoxic T-cells are generated against cells (e.g. virally infected) which have intracellularly derived peptide associated with surface MHC class I.
• T-cell mediated inflammation is strongly downregulated by IL-10.

### Proliferation of B-cell responses is mediated by cytokines

• Early proliferation is mediated by IL-4 which also aids IgE synthesis.
• IgA producers are driven by TGFβ and IL-5.
• IL-4 plus IL-5 promotes IgM and IL-4/5 and 6 plus IFNγ stimulate IgG synthesis.

### Events in the germinal center

• There is clonal expansion, isotype switch and mutation in the dark zone centroblasts.
• The B-cell centroblasts die through apoptosis unless rescued by certain signals which upregulate bcl-2. These include (i) cross-linking of surface Ig by complexes on follicular dendritic cells, (ii) engagement of the CD40 receptor which drives the cell to the memory compartment, and (iii) soluble CD23 plus IL-1α which stimulates antibody formation.

• The selection of mutants by antigen guides the development of high affinity B-cells.

### The synthesis of antibody

• mRNA for variable and constant regions are spliced together before leaving the nucleus.
• Differential splicing allows coexpression of IgM and IgD with identical V regions on a single cell and the switch from membrane-bound to secreted IgM.

### Ig class-switching occurs in individual B-cells

• IgM produced early in the response switches to IgG, particularly with thymus-dependent antigens. The switch is largely under T-cell control.
• IgG, but not IgM, responses improve on secondary challenge.

### Antibody affinity during the immune response

• Low doses of antigen tend to select high affinity B-cells and hence antibodies since only these can be rescued in the germinal center.
• For the same reasons, affinity matures as antigen concentration falls during an immune response.

### Memory cells

• Activated memory cells are sustained by recurrent stimulation with antigen.
• This must occur largely in the germinal centers since only the complexes on the surface of follicular dendritic cells are the long-term source of antigen.
• Memory cells have higher affinity than naive cells, in the case of B-cells through somatic mutation, and in the case of T-cells through selective proliferation of cells with higher affinity receptors and through upregulated expression of association molecules such as CD2 and LFA-1, which increase the avidity (functional affinity) for the antigen-presenting cell.
• Activated memory and naive T-cells are distinguished by expression of CD45 isoforms; the former having the CD45RO phenotype, the latter CD45RA. It seems likely that a proportion of the CD45RO population reverts to a CD45RA pool of resting memory cells.

## FURTHER READING

Capra J.D. (1996) Germinal centers: a new lease of life for B-cells and 'B-cell-ologists'. *The Immunologist* 4(3), 84.
Gazzinelli R.T. (1996) Molecular and cellular basis of interleukin 12 activity in prophylaxis and therapy against infectious diseases.
*Molecular Medicine* 2(6), 258.
Griffiths G.M. (1995) The cell biology of CTL killing. *Current Opinion in Immunology* 7, 343.
Jacob J., Kelsoe G., Rajewsky K. & Weiss U. (1991) Intraclonal

generation of antibody mutants in germinal centres. *Nature* **354**, 389.

Lebman D.A. & Coffman R.L. (1988) The effects of IL-4 and IL-5 on the IgA response by murine Peyer's patch B-cell subpopulations. *Journal of Immunology* **141**, 2050.

Mitchison N.A. & O'Malley C. (1987) Three-cell-type clusters of T-cells with antigen-presenting cells best explain the epitope linkage and non-cognate requirements of the *in vivo* cytolytic response. *European Journal of Immunology* **17**, 1579.

Raynaud C.-A. & Weill J.-C. (eds) (1996) Somatic mutation: mechanisms and signals. *Seminars in Immunology* **8**, 125.

Stout R.D. & Suttles J. (1996) The many roles of CD40 in cell-mediated inflammatory responses. *Immunology Today* **17**, 487–492.

Swain S.L. & Cambier J.C. (eds) (1996) Lymphocyte activation and effector functions. *Current Opinion in Immunology* **8**, 309–418.

Vicari A.P. & Zlotnik A. (1996) Mouse NK1.1+ T-cells: a new family of T-cells. *Immunology Today* **17**, 71.

# CONTROL MECHANISMS

### CONTENTS

## ANTIGEN IS A MAJOR FACTOR IN CONTROL

The acquired immune response evolved so that it would come into play when contact with an infectious agent was first made. The appropriate antigen-specific cells expand, the effectors eliminate the antigen and then the response quietens down and leaves room for reaction to other infections. Feedback mechanisms must operate to limit antibody production, otherwise, after antigenic stimulation, we would become overwhelmed by the responding clones of antibody-forming cells and their products — obviously an unwelcome state of affairs, as may be clearly seen in multiple myeloma, where control over lymphocyte proliferation is lost. It makes sense for

antigen to be a major regulatory factor and for antibody production to be driven by the presence of antigen, falling off in intensity as the antigen concentration drops (figure 11.1). There is abundant evidence to support this view. Antigens can stimulate lymphocytes through their surface receptors directly, as witnessed by proliferation of T-cell clones presented with antigen *in vitro* and formation of a clone of antibody-forming cells from a single B-cell precursor cultured with antigen and T-cell soluble factors under limiting-dilution conditions. Furthermore, clearance of antigen by injection of excess antibody during the course of an immune response leads to a dramatic drop in antibody synthesis and the number of antibody-secreting cells.

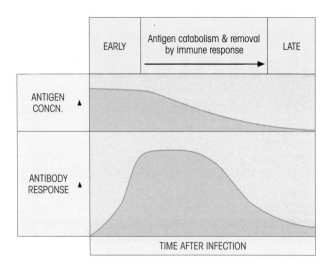

**Figure 11.1. Antigen drives the immune response.** As the antigen concentration falls due to catabolism and elimination by antibody, the intensity of the immune response declines but is maintained for some time at a lower level by antigen trapped on the follicular dendritic cells of the germinal centers.

## Antigens can interfere with each other

The presence of one antigen in a mixture of antigens can drastically diminish the immune response to the others. This is true even for epitopes within a given molecule; for example the response to epitopes on the Fab fragment of IgG is far greater when the Fab rather than whole IgG is used for immunization due to the inhibitory nature of the Fc region. The mechanism of this effect lies at the level of competition of processed

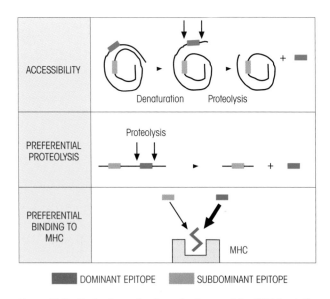

**Figure 11.2. Mechanisms of epitope dominance at the MHC level.** The other factor which can influence dominance is the availability of reactive T-cells; if these have been eliminated, e.g. through tolerization by cross-reacting self-antigens, a peptide which may have dominated the MHC groove would be unable to provoke an immune response.

antigenic peptides for the major histocompatibility complex (MHC) groove. There is a clear hierarchy of epitopes with respect to this competitive binding based on differential accessibility to proteases as the molecule unfolds, and the presence or absence of particular amino acid sequences which facilitate breakdown to yield peptides in high abundance and with relatively high affinity for the MHC groove (figure 11.2). Thus, Sercarz envisages **dominant epitopes,** which bag the lion's share of the available MHC grooves, **subdominant epitopes,** which are less successful, and **cryptic epitopes,** which generate miserably low concentrations of MHC complex which are ignored by potentially reactive naive T-cells.

Clearly the possibility that certain antigens in a mixture, or particular epitopes in a given antigen, may block a desired protective immune response has obvious implications for vaccine design. Contrariwise, the identification of inhibitory peptides with a predatory affinity for the MHC groove(s) should provide therapeutic agents to squash unwanted hypersensitivity reactions.

## ANTIBODY EXERTS FEEDBACK CONTROL

A useful control mechanism is to arrange for the product of a reaction to be an inhibitor and this type of negative feedback is seen with antibody. Thus we see examples of antibody diverting antigen to immunogenically inoffensive sites in the body to prevent primary sensitization in the protection against rhesus immunization afforded by administration of anti-D to mothers at risk (see p. 339), and the inhibitory effect of maternal antibody on the peak titers obtained on vaccinating infants. Removal of circulating antibody by plasmapheresis during an on-going response leads to an increase in synthesis, whereas injection of preformed IgG antibody markedly hastens the fall in the number of antibody-forming cells (figure 11.3) consistent with feedback control on overall synthesis. It is unlikely that this is achieved by simple neutralization of antigen since whole IgG is so much more effective than its F(ab')$_2$ fragment in switching off the reaction, even allowing for the longer half-life of the complete immunoglobulin. A clue to the underlying mechanism comes from the finding that cross-linking of IgM on the resting B-cell surface by an IgG anti-μ has no discernible effect, whereas the F(ab')$_2$ fragment of this anti-μ induces proliferation (figure 11.4a and b). The current view is that a complex of antigen with IgG antibody could block the productive phase of the T-dependent B-cell response by **cross-linking the antigen and Fcγ surface receptors** (figure 11.4c).

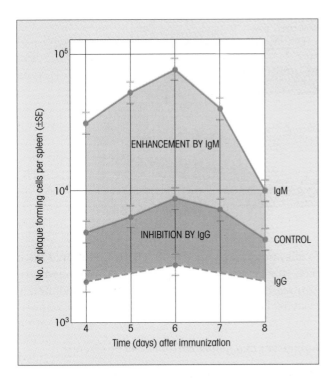

**Figure 11.3.** **Time-course of enhancement of antibody response to sheep red blood cells (SRBC) due to injection of preformed IgM, and of suppression by preformed IgG antibodies.** Mice received medium containing monoclonal IgM anti-SRBC, IgG anti-SRBC or medium alone intravenously 2 hours prior to immunization with $10^5$ SRBC. (Data provided by J. Reiter, P. Hutchings, P. Lydyard and A. Cooke.)

In complete contrast, injection of IgM antibodies enhances the response (figure 11.3), presumably by cross-linking antigen bound to the sIgM receptors without activating the Fcγ inhibitory receptor. Since antibodies of this isotype appear at an early stage after antigen challenge, they would be useful in boosting the initial response.

# T-CELL REGULATION

## T-helper cells

We have deliberated at length on the role of T-helper (TH) cells in the facilitation of cytotoxic T-cell (Tc) and B-cell responses, and in the production of class-switching and memory responses. We should perhaps note that the TH cells do not expand B-cell and Tc clone sizes indefinitely since the maturation factors inhibit the action of the proliferative lymphokines.

Different T-cells have surface receptors for the Fc regions of the various Ig classes, and a role for these in isotype-specific help has been sought. CD4 TH2 helpers can use their Fcμ receptors to bind to the surface IgM on B-cells, so contributing to the formation of antigen-specific MHC restricted T–B cytoconjugates, i.e. they act as additional accessory adhesion molecules to target IgM-positive B-cells and maybe augment activation of the helper cell. T-cell lines from Peyer's patches produced many more IgA-producing B-cells from Peyer's patch precursors than did splenic T-cell lines. However, the bias was for help to IgA-precommitted B-cells rather than inducing a class-switch to IgA, since Peyer's patch T-cells did not markedly enhance IgA production by splenic B-cells. Evidence for the production of IgE-binding factors from Fcε–receptor bearing T-cells which enhance B-cell secretion of IgE has been obtained; intriguingly, lipocortin produced by CD8 T-cells under the influence of steroids, or following immunization with mycobacteria is said to block glycosylation of the IgE-binding factor so that it now becomes a *suppressor* of IgE synthesis.

As one might anticipate, there is a built-in braking system on T-cell expansion in the form of fas-

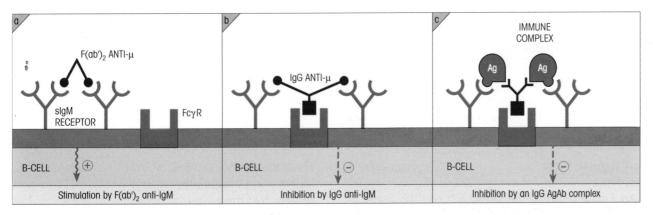

**Figure 11.4 Cross-linking of surface IgM antigen receptor and IgG Fc receptor leads to inhibition of B-cell function.** This can be observed at the level of c-*myc* induction (cf. p. 385). IL-4 blocks this effect. Cross-linking of sIgM through IgM complexed to antigen would be expected to stimulate, since the Fcγ receptor would not be engaged.

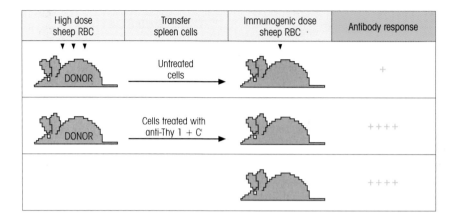

| High dose sheep RBC | Transfer spleen cells | Immunogenic dose sheep RBC | Antibody response |
|---|---|---|---|
| DONOR | Untreated cells | | + |
| DONOR | Cells treated with anti-Thy 1 + C' | | + + + + |
| | | | + + + + |

**Figure 11.5. Demonstration of T-suppressor cells.** Spleen cells from a donor injected with a high dose of antigen depress the antibody response of a syngeneic animal to which they have been transferred. The effect is lost if the spleen cells are first treated with a T-cell specific antiserum (anti-Thy 1) plus complement, showing that the suppressors are T-cells. (After Gershon R.K. & Kondo K. (1971) *Immunology* **21**, 903.)

mediated apoptosis of activated mature cells. Both fas and fas-ligand are expressed and this can lead to suicide or mutual homicide, particularly between the daughter cells of mitotic division. Furthermore, although nitric oxide (NO) at constitutive levels is necessary for normal T-cell proliferation, TH1 cells, but not TH2, produce high levels of NO which act as feedback inhibitors to limit production of TH1 progeny.

## T-cell suppression

We raised the question of suppression as distinct from help and perhaps it is inevitable that Nature, having evolved a functional set of T-cells which promote immune responses, should also develop a regulatory set whose job would be to modulate the helpers. T-cell suppression was first brought to the serious attention of the immunological fraternity by a phenomenon colorfully named by its discoverer, 'infectious tolerance'. Quite surprisingly it was shown that if mice were made unresponsive by injection of a high dose of sheep red cells (SRBC), their T-cells would suppress specific antibody formation in normal recipients to which they had been transferred (figure 11.5). It may not be apparent to the reader why this result was at all surprising, but at that time antigen-induced tolerance was regarded essentially as a negative phenomenon involving the depletion or silencing of clones rather than a state of active suppression. Over the years, T-cell suppression has been shown to modulate a variety of humoral and cellular responses, the latter including delayed-type hypersensitivity, cytotoxic T-cells and antigen-specific T-cell proliferation. However, the existence of dedicated professional T-suppressor cells is a question which has generated a great deal of heat.

### Suppressor and helper epitopes can be discrete

Detailed analysis of murine responses to antigens such as hen egg-white lysozyme tells us that certain determinants can evoke very strong suppressor rather than helper responses depending on the mouse strain, and also, that T-suppressors directed to one determinant can switch off helper and antibody responses to other determinants on the same molecule. Thus mice of *H-2b* haplotype respond poorly to lysozyme because they develop dominant suppression; however, if the three N-terminal amino acids are removed from the antigen, H-2b mice now make a splendid response showing that the T-suppression directed against the determinant associated with the N-terminal region had switched off the response to the remaining determinants on the antigen. Similar results have been obtained in several other systems. This must imply that the antigen itself must act as a form of bridge to allow communication between T-suppressor and cells reacting to the other determinants, as might occur through these cells binding to an antigen-presenting cell expressing several different processed determinants of the same antigen on its surface (figure 11.6).

### Characteristics of suppression

There are many examples of immune responses, e.g. *Leishmania*, polyglutamyl-alanyl-tyrosyl peptide and lactate dehydrogenase β, where T-suppression has been linked to the *H-2E* haplotype and this, together with the fact that most, but by no means all, TH clones are H-2A rather than H-2E restricted, has led to

205

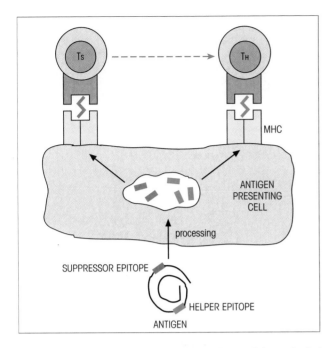

**Figure 11.6. Possible mechanism to explain the need for a physical linkage between suppressor and helper epitopes.** The helper and putative suppressor cells can interact by binding close together on the surface of an antigenpresenting cell which processes the antigen and displays the different epitopes on separate MHC molecules on its surface.

Klein's suggestion that in the majority of cases (but not necessarily in all) TH use H-2A and suppressors H-2E. Strands of evidence which accord with this hypothesis derive from the enhancement of antigen-specific proliferation of putatively suppressed T-cells resulting from addition of anti-H-2E, as with the mouse liver F-protein and lactate dehydrogenase responses (figure 11.7). The human disease, lepromatous leprosy, is very informative in this respect. These patients carry large numbers of bacteria in their tissues, make buckets of useless antibodies and manifest a selective T-cell unresponsiveness to *Mycobacterium leprae* but not to *M. tuberculosis*. In 10% of lepromatous patients addition of anti-HLA-DQ (a human class II molecule) to the culture medium resulted in a greatly improved proliferative response to *M. leprae*, suggesting the release of cells from the grip of DQ-mediated suppression. The fact that DQ is structurally homologous with H-2A rather than H-2E is a slight hiccup for the hypothesis unless there was a flip over from DR to DQ for suppressor purposes during evolution, but the main point is that the overall class II restriction of the phenomenon remains a dominant feature.

What of the effectors of suppression? In a number of experimental systems the cells which mediate suppression are far more vulnerable than helpers to adult

thymectomy, X-irradiation and cyclophosphamide. For example, adult thymectomy in the mouse has little effect on the TH population but does lead to a fall in the T-suppressors, thereby increasing the response to T-independent antigens and preventing the fall-off in IgE antibody to haptens coupled with *Ascaris* extracts which occurs in intact animals.

The effectors are classically said to be of the CD8+ phenotype in the mouse and belong to the CD8+ subset in the human. To look at some examples, the B10.A (2R) mouse strain has a low immune response to lactate dehydrogenase β (LDHβ) associated with the possession of the *H-2Eβ* gene of *k* rather than *b* haplotype. Lymphoid cells taken from these animals after immunization with LDHβ proliferate poorly *in vitro* in the presence of antigen but if CD8+ cells are depleted, the remaining CD4+ cells give a much higher response (figure 11.7). Adding back the CD8+ cells reimposed the active suppression. Another example is malaria in the unresponsive C3H/HeN mouse strain where the nonproliferative status induced by immunization with sporozoites is rapidly reversed by injection of monoclonal anti-CD8.

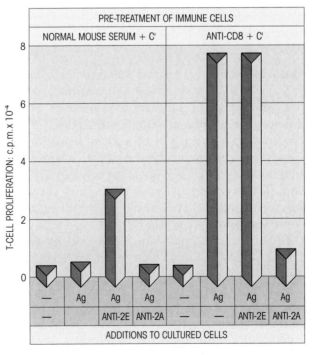

**Figure 11.7. Low responsiveness to lactate dehydrogenase β in B10.A (2R) mice is due to active suppression** by H-2E restricted, CD8+ T-suppressors. Left: lymph node cells from immunized animals showed increased proliferation to antigen when cultured in the presence of anti-H-2E. Right: removal of CD8 cells prior to culture revealed a high proliferative response to antigen which was restricted to H-2A. (Data from Baxevanis C.V., Nagy Z.A. & Klein J. (1981) *Proceedings of the National Academy of Sciences (USA)* **78**, 3809.)

In a study of human populations in Japan who were either spontaneously or deliberately exposed to streptococcal cell wall, *M. leprae*, cedar pollen and hepatitis B surface antigens, low responsiveness was linked to HLA class II and was inherited dominantly, indicative of active suppression; supportive evidence was obtained from the demonstration that depletion of CD8 cells increased the T-cell response to antigen of peripheral blood cells *in vitro*.

A series of lepromin-specific CD8 suppressor clones have been established using lymphocytes from the lesions or blood of immunologically unresponsive lepromatous leprosy patients. Antigen-specific CD4 T-cell clones exposed to these suppressor cells plus antigen *in vitro*, become unresponsive to antigen for at least 10 days, although they proliferate normally to interleukin-2 (IL-2). All these CD8 clones expressed αβ receptors, restricted to HLA-DQ (strange for a CD8 cell!) and produced TH2 type cytokines, especially IL-4. In sharp contrast, alloreactive CD8 HLA-B27 specific cytolytic T-cell clones produce γ-interferon (IFNγ) and no IL-4. This obviously bears comparison with the cytokine patterns of TH1 and TH2 subsets and has led to the suggestion that **parallel T1/T2 subsets exist within the CD8 population**.

### Suppression due to T–T interaction on antigen-presenting cells

Can we see a rational basis for the phenomena of suppression? We have already entertained the idea that antigen-linked T–T interactions can occur on the surface of an antigen-presenting cell (figure 11.6) and the concept of T1 and T2 CD8 subsets paralleling the TH1/TH2 dichotomy. Furthermore, the evidence for mutual antagonism (suppression) between TH1 and TH2 cells is very strong indeed. Gathering everything together as a coherent scheme, one could postulate downregulation of TH1 cells by type 2 IL-4 producing CD8 cells, and suppression of TH2 cells by type 1 IFNγ-producing cytolytic CD8 cells, all interacting on the surface of an antigen-presenting cell (figure 11.8). On this model, when the immune response has locked onto a particular mode, e.g. TH1-mediated cellular immunity, other types of response such as T–B collaboration are restricted through a cytokine inhibitory effect. Although these cells mediate T-suppression they would not be called dedicated professional suppressors since, in a sense, their suppressive powers are a by-product of their main defensive function. It remains to be seen whether the type 2 IL-4 producing CD8 cells have an identifiable role in defense, or whether these are really dedicated T-suppressors

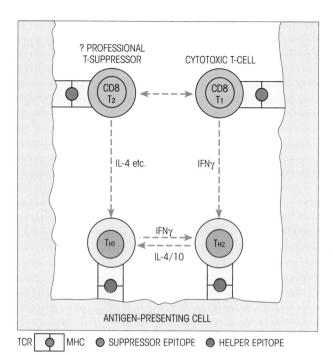

**Figure 11.8. Mutual antagonisms between T-cell subsets** linked indirectly by processed antigen on an antigen-presenting cell lead to functionally distinct modes of suppression. (Leaning heavily on Bloom B.R., Salgame P. & Diamond B. (1992) Revisiting and revising suppressor T-cells. *Immunology Today* **13**, 131.) Yet another mechanism may prove to be important. Unlike the mouse, many other mammalian species can express MHC class II on a proportion of their activated T-cells; presentation of processed peptide by these cells can induce CD4-positive cytolytic cells with suppressor potential. We also need to know more about the circumstances leading to production of TGFβ by suppressors since this cytokine inhibits T-cell proliferation.

after all. Perhaps we need these cells to prevent TH2 cells getting out of hand by excessive proliferation, just as IgG holds back the B-cells by feedback control. There is indeed abundant evidence for such a regulatory mechanism in which suppressors are induced by TH1 cells. This would also account for the involvement of class II and CD8 T-cells in suppression (figure 11.7), although the unusual observations of the lepromin HLA-DQ (class II) restricted CD8 T-cell clones could account for this (remember that normally CD8 cells are class I restricted).

The nature of the antigen-presenting cell upon whose surface these interactions are thought to occur, may influence the type of cells involved and the outcome. It may be recalled that dendritic cells, macrophages, B-cells, activated T-cells and even epithelial cells with upregulated class II can all act as antigen-presenters. Of interest is the finding that irradiation with UVB light inactivates dendritic cells and stimulates T-suppression; IL-2 and IFNγ are downregulated and IL-4 production is increased.

Other issues which require solution are, the mechanism by which high-dose antigen induces suppression, the role of *cytotoxic* CD4 and CD8 T-cells in these phenomena, the generation of the suppressive cytokine transforming growth factor β (TGFβ) and the extent to which idiotype-specific T-suppressors contribute.

It is important not to lose track of the so-called 'natural suppressor cells' such as those provoked by total lymph node irradiation (cf. p. 364), and I would like to draw attention to a report that natural killer (NK) cells can inhibit the one-way mixed lymphocyte reaction (see p. 356) or the primary IgM response to sheep cells *in vitro*, by suppressing dendritic cells which have already reacted with the antigen; this offers a further opportunity for feedback control since IFNγ and IL-2 produced by Tн can activate NK cells.

Make no mistake, suppression is still a murky area, and is not for the unwary, but the light at the end of the tunnel is beckoning.

### Effector T-cells are guided to the appropriate target by MHC surface molecules

Not only do MHC molecules signal that they are on the surface of a cell bearing a tell-tale peptide which reveals the presence of an intracellular precursor (cf. p. 95, Chapter 5), they also have to make sure that the T-cell makes contact with antigen on the surface of the appropriate target cell.

Let us explore this point by looking at the role of Tc in viral infection. When a cell is first infected with virus, there is an eclipse phase during which the machinery of the cell is being switched for viral replication and the only marker of the complete microbe is the processed viral antigen peptide on the cell surface. At this stage, killing of the cell by a cytotoxic T-cell will prevent viral replication. The killer T-cell knows it has reached its target when it recognizes the surface viral peptide in association with class I MHC molecules which are present on nearly every cell in the body and can therefore be used as markers for cells as such. Thus the killer cell operates on the basis that processed viral antigen is the code for '**viral infection**' and class I molecules are the code for '**cell**' (cf. figure 5.25).

The situation is quite different with intracellular bacteria and protozoa which do not go through an eclipse phase after phagocytosis by macrophages but are held as infectious entities; lysis by cytotoxic T-cells will merely release the organisms, not kill them. A separate strategy utilizing the delayed-type hypersensitivity T-cell population is required and, in this case, the effector Tн1-lymphocyte recognizes the

Table 11.1. Guidance of T subpopulations to appropriate target cell by MHC molecules.

| Function | Cell interaction | MHC marker on target cell |
|---|---|---|
| T-cell priming | T–APC | II (+*B7/CD28) |
| T-helper (Tн1) | T–macrophage | II (+peptide) |
| T-helper (Tн2) | T–B | II (+*CD40L/CD40) |
| T-suppressor | T–T | ? |
| T-cytotoxic | T–target cell | I |

* Costimulatory molecular and their ligand.

infected macrophage by the presence of microbial antigen on the surface in association with a class II molecule which is now a code for 'macrophage'. This interaction triggers the release of macrophage-stimulating lymphokines, dominant among which are IFNγ and macrophage inhibitory factor (MIF) which activate multiple microbicidal mechanisms including formation of reactive oxygen intermediates and synthesis of NO, to the detriment of the intracellular parasites (see p. 269). Similarly, in T–B cooperation, the **B-cell** is recognized through its class II molecule associated with the foreign antigen, although in this case costimulatory signals through CD40L–CD40 interactions are required for activation. T-cells mediating **suppression** also utilize MHC molecules but the mechanisms are unclear. In summary, each antigen-specific T-lymphocyte subset has to communicate with a particular cell type in order to make the appropriate immune response and it does so by recognizing not only processed foreign antigen but also the particular MHC molecule used as a marker of that cell (table 11.1).

## IDIOTYPE NETWORKS

### Jerne's network hypothesis

The hypervariable loops on the immunoglobulin molecule which go to form the antigen combining site have individual characteristic shapes which can be recognized by the appropriate antibodies as idiotypic determinants (cf. p. 49). There are hundreds of thousands, if not more, of different idiotypes in one individual.

Jerne reasoned brilliantly that the great diversity of idiotypes would to a considerable extent mirror the diversity of antigenic shapes in the external world. Thus, he said, if lymphocytes can recognize a whole range of foreign antigenic determinants, they should be able to recognize the idiotypes on other lymphocytes. They would therefore form a large network or series of networks depending upon **idiotype–**

| Ab$_{2\beta}$ | Ab$_1$ | Ab$_{2\alpha}$ | Ab$_3$ |
|---|---|---|---|
| ANTI-IDIOTYPE (internal image) | IDIOTYPE | ANTI-IDIOTYPE | ANTI-ANTI-IDIOTYPE |

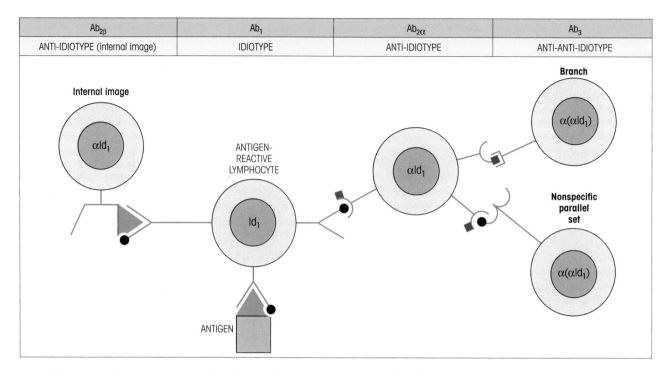

**Figure 11.9. Elements in an idiotypic network** in which the antigen receptors on one lymphocyte reciprocally recognize an idiotype on the receptors of another. T-helper, T-suppressor and B-lymphocytes interact through idiotype–anti-idiotype reactions producing either stimulation or suppression. T–T interactions could occur through direct recognition of one T-cell receptor (TCR) by the other, or more usually by recognition of a processed TCR peptide associated with MHC. One of the anti-idiotype sets, Ab$_{2\beta}$, may bear an idiotype of similar shape to (i.e. provides an **internal image** of) the antigen. The same idiotype (●) may be shared by receptors of different specificity, the nonspecific parallel set (since the several hypervariable regions provide a number of potential idiotypic determinants and a given idiotype does not always form part of the epitope binding site, i.e. the paratope), so that the anti-(anti-Id$_1$) does not necessarily bind the original antigen. (The following abbreviations are often employed: α as a prefix = anti; Id = idiotype; Ab$_1$ = Id; Ab$_2$α = αId not involving the paratope; Ab$_{2\beta}$ = internal image αId involving the paratope; Ab$_3$ = α(αId).)

**anti-idiotype recognition** between lymphocytes of the various T- and B-subsets (figure 11.9) and the response to an external antigen perturbing this network would be conditioned by the state of the idiotypic interactions.

## Evidence for idiotypic networks

### Anti-idiotype can be induced by autologous idiotypes

There is no doubt that the elements which can form an idiotypic network are present in the body. Individuals can be immunized against idiotypes on their own antibodies, and such autoanti-idiotypes have been identified during the course of responses induced by antigens. For example, when certain strains of mice are injected with pneumococcal vaccines, they make an antibody response to the phosphorylcholine groups in which the germ-line-encoded idiotype T15 dominates. If the individual antibody-forming cells are examined by plaque assays at different times after immunization, waves of T15$^+$ and of anti-T15 (i.e. autoanti-idiotype) cells are demonstrable. Similarly, immunization with the acetylcholine agonist BISQ followed by fusion of the spleen cells to produce hybridomas, yielded a series of anti-BISQ monoclonals (idiotypes) and a smaller number of anti-idiotypic monoclonals, of which a surprising proportion behaved as internal images of BISQ in their ability to stimulate acetylcholine receptors (figure 11.10).

### A network is evident in early life

If the spleens of fetal mice which are just beginning to secrete immunoglobulin are fused with myeloma cells to produce hybridomas, an unusually high proportion are interrelated as idiotype–anti-idiotype pairs. This high level of idiotype connectivity is not seen in later life and suggests that these early cells, largely the **B1 subset** (cf. p. 237), most of which bear the T-cell marker CD5, are programmed to synthesize germ-line gene specificities which have network relationships.

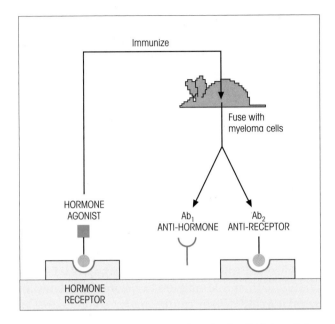

**Figure 11.10. The spontaneous production of autoanti-idiotype during immunization with a hormone agonist.** Hybridomas obtained from the immunized mouse secrete anti-hormone and anti-idiotype which reacts with the hormone receptor; this indicates a close relationship between hormone, receptor, anti-hormone and anti-idiotype, implying some connection between autoantibodies within the idiotype network and hormone systems.

*T-cells can also do it*

It seems likely that similar interactions will be established for early T-cells, possibly linking with the B-cell network. Certainly, anti-idiotypic reactivity can be demonstrated in T-cell populations. For example, let us divide a sample of T-cells from the peripheral blood of individual X into two; one half is cultured with irradiated lymphocytes from individual Y of the same species and gives rise to proliferating T-cell blasts directed against the allogeneic MHC class II of Y. If these blasts are now added back to the remaining (resting) half of X's cells, they induce a T-cell proliferation, i.e. the resting cells contain a population of T-cells which spontaneously recognize the idiotype of the expanded autologous T-blasts. Take another interesting experiment: a T-cell population which has been polyclonally activated (e.g. by concanavalin A which stimulates T-cells independently of their antigen specificity) can be analysed by limiting dilution (cf. p. 140) for the frequency of cells reacting to specified antigens. In wells with relatively small numbers of T-cells, a surprising degree of degeneracy in the recognition of antigen was uncovered in that for every antigen tested, the frequency of specific clones approached 1%. This is startling and has interesting implications, but the relevant point comes next. As

the number of cells in each well was increased, antigen reactivity was largely lost. The interpretation is that the population of T-cells contains naturally occurring anti-idiotype suppressors which are likely to be present together with the antigen-reactive cell in wells with high T-cell numbers, whereas at low cell numbers it is likely that wells containing single antigen-specific lymphocytes will be unaccompanied by suppressors.

## Preoccupation of networks with self

Paradoxically, there is increasing evidence that preformed idiotype networks have, what might seem at first sight, a somewhat unhealthy interest in self-antigens. The CD5 IgM hybridomas produced from fetal mouse spleen with high idiotype connectivity have specificities very similar to those of the '**natural antibodies**' which appear spontaneously in germ-free animals not exposed to exogenous antigens. Not only are many of them directed to polysaccharide antigens of common pathogens, e.g. phosphorylcholine, but it is noteworthy that several have low affinity for self components such as DNA, IgG, heat-shock proteins and cytoskeletal elements. The concept of a largely CD5 B-1 cell population forming an inward-looking world in which the component cells recognize and stimulate each other ceaselessly through their idiotypic receptor interactions to produce a range of IgM antibodies which provide an early defense against infection is most plausible. But the self-reactivity of many of these cells is enigmatic. Preset regulatory T-cell networks may also involve certain dominant autoantigens such as heat-shock protein hsp65 and myelin basic protein from the nervous tissue. Is recognition of self as important as non-self?

Irun Cohen has proposed the intriguing notion of an **immunological homunculus** (little man) in which a functional picture of the body is encoded within the immune system by regulatory network committees of B- and T-cells which recognize certain dominant self-antigens representing the major organs in the body. (The analogy is with the neurological homunculus, a functional picture of the body in which the space occupied by a given neural network is directly related to the neurological importance of the organ it encodes, e.g. human visual and speech organs and canine olfactory organs are prominently represented.) The relevance of these ideas to the control of autoimmunity will be discussed in Chapter 19, but here we can speculate on how they might also relate to the response to infection. Consider a dominant microbial antigen such as heat-shock protein hsp65 which is very highly conserved in nature and bears several potential epitopes identical with the self homolog. In an infection, B1-cells bearing surface receptors for self-hsp65 will selectively focus the bacterial hsp65 onto their surface receptors (making it dominant over other bacterial antigens) and process it. The self-epitopes will be recognized by autoreactive T-cells which are highly regulated within the homunculus, whereas T-cells specific for the non-self hsp epitopes are not so constrained and will generate an effective immune response (figure 11.11).

## Idiotypic regulation of immune responses

There has been a series of investigations based on the following cascade protocol. Antigen is injected into $animal_1$ and the antibody produced, $Ab_1$ (idiotype), is purified and injected into $animal_2$. $Ab_2$ (anti-idiotype) so formed is purified and used to immunize $animal_3$ and so on (figure 11.12). Consistently, it is found that

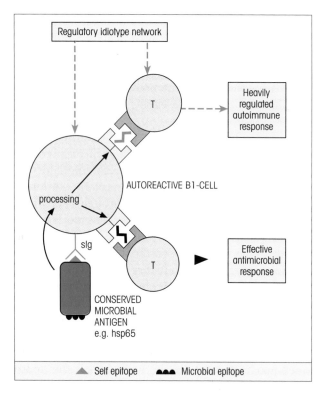

**Figure 11.11. Speculation on the role of self-reacting CD5 B1-cells in microbial infection.** The surface immunoglobulin (sIg) receptor selectively captures the cross-reacting conserved bacterial antigen (in this case heat-shock protein hsp65) and after processing presents self and microbe-specific epitopes associated with MHC class II. The autoreactive T-cell is heavily controlled by the idiotype regulatory network since (*ex hypothesi*) important self-antigens are dominantly encoded within the 'immunological homunculus' but the antimicrobial T-cell is free to mount a vigorous response. This accounts for the dominance of conserved antigens. (Based upon Cohen I.R. & Young D.B. (1991) *Immunology Today* **12**, 105.)

$Ab_2$ (anti-$Id_1$) recognizes an idiotype ($Id_1$) on $Ab_1$ which is also strongly present in $Ab_3$. $Ab_4$ behaves like $Ab_2$ in seeing the common idiotype on $Ab_1$ and $Ab_3$. Nonetheless, although $Ab_1$ and $Ab_3$ share idiotypes, only a small fraction of $Ab_3$ reacts with the original antigen. This is the result one would expect if the idiotype was a cross-reacting Id (public Id) present on a variety of antibodies (and by implication B-cell receptors) of different specificities. As may be seen in figure 11.12, the anti-$Id_1$ ($Ab_2$), when injected into $animal_3$, would react with all B-cells bearing $Id_1$ and presumably trigger them to produce $Id_1$ antibodies, only a fraction of which have specificity for the original antiserum.

Such frequently occurring and usually germline-encoded idiotypes seem to be provoked fairly readily with anti-Id and are therefore candidates for **regulatory Id** which can be under some degree of control by a limited idiotypic network. Germane to this idea are the observations that, late in immunization, antibodies with utterly distinct specificities, directed against totally different epitopes on the same antigen, often bear a common or cross-reacting idiotype. Presumably, the first clone of B-cells to be expanded which bears a dominant cross-reacting Id can generate a population of regulatory TH cells which recognize this Id as well as antigen. Processing of internalized Ig receptor plus antigen leads to expression of peptides derived from the idiotype and antigen in association with MHC class II; these B-cells can then access the full repertoire of antigen-specific and idiotype-specific TH cells. The latter may be of two types, one recognizing the native receptor idiotype (non-MHC-restricted) and the other, processed idiotype (MHC-restricted) (figure 11.13). From the complex mixture of B-lymphocytes activated by the other epitopes on the antigen, these TH cells will selectively recruit those with Id-positive receptors. We can now see how the antigen- and idiotype-specific TH synergize in the antibody response, the latter expanding Id-positive clones induced by the former.

While there would be a large measure of agreement with the view that relatively closed Id anti-Id circuits involving major germ-line idiotypes contribute to a regulatory system, there is probably much less support for a full 'Jernerian' network extending functionally to the myriad **private** idiotypes. Given that regulation can occur through interaction with public or cross-reactive idiotypes, what is its importance relative to exogenous antigen-mediated control? Although the answer will vary with different antigens, it may turn out that in general the antigen-

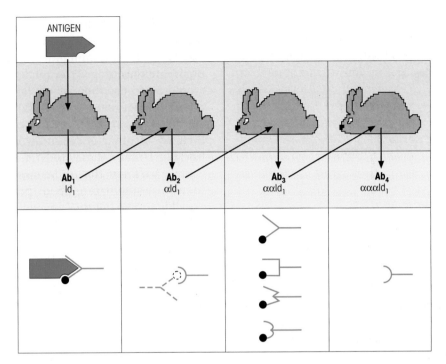

**Figure 11.12. An idiotype cascade.** $Ab_1$ produced by the antigen is injected into a second animal to produce $Ab_2$; this in turn is purified and injected into animal$_3$ and so on. $Ab_2$ and $Ab_4$ both react with an idiotype (●) on $Ab_1$ and $Ab_3$ but only a fraction of $Ab_3$ reacts with the original antigen. Bona & Paul (*Immunology Today* 1982, **3**, 230) interpret the results in terms of a common regulatory idiotype $Id_1$ shared by many antibodies other than those reacting with the original antigen but recruited by the injection of anti-$Id_1$ ($Ab_2$) which stimulates the range of lymphocytes whose receptors bear this common or cross-reacting idiotype. On this basis, one can understand the paradoxical finding of Oudin & Cazenave that not all the Ig molecules bearing a given Id in response to an antigen can function as specific antibody since they belong to the nonspecific parallel set. The presence of large amounts of $Id_1$ in $Ab_3$ also suggests that the linear relationship through the cross-reacting $Id_1$ is dominant, with relatively insignificant branching through the variety of 'private' idiotypes on $Ab_2$ molecules (cf. figure 11.9) because of the low frequency of such idiotypes and their anti-idiotypes.

directed systems will dominate, with idiotypic networks providing accessory amplification and suppressive loops, since (i) it seems most likely that antigen recognition and elimination were the driving forces behind the evolutionary selection for an adaptive immune response and therefore one wants the system to be sensitive to the presence and concentration of antigen, and (ii) there would seem to be little point in Id and anti-Id squabbling about control of the response after antigen had been eliminated. The Id network could allow the response to 'tick over' for extended periods and maintain the memory-cell population, while the presence of primed TH cells directed against a common Id on the various memory B-cells specific for a given antigen would increase their rate of mobilization during a secondary response. Possibly these functions are secondary to a primary role in controlling autoimmunity in the manner we have already discussed. The self-reactive bias of the germ-line idiotypic network may also help to maintain the *V* gene repertoire and determine the initial state of the immune system before the encounter with antigen, as we shall discuss in the next chapter.

## Manipulation of the immune response through idiotypes

Quite low doses of anti-idiotype, of the order of nanograms, can greatly enhance the expression of the idiotype in the response to a given antigen, whereas doses in the microgram range lead to a suppression (figure 11.14). Thus the idiotypic network provides interesting opportunities to manipulate the immune response, particularly in hypersensitivity states such as autoimmune disease, allergy and graft rejection. However, the B-cell response is normally so diverse, suppression by anti-Id is likely to prove difficult; even when the response is dominated by a public Id and that Id is suppressed, compensatory expansion of Id-negative clones ensures that the fall in the total antibody titer is relatively undramatic (cf. figure 11.14). Perhaps ways can be developed to restrict this Id-negative compensation, particularly if the total number of idiotypes is small, as might perhaps be the case with IgE antibody synthesis in patients with atopic allergy. Conceivably, TH cells may express a narrow spectrum of idiotypes, thereby being more susceptible to suppression by Id autoimmunization,

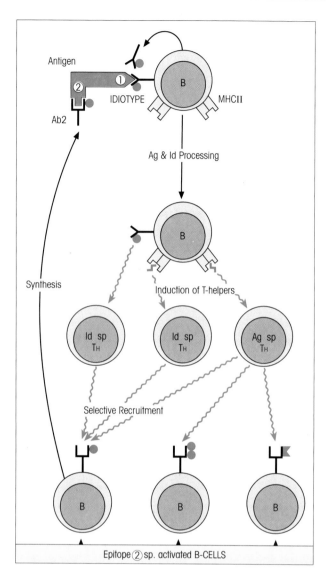

**Figure 11.13. Role of anti-idiotypic T-helpers (T$_H$) in recruiting antibodies** with specificities for the different epitopes on an antigen but bearing the same public or cross-reacting idiotype. The first expanded B-cell clone producing antibodies (Ab$_1$) specific for epitope (1) and bearing a cross-reacting Id ( ● ) induces antigen-specific plus idiotype-specific T$_H$ recognizing either native or processed Id. These are assumed selectively to recruit Id+ B-cells already activated by antigen which then synthesize Id+ antibodies (Ab$_2$) directed to a different epitope; if resting Id+ cells were recruited, the amount of nonspecific Ig synthesized might be wastefully high. It is also possible that recruitment might operate via anti-idiotypic *antibodies* which could act on Id+ B-cells to increase their surface class II and improve their 'cooperability' with T$_H$. It is worth considering whether memory αId T$_H$ cells could be responsible for the phenomenon of '**original antigenic sin**' in which a second infection with influenza virus involving an antigenically related but not identical strain generates antibodies with a higher titer for the strain which produced the first infection.

which, in any case, may produce far more widespread effects within the internal network than treatment with anti-Ids from other species, which may see only a small part of the system. In this respect, reports that

'vaccination' with irradiated lines of T$_H$ cells specific for brain or thyroid antigens prevents the induction of experimental autoimmunity against the relevant organ are encouraging. A totally different approach would be to use monoclonal anti-Id of the 'antigen internal image' set (figure 11.9) to stimulate antigen-specific T-suppressors capable of turning off B-cells directed to other epitopes on the antigen through bridging by the antigen itself (cf. figure 11.6).

Since we know that under suitable conditions anti-Id can also stimulate antibody production, it might be possible to use 'internal image' monoclonal anti-Ids as 'surrogate' antigens for immunization in cases where the antigen is difficult to obtain in bulk — for example, antigens from parasites such as filaria or the weak embryonic antigens associated with some cancers. Another example is where protein antigens obtained by chemical synthesis or gene cloning fail to fold into the configuration of the native molecule; this is not a problem with the anti-Id which by definition has been selected to have the shape of the antigenic epitope.

At this stage, if the reader is feeling a little groggy, try a glance at figure 11.15 which attempts a summary of the main factors currently thought to modulate the immune response.

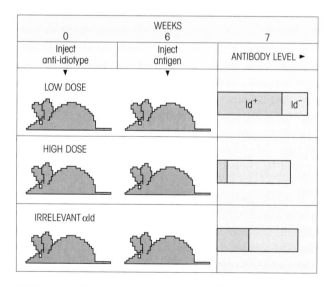

**Figure 11.14. Modulation of a major idiotype in the antibody response to antigen by anti-idiotype.** In the example chosen, the idiotype is present in a substantial proportion of the antibodies produced in controls injected with irrelevant anti-Id plus antigen (i.e. this is a public or cross-reacting Id; see p. 50). Pretreatment with 10 ng of a monoclonal anti-Id greatly expands the Id+ antibody population, whereas prior injection of 10 μg of anti-Id completely (or almost completely) suppresses expression of the idiotype without having any substantial effect on total antibody production due to a compensatory increase in Id antibody clones.

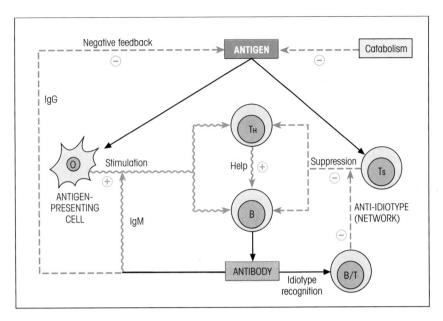

**Figure 11.15. Regulation of the immune response.** T$_H$=T-helper cell; T$_S$=T-suppressor cell. T-help for cell-mediated immunity will be subject to similar regulation. Some of these mechanisms may be interdependent; for example, one could envisage anti-idiotypic antibody acting in concert with a suppressor T-cell by binding to its Fc receptor, or suppressor T-cells with specificity for the idiotype on T$_H$, or B-cells. To avoid too many confusing arrows, I have omitted the recruitment of B-cells by anti-idiotypic T$_H$ cells and direct activation of anti-idiotype T-suppressors by idiotype-positive T$_H$ cells.

## THE INFLUENCE OF GENETIC FACTORS

### Some genes affect general responsiveness

Mice can be selectively bred for high or low antibody responses through several generations to yield two lines, one of which consistently produces high-titer antibodies to a variety of antigens, and the other, antibodies of relatively low titer (figure 11.16; Biozzi & colleagues). Out of the ten or so different genetic loci involved, some gave rise to a higher rate of B-cell proliferation and differentiation, while one or more affect macrophage behavior. The two lines are comparable in their ability to clear carbon particles or sheep erythrocytes from the blood by phagocytosis, but macrophages from the high responders present antigen more efficiently (cf. p. 163). On the other hand, the low responders survive infection by *Salmonella typhimurium* better and their macrophages support much slower replication of *Listeria* (cf. p. 267) indicative of an inherently more aggressive microbicidal ability.

### Immune response linked to immunoglobulin genes

A large proportion of the antibodies made by the A/J strain of mice in response to the hapten *p*-azophenylarsonate, bear a major cross-reacting idiotype (CRI$_A$) somewhat coarsely referred to often as the ARS idiotype. Breeding experiments have shown that the capacity to produce this idiotype is inherited and is linked to the genetic markers for the immunoglobulin constant region, i.e. as might be expected, the gene encoding the idiotype occurs on the chromosome carrying the genes for the constant region. Thus, since we inherit genes which enable us to make particular antibodies, one might suppose that the capacity to produce an antibody response would be limited by the repertoire of specificities encoded by the genes on this chromosome. However, since the mechanisms for generating antibody diversity from the available genes are so powerful, immunodeficiency is unlikely to occur as a consequence of a poor Ig variable region gene repertoire. Just occasionally we see holes in the repertoire due to absence of a gene; failure to respond to the sugar polymer α1–6, dextran is a feature of animals without the $V_{dex}$ gene and mice lacking the $V\alpha_2$ T-cell receptor gene cannot mount a cytotoxic T-cell response to the male (H-Y) antigen.

### Immune response can be influenced by the MHC

There was much excitement when it was first discovered that the antibody responses to a number of thymus-dependent antigenically simple substances are determined by genes mapping to the MHC. For example, mice of the *H-2$^b$* haplotype respond well

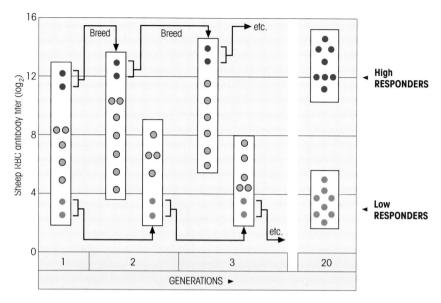

**Figure 11.16. Bidirectional selective breeding of high and low antibody responders** (after Biozzi and colleagues). A foundation population of wild mice (with crazy mixed-up genes and great variability in antibody response) are immunized with sheep red blood cells (SRBC), a multideterminant antigen. The antibody titer of each individual mouse is shown by a circle. The male and female giving the highest titer antibodies (⬤) were bred and their litter challenged with antigen. Again, the best responders were bred together and so on for 20 generations when all mice were high responders to SRBC and a variety of other antigens. The same was done for the poorest responders (⬤), yielding a strain of low-responder animals.

to the synthetic branched polypeptide (T,G)-A–L, whereas $H\text{-}2^k$ mice respond poorly (table 11.2).

It was said that mice of the $H\text{-}2^b$ haplotype (i.e. a particular set of H-2 genes) are **high responders** to (T,G)-A–L because they possess the appropriate immune response (Ir) gene. With another synthetic antigen, (H,G)-A–L, having histidine in place of tyrosine, the position is reversed, the 'poor (T,G)-A–L responders' now giving a good antibody response and the 'good (T,G)-A–L responders' a weak one, showing that the capacity of a particular strain to give a high or low response varies with the individual antigen (table 11.2). These relationships are only apparent when antigens of highly restricted structure are studied because the response to each single determinant is controlled by an Ir gene and it is less likely that the different determinants on a complex antigen will all be associated with consistently high or consistently low responder Ir genes; however, although one would expect an average of randomly high and low responder genes since the various determinants on most thymus-dependent complex antigens are structurally unrelated, the outcome will be biased by the dominance of one or more epitopes (cf. p. 202). Thus H-2 linked immune responses have been observed not only with relatively simple polypeptides, but also with transplantation antigens from another strain and autoantigens where merely one or two determinants are recognized as foreign by the host. With complex antigens, in most but not all cases, H-2 linkage is usually only seen when the dose administered is so low that just one immunodominant determinant is recognized by the immune system. In this way, reactions controlled by Ir genes are distinct from the overall responsiveness to a variety of complex antigens which is a feature of the Biozzi mice (above).

### The Ir genes map to the H-2I region and control T–B cooperation

Table 11.3 gives some idea of the type of analysis used to map the Ir genes. The three high responder strains have individual H-2 genes derived from prototypic pure strains which have been interbred to produce recombinations within the H-2 region. The only genes they have in common are $A^k$ and $D^b$; since the B.10 strain bearing the $D^b$ gene is a low responder, high response must be linked in this case to possession of

**Table 11.2. H-2 haplotype linked to high, low and intermediate immune responses to synthetic peptides.** (TG)-A–L = polylysine with polyalanine side chains randomly tipped with tyrosine and glutamine; (HG)-A–L = the same with histidine in place of tyrosine.

| ANTIGEN | H-2 HAPLOTYPE | | | | |
|---|---|---|---|---|---|
| | b | k | d | a | s |
| (TG)-A–L | Hi | Lo | Int | Lo | Lo |
| (HG)-A–L | Lo | Hi | Int | Hi | Lo |

**Table 11.3. Mapping of the *Ir* gene for (H,G)-A–L responses by analysis of different recombinant strains.**

| Strain | H-2 region | | | | | (H,G)-A–L |
|---|---|---|---|---|---|---|
| | K | A | E | S | D | Response |
| A | k | **k** | k | b | b | Hi |
| A.TL | s | **k** | k | k | b | Hi |
| B.IO.A (4R) | k | **k** | b | b | b | Hi |
| B.IO | b | b | b | b | b | Lo |
| A.SW | s | s | s | s | s | Lo |

$A^k$. The I-region molecules must almost certainly represent the *Ir* gene product since a point mutation in the H-2A subregion in one strain led to a change in the class II molecule at a site affecting its polymorphic specificity and changed the mice from high to low responder status with respect to their thymus-dependent antibody response to antigen *in vivo*. The mutation also greatly reduced the proliferation of T-cells from immunized animals when challenged *in vitro* with antigen plus appropriate presenting cells, and there is a good correlation between antigen-specific T-cell proliferation and the responder status of the host. The implication that **responder status may be linked to the generation of Tн cells** is amply borne out by adoptive transfer studies showing that irradiated (H-2$^b$×H-2$^k$) F1 mice make good antibody responses to (T,G)-A–L when reconstituted with antigen-primed B-cells from another F1 plus T-cells from a primed H-2$^b$ (high responder); T-cells from the low responder H-2$^k$ mice only supported poor antibody responses. This also explains why these *H-2* gene effects are seen with thymus-dependent but not T-independent antigens.

Three mechanisms have been proposed to account for class-II-linked high and low responsiveness.

*1 Defective presentation.* In a high responder, processing of antigen and its recognition by a corresponding T-cell leads to lymphocyte triggering and clonal expansion (figure 11.17a). Although there is (and has to be) considerable degeneracy in the specificity of the class II groove for peptide binding, variation in certain key residues can alter the strength of binding to a particular peptide (cf. p. 97) and convert a high to a low responder because the MHC fails to present antigen to the reactive T-cell (figure 11.17b). Sometimes the natural processing of an antigen in a given individual does not produce a peptide which fits well into their MHC molecules. A recent study showed that a cytotoxic T-cell clone restricted to HLA-A2, which recognized residues 58–68 of influenza A virus

matrix protein, could cross-react with cells from an Aw69 subject pulsed with the same peptide; nonetheless, the clone failed to recognize Aw69 cells *infected* with influenza A virus. Interestingly, individuals with

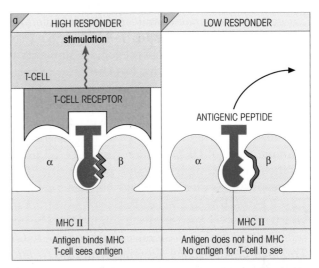

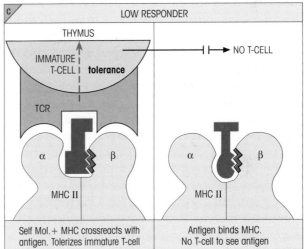

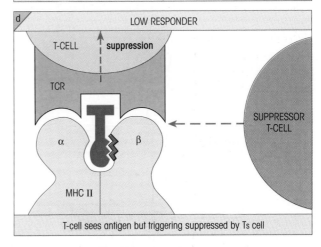

**Figure 11.17. Different mechanisms can account for low T-cell response to antigen in association with MHC class II.**

the HLA–Aw69 class I MHC develop immunity to a different epitope on the same protein.

*2 Defective T-cell repertoire.* It is now accepted that T-cells with moderate to high affinity for self-MHC molecules and their complexes with processed self-antigens, will be rendered unresponsive (cf. tolerance induction, p. 231), so creating a 'hole' in the T-cell repertoire. If there is a cross-reaction, i.e. similarity in shape at the T-cell recognition level between a foreign antigen and a self-molecule which has already induced unresponsiveness, the host must lack T-cells specific for the foreign antigen and will therefore be a low responder (figure 11.17c). To take a concrete example, mice of DBA/2 strain respond well to the synthetic peptide polyglutamyl, polytyrosine (GT), whereas BALB/c do not, although both have identical class II genes. BALB/c B-cell blasts express a structure which mimics GT and the presumption would be that self-tolerance makes these mice unresponsive to GT. This was confirmed by showing that DBA/2 mice made tolerant by a small number of BALB/c hematopoietic cells were changed from high to low responder status. To round off the story in a very satisfying way, DBA/2 mice injected with BALB/c B-blasts, induced by the polyclonal activator lipopolysaccharide, were found to be primed for GT.

*3 T-suppression.* I would like to refer again to the MHC class II-restricted low responsiveness to relatively complex antigens occurring within families (see p. 206), since it illustrates the notion that low responder status can arise as an expression of CD8 T-suppressor activity (figure 11.17d). Low response was dominant in class II heterozygotes, indicating that suppression can act against TH restricted to any other

class II molecule. In this it differs from models 1 and 2 above where high response is dominant in a heterozygote because the factors associated with the low-responder gene cannot influence the activity of the high responder. Overall, it seems likely that each of the three models may provide the basis for class II-linked *Ir* gene phenomena in different circumstances.

Factors influencing the genetic control of the immune response are summarized in figure 11.18.

## ARE THERE REGULATORY IMMUNONEURO-ENDOCRINE NETWORKS?

There is a danger, as one focuses more and more on the antics of the immune system, of looking at the body as a collection of myeloid and lymphoid cells roaming around in a big sack and of having no regard to the integrated physiology of the organism. ('Are there really people who are so myopic?' I can hear you say.) Within the wider physiological context, attention has been drawn increasingly to interactions between immunological and neuroendocrine systems.

Immunological cells have the receptors which enable them to receive signals from a whole range of hormones: corticosteroids, insulin, growth hormone, estradiol, testosterone, β-adrenergic agents, acetylcholine, endorphins and enkephalins. There is an extensive literature concerning their influence on immune function, but by and large, glucocorticoids and androgens depress immune responses, whereas estrogens, growth hormone, thyroxine and insulin do the opposite.

### A neuroendocrine feedback loop affecting immune responses

The secretion of **glucocorticoids** is a major response to stresses induced by a wide range of stimuli such as extreme changes of temperature, fear, hunger and physical injury. They are also released as a consequence of immune responses and limit those responses in a neuroendocrine feedback loop. Thus, IL-1 (figure 11.19), IL-6 and α-tumor necrosis factor (TNFα) are capable of stimulating glucocorticoid synthesis and do so through the hypothalamic–pituitary–adrenal axis. This, in turn, leads to down-regulation of TH1 and macrophage activity so completing the negative feedback circuit (figure 11.20).

To take an example, adrenalectomy prevents spontaneous recovery from experimental allergic encephalomyelitis (EAE), a demyelinating disease

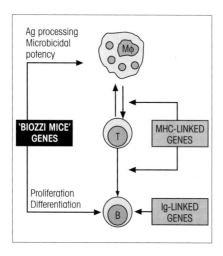

**Figure 11.18. Genetic control of the immune response.**

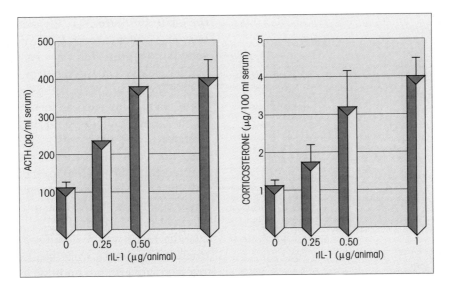

**Figure 11.19. Enhancement of ACTH and corticosterone blood levels in C3H/HeJ mice** 2 hours after injection of recombinant IL-1 (values are means ± SEM for groups of seven or eight mice). The significance of the mouse strain used is that they lack receptors for bacterial lipopolysaccharide (LPS) so the effects cannot be attributed to LPS contamination of the IL-1 preparation. (Reprinted from Besedovsky H., del Rey A., Sorkin E. & Dinarello C.A. (1986) *Science* **233**, 652, with permission. Copyright 1986 by the AAAS.)

with progressive paralysis produced by myelin basic protein in complete Freund's adjuvant which, however, can be blocked by implants of corticosterone. Spontaneous recovery from EAE in intact animals is associated with a dominance of TH2 autoantigen-specific clones indicative of the widely held view that glucocorticoids suppress TH1 and may augment TH2 cells. Individuals with a genetic predisposition to high levels of stress-induced glucocorticoids would be expected to have increased susceptibility to infections with intracellular pathogens such as *M. leprae* which require effective TH1 cell-mediated immunity for their eradication.

## Sex hormones come into the picture

Estrogen is said to be the major factor influencing the more active immune responses in females relative to males. They have higher serum Ig and secreted IgA levels, a higher antibody response to T-independent antigens, relative resistance to T-cell tolerance and greater resistance to infections. Females are also far more susceptible to autoimmune disease, an issue that will be discussed in greater depth in Chapter 19, but here let us note that oral contraceptives can induce flares of the autoimmune disorder systemic lupus erythematosus (SLE; see p. 403) and the mildly androgenic adrenal hormone, **dehydroepiandrosterone (DHEA)**, can significantly prolong the lifespan of (NZB×W) F1 females with the murine model of SLE. DHEA has positive effects on TH1 at the

expense of TH2 cells and can clearly antagonize the inhibitory effects of cortisol on thymocytes and T-cell proliferation. As they say in the tabloids, watch this space.

## Inching towards 'psychoimmunology'

There are even more interrelationships between the immune, endocrine and neurological systems. Immunological organs are innervated by autonomic and primary sensorial neurons, and neonatal (but not adult) sympathectomy with 6-hydroxydopamine and surgical denervation of the spleen enhance immune responses. Mast cells and nerves often have an intimate anatomical relationship and nerve growth factor causes mast cell degranulation. The gastrointestinal tract also has extensive innervation and a high number of immune effector cells. In this context, the ability of substance P to stimulate, and of somatostatin and vasoactive intestinal peptide (VIP) to inhibit, proliferation of Peyer's patch lymphocytes may prove to have more than a trivial significance. The pituitary hormone prolactin has been brought to our attention from the experimental observation that inhibition of prolactin secretion by bromocriptine suppresses TH activity.

There seems to be an interaction between inflammation and nerve growth in regions of wound healing and repair. Mast cells are often abundant, IL-6 induces neurite growth and IL-1 enhances production of nerve growth factor in sciatic nerve explants. IL-1 also

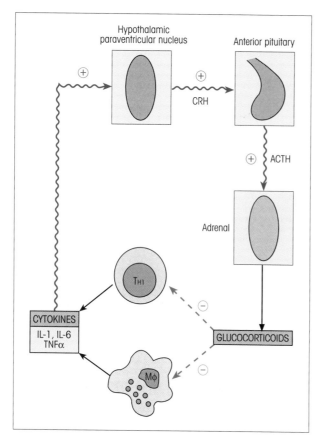

**Figure 11.20. Glucocorticoid negative feedback on cytokine production.**
CRH = corticotropin-releasing hormone; ACTH = adrenocorticotropic hormone. Evidence for another type of circuit encompassing hormone receptor, hormone, anti-hormone and internal image anti-idiotype was presented in figure 11.10 and may be of relevance to the pathogenesis of autoimmune disorders directed against hormone receptors (see p. 407). More generally, cells of the immune system in both primary and secondary lymphoid organs can produce hormones and neuropeptides, while classical endocrine glands as well as neurones and glial cells can synthesize cytokines and appropriate receptors. Production of prolactin and its receptors by peripheral lymphoid cells and thymocytes is worthy of attention. Lymphocyte expression of the prolactin receptor is upregulated following activation and in autoimmune disease, witness the beneficial effects of bromocriptine, an inhibitor of prolactin synthesis, in the NZB x W model of murine SLE (cf. p. 406).

increases slow-wave sleep when introduced into the lateral ventricle of the brain and both IL-1 and interferon produce pyrogenic effects through their action on the temperature-controlling center. The significance of IgFc binding to pituitary adrenocorticotropic hormone (ACTH)-producing cells has still not been revealed.

It is not easy at this stage to see just how these diverse neuro-endocrine effects fit into the regulation of immune responses but at a more physiological level, stress and circadian rhythms modify the functioning of the immune system and there is a very popular observation concerning modulation of the delayed-type hypersensitivity Mantoux reaction in the skin by hypnosis. Elegant demonstration of nervous system control is provided by studies showing suppression of conventional immune responses and enhancement of NK cell activity by Pavlovian conditioning. In the classic Pavlovian paradigm, a stimulus such as food that unconditionally elicits a particular response, in this case salivation, is repeatedly paired with a neutral stimulus that does not elicit the same response. Eventually the neutral stimulus becomes a conditional stimulus and will elicit salivation in the absence of food. Rats were given cyclophosphamide as unconditional and saccharin as the conditional stimulus repeatedly; subsequently, there was a depressed antibody response when the animals were challenged with antigen together with just the conditional stimulus, saccharin.

Let's get down to personality; even rats have it. Compared with control strains such as F344 and PVG, the Lewis rat is extraordinarily susceptible to a broad array of experimentally induced autoimmune diseases, such as collagen arthritis and allergic encephalomyelitis (cf. p. 406), and readily develops more severe acute inflammation to almost any irritant. These animals have a profound defect in their hypothalamic paraventricular nucleus involving synthesis and secretion of corticotropin releasing hormone. Here is the point: Lewis rats are docile, non-aggressive, serene and hypoarousable (i.e. type B personality). They are also more prone to addiction to alcohol, morphine and cocaine. In contrast, F344s have a type A personality being easily aroused, nervous and potentially aggressive. These fascinating models, the increasing understanding of immunoneuroendocrine interactions and the numerous investigations alleging an adverse effect of psychological factors such as bereavement upon immune function in the human, are leading us with tiny faltering steps to a new age of 'psychoimmunology'.

## EFFECTS OF DIET, EXERCISE, TRAUMA AND AGE ON IMMUNITY

### Malnutrition diminishes the effectiveness of the immune response

The greatly increased susceptibility of undernourished individuals to infection can be attributed to many factors: poor sanitation and personal hygiene, overcrowding and inadequate health education. But in addition there are gross effects of **protein–calorie malnutrition** on immunocompetence. The widespread atrophy of lymphoid tissues and the 50% reduction in circulating CD4 T-cells underlies **serious impairment of cell-mediated immunity**. Antibody responses may be intact but they are of lower affinity; phagocytosis of bacteria is relatively normal but the subsequent intracellular destruction is defective.

Deficiencies in pyridoxin, folic acid, and vitamins A, C and E result in generally impaired immune responses. **Vitamin D is an important regulator**. It is produced not only by the UV-irradiated dermis but also by activated macrophages, the hypercalcemia associated with sarcoidosis being attributable to production of the vitamin by macrophages in the active granulomata. The vitamin is a potent inhibitor of T-cell proliferation and of cytokine production by $T_{H}1$ cells. This generates a neat feedback loop at sites of inflammation where macrophages activated by IFNγ produce vitamin D which suppresses the T-cells making the interferon. It also downregulates antigen presentation by macrophages and promotes multinucleated giant cell formation in chronic granulomatous lesions. Nonetheless, in further emphasis of the potential duality of the CD4 helper subsets, it promotes $T_{H}2$ activity, especially at mucosal surfaces: quite a busy little vitamin. Zinc deficiency is rather interesting; this greatly affects the biological activity of thymus hormones and has a major effect on cell-mediated immunity, perhaps as a result. Iron deficiency impairs the oxidative burst in neutrophils since the flavocytochrome NADP oxidase is an iron-containing enzyme.

Of course there is another side to all this in that moderate restriction of total calorie intake and/or marked reduction in fat intake, ameliorates age-related diseases such as autoimmunity. Oils with an n-3 double bond, such as fish oils, are also protective, perhaps due to increased synthesis of immunosuppressive prostaglandins.

Given the overdue sensitivity to the importance of environmental contamination, it is important to monitor the nature and levels of pollution that may influence immunity. Here is just one example: polyhalogenated organic compounds (such as polychlorinated biphenyls) steadily pervade the environment and, being stable and lipophilic, accumulate readily in the aquatic food chain where they largely resist metabolic breakdown. It was shown that Baltic herrings with relatively high levels of these pollutants, as compared with uncontaminated Altantic herrings, were immunotoxic when fed to captive harbour seals, suggesting one reason why seals along the coasts of northwestern Europe succumbed so alarmingly to infection with the otherwise nonvirulent phocine distemper virus in 1988.

## Other factors

**Exercise**, particularly severe exercise, induces stress and raises plasma levels of cortisol, catecholamines, IFNα, IL-1, β-endorphin and metenkephalin. It can lead to reduced IgA levels, immune deficiency and increased susceptibility to infection. Maniacal joggers and other such like masochists — you have been warned!

**Multiple traumatic injury**, surgery and major burns are also immunosuppressive and so contribute to the increased risk of sepsis. Corticosteroids produced by stressful conditions, the immunosuppressive prostaglandin $E_2$ released from damaged tissues and bacterial endotoxin derived from disturbance of gut flora, are all factors which influence the outcome after trauma. A novel suppressive peptide, SAP, appears in serum within hours of a burn and awaits characterization.

Accepting that the problem of understanding the mechanisms of **aging** is a tough nut to crack, it is a trifle disappointing that the easier task of establishing the influence of age on immunological phenomena is still not satisfactorily accomplished. Perhaps the elderly population is skewed towards individuals with effective immune systems which give a survival advantage. Be that as it may, there is a general belief that IL-2 production by peripheral blood lymphocytes (figure 11.21) and T-cell-mediated functions such as delayed-type hypersensitivity reactions to common skin test antigens decline with age and so, it is thought, does T-suppression, although this is a notoriously elusive function to measure.

Most B-cell responses to exogenous antigens are not dramatically changed with the passage of time, but one of the few well-founded observations concerns the relative increase in agalactosyl oligosaccharides

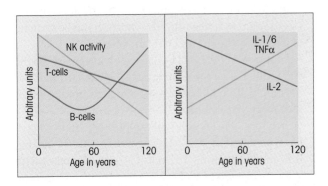

**Figure 11.21. Age trends in some immunological parameters.** (Based on Franceschi C., Monti D., Sansoni P. & Cossarizza A. (1995) *Immunology Today* **16**, 12.)

on the Cγ2 domains of IgG (cf. p. 433) in parallel with a rise in IL-6 in the older age groups (figure 11.21). This is accompanied by a decrease in DHEA and it may be significant that injection of the androgen into elderly mice leads to a fall in circulating IL-6 concentrations. Do these studies provide us with a clue to the increased prevalence of autoantibodies in our senior citizens?

## SUMMARY

### Control by antigen

• Immune responses are largely antigen driven and as the level of exogenous antigen falls, so does the intensity of the response.
• Antigens can compete with each other: this is a result of competition between processed peptides for the available MHC grooves.

### Feedback control by antibody

• Early IgM antibodies boost antibody responses.
• IgG antibodies inhibit responses via the Fcγ receptor on B-cells.

### T-cell regulation

• TH cells may use their surface receptors for Ig isotypes to augment the expansion of B-cells expressing the related isotype.
• Activated T-cells express fas and fasL which can restrain unlimited clonal expansion.
• At high levels of antigen, T-cells which suppress T-helpers emerge presumably as feedback control of excessive TH expansion.
• Suppressor and helper epitopes on the same molecule can be discrete.
• In some instances of suppression, the effectors are CD8 T-cells restricted either directly (which would be strange) or indirectly through a CD4 intermediary.
• Suppression may well be due to T–T interaction on the surface of antigen-presenting cells. Just as TH1 and TH2 cells mutually inhibit each other through production of their respective cytokines IFNγ and IL-4/10, so there may be two types of CD8 cells with suppressor activity; one of the type found in lepromatous leprosy patients making IL-4 and suppressing TH1 cells (T1), and the other with cytolytic phenotype making IFNγ capable of suppressing TH2 cells (T2).

### Idiotype networks

• Antigen-specific receptors on lymphocytes can interact with the idiotypes on the receptors of other lymphocytes to form a network (Jerne).
• Anti-idiotypes can be induced by autologous idiotypes.
• An idiotype network involving mostly CD5 B1-cells is evident in early life.
• T-cell idiotypic interactions can also be demonstrated.
• Preset idiotypic networks involve a number of lymphocytes with self-reactivity for dominant autoantigens. It is speculated that this preoccupation with self helps to regulate unwanted autoimmune reactions and may help to target the response to infectious agents on dominant conserved antigens like heat-shock protein hsp65 which cross-react with self.
• Idiotypes which occur frequently and are shared by a multiplicity of antibodies (public or cross-reacting Id) are targets for regulation by anti-idiotypes in the network, thus providing a further mechanism for control of the immune response.
• The network offers the potential for therapeutic intervention to manipulate immunity.

### Genetic factors influence the immune response

• Approximately ten genes control the overall antibody response to complex antigens: some affect macrophage antigen processing and microbicidal activity and some the rate of proliferation of differentiating B-cells.
• Genes coding for antibodies of given specificities may be inherited together with (i.e. linked to) genetic markers for the heavy chain.
• Immune response genes linked to the major histocompatibility locus define the class II products on the T- and B-cells and antigen-presenting cells which control the interactions required for T–B collaboration.
• Class II-linked high and low responsiveness may be

*(Continued)*

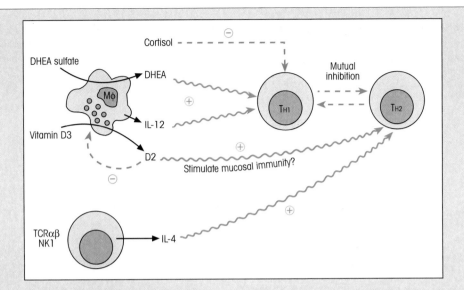

**Figure 11.22. Summary of major factors affecting TH1/TH2 balance.** Evidence for preferential stimulation of mucosal antibody synthesis by vitamin D is still accumulating. By downregulating macrophage activity, TH1 effectiveness is decreased. Cortisol and dehydroepiandrosterone (DHEA) are products of the adrenal and have opposing effects on the T1 subset. A relative deficiency of DHEA will lead to poor TH1 performance.

due to defective presentation by MHC, a defective T-cell repertoire caused by tolerance to MHC+self peptides and T-suppression.

### Immunoneuroendocrine networks

• Immunological, neurological and endocrinological systems can all interact.
• Regulatory interdependent circuits are being described, of which the feedback by cytokines augmenting the production of corticosteroids is important because this shuts down TH1 and macrophage activity.
• Estrogens may be largely responsible for the more active immune responses in females relative to males. The male hormone, DHEA, prolongs life in females with the murine equivalent of the human autoimmune disease SLE.

• Increasing understanding of immunoneuroendocrine relationships and the identification of different rat strains, with type A and B 'personalities' should provide a basis for studying psychoimmunology.

### Effects of diet and other factors on immunity

• Protein-calorie malnutrition grossly impairs cell-mediated immunity and phagocyte microbicidal potency.
• Exercise, trauma, age and environmental pollution can all act to impair immune mechanisms. The pattern of cytokines produced by peripheral blood cells changes with age, IL-2 decreasing and TNFα, IL-1 and IL-6 increasing; the latter associated with a lowered DHEA level.

### Factors influencing the bias between TH1 and TH2 subsets

• These have figured with some prominence in this chapter and a summary of some of the major influences on the balance between TH1 and TH2 responses is presented in figure 11.22.

## FURTHER READING

Bloom B.R., Salgame P. & Diamond B. (1992) Revisiting and revising suppressor T-cells. *Immunology Today* **13**, 131.

Chandra R.K. (1992) Nutrition and the immune system. In Roitt I.M. & Delves P.J. (eds) *Encyclopedia of Immunology*, p. 1369. Academic Press, London. (See also other relevant articles in the *Encyclopedia*: 'Aging and the immune system', p. 45; 'Behavioural regulation of immunity', p. 228; 'Vitamin D', p. 1567.)

Cohen I.R. & Young D.B. (1991) Autoimmunity, microbial immunity and the immunological homunculus. *Immunology Today* **12**, 105.

Goetz H. (1994) Exercise and the immune system: a model of the stress response. *Immunology Today* **15**, 382.

Havran W. (ed.) (1996) Dendritic epithelial T cells. *Seminars in Immunology* **8**, 313.

Male D.K., Champion B., Cooke A. & Owen M. (1996) *Advanced Immunology*, 3rd edn. Times Mirror International Publishers Ltd, London.

Mason D. (1991) Genetic variation in the stress-response: susceptibility to experimental allergic encephalomyelitis and implications for human inflammatory disease. *Immunology Today* **12**, 57.

Mitchison N.A. (1992) Specialization, tolerance, memory, competition, latency and strife among T-cells. *Annual Review of Immunology* **10**, 1.

Sercarz E. & Krzych U. (1991) The distinctive specificity of antigen-specific suppressor T-cells. *Immunology Today* **12**, 111.

Swain S.L. & Cambier J.C. (eds) (1996) Lymphocyte activation and effector functions. *Current Opinion in Immunology* **8**, 309–418.

Talal N. (1992) Sex hormones and immunity. In Roitt I.M. & Delves P.J. (eds) *Encyclopedia of Immunology*, p. 1369. Academic Press, London.

# ONTOGENY AND PHYLOGENY

## THE MULTIPOTENTIAL HEMATOPOIETIC STEM CELL GIVES RISE TO THE FORMED ELEMENTS OF THE BLOOD

Hematopoiesis originates in the early yolk sac but as embryogenesis proceeds, this function is taken over by the fetal liver and finally by the bone marrow where it continues throughout life. The hematopoietic stem cell which gives rise to the formed elements of the blood (figure 12.1) can be shown to be multipotent, to seed other organs and to have a relatively unlimited capacity to renew itself through the creation of further stem cells. Thus an animal can be completely protected against the lethal effects of high doses of irradiation by injection of bone marrow cells which will repopulate its lymphoid and myeloid systems. The capacity for self-renewal is not absolute and declines with age in parallel with a shortening of

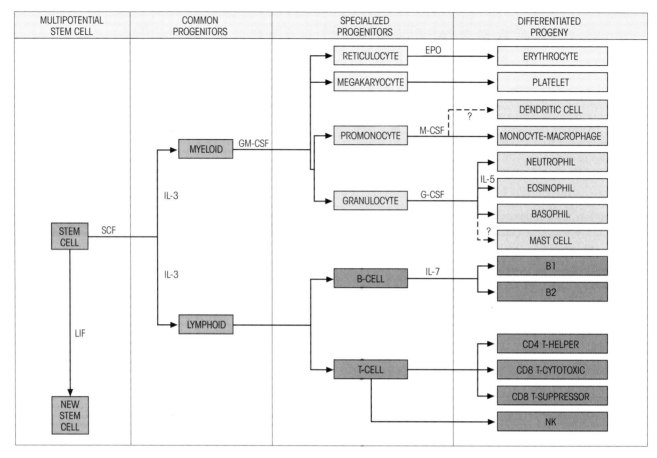

**Figure 12.1. The multipotential hematopoietic stem cell and its progeny** which differentiate under the influence of a series of growth factors within the microenvironment of the bone marrow. The *Ikaros* gene encodes a family of zinc-fingered DNA binding proteins acting as transcription factors which are critical for driving the development of a common myeloid/lymphoid precursor into a bipotential lymphoid restricted progenitor giving rise to T- and B-cells. There is a selective requirement for the transcription factor E2A for B-cell development and homozygous E2A mutant mice specifically lack B-lineage cells, there being a block to $D_H/_H$ rearrangement in the Ig heavy chain locus plus severe reduction in μ-chain, Rag-1, mb-1, CD19 and λ5 transcripts (see section below on development of B-cell specificity). SCF = stem cell

factor; LIF = leukemia inhibitory factor; IL-3 = interleukin-3, often termed the multi-CSF because it stimulates progenitors of platelets, mast cells and all the other types of myeloid and erythroid cells; GM–CSF = granulocyte–macrophage colony-stimulating factor, so called because it promotes the formation of mixed colonies of these two cell types from bone marrow progenitors either in tissue culture or on transfer to an irradiated recipient where they appear in the spleen; G-CSF = granulocyte colony-stimulating factor; M-CSF = monocyte colony-stimulating factor; EPO = erythropoietin; the dendritic cells present antigen to T-cells in contrast with the germinal center follicular dendritic cells which interact with B-cells.

the telomeres and a reduction in telomerase, the enzyme which repairs the shortening of the ends of chromosomes which would otherwise occur at every round of cell division.

The stem cells differentiate within the microenvironment of sessile stromal cells which produce various growth factors such as IL-3, 4, 6 and 7, GM-CSF, and so on. The importance of this interaction between undifferentiated stem cells and the microenvironment which guides their differentiation is clearly shown by studies on mice homozygous for mutations at the *w* or the *sl* loci which, amongst other defects, have severe macrocytic anemia. Bone marrow stromal cells produce a stem cell factor (SCF) which remains associated with the extracellular matrix and

acts on primitive stem cells through a tyrosine kinase membrane receptor, c-kit. *sl/sl* mutants have normal stem cells but defective stromal production of SCF which can be corrected by transplantation of a normal spleen fragment; *w/w* mutant myeloid progenitors lack the c-kit surface receptor for SCF so can be restored by injection of normal bone marrow cells (figure 12.2).

We have come a long way towards the goal of isolating highly purified populations of hematopoietic stem cells, although not all agree that we have yet achieved it. In the mouse, the most likely candidate, at least a *very* early progenitor, is the cell with the following surface phenotype: high expression of major histocompatibility complex (MHC), low positivity for

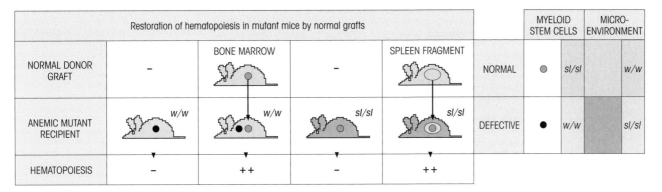

**Figure 12.2. Hematopoiesis requires normal bone marrow stem cells differentiating in a normal microenvironment.** The W locus codes for the c-*kit* oncogene, a stem cell tyrosine kinase membrane receptor for the stem cell growth factor (SCF) encoded by the *sl* locus. Mice which are homozygous for mutant alleles at these loci develop severe macrocytic anemia which can be corrected by transplantation of appropriate normal cells. The experiments show that the w/w mutant lacks normal stem cells and the sl/sl mutant lacks the environmental factor needed for their development.

Thy1, clearly positive for Sca-1 (recognized by a monoclonal antibody reacting with stem cells) and for the adhesion molecule PGP-1, but negative for B220, Mac-1, Gr-1 and CD8 (markers for B-cells, macrophages, granulocytes and cytotoxic T-cells respectively). Impressively, less than 100 of such cells can prevent death in a lethally irradiated animal. In the human, CD34 is a marker of an extremely early cell but again, there is some debate as to whether this identifies the holy pluripotent stem cell itself.

Mice with severe combined immunodeficiency (SCID) provide a happy environment for fragments of human fetal liver and thymus which, if implanted contiguously, will produce formed elements of the blood for 6 to 12 months. We already know that fetal liver is a source of hematopoietic stem cells; what is the role of the thymus?

## THE THYMUS PROVIDES THE ENVIRONMENT FOR T-CELL DIFFERENTIATION

The gland is organized into a series of lobules based upon meshworks of epithelial cells derived embryologically from an outpushing of the gut endoderm of the third pharyngeal pouch and which form well-defined cortical and medullary zones (figure 12.3). Monoclonal antibodies raised against thymic epithelial cells reveal six staining patterns by immunofluorescence, which show marked species consistency. There is shared antigen expression between subcapsular, perivascular and medullary epithelium and distinct antigens in the cortical epithelial cells, one of which is the IL-4 receptor. This framework of cells provides the microenvironment for T-cell differentiation. There are subtle interactions between the extra-

cellular matrix proteins and a variety of integrins on different lymphocyte subpopulations produced by differential splicing and posttranslational glycosylation; current musings are that the expression of these integrins plays a role in the homing of progenitors to the thymus and their subsequent migration within the gland. In addition, the epithelial cells produce a series of peptide hormones which mostly seem capable of promoting the appearance of T-cell differentiation markers and a variety of T-cell functions on culture with bone marrow cells *in vitro*. Four have been well characterized and sequenced: thymulin, $\alpha_1$- and $\beta_4$-thymosin, and thymopoietin (and its active pentapeptide TP-5). Of these only thymopoietin and thymulin are of exclusively thymic origin. The zinc-dependent nonapeptide, thymulin, tends to normalize the balance of immune responses: it restores antibody avidity and antibody production in aged mice and yet stimulates suppressor activity in animals with autoimmune hemolytic anemia induced by cross-reactive rat red cells (cf. p. 418). It may be looked upon as a true hormone acting at a distance from the thymus as a fine physiological immunoregulator contributing to the maintenance of T-cell subset homeostasis.

The specialized large epithelial cells in the outer cortex are known as 'nurse' cells because they can each be associated with large numbers of lymphocytes which do appear to be lying within their cytoplasm. The epithelial cells of the deep cortex have branched dendritic processes rich in class II MHC. They connect through desmosomes to form a network through which cortical lymphocytes must pass on their way to the medulla (figure 12.3). The cortical lymphocytes are densely packed compared with those in the medulla, many are in division and a sur-

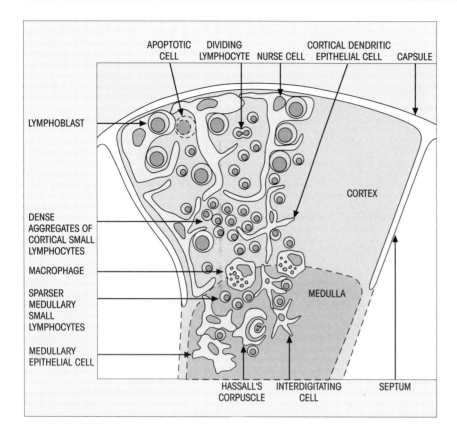

**Figure 12.3. Cellular features of a thymus lobule.** See text for description. (Adapted from Hood L.E., Weissman I.L., Wood W.B. & Wilson J.H. (1984) *Immunology*, 2nd edn. p. 261. Benjamin Cummings, California.)

prising number are in the throes of dying as evidenced by their pyknotic nuclei. On their way to the medulla, the lymphocytes pass a cordon of 'sentinel' macrophages at the cortico-medullary junction. A number of bone marrow-derived interdigitating dendritic cells are present in the medulla and the epithelial cells have broader processes than their cortical counterparts and express high levels of both class I and class II MHC. Whorled, possibly degenerate aggregates of epithelial cells form the highly characteristic Hassall's corpuscles beloved of histopathology examiners.

A fairly complex relationship with the nervous system awaits discovery; the thymus is richly innervated with both adrenergic and cholinergic fibers, while the neurotransmitter oxytocin, vasopressin and neurophysin are synthesized endogenously by subcapsular, perivascular and medullary epithelial cells and nurse cells. Acute stress leads to an indecently rapid loss of cortical thymocytes and an increase in epithelial cells expressing both cortical and medullary markers — surely intrathymic epithelial stem cells? The destruction of cortical thymocytes is at least partly due to the cytolytic action of steroids, the relative invulnerability of the medullary lymphocytes being attributable to their possession of a 20α-hydroxyl steroid dehydrogenase. The distinctive

nature of the two main compartments in the gland is emphasized by the selective atrophy induced by a number of agents; thus the primary target of organotin is the immature cortical thymocyte. Dioxin interacts with a receptor on cortical epithelial cells, while the immunosuppressive drug cyclosporin A causes atrophy of all the medullary elements, thereby blocking differentiation of cortical to medullary thymocyte with intriguing consequences.

In the human, thymic involution commences within the first 12 months of life, reducing by around 3% a year to middle age and by 1% thereafter. The size of the organ gives no clue to these changes because there is replacement by adipose tissue. In a sense, the thymus is progressively disposable because, as we shall see, it establishes a long-lasting peripheral T-cell pool which enables the host to withstand loss of the gland without catastrophic failure of immunological function, witness the minimal effects of thymectomy in the adult compared with the **dramatic influence in the neonate** (Milestone 12.1).

## Bone marrow stem cells become immunocompetent T-cells in the thymus

The evidence for this comes from experiments on the reconstitution of irradiated hosts. An irradiated

## Milestone 12.1—The Immunological Function of the Thymus

Ludwig Gross had found that a form of mouse leukemia could be induced in low-leukemia strains by inoculating filtered leukemic tissue from high-leukemia strains provided this were done in the immediate neonatal period. Since the thymus was known to be involved in the leukemic process, Jacques Miller decided to test the hypothesis that the Gross virus could only multiply in the neonatal thymus, by infecting neonatally thymectomized mice of low-leukemia strains. The results were consistent with his hypothesis, but strangely, animals of one strain died of a wasting disease which Miller deduced could have been due to susceptibility to infection, since fewer mice died when they were moved from the converted horse stables which served as an animal house to 'cleaner' quarters.

Autopsy showed the animals to have atrophied lymphoid tissue and low blood lymphocyte levels and Miller therefore decided to test their immunocompetence before the onset of wasting disease. To his astonishment, skin grafts, even from rats (figure M12.1.1) as well as from other mouse strains, were fully accepted. These phenomena were not induced by thymectomy later in life and in

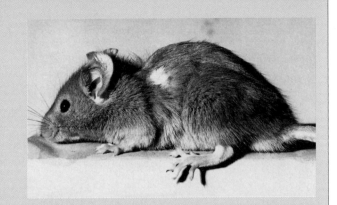

**Figure M12.1.1.** Acceptance of a rat skin graft by a mouse which had been neonatally thymectomized.

writing up his preliminary results in 1961 (Miller J.F.A.P. *Lancet* **ii**, 748) Miller opined that 'during embryogenesis the thymus would produce the originators of immunologically competent cells, many of which would have migrated to other sites at about the time of birth'. All in all a superb example of the scientific method and its application by a top-flight scientist.

animal is restored by bone marrow grafts through the immediate restitution of granulocyte precursors; in the longer term also through reconstitution of the T- and B-cells destroyed by irradiation. However, if the animal is thymectomized before irradiation, bone marrow cells will not reconstitute the T-lymphocyte population (cf. figure 7.14).

By day 11–12 in the mouse embryo, lymphoblastoid stem cells from the bone marrow begin to colonize the periphery of the epithelial thymus rudiment. If the thymus is removed at this stage and incubated in organ culture, a whole variety of mature T-lymphocytes will be generated. This is not seen if 10-day thymuses are cultured and shows that the lymphoblastoid colonizers give rise to the immunocompetent small-lymphocyte progeny.

## T-CELL ONTOGENY

### Differentiation is accompanied by changes in surface markers

The incoming thymic lymphoid progenitor attracted to the thymus by some chemotactic factor, stains positively for CD34 and the enzyme terminal deoxynu-

cleotidyl transferase (TdT) (figure 12.4) which is thought to be involved in the insertion of nucleotide sequences at the N-terminal region of D and J variable region segments to increase diversity of the T-cell receptors (TCRs) (cf. p. 69). They also express high levels of CD44 (Pgp-1) and CD117, the stem cell factor receptor, c-kit (p. 224). Under the influence of IL-1 and TNF they differentiate into prothymocytes, committed to the T-lineage and these now undergo IL-7-mediated proliferation to form a population of CD44⁻ CD117⁻ pre-T-cells. At this stage the cells begin to express various TCR chains and are then expanded, ultimately synthesizing CD3, the invariant signal transducing complex of the TCR and becoming **double-positive** for CD4⁺, CD8⁺, the markers of the helper and cytotoxic/suppressor subsets respectively. Finally the cells traverse the cortico-medullary junction to the medulla as the CD4 and CD8 markers segregate in parallel with differentiation into separate immunocompetent populations of **single-positive CD4⁺ T-helpers** and **CD8⁺ cytotoxic T-cell precursors** (figure 12.4). The γδ cells remain double-negative, i.e. CD4⁻8⁻, except for a small subset which express CD8.

The precise lineage of NK cells is still in doubt. They express the markers CD2, 3 and 8 which are normally

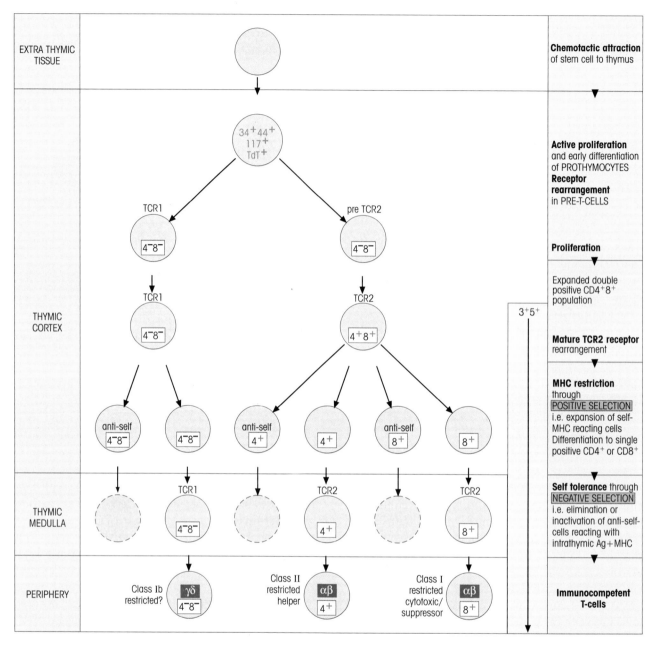

**Figure 12.4. Differentiation of T-cells within the thymus gland.** Numbers refer to CD designation. TCR1 = γδ receptors; 'pre-TCR2' = pre-Tαβ receptor; TCR2 = mature αβ; TdT = terminal deoxynucleotidyl transferase. Negatively selected cells in gray. The diagram is partly simplified for the sake of clarity. Autoreactive cells with specificity for self-antigens not expressed in the thymus may be tolerized by extrathymic peripheral contact with antigen. Some γδ cells are restricted by nonclassical MHC class Ib, some by class II and others by antigen. A significant population of slowly expanding, acti-

vated, double-negative (CD4–8–) or CD4–8lo αβ T-cells is present in the periphery and might be generated in the thymus; their function is unknown but such cells bearing a transgenic autoreactive TCR were not downregulated and this raises the possibility that they represent the T-cell analog of the self-reactive B-1-cell which participates in an idiotype network. The developmental pathway of the relatively primitive αβ T-cells bearing the NK1 marker and frequently CD4 (cf. p. 100) is restricted by CD1.

restricted to T-cells, they have IL-2 receptors and are driven to proliferate by IL-2, and they can produce IFNγ. Their T-receptor *V* genes are not rearranged but they must be related to T-cells in some way.

## Receptor rearrangement

The rearrangement of *V*, *D* and *J* region genes

required to generate the TCR (see p. 67) has not yet taken place at the prothymocyte stage. The *Lyf-1* gene for TdT and the recombinase activator genes, *RAG-1* and *RAG-2*, are transcribed at the pre-T stage and, by day 15, cells with the γδ TCR1 can be detected in the mouse thymus followed soon by the appearance of a **'pre-TCR2'**.

## The development of αβ receptors

The $V_\beta$ is first rearranged in the double-negative CD4⁻8⁻ cells and associates with a conserved pre-α-chain, pTα to form a single 'pre-TCR2' (figure 12.4). This early receptor is signaled by an as yet unidentified ligand and drives the pre-T-cells in a further frenetic burst of proliferation controlled by thymic epithelial cells and fibroblasts, to the double-positive CD4⁺8⁺ stage. Further development now requires rearrangement of the $V_\alpha$ gene segments so allowing formation of the mature αβ TCR2. The cells are now ready for subsequent bouts of positive and negative receptor editing as will be discussed shortly.

Rearrangement of the $V_\beta$ genes on the sister chromatid is suppressed (remember each cell contains two chromosomes for each α and β cluster). Thus each cell only expresses a single TCR β chain and the process by which the homologous genes on the sister chromatid are suppressed is called **allelic exclusion** (cf. p. 240). The α chains are *not* allelically excluded so each cell has two antigen-specific receptors, each with their own α chain but sharing a common β chain. Curiously, the receptors on CD8 T-cells in gut epithelium which are generated extrathymically are αα homodimers in contrast to the αβ heterodimers of conventional thymic T-cells.

The T-cell repertoires in neonatal and adult mice differ. Fetal T-cells exploit more 3'-V and 5'-J segments, while adults utilize a broader spectrum with some bias towards 5'-V and 3'-J. There are also far more N-nucleotide insertions in the adult, indicative perhaps of new waves of precursors entering the thymus later in life.

## The development of γδ receptors

The γδ lineage do not produce a 'pre-receptor' and this may account for their smaller numbers relative to the αβ TCR2 population, which utilize their pTαβ receptor to expand the CD4⁻8⁻ cells. Mice expressing rearranged γ and δ transgenes do not rearrange any further γ or δ gene segments, indicating allelic exclusion of sister chromatid genes. Furthermore, they produce normal numbers of αβ T-cells in which γδ transcripts are undetectable. That this is due to transcriptional silencing in the αβ cells seems likely since γδ transgenic mice in which the downstream silencer element was deleted from the transgene construct, failed to develop αβ cells. Presumably progenitor cells split into two lineages depending on whether the γ-silencer is switched on or off.

γδ-T-cells in the mouse, unlike the human, predominate in association with epithelial cells. A curious feature of the cells leaving the fetal thymus is the restriction in *V* gene utilization. Thus virtually all of the first wave of fetal γδ cells express the same *V* genes and colonize the skin; the second wave use the same δ-gene combination but a different γ *V-J* pair and they seed the female reproductive organs. In adult life, there is far more receptor diversity due to a high degree of junctional variation (cf. p. 69), although the intraepithelial cells in the intestine and those in encapsulated lymphoid tissue form two distinct groups with respect to single *V* gene usage.

The Vγ set in the skin readily proliferate and secrete IL-2 on exposure to heat-shocked keratinocytes implying a role in the surveillance of trauma signals. The Vγ4 cells in peripheral lymphoid tissue respond well to the tuberculosis antigen PPD and to conserved residues 180–196 from mycobacterial and self heat-shock protein hsp65.

Two major γδ subsets predominate in the human, Vγ9,Vδ2 and Vγ1,Vδ2. The Vγ9 set rise from 25% of the total γδ cells in cord blood to around 70% in adult blood; at the same time the proportion of Vγ1 falls from 50% to less than 30%. The majority of the Vγ9 set have the activated memory phenotype CD45RO, probably as a result of stimulation by common ligands for the Vγ9,Vδ2 TCR such as components of mycobacteria, *Plasmodium falciparum*, and the superantigen staphylococcal enterotoxin A. Vγ9 subsets of extremely limited junctional diversity were observed in the blood and bronchoalveolar lavage of two patients with sarcoidosis, a granulomatous disease with mycobacterial involvement. The conclusion that these two major γδ subpopulations are selected by powerful antigens seems inescapable.

## Cells are positively selected for self-MHC restriction in the thymus

The ability of T-cells to recognize antigenic peptides in association with self-MHC is developed in the thymus gland. If an (H-2ᵏ×H-2ᵇ) F1 animal is sensitized to an antigen, the primed T-cells can recognize that antigen on presenting cells of either *H-2ᵏ* or *H-2ᵇ* haplotype, i.e. they can use either parental haplotype as a recognition restriction element. However, if bone marrow cells from the (H-2ᵏ×H-2ᵇ) F1 are used to reconstitute an irradiated F1 which had earlier been thymectomized and given an H-2ᵏ thymus, the subsequently primed T-cells can only recognize antigens in the context of H-2ᵏ, not of H-2ᵇ (figure 12.5). Thus it is **the phenotype of the thymus that imprints H-2 restriction** on the differentiating T-cells.

It will also be seen in figure 12.5 that incubation of the thymus graft with deoxyguanosine, which

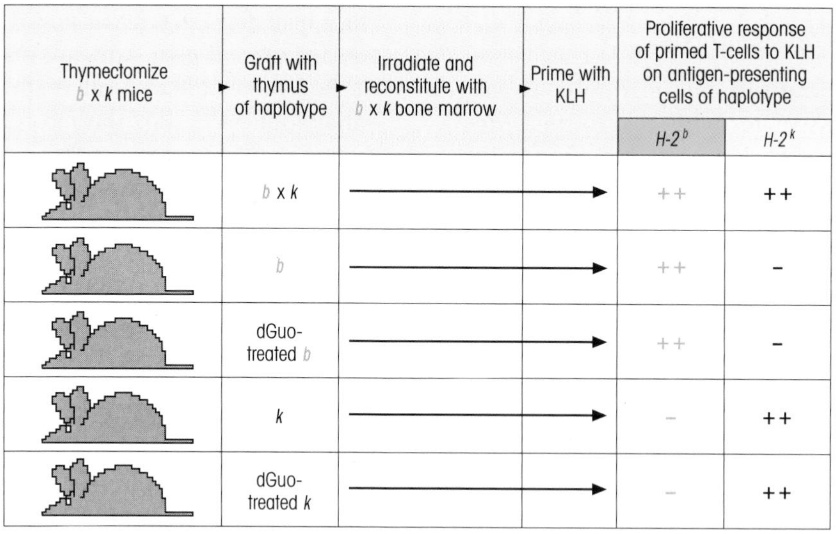

| Thymectomize *b* x *k* mice | Graft with thymus of haplotype | Irradiate and reconstitute with *b* x *k* bone marrow | Prime with KLH | Proliferative response of primed T-cells to KLH on antigen-presenting cells of haplotype | |
|---|---|---|---|---|---|
| | | | | *H-2*$^b$ | *H-2*$^k$ |
| | *b* x *k* | ⟶ | | + + | + + |
| | *b* | ⟶ | | + + | – |
| | dGuo-treated *b* | ⟶ | | + + | – |
| | *k* | ⟶ | | – | + + |
| | dGuo-treated *k* | ⟶ | | – | + + |

**Figure 12.5. Imprinting of H-2 T-helper restriction by the haplotype of the thymus.** Host mice were F1 crosses between strains of haplotype *H-2*$^b$ and *H-2*$^k$. They were thymectomized and grafted with 14-day fetal thymuses, irradiated and reconstituted with F1 bone marrow. After priming with the antigen keyhole limpet hemocyanin (KLH), the proliferative response of lymph node T-cells to KLH on antigen-presenting cells of each parental haplotype was assessed. In some experiments the thymus lobes were cultured in deoxyguanosine (dGuo), which destroys intrathymic cells of macrophage/dendritic cell lineage, but this had no effect on positive selection. (From Lo D. & Sprent J. (1986) *Nature* **319**, 672.)

destroys the cells of macrophage and dendritic cell lineage, has no effect on imprinting, suggesting that this function is carried out by epithelial cells. Confirmation of this comes from a recent study showing that lethally irradiated H-2$^k$ mice reconstituted with (b×k)F1 bone marrow and then injected intrathymically with an H-2$^b$ thymic epithelial cell line, developed T-cells restricted by the *b* haplotype. The epithelial cells are rich in surface MHC molecules and the current view is that double-positive (CD4$^+$8$^+$) T-cells bearing receptors which recognize self-MHC on the epithelial cells are positively selected for differentiation to CD4$^+$8$^-$ or CD4$^-$8$^+$ single-positive cells. The evidence for this comes largely from transgenic mice in which the appropriate genes are introduced artificially into fertilized eggs. Since this is a very active area, I would like to cite some experimental examples; nonprofessionals may need to hang on to their haplotypes, put on their ice-packs and concentrate.

One highly sophisticated study starts with a cytotoxic T-cell clone raised in H-2$^b$ females against male cells of the same strain. The clone recognizes the male antigen, H-Y, and this is seen in association with the H-2D$^b$ self-MHC molecules, i.e. it reacts with the H-2$^b$/Y complex. The α- and β-peptides forming the T-cell receptor of this clone are now introduced as transgenes into SCID mice which lack the ability to rearrange their own germ-line variable region receptor genes; thus the only TCR which could possibly be expressed is that encoded by the transgenes, provided of course, we are looking at females rather than males, in whom the clone would be eliminated by self-reactivity. If the transgenic SCID females bear the original *H-2*$^b$ haplotype (e.g. F1 hybrids between *b*×*d* haplotypes), then the anti-H-2$^b$/Y receptor is amply expressed on CD8$^+$ cytotoxic precursor cells (table 12.1a), whereas H-2$^d$ transgenics lacking H-2$^b$ produce only double CD4$^+$8$^+$ thymocytes with no single CD4$^+$8$^-$ or CD4$^-$8$^+$ cells. Thus as CD4$^+$8$^+$ cells express their TCR transgene, they only differentiate into CD8$^+$ immunocompetent cells if they come into contact with thymic epithelial cells of the MHC haplotype recognized by their receptor. We say that such self-recognizing thymocytes are being **positively selected**. Positive intracellular events accompany the positive selection process since the protein tyrosine kinases fyn and lck are activated in double-positive CD4$^+$8$^+$ thymocytes maturing to single-positive CD8$^+$ cells in the *b* haplotype background, but low in cells which fail to differentiate into mature cells in the non-selective *d* haplotype.

In another example, genes coding for an αβ-receptor from a T-helper clone (2B4) which responds to moth cytochrome *c* in association with the class II molecule H-2Eα$^k$,β$^b$ (remember H-2E has an α and β chain), are transfected into H-2$^k$ and H-2$^b$ mice. For irrelevant reasons, H-2$^k$ express the H-2E molecule on the surface of their antigen-presenting cells, but H-2$^b$ do not. In the event, the frequency of circulating CD4$^+$

**Table 12.1. Positive and negative selection in SCID transgenic mice** bearing the αβ receptors of an H-2Dᵇ T-cell clone cytotoxic for the male antigen H-Y, i.e. the clone is of *H-2ᵇ* haplotype and is female anti-male. (a) The only T-cells are those bearing the already rearranged transgenic TCR, since SCID mice cannot rearrange their own *V* genes. The clones are only expanded beyond the CD4+8+ stage when positively selected by contact with the MHC haplotype (*H-2ᵇ*) recognized by the original clone from which the transgene was derived. Also, since the receptor recognized class I, only CD8+ cells were selected. (b) When the anti-male transgenic clone is expressed on intrathymic T-cells in a male environment, the strong engagement of the TCR with male antigen-bearing cells eliminates them. (Based on data from von Boehmer H. *et al.* (1989) In Melchers F. *et al.* (eds), *Progress in Immunology* **7**, p. 297. Springer-Verlag, Berlin.)

| Phenotype of thymocytes | a / Positive selection | | b / Negative selection | |
|---|---|---|---|---|
| | Haplotype of transgenic females | | Transgenic H-2ᵇ mice | |
| | *H-2ᵇ/ᵈ* | *H-2ᵈ/ᵈ* | Males | Females |
| CD4⁻8⁻ TCR⁻ | + | ++ | +++ | + |
| CD4⁺8⁺ TCR± | ++ | + | − | +++ |
| CD4⁻8⁺ TCR⁺⁺ | + | − | − | + |
| CD4⁺8⁻ TCR⁺⁺ | − | − | − | − |

+ = crude measure of the relative numbers of T-cells in the thymus having the phenotype indicated.

T-cells bearing the 2B4 receptor was 10 times greater in the H-2ᵏ relative to H-2ᵇ strains, again speaking for positive selection of double-positive thymocytes which recognize their own thymic MHC. In a further twist to the story, positive selection only occurred in mice manipulated to express H-2E on their cortical rather than their medullary epithelial cells, showing that this differentiation step is effected before the developing thymocytes reach the medulla. ('Read it again Sam' as Humphrey Bogart might have said!)

# T-CELL TOLERANCE

## The induction of immunological tolerance is necessary to avoid self-reactivity

In essence, lymphocytes recognize foreign antigens through complementariness in shape mediated by the intermolecular forces we have described previously (see p. 86). To a large extent the building blocks used to form microbial and host molecules are the same, so it is the assembled shapes of *self* and *non-self* molecules which must be discriminated by the immune system if potentially disastrous autoreactivity is to be avoided. The restriction of each lymphocyte to a single specificity makes the job of establishing self-tolerance that much easier, simply because it just requires a mechanism which functionally deletes self-reacting cells and leaves the remainder of the reper-

toire unscathed. The most radical difference between self and nonself molecules lies in the fact that, in early life, the developing lymphocytes are surrounded by self and normally only meet nonself antigens at a later stage and then within the context of the adjuventicity and cytokine release usually associated with infection. With its customary efficiency, the blind force of evolution has exploited these differences to establish the mechanisms of **immunological tolerance to host constituents** (Milestone 12.2).

## Self-tolerance can be induced in the thymus

Since developing T-cells are to be found in the thymus gland, one might expect this to be the milieu in which exposure to self-antigens on the surrounding cells would induce tolerance. The expectation is reasonable. If stem cells in bone marrow of *H-2ᵏ* haplotype are cultured with fetal thymus of H-2ᵈ origin, the maturing cells become tolerant to H-2ᵈ, as shown by their inability to give a mixed lymphocyte proliferative response when cultured with stimulators of H-2ᵈ phenotype; third-party responsiveness is not affected. Further experiments with deoxyguanosine-treated thymuses showed that the cells responsible for tolerance induction were deoxyguanosine-sensitive, bone-marrow-derived macrophages or dendritic cells which are abundant at the cortico-medullary junction (table 12.2).

## Intrathymic clonal deletion leads to self-tolerance

There seems little doubt that self-reactive T-cells can be physically deleted within the thymus gland. If we look at the experiment in table 12.1b, we can see that SCID males bearing the rearranged transgenes coding for the αβ receptor reacting with the male H-Y antigen

**Table 12.2. Induction of tolerance in bone marrow stem cells** by incubation with deoxyguanosine (dGuo)-sensitive macrophages or dendritic cells in the thymus. Clearly the bone marrow cells induce tolerance to their own haplotype. Thus the thymic tolerance-inducing cells can be replaced by progenitors in the bone marrow inoculum (Jenkinson E.J., Jhittay P., Kingston R. & Owen J.J. (1985) *Transplantation* **39**, 331) or by adult dendritic cells from spleen showing that it is the stage of differentiation of the immature T-cell rather than any special nature of the thymic antigen-presenting cell which leads to tolerance (Matzinger P. & Guerder S. (1989) *Nature* **338**, 74).

| Bone marrow cells | Incubate with H-2ᵈ thymus | Tolerance induction to *H-2* haplotype | | |
|---|---|---|---|---|
| | | k | d | b |
| k | Untreated | + | + | − |
| k | dGuo-treated | + | − | − |
| k + d | dGuo-treated | + | + | − |

# Milestone 12.2—The Discovery of Immunological Tolerance

Over 40 years ago Owen made the intriguing observation that nonidentical (dizygotic) twin cattle, which shared the same placental circulation and whose circulations were thereby linked, grew up with appreciable numbers of red cells from the other twin in their blood; if they had not shared the same circulation at birth, red cells from the twin injected in adult life would be rapidly eliminated by an immunological response. From this finding Burnet and Fenner conceived the notion that potential antigens which reach the lymphoid cells during their developing immunologically immature phase can in some way specifically suppress any future response to that antigen when the animal reaches immunological maturity. This, they considered, would provide a means whereby unresponsiveness to the body's own constituents could be established and thereby enable the lymphoid cells to make the important distinction between 'self' and 'nonself'. On this basis, any foreign cells introduced into the body during immunological development should trick the animal into treating them as 'self' components in later life, and the studies of Medawar and his colleagues have shown that **immunological tolerance**, or unresponsiveness, can be artificially induced in this way. Thus neonatal injection of CBA mouse cells into newborn A strain animals suppresses their ability to reject a CBA graft immunologically in adult life (figure M12.2.1). Tolerance can also be induced with soluble antigens; for example, rabbits injected with bovine serum albumin without adjuvant at birth fail to make antibodies on later challenge with this protein.

Persistence of antigen is required to maintain tolerance. In Medawar's experiments the tolerant state was long lived because the injected CBA cells survived and the animals continued to be chimeric (i.e. they possessed both A and CBA cells). With nonliving antigens, such as soluble bovine serum albumin, tolerance is gradually lost; the most likely explanation being that, in the absence of antigen, newly recruited immunocompetent cells which are being generated throughout life are not being rendered tolerant. Since recruitment of newly competent T-lymphocytes is drastically curtailed by removal of the

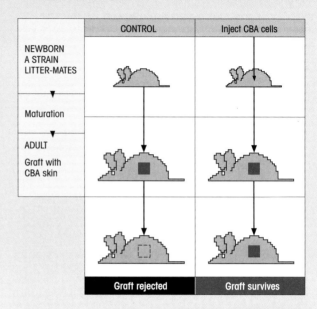

**Figure M12.2.1. Induction of tolerance to foreign CBA skin graft in A strain mice by neonatal injection of antigen.** The effect is antigen specific since the tolerant mice can reject third-party grafts normally. (After Billingham R., Brent L. & Medawar P.B. (1953) *Nature* **172**, 603.)

thymus, it is of interest to note that the tolerant state persists for much longer in thymectomized animals.

The vital importance of the experiments by Medawar and his team was their demonstration that a state of immunological tolerance can result from exposure to an antigen. Recent studies, however, suggest that the concept of a *neonatal window* for tolerance induction is more apparent than real and stems from the relatively low number of peripheralized immunocompetent T-cells, which do not differ in behaviour from resting T-cells in the adult in their tolerizability or capacity for an immune response (see papers in *Science* (1996) **271**, pp. 1723, 1726 & 1728) albeit that resting T-cells are more readily tolerizable than memory cells. As will be discussed in the text, there is a window of susceptibility to clonal deletion of self-reacting T-lymphocytes at an immature phase in their ontogenic development within the thymus (and in the case of B-cells within the bone marrow).

do not possess any immunocompetent thymic cells expressing this receptor, whereas the females which lack H-Y do. Thus, when the developing T-cells react with self antigen in the thymus, they are deleted. In other words, self-reactive cells undergo a **negative selection** process in the thymus. A similar phenom-enon is seen when the thymic cells bear certain self-components which act as superantigens (cf. p. 100) by reacting with a whole family of Vβ receptors through recognition of nonvariable structures on a Vβ segment. An example is the H-2E molecule which reacts with receptors belonging to the Vβ17a family;

strains which cannot express H-2E because of a defect in the *Ea* gene, possess mature T-cells utilizing Vβ17a, whereas strains which express H-2E normally delete their Vβ17a positive T-cells. Likewise mice of the *Mls*$^\alpha$ genotype delete Vβ6-bearing cells, the *Mls* being a locus encoding a B-cell superantigen which induces strong proliferation in Vβ6 T-cells from a strain bearing a different *Mls* allele (cf. p. 100). Even exogenous superantigens, such as staphylococcal enterotoxin B which activates the Vβ3 and Vβ8 T-cell families in the adult, will eliminate these cells when incubated with early immature thymocytes. Even more enlightening is the fact that, under these circumstances, the Vβ3 and Vβ8 thymocytes can actually be seen to undergo programmed cell death (apoptosis, cf. p. 19).

## Factors affecting positive or negative selection in the thymus

It is established that engagement of TCR by MHC/peptide complex on some type of antigenpresenting cell underlies both positive and negative selection. But how can the same MHC/peptide signal have two totally different outcomes? Well, positive and negative selection may occur at low and high degrees of TCR ligation respectively. For example, corticosteroids or high concentrations of antibody to the TCR induce apoptosis in thymocytes (figure 12.6); however, low concentrations of anti-TCR will rescue the cells from killing by corticosteroids. Furthermore, many examples have been published showing that the same peptide will induce positive selection at low concentration and negative selection at high (see legend figure 12.7). This has led to the avidity model, which postulates that a functionally low avidity interaction between T-cell and peptide/MHC involving a relatively low number of TCRs will positively select double-positive CD4$^+$8$^+$ thymocytes, while a high avidity interaction will lead to clonal deletion (figure 12.7). Since the overall avidity of the T-cell interaction will be *inter alia* a function of ligand density × TCR density × affinity, an increase in peptide concentration will increase ligand density and hence avidity. One problem will be immediately apparent to the discerning reader in that a given peptide ligand giving a low avidity initial stimulus for positive selection, should give a negative signal as the thymocyte differentiates and the density of TCRs increases with the change from double- to single-positive cells. This has led to the suggestion that thymic cortical cells progressively desensitize the maturing thymocyte so that it resists the more powerful stimulus of the macrophages and

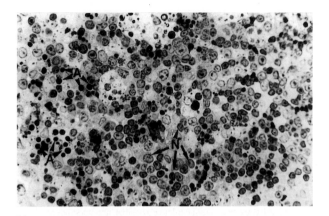

(a)

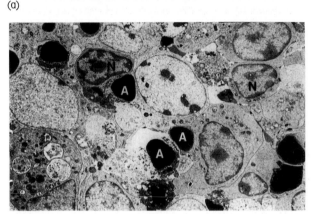

(b)

**Figure 12.6. Histological appearance of cells induced to undergo apoptosis in intact fetal thymus lobes after short-term exposure to anti-CD3.** (a) Toluidine blue-stained 1 μm sections. (b) Electron micrograph taken from the same anti-CD3-treated culture as in (a). A and N indicate representative apoptotic and normal lymphocytes respectively. Note the highly condensed state of the nuclei of the apoptotic lymphocytes. (Photographs kindly donated by Professor J.J.T. Owen, from Smith *et al.* (1989) *Nature* **337**, 181. Reproduced by permission from Macmillan Journals Ltd, London.)

medullary dendritic cells, which would otherwise induce apoptosis.

To pause for a moment, we seem to be saying that engagement of the TCR of differentiating double-positive CD4$^+$8$^+$ thymocytes with self-MHC on cortical epithelial cells leads to expansion and positive selection for clones which recognize self-MHC, perhaps with a whole range of affinities, but that engagement of the TCR with high affinity for self MHC (+ self peptide) on bone marrow-derived medullary cells will lead to elimination and hence negative selection. Although still not fully worked out, there are also obvious differences in the biochemical pathways used for positive and negative signaling. Positive selection is cyclosporin A-sensitive and dependent on p21 ras and MAP kinase pathways, whereas negative selection is cyclosporin A-resistant and independent of p21 ras and MAP kinase. Further-

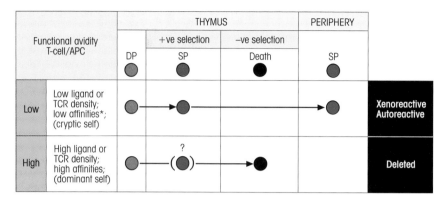

| Functional avidity T-cell/APC | | THYMUS | | | PERIPHERY |
|---|---|---|---|---|---|
| | | | +ve selection | −ve selection | |
| | | DP | SP | Death | SP |
| | | ● | ● | ● | ● |
| Low | Low ligand or TCR density; low affinities*; (cryptic self) | ● → | ● → | | → ● | **Xenoreactive Autoreactive** |
| High | High ligand or TCR density; high affinities; (dominant self) | ● — | ? (●) → | ● | **Deleted** |

**Figure 12.7. The avidity model of thymic positive and negative selection.** It is postulated that a low avidity interaction between the T-cell and antigen-presenting cell (APC) will give positive selection and high avidity deletion. DP = double-positive CD4+8+; SP = single-positive CD4+ or CD8+; *refers to affinity of peptide for the MHC or of the MHC/peptide complex for the TCR.

When Tap-1 mutant mice (cf. p. 92) are mated with mice bearing the transgenes for the TCR specific for a complex of H-2Dᵇ with an LCM virus peptide, the positive selection of the transgenic T-cells is impaired because of lack of MHC/peptide. However, low concentrations of the peptide added to fetal organ cultures of these mice selected the transgenic T-cells positively, while higher concentrations gave negative selection (Ljunggren H.G. & Kaer L. van (1995) *The Immunologist* **3**, 136). 'Cryptic self' peptides (cf. p. 202) are presented at very low concentrations and will not delete potentially autoreactive clones, which may therefore escape to the periphery.

more, negative signaling requires coreceptors but at the time of writing there is little agreement on their identity. Let us finish on a cautionary note: the avidity model may be substantially correct but it could be an oversimplification. For instance, certain superantigens which can cause clonal deletion of certain Vβ families, fail to expand them even at very low concentrations when the model would have indicated positive selection. This has spawned other models involving conformational changes, and given the complex interactions of peptides behaving as agonists, partial agonists and antagonists (cf. p. 173), the last word has not yet been spoken (not that it ever is in science!).

Looking again at figure 12.7, the specificities of the T-cells entering the periphery from the thymus must be moulded by the self-peptides, which drive positive selection, since normally the only peptides around must be derived from self. It is satisfying to note therefore that the T-cell repertoire tends to be biased towards peptides from extrinsic antigens which resemble self; thus, T-cell epitopes recognized on immunization with xenogeneic lysozyme corresponded with sequences having the highest homology to the syngeneic protein.

### T-cell tolerance can be due to clonal anergy

We have already entertained the idea that engagement of the TCR plus a costimulatory signal from an antigen-presenting cell are both required for T-cell stimulation, but when the costimulatory signal is lacking, the T-cell becomes tolerized or anergic, or if you prefer, paralysed.

Thus, anergy can be induced in **extrathymic T-cells** by peripheral antigens *in vivo* when presented by cells lacking costimulatory molecules. If a transgene construct of H-2Eᵇ attached to an insulin promoter is introduced into a mouse which normally fails to express H-2E, the H-2Eᵇ transgene product appears on the β-cells of the pancreas and induces tolerance to itself. Whereas the expression of H-2E on bone-marrow-derived cells in the thymic medulla deletes T-cells bearing Vβ17a receptors, these cells are not lost in the tolerant transgenic mouse expressing pancreatic H-2E, i.e. there is a state of clonal anergy, not deletion. The altered immunological status of these cells is revealed by their inability to proliferate when their receptors are cross-linked by an antibody to Vβ17a.

It is unlikely that these results are due to low level expression of antigen in the thymus. Similar experiments with mice expressing influenza hemagglutinin on the pancreatic β-islets also became tolerant irrespective of whether the transgenic thymus was replaced by a normal gland or not. Nonetheless, anergic cells can also be generated within the thymic population as seen in mice transgenic for both an anti-Kᵇ TCR and a *Kᵇ* gene controlled by a truncated fragment of a keratin IV promoter which allowed expression on thymic medullary cells.

Peripheral T-cell anergy can occur at different levels depending upon the circumstances of antigen exposure. If the above double transgenic experiment is repeated with a full keratin IV promoter, the Kᵇ antigen is expressed on keratinocytes and induces full tolerance, even though the same high frequency of cytotoxic T-cell precursors with the transgene TCR is

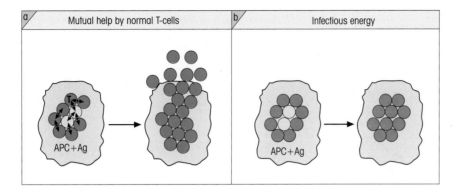

**Figure 12.8. Infectious anergy.** (a) Clusters of normal T-cells (green) around newly immunocompetent cells (gray) reacting with the same APC, mutually support activation and proliferation. (b) Newly immunocompetent cells surrounded by anergic T-cells (red) receive no stimulatory signals from their neighbors and are themselves rendered anergic.

seen as in single transgenic animals lacking $K^b$. If $K^b$ is expressed on cells of neuroectodermal origin or hepatocytes, again the double transgenic mice are tolerant but there is dramatic downregulation of TCR and CD8 molecules; in the former but not the latter case, downregulation of TCR could be reversed by exposure to antigen *in vitro*. In some experimental models, tolerance can be abrogated by IL-2. To recapitulate, autoreactive T-cells leaving the thymus can be rendered anergic in the periphery and can display different degrees of potentially reversible unresponsiveness.

*Infectious anergy*

If a clone of T-helpers is subject to a limiting dilution experiment (p. 140), the minimal unit of proliferation in response to peptide on an APC is usually several cells not just one. This implies that triggering only occurs in small groups or clusters of cells and suggests that paracrine or multicellular interactions between potential responders bound to a single APC are needed to drive the cells into division (figure 12.8a). It will be appreciated that if a newly arising extrathymic naive T-cell binds to its antigen, even on a professional APC, it will not be stimulated if its neighbours in the cluster have already been made anergic. Indeed instead of being triggered, it will itself become anergic, so perpetuating the infectious anergic process (figure 12.8b). We shall see later in Chapter 17 that the induction of transplantation immunosuppression with a nondepleting anti-CD4 can be long-lasting because the production of anergic cells prevents the priming of newly immuno-

competent T-lymphocytes by the transplantation antigen(s).

These anergic cells are really acting as suppressors. So far in our discussions, we have not asked the question: do dedicated T-suppressors contribute to self-tolerance? Frankly, another gray area, but experimentally we can demonstrate that if autoimmunity is induced in a normal animal, either actively, by injection of an antigen cross-reacting with self, or passively, by injection of autoreactive T-cells (cf. pp. 418 & 437), the self-reacting clones are usually squashed by idiotype or antigen-specific T-suppression. In a nutshell, suppressors probably do not prevent autoimmunity but they may reverse it.

## Lack of communication can cause unresponsiveness

It takes two to tango: if the self-molecule cannot engage the TCR, there can be no response. The anatomical isolation of molecules like the lens protein of the eye and myelin basic protein in the brain virtually precludes them from contact with lymphocytes, except perhaps for minute amounts of breakdown metabolic products which leak out and may be taken up by antigen-presenting cells, but at concentrations way below that required to trigger the corresponding naive T-cell.

Even when a tissue is exposed to circulating lymphocytes, the concentration of processed peptide on the cell surface in the absence of costimulatory B7 may be insufficient to attract attention from a potentially autoreactive cell. This was demonstrated rather elegantly in animals bearing two transgenes: one for the TCR of a CD8 cytotoxic T-cell specific for LCM virus glycoprotein, and the other for the glycoprotein itself expressed on pancreatic β-cells through the insulin promoter. The result? A deafening silence: the T-cells were not deleted or tolerized, neither were the β-cells attacked. If these mice were then infected

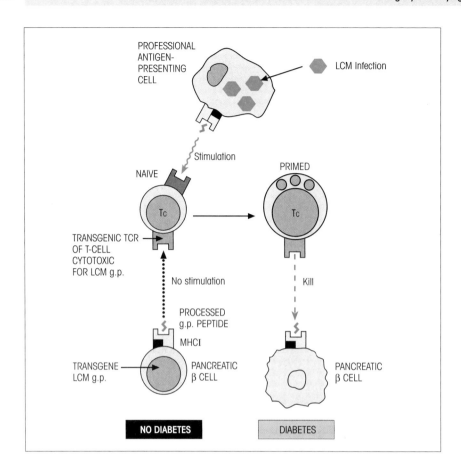

**Figure 12.9. Mutual unawareness of a naive cytotoxic precursor T-cell and its B7 negative cellular target-bearing epitopes present at low concentrations**. Priming of the naive cell by a natural infection and subsequent attack by the higher avidity primed cells on the target tissue. LCM = lymphocytic choriomeningitis virus. (From Ohashi *et al.* (1991) *Cell* **65**, 305.)

with LCM virus, the naive transgenic T-cells were presented with adequate concentrations of the processed glycoprotein within the adjuvant context of a true infection and were now stimulated. Their *primed* progeny, having an increased avidity (cf. p. 393) and thereby being able to recognize the low concentrations of processed glycoprotein on the β-cells, attacked their targets even in the absence of B7 and caused diabetes (figure 12.9). This may sound a trifle tortuous but the principle could have important implications for the induction of autoimmunity by cross-reacting T-cell epitopes (cf. p. 415).

Molecules that are specifically restricted to particular organs which do not normally express MHC class II represent another special case, since they would not have the opportunity clonally to delete or paralyse organ-specific CD4 T-helper cells.

Immunological silence would also result if an individual has no genes coding for lymphocyte receptors directed against particular self-determinants; analysis of the experimentally induced autoantibody response to cytochrome suggests that only those parts of the molecule which show species variation are autoantigenic, whereas the highly conserved regions where the genes have not altered for a much

longer time appear to be silent, supposedly because the autoreactive specificities have had time to disappear.

## B-CELLS DIFFERENTIATE IN THE FETAL LIVER AND THEN IN BONE MARROW

The B-lymphocyte precursors, pro-B-cells, are present among the islands of hematopoietic cells in fetal liver by 8–9 weeks of gestation in man and 14 days in the mouse. Production of B-cells wanes and is mostly taken over by the bone marrow for the remainder of life. Using the modified culture conditions introduced by Whitlock and Witte, it is now possible to grow bone marrow cells *in vitro* and achieve the differentiation of B-cells and their precursors. Stromal reticular cells which express adhesion molecules and secrete IL-7, extend long dendritic processes making intimate contact with IL-7 receptor positive B-cell progenitors. Although early B-cells comprise only a minor subpopulation of the cells in those cultures, it is possible to analyse the different stages in their development by rescue with the Abelson murine leukemia virus (A-MuLV), a replication-defective retrovirus capable of transforming pre-B cells at various points in their

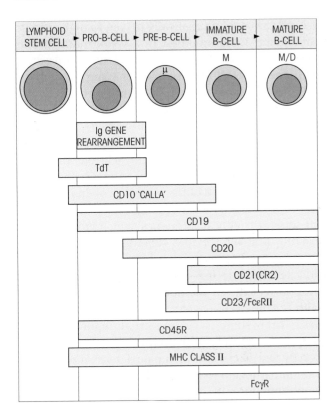

**Figure 12.10. Some of the differentiation markers of developing B-cells.** The boxes show the time of appearance of the surface markers, many of them defined by monoclonal antibodies (see table 8.1 for list of CD members.)

development into clones. A series of differentiation markers associated with B-cell maturation have now been established (figure 12.10).

## B-1 AND B-2 CELLS REPRESENT TWO DISTINCT POPULATIONS

We have previously drawn attention to the subpopulation of B-cells which, in addition to surface IgM, express the T-cell marker CD5 (cf. p. 208). The progenitors of this subset move from the fetal liver to the peritoneal cavity fairly early in life, at which stage they are the most abundant B-cell type and predominate in their contribution to the idiotype network and to the production of low-affinity, multispecific IgM autoantibodies and the so-called 'natural' antibodies to bacterial carbohydrates which seemingly arise slightly later in the neonatal period without obvious exposure to conventional antigens.

The **B-1 phenotype viz. high surface IgM, Mac-1+ and CD23−** is shared by a minority subpopulation which are however CD5−, and it has now been decided that these should be labeled B-1a and B-1b respectively (figure 12.11). The **phenotype** of the pool of conventional **B-2 cells, low surface IgM, CD5−,**

**Mac-1− and CD23+**, reflects the fact they represent a separate developmental lineage (figure 12.11) and many of the salient points for comparison of these two subsets are made in table 12.3. Some general comments may be in order. The B-1 and B-2 lineages replenish themselves but not each other. The B-1 cells maintain their numbers by self-replenishment and limit their *de novo* production from progenitors by feedback regulation. They can express both CD5 and its ligand CD72 on their surface, which should encourage mutual interaction, but a major factor influencing self-renewal could be the constitutive production of IL-10 since treatment of mice with anti-IL-10 from birth virtually wipes out the B-1 subset.

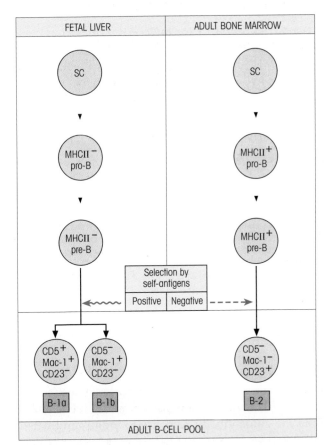

**Figure 12.11. The development of separate B-cell subpopulations.** The B-1 phenotype is also characterized by high surface IgM, while B-2 cells have low IgM. It is presumed that B-1 cells of sufficiently high avidity for, say, self-surface antigens are eliminated leaving lower affinity specificities for soluble self antigens and the spectrum of 'natural' anti-B-1 cells. Evidence that self-antigens drive B-1 cell proliferation is provided by mice made transgenic for $V_H81X$ (the most D-proximal $V_H$ gene which is preferentially rearranged in the perinatal period). Self-reactive B-1 cells expressing the $V_H81X$ transgene linked to a particular κ light chain, remain at low levels if the mice are constantly infused with antibody of the same specificity, the implication being that the autoantigen which is the natural ligand, was being prevented from expanding that particular B-1 cell clone. SC = stem cell; Mac-1 = CD11b.

**Table 12.3. Comparison of two mouse B-cell subsets.** (Developed from Herzenberg L.A., Stall A., Melchers F. et al. (eds) (1989) *Progress in Immunology* **7**, 409. Springer-Verlag, Berlin.)

| | B1 | B2 |
|---|---|---|
| **PHENOTYPE** | | |
| IgM | +++ | + |
| IgD | + | +++ |
| B220 | + | +++ |
| CD5 | + or − | − |
| CD23 | − | + |
| Mac-1 | + | − |
| Size | large | small |
| **MAIN LOCATION** | Peritoneal cavity | Lymphoid organs |
| **ONTOGENY** | Arise first in fetal liver | Arise later in adult bone marrow |
| **LIFESPAN** | Self-renewing Constitutive production IL-10 | Replaced by IgM⁻ precursors in bone marrow |
| **GROWTH** | Propensity to expansion | Die easily |
| **IMPAIRED DEVELOPMENT** | Xid (CBA/N)[1] | me^v (motheaten)[2] |
| **Ig GENES** | Remain germ-line, little N-nucleotide insertion | Mutate, common N-nucleotide insertion |
| **ANTIBODY PRODUCTION** | | |
| Serum IgM, IgG3 | +++ | + |
| IgG1 | + | +++ |
| IgG2a, IgG2b | + to ++ | ++ to +++ |
| IgM autoantibody | +++ | ? |
| IgM anti-Id | +++ | ? |
| IgM anti-bacterial Ab | +++ | + to +++ |
| Anti-hapten/protein | ? | +++ |
| T-dependence | − | ++ |
| Affinity maturation | − | ++ |

1 CBA/N mice have an X-linked immunodeficiency gene (Xid) producing a defect in the Bruton tyrosine kinase (btk) associated with poor B-1 cell maturation and inadequate responses to type II T-independent antigens.
2 Motheaten mice have the me^v mutation affecting the protein tyrosine phosphatase 1C (*PTP-1C*) gene which dramatically alters the threshold for antigen and strongly biases development toward the B-1 subpopulation. The mice have widespread autoimmunity and most of their B-cells are B-1.

The predisposition for self-renewal may underlie their undue susceptibility to become leukemic.

B-1 cells tend to use particular germ-line *V* genes and the autoantibody response to bromelain-treated erythrocytes is restricted to this subset which utilize the rather diminutive $V_{H11}$ and $V_{H12}$ families. Clonal expansion seems to be driven by reaction with self-antigens (see legend figure 12.11). They tend to respond to type 2 thymus-independent antigens (cf. p. 173) and, unlike the B-2 population, they do not enter into liaisons with thymus-dependent antigens, do not enter germinal centers and hence do not undergo somatic mutation or form high affinity antibodies. This may be just as well if the harmless low affinity autoantibodies which are produced by many

B-1 cells are not automatically driven to high affinity pathogenic autoantibodies. In a weak moment one sometimes hears of 'good' and 'bad' autoantibodies, with the 'good guys' possibly having the job of sweeping up broken down self-components as envisaged by dear Pierre Grabar many years ago when he thought of them as *globulines transporteurs*.

Other functions may be the generation of an idiotype network concerned in self-tolerance, the response to conserved microbial antigens, and possibly the maintenance of the *V* gene pool and the idiotypic regulation of B-2 responses. They are certainly the source of 'natural antibodies' which provide a pre-existing first line of IgM defense against common microbes, and recently it has been shown that a fraction develop into IgA-producing cells in the lamina propria which coat the normal microflora of the gut with IgA. Ideas now get a little cloudy but one view has it that in some, as yet mysterious manner, this stabilizes the normal gut flora which prevent colonization by new bacteria as an innate defense mechanism. Should pathogenic bacteria penetrate the gut then we would pin our faith in the production of high affinity narrowly tuned IgA produced by the conventional B-2 cells derived from Peyer's patches. Yet another cunning strategy would be for the B-1 antibodies with their wide-ranging multispecificities, to form immune complexes with a newly encountered antigen in a previously unsensitized animal which could be captured by the surface receptors on follicular dendritic cells and help to initiate germinal center formation. There truly seem to be no shortage of suggestions for this interesting subpopulation.

## DEVELOPMENT OF B-CELL SPECIFICITY

### The sequence of immunoglobulin gene rearrangements

By analysis of Abelson-MuLV-transformed clones of pre-B cells, it has proved possible to unravel the orderly cascade of Ig gene rearrangements which occur during differentiation.

**Stage 1.** Initially, the *D-J* segments on both heavy chain coding regions (one from each parent) rearrange (figure 12.12).

**Stage 2.** A *V–DJ* recombinational event now occurs on one heavy chain. If this proves to be a *nonproductive* rearrangement (i.e. adjacent segments are joined in an incorrect reading frame or in such a way as to generate a termination codon downstream from the splice point), then a second *V–DJ* rearrangement will occur on the sister heavy chain region. If a productive

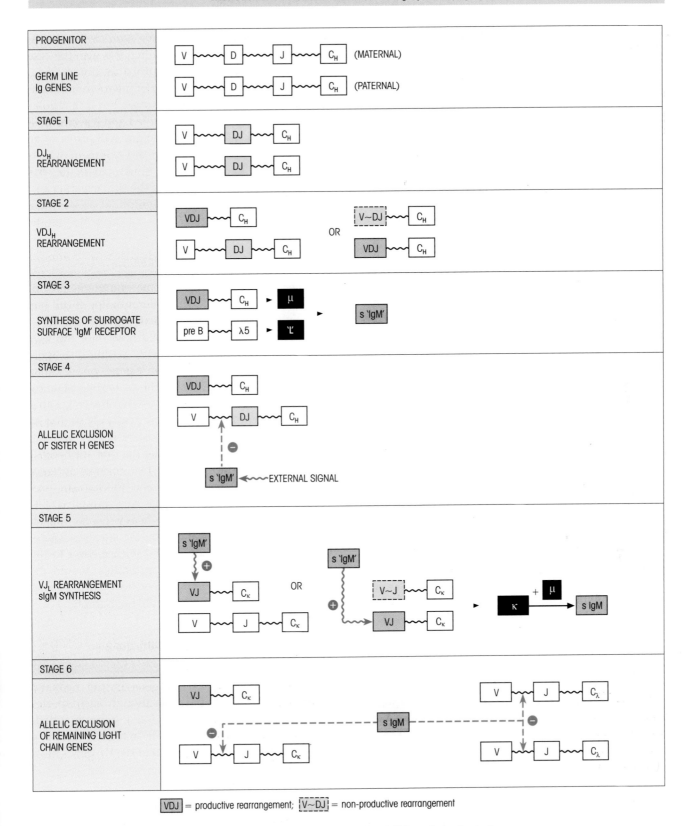

VDJ = productive rearrangement; V~DJ = non-productive rearrangement

**Figure 12.12. Postulated sequence of B-cell gene rearrangements and mechanism of allelic exclusion** (see text).

rearrangement is not achieved, we can wave the pre-B-cell a fond farewell.

**Stage 3.** Assuming a productive rearrangement is made, the pre-B-cell can now synthesize μ chains. At around the same time, two genes $V_{preB}$ and $\lambda_5$ with homology for the $V_L$ and $C_L$ segments of λ-light chains respectively are temporarily transcribed to form a 'pseudo light chain' which associates with the μ chains to generate a surface surrogate 'IgM' receptor together with the IgM-α and Ig-β chains conventionally required to form a functional B-cell receptor. Expression of this receptor is absolutely essential for further differentiation of the B-lymphocytes since disruption of the membrane exon of the μ chain or of the $\lambda_5$ gene by homologous recombination of embryonic stem cells (cf. p. 144) arrests development at the pre-B stage and the animal is devoid of mature B-cells. This surrogate receptor closely parallels the pre-Tα/β receptor on pre-T-cell precursors of native TCR2 bearing cells.

**Stage 4.** The surface receptor is signaled, perhaps by a stromal cell, to suppress any further rearrangement of heavy chain genes on a sister chromatid. This is termed **allelic exclusion** and was first discussed in relation to the rearrangement of TCR β-chains (see p. 229).

**Stage 5.** It is presumed that the surface receptor now initiates the next set of gene rearrangements which occur on the κ light chain gene loci. These involve $V–J$ recombinations on first one and then the other κ allele until a productive $V_\kappa–J$ rearrangement is accomplished. Were that to fail, an attempt would be made to achieve productive rearrangement of the λ alleles. Synthesis of conventional sIgM now proceeds.

**Stage 6.** The sIgM molecule now prohibits any further gene shuffling by allelic exclusion of any unrearranged light chain genes.

At the next stage of differentiation, the cell develops a commitment to producing a particular antibody class and either bears surface IgM alone or in combination with IgA or IgG. The further addition of surface IgD now marks the readiness of the virgin B-cell for priming by antigen. Some cells, therefore, bear surface Ig of three different classes: M, G and D or M, A and D, but all Ig molecules on a single cell have the same idiotype and therefore are derived from the same $V_H$ and $V_L$ genes, presumably by splicing of a long RNA transcript. IgD is lost on antigenic stimulation so that memory cells lack this Ig. At the terminal stages in the life of a fully mature plasma cell, virtually all surface Ig is shed. Injection of anti-μ (anti-IgM heavy chain) into chick embryos prevents the subsequent maturation of IgM and IgG antibody-producing cells, whereas anti-γ inhibits only IgG

development. Although we have seen earlier that T-helpers can induce class-switching, it is also the case that some isotype switching probably occurs independently of antigen as a result of microenvironmental factors. In the embryonic chicken bursa, a regular switch from IgM to IgG is observed and it seems possible that local influences in the gut will prove to be responsible for the predominant development of IgA-bearing cells. These cells are generated in Peyer's patches, pass into the blood via the thoracic duct and return to populate the diffuse lymphoid tissue in the lamina propria of the gut.

## The importance of allelic exclusion

Since each cell has chromosome complements derived from each parent, the differentiating B-cell has four light- and two heavy-chain gene clusters to choose from. We have described how once the $VDJ$ DNA rearrangement has occurred within one light- and one heavy-chain cluster, the $V$ genes on the other four chromosomes are held in the embryonic state by an allelic exclusion mechanism so that the cell is able to express only one light and one heavy chain. This is essential for clonal selection to work since the cell is then only programmed to make the one antibody it uses as a cell surface receptor to recognize antigen. Furthermore, this gene exclusion mechanism prevents the formation of molecules containing two different light or two different heavy chains which would have nonidentical combining sites and therefore be functionally monovalent with respect to the majority of antigens; such antibodies would be nonagglutinating and tend to have low avidity as the bonus effect of multivalency could not operate.

## Different specific responses can appear sequentially

The responses to given antigens in the neonatal period appear sequentially, as though each species were programmed to rearrange its $V$ genes in a definite order (figure 12.13). Early in ontogeny there is a bias favoring the rearrangement of the $V_H$ genes most proximal to the $DJ$ segment.

# THE INDUCTION OF TOLERANCE IN B-LYMPHOCYTES

## Tolerance can be caused by clonal deletion and clonal anergy

Just as for T-cells, so both mechanisms can operate on

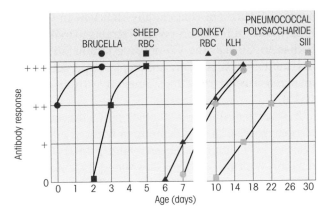

Figure 12.13. Sequential appearance of responsiveness to different antigens in the neonatal rat. RBC = red blood cell; KLH = keyhole limpet hemocyanin.

B-cells to prevent the reaction to self. Excellent evidence for deletion comes from mice bearing transgenes coding for IgM which binds to H-2K molecules of all *H-2* haplotypes except *d* and *f*. Mice of *H-2ᵃ* haplotype express the transgenic IgM abundantly in the serum, while 25–50% of total B-cells bear the transgenic idiotype. (*d* × *k*)F1 crosses completely failed to express the transgene, either in the serum or on B-cells, i.e. B-cells programmed for anti-H-2Kᵏ were expressed in *H-2ᵈ* mice but deleted in mice positive for H-2Kᵏ which in these circumstances acts as an autoantigen.

Tolerance through B-cell anergy was clearly demonstrated in another study in which double transgenic mice were made to express both lysozyme and a high-affinity antibody to lysozyme. The animals were completely tolerant and could not be immunized to make anti-lysozyme; nor did the transgenic antibody appear in the serum although it was abundantly present on the surface of B-cells. These anergic cells could bind antigen to their surface receptors but could not be activated. Like the aged roué, wistfully drinking in the visual attractions of some young belle, these tolerized lymphocytes can 'see' the antigen but lack the ability to do anything about it.

Whether deletion or anergy is the outcome of the encounter with self probably depends upon concentration and ability to cross-link Ig receptors. In the first of the two B-cell tolerance models above, the H-2Kᵏ autoantigen would be richly expressed on cells in contact with the developing B-lymphocytes and could effectively cause cross-linking. In the second case, the lysozyme, masquerading as a 'self' molecule, is essentially univalent with respect to the receptors on an anti-lysozyme B-cell and would not readily bring about cross-linking. The hypothesis was tested by stitching a transmembrane hydrophobic segment

onto the lysozyme transgene so that the antigen would be inserted into the cell membrane. Result? B-cells expressing the high affinity anti-lysozyme transgene were eliminated.

Another self-censoring mechanism termed 'receptor editing' may come into play. This can best be explained by an example. If the heavy- and light-chain Ig genes encoding a high affinity anti-DNA autoantibody are introduced as transgenes into a mouse, a variety of light chains is produced by genetic reshuffling until a combination with the heavy chain is achieved which no longer has anti-DNA activity, i.e. the autoreactivity has been edited out in some way.

Most peripheral B-cells in mice are ligand selected as revealed by analysis of the $V_H$ repertoire at the cDNA level of bone marrow pre-B-cells compared with mature spleen B-cells. Once peripheralized, the bulk of the B-cell pool is stable; lymph node B- (and T-) cells from unprimed mice survived comfortably for at least 20 months on transfer to H-2 identical SCID animals.

## Tolerance may result from helpless B-cells

With soluble proteins at least, T-cells are more readily tolerized than B-cells (figure 12.14) and, depending upon the circulating protein concentration, a number of self-reacting B-cells may be present in the body which cannot be triggered by T-dependent self-components since the T-cells required to provide the

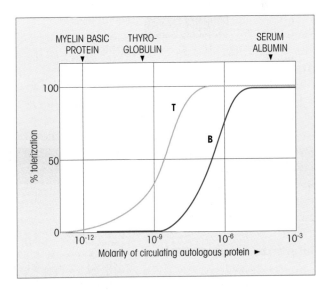

Figure 12.14. Relative susceptibility of T- and B-cells to tolerance by circulating autologous molecules. Those circulating at low concentration induce no tolerance; at intermediate concentration, e.g. thyroglobulin, T-cells are moderately tolerized; molecules such as albumin which circulate at high concentrations tolerize both B- and T-cells.

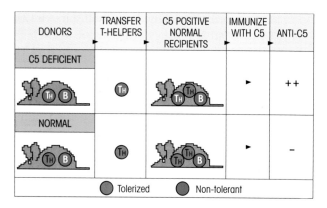

| DONORS | TRANSFER T-HELPERS | C5 POSITIVE NORMAL RECIPIENTS | IMMUNIZE WITH C5 | ANTI-C5 |
|---|---|---|---|---|
| C5 DEFICIENT | | | | |
| | TH | | ▶ | ++ |
| NORMAL | | | | |
| | TH | | ▶ | − |
| | ● Tolerized | ● Non-tolerant | | |

**Figure 12.15. Circulating C5 tolerizes T- but not B-cells leaving them helpless.** Animals with congenital C5 deficiency do not tolerize their T-helpers and can be used to break tolerance in normal mice.

necessary T–B help are already tolerant — you might describe the B-cells as helpless. If we think of the determinant on a self-component which combines with the receptors on a self-reacting B-cell as a hapten and another determinant which has to be recognized by a T-cell as a carrier (cf. figure 9.8), then tolerance in the T-cell to the carrier will prevent the provision of T-cell help and the B-cell will be unresponsive. Take C5 as an example; this is normally circulating at concentrations which tolerize T- but not B-cells. Some

strains of mice are congenitally deficient in C5 and their T-cells can help C5-positive strains to make antibodies to C5, i.e. the C5-positive strains still have inducible B-cells but they are helpless and need non-tolerized T-cells from the C5-negative strain (figure 12.15).

It is worth noting a recent observation that injection of high doses of a soluble antigen without adjuvant, even when given several days after primary immunization with that antigen, prevented the emergence of high affinity mutated antibodies. Transfer experiments showed the T-cells to be tolerant. This tells us that even when an immune response is well underway, T-helpers in the germinal center are needed to permit the mutations which lead to affinity maturation of antibody, and as a further corollary, that soluble self antigens in the extracellular fluids can act to switch off autoreactive B-cells arising in the germinal centers by hypermutation.

Presumably, self-tolerance in both B- and T-cells involves all the mechanisms we have discussed to varying degrees and these are summarized in figure 12.16. Remember that throughout the life of an animal, new stem cells are continually differentiating into immunocompetent lymphocytes and what is early in ontogeny for them can be late for the host; this means that self-tolerance mechanisms are still acting

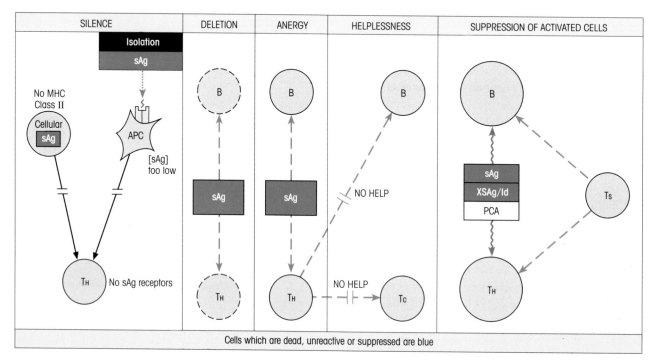

**Figure 12.16. Mechanisms of self-tolerance** (see text). sAg = self antigen; XS Ag/Id = cross-reacting antigen or idiotype; PCA = polyclonal activator; APC = antigen-presenting cell; TH = T-helper; Ts = T-suppressor; Tc = cytotoxic T-cell precursor.

on early lymphocytes even in the adult, although it is always comforting to note that the threshold concentration for tolerance induction is very much lower for pre-B relative to mature B-cells.

## THE OVERALL RESPONSE IN THE NEONATE

Lymph node and spleen remain relatively underdeveloped in the human, even at birth, except where there has been intrauterine exposure to antigens as in congenital infections with rubella or other organisms. The ability to reject grafts and to mount an antibody response is reasonably well developed by birth but the immunoglobulin levels, with one exception, are low, particularly in the absence of intrauterine infection. The exception is IgG which is acquired by placental transfer from the mother, a process dependent upon Fc structures specific to this Ig class. This material is catabolized with a half-life of approximately 30 days and there is a fall in IgG concentration over the first 3 months accentuated by the increase in blood volume of the growing infant. Thereafter the rate of synthesis overtakes the rate of breakdown of maternal IgG and the overall concentration increases steadily. The other immunoglobulins do not cross the placenta and the low but significant levels of IgM in

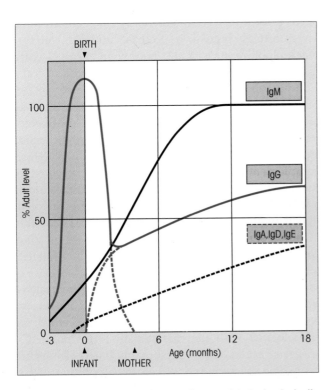

**Figure 12.17. Development of serum immunoglobulin levels in the human.** (After Hobbs J.R. (1969) In Adinolfi M. (ed.) *Immunology and Development*, p. 118. Heinemann, London.)

cord blood are synthesized by the baby (figure 12.17). IgM reaches adult levels by 9 months of age. Only trace levels of IgA, IgD and IgE are present in the circulation of the newborn.

## THE EVOLUTION OF THE IMMUNE RESPONSE

### Recognition of self is fundamental for multicellular organisms

The multiplicity of life forms which inhabit our planet have arisen from selective forces operating on 'selfish genes' driven by the chance establishment of mechanisms which optimized their replication and survival. As an example of the stringency of such mechanisms we have only to look at bacteria which use restriction endonucleases to cleave the DNA of invading viruses; they protect their own DNA by methylating the specific nucleotide sequences recognized by the enzyme. Primitive discriminatory processes must come into play when amebocytes, which are so widespread throughout invertebrate phylogeny, feed by recognizing nonself material for phagocytosis and digestion. Where survival of cellular DNA is increased by organized aggregation of identical cells into a multicellular organism, it is essential that each such colony maintains its individuality. It is not surprising, therefore, that mechanisms for the recognition and subsequent rejection of nonself can be identified in invertebrates such as the earthworm (figure 12.18b) and even as far down the evolutionary scale as the sponges, commonly regarded as the most primitive of present-day animals (figure 12.18a). A like phenomenon has been studied in more detail in the colonial tunicate *Botryllus schosseri*, which occur as subtidal individual cells or colonies, which on meeting fuse or reject, the fusion resulting in establishment of a parabiotic multi-individual colony. Genetically identical members fuse and establish a common blood supply, but when different individuals fuse, although an initial vascular anastomosis is formed, this is rapidly plugged by inflammatory blood cells, both within the blood vessel and in the perivascular tunic. Cytotoxic cells, macrophages and other blood cells stream in and pinch off the blood vessel—truly transplantation in the wild! Rejection is controlled by a single gene locus with many alleles and if a homozygous colony (say of genotype *AA*) fuses with a heterozygote (AB), it is the homozygote which is preferentially absorbed. This contributes to an impressive polymorphism and contrasts with the rules of graft rejection in vertebrates, where the homozygote would react against

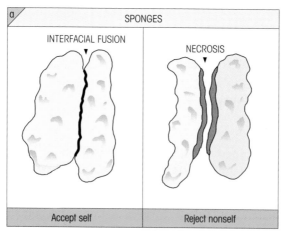

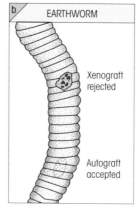

**Figure 12.18. Recognition and rejection of nonself.** (a) Parabiosed fingers of sponge from the same colony are permanently united but members of different colonies reject each other by 7–9 days. (b) A xenograft of body wall tissue from the earthworm *Eisenia* onto the earthworm *Lumbricus* is completely destroyed by 50 days.

the heterozygote. There is little evidence in these responses for allele-specific memory and it is seriously questionable whether this and related phenomena in the lower animal orders are true precedents of T-cell-mediated reactions in vertebrates.

## Invertebrates have microbial defense mechanisms

These rejections are mediated by coelomocytes which kill by direct contact. They are also powerfully phagocytic cells emphasizing the mainstream importance of this activity throughout the animal kingdom (cf. Milestone 1.1, Chapter 1). Thus starfish coelomocytes respond mitogenically to IL-1 and make it themselves. Also they are chemotactically attracted to bacteria.

In many phyla, phagocytosis is augmented by coating with agglutinins and bactericidins in the body fluids of nonimmunized hosts; these are capable of lectin-like binding to carbohydrate patterns on the microbial surface so providing the basis for recognition of 'nonself'. Ever sensitive to phylogenetically widespread mechanisms, we now find echoes of the mammalian acute phase reaction (cf. p. 16) in the insect world. It is notable that **infection very rapidly induces the synthesis of an impressive battery of antimicrobial peptides** in the fat body of higher insects following activation of transcription factors which bind to promoter sequence motifs homologous to regulatory elements involved in the mammalian acute phase response. Close to 100 insect polypeptides have so far been characterized and they fall into two classes: cyclic peptides containing disulfide bridges and linear peptides. Prominent in the former category are the 4 kDa anti-Gram-positive

defensins and the 5 kDa antifungal peptide, drosomycin. The linear peptides inducible by infection include the cecropins and a series of anti-Gram-negative glycine- or proline-rich polypeptides. Cecropins, which have also been identified in mammals, are 4 kDa strongly cationic amphipathic α-helices causing immediate and lethal disintegration of bacterial membranes, possibly by creating ion channels but more probably through acting as quaternary detergents.

One might also expect to find provocative elements of a primordial complement system among the lower orders. Indeed, a protease inhibitor, an $\alpha_2$-macroglobulin structurally homologous to C3 with internal thiolester, is present in the horseshoe crab. Conceivably this might represent an ancestral version of C3 which is activated by proteases released at a site of infection, deposited onto the microbe and recognized there as a ligand for the phagocytic cells. During evolution one could envisage the alternative complement pathway arising through a critical gene fusion which created a protease with a binding site for ancestral C3b; in other words, a prototype Factor B which would amplify the protease released at the infection site and hence further C3b deposition. The complement receptor CR3 is an integrin, and related integrins in insects may harbor common ancestors. Mention of the horseshoe crab may have stirred a neuronal network in readers with good memories, to recall its synthesis of limulin (cf. p. 17) which is homologous with the mammalian acute phase C-reactive protein (CRP); presumably it acts as a lectin to opsonize bacteria and is likely to be a product of the evolutionary line leading ultimately to C1q, mannose binding protein and lung surfactant.

The other major strategy effectively deployed by

invertebrates is to wall off an invading microorganism. This is achieved through proteolytic cascades (cf. complement and blood clotting amplifying cascades, p. 11), which produce a coagulum of 'gelled' hemolymph around the offender, or activate the phenoloxidase system leading to melanotic encapsulation of the invading microbe and associated generation of toxic quinone metabolites.

Please do not let us overlook plants. Higher plants develop an 'immune state' of **systemic acquired resistance** (SAR), which can be established following a localized infection with pathogens that induce lesions involving host cell death. SAR persists for several weeks and extends to a broad range of bacterial, viral and fungal pathogens beyond the initiating infective agent. A series of SAR genes encode a wide variety of microbicidal proteins which can be induced through endogenous chemical mediators such as salicylic acid (remember the acetyl ester is aspirin — probably an irrelevant observation) and methyl-2,6-dichloroisonicotinic acid. One function of salicylic acid is to bind to a protein with catalase activity, thereby increasing $H_2O_2$, but while this may contribute to an acute defensive response, other mechanisms are thought to be concerned in the induction of SAR.

## Adaptive immune responses appear with the vertebrates

### Lower vertebrates

Lymphocytes and genuine adaptive T- and B responses do not emerge in the phylogenetic tree until we reach the vertebrates, although neither can be elicited in the lowliest vertebrate studied — the California hagfish. This unpleasant cyclostome (which preys upon moribund fish by entering their mouths and eating the flesh from the inside) was originally considered 'the negative hero of the phylogeny of immunity' since it appeared incapable of reacting immunologically. It then transpired that the fish could make some response to hemocyanin provided they were maintained at temperatures approaching 20°C (in general, poikilotherms make antibodies better at higher temperatures). However this was a false dawn for the hagfish, since true immunoglobulins were not involved and its rather dubious 'heroic' status has been restored. Further up the evolutionary scale in the cartilaginous fishes, well-defined 18*S* and 7*S* immunoglobulins with heavy and light chains have now been defined but the responses are T-independent.

### T-cells appear

The toad, *Xenopus*, is a pliable, if unlovely, species for study since it is possible to make transgenics and cloned tadpoles fairly readily and it has a less complex lymphoid system than mammals, characterized by a small number of lymphocytes and a restricted antibody repertoire not subject to somatic mutation. Furthermore, positive and negative thymic selection have been demonstrated in frogs and I must say that if I belonged to an immunological laboratory which was strapped for funds, I would give serious consideration to the possibility of working with amphibian systems for certain problems.

The emergence of an honest-to-God thymus in the teleosts (bony fishes), amphibians, reptiles, birds and mammals was of course associated with MHC molecules, cell-mediated immunity, cytotoxic T-cells and allograft rejection. It could be argued that we also see phylogenetically more ancient, T-independent B-1 (CD5 positive) cells joined by a new T-dependent B-2 population.

However, T-dependent high-affinity, heterogeneous, rapid secondary antibody responses are only seen with warm-blooded vertebrates such as birds and mammals and these are linked directly with the evolution of the **germinal center** (table 12.4). I make no apologies for extolling the virtues of this rather fascinating structure in enhancing the quality of anamnestic antibody responses yet again. No doubt the reader, knowing that *Shigella dysenteriae* toxin selectively kills germinal center B-cells, will nod his or her head in appreciation of the finding that the toxin cannot induce isotype switch nor rapid secondary responses. It has been speculated that warm-blooded

**Table 12.4.** Relation of germinal centers to enhanced antibody formation in warm vs cold-blooded animals. (Based on Nahm M.H., Kroese, F.G.M. & Hoffmann J.W. (1992) The evolution of immunology and germinal centers. *Immunology Today* **13**, 438.)

| Vertebrate species | Somatically mutated Ab | Anamnestic (secondary) Ab response | Ab affinity LM⁻¹ (average) | Germinal center |
|---|---|---|---|---|
| Poikilothermic (cold-blooded) | | | | |
| Shark | − | slow | $10^5$ | − |
| Bony fish | − | slow | $10^6$ | − |
| Frog | − | slow | $10^6$ | − |
| Homoiothermic (warm-blooded) | | | | |
| Chicken | + | Rapid | $10^7$ | + |
| Mouse | + | Rapid | $10^8$ | + |
| Rabbit | + | Rapid | $10^9$ | + |
| Human | + | Rapid | $10^9$ | + |

**Table 12.5. Effect of neonatal bursectomy and thymectomy on the development of immunologic competence in the chicken.** (From Cooper M.D., Peterson R.D.A., South M.A. & Good R.A. (1966) *Journal of Experimental Medicine* **123**, 75, with permission of the editors.)

| All X-irradiated after birth | Peripheral blood lymphocyte count | Ig conc. | Antibody | Delayed skin reaction to tuberculin | Graft rejection |
|---|---|---|---|---|---|
| Intact | 14 800 | ++ | +++ | ++ | +++ |
| Thymectomized | 9 000 | ++ | + | – | + |
| Bursectomized | 13 200 | – | – | + | + |

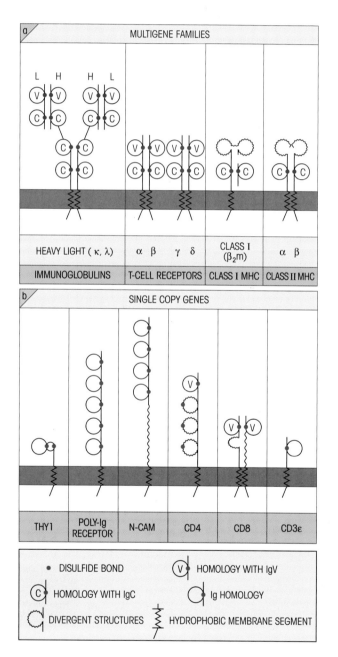

**Figure 12.19. The immunoglobulin gene superfamily,** a series of surface molecules involved in cell–cell recognition which all share a common structure, the immunoglobulin homology unit, suggesting evolution from a single primordial ancestral gene. (a) Multigene families involved in antigen recognition (the single copy $\beta_2$-microglobulin is included because of its association with class I). (b) Single copy genes. Thy 1 is present on T-cells and neurons. Poly-Ig transports IgA across mucosal membranes. N-CAM is an adhesion molecule binding neuronal cells together. Other molecules now included in this superfamily are $\alpha_1$B glycoprotein, a human plasma protein; neurocytoplasmic protein 3 (NP3), a brain-specific molecule; OX-2, of unknown function present on lymphocytes and neurons; and the CD3 $\delta$ chain. (Reprinted by permission from *Nature* **323**, 15. © 1986, Macmillan Magazines Limited with some updating.)

animals acquired this new lymphoid structure under selection pressure from the rapid growth of pathogens which had adapted to their high and constant temperature. A rapid response and a high affinity which ensures that effective antibody defenses can still be provided as the concentration falls to relatively low levels, would both be advantageous for survival.

*Generation of antibody diversity*

Mechanisms for the generation of antibody diversity receive quite different emphasis as one goes from one species to another. We are already familiar with the mammalian system where multiple *V* genes are greatly amplified by a variety of recombinational events involving multiple *D* and *J* segments. The horned shark also has many *V* genes but the opportunities for combinatorial joining are tightly constrained by close linkage between individual, *V, D, J* and *C* segments and this may be a factor in the restricted antibody response of this species. In sharp contrast, there seems to be only one operational *V* gene at the light chain locus in the chicken but this undergoes extensive somatic diversification, possibly utilizing nonfunctional adjoining *V* pseudogenes in a somatic gene-conversion-like process. Camel-lovers should note that not only do they get by on little water, they also survive on antibodies which lack light chains.

## THE EVOLUTION OF DISTINCT B- AND T-CELL LINEAGES WAS ACCOMPANIED BY THE DEVELOPMENT OF SEPARATE SITES FOR DIFFERENTIATION

The differential effects of neonatal thymectomy and bursectomy in the chicken on subsequent humoral and cellular responses paved the way for our eventual recognition of the separate lymphocyte lineages which subserve these functions. Like the thymus, the bursa of Fabricius develops as an embryonic outpushing of the gut endoderm, this time from hind- as distinct from fore-gut, and provides the microenvironment to cradle incoming stem cells and direct their differentiation to immunocompetent B-lymphocytes. As may be seen from table 12.5, neonatal bursectomy had a profound effect on humoral antibody synthesis, but did not unduly influence the cell-mediated reactions responsible for tuberculin skin reactivity and graft rejection. On the other hand, thymectomy grossly impaired cell-mediated reactions and inhibited antibody production to most protein antigens.

The distinctive anatomical location of the B-cell differentiation site in a separate lymphoid organ in the chicken was immensely valuable to progress in this field because it allowed such experiments to be carried out. However, many years went by in a fruitless search for an equivalent bursa in mammals before it was realized that the primary site for B-cell generation was in fact the bone marrow itself (a nameless immunologist regularly used to slay his students by recalling that 'the bursa is strictly for the birds').

## CELLULAR RECOGNITION MOLECULES EXPLOIT THE IMMUNOGLOBULIN GENE SUPERFAMILY

When nature fortuitously chances upon a protein structure ('motif' is the buzz word) which successfully mediates some useful function, the selective forces of evolution make sure that it is widely exploited. Thus, all the molecules involved in antigen recognition which we have described at such (painful!) length in Chapters 3 and 4 are members of a gene superfamily related by sequence and presumably a common ancestry. All polypeptide members of this family which includes heavy and light Ig chains, T-cell receptor $\alpha$ and $\beta$ chains, MHC class I and class II peptides and $\beta_2$-microglobulin, are composed of one or more immunoglobulin homology units. Each unit is roughly 110 amino acids in length and is characterized by certain conserved residues around the two cysteines found in every domain and the alternating hydrophobic and hydrophilic amino acids which give rise to the familiar anti-parallel $\beta$-pleated strands with interspersed short variable lengths having a marked propensity to form reversed turns — the 'immunoglobulin fold' in short (cf. p. 50).

Attention has been drawn to a very important feature of the Ig domain structure, namely the mutual complementarity which allows strong interdomain noncovalent interactions such as those between $V_H$ and $V_L$ and the two $C_H3$ regions which form the IgG pFc' fragment. Gene duplication and diversification can create mutual families of interacting molecules such as TCRs with MHC, and IgA with the poly-Ig receptor (figure 12.19). On this basis, it is not surprising that the domain homology units are turning up in other surface molecules concerned in cell–cell interactions, such as CD8 which associates with class I MHC, and CD4 which helps focus the helper cell onto target class II MHC. Likewise the intercellular adhesion molecules ICAM-1 and N-CAM (figure 12.19) are richly endowed with these domains and the long evolutionary history of N-CAM strongly suggests that these structures made an early appearance in phylogeny as mediators of intercellular recognition (mediating sponge cell rejection?). A recent trawl of the protein sequence database revealed hundreds of known members of the Ig superfamily. Some family!

The **integrins** form another structural superfamily which includes a number of hematopoietic cell-surface molecules concerned with adhesion to extracellular matrix proteins, their function is to direct these cells to particular tissue sites (see discussion p. 225).

# SUMMARY

## Multipotential stem cells from the bone marrow give rise to all the formed elements of the blood

- Expansion and differentiation is driven by soluble growth (colony-stimulating) factors and contact with reticular stromal cells.

## The differentiation of T-cells occurs within the microenvironment of the thymus

- Bone marrow stem cells become immunocompetent T-cells in the thymus.

## T-cell ontogeny

- Differentiation to immunocompetent T-cell subsets is accompanied by changes in the surface phenotype which can be recognized with monoclonal antibodies.
- TCR genes rearrange in the thymus cortex, TCR1 $\gamma\delta$ and a pre-TCR2 consisting of an invariant pre-T$\alpha$ associated with a conventional V$\beta$, before final rearrangement of the V$\alpha$ to generate the mature TCR2 $\alpha\beta$.
- Double-negative CD4$^-$8$^-$ pre-T-cells are driven and expanded by the pre-receptor to become double-positive CD4$^+$8$^+$.
- The thymus epithelial cells **positively select** CD4$^+$8$^+$ T-cells with avidity for their MHC haplotype so that single-positive CD4$^+$ or CD8$^+$ T-cells develop that are restricted to the recognition of antigen in the context of the epithelial cell haplotype.

## T-cell tolerance

- The induction of immunological tolerance is necessary to avoid self-reactivity.
- High avidity T-cells which react with self-antigens presented by cortico-medullary macrophages and interdigitating dendritic cells are eliminated by **negative selection**. The paradigm that low avidity binding to MHC/peptide produces positive selection and high avidity negative, is probably broadly true but may need some amendment.
- Self-tolerance can also be achieved by paralysis (anergy) and furthermore, newly arising immunocompetent cells within a cluster of anergic cells, are themselves rendered anergic.
- A state of what is effectively self-tolerance also arises when there is a failure to adequately present a self-antigen to lymphocytes, either because of compartmen-

talization, lack of class II on the antigen-presenting cell or low concentration of peptide/MHC (cryptic self).
- T-suppression is probably more concerned in reversing autoimmunity rather than preventing it.

## B-cells differentiate in the fetal liver and then in the bone marrow

- They become immunocompetent B-cells after passing through pre-B and immature B-cell stages.

## B-1 and B-2 represent two distinct subpopulations of B-cells

- B-1 cells represent a minor population expressing the phenotype: sIgM$^{hi}$, Mac-1$^+$, CD23$^-$. B-1a cells are CD5$^+$, B-1b, CD5$^-$. The majority of conventional B-cells, the B-2 population, are sIgM$^{lo}$, Mac-1$^-$, CD23$^+$. The B-1 population predominates in early life, shows a high level of idiotype–anti-idiotype connectivity, produces low affinity, IgM polyreactive antibodies, many of them auto-antibodies, and is responsible for the T-independent 'natural' IgM antibacterial antibodies which appear spontaneously.

## Development of B-cell specificity

- The sequence of Ig variable gene rearrangements is *DJ* and then *VDJ*.
- *VDJ* transcription produces $\mu$ chains which associate with $V_{preB} \cdot \lambda_5$ chains to form a surrogate surface IgM-like receptor.
- This receptor signals allelic exclusion of unrearranged heavy chains and initiates rearrangement of $V$-$J_k$ (in the mouse) and, if unproductive, $V$-$J_\lambda$.
- If the rearrangement at any stage is unproductive, i.e. does not lead to an acceptable gene reading frame, the allele on the sister chromosome is rearranged.
- The mechanisms of allelic exclusion ensure that each lymphocyte is programmed for only one antibody. Responses to different antigens appear sequentially with age.

## The induction of tolerance in B-lymphocytes

- B-cell tolerance is induced by clonal deletion, clonal anergy, receptor editing and 'helplessness' due to preferential tolerization of T-cells needed to cooperate in B-cell stimulation.

*(Continued)*

## The overall response in the neonate

• Maternal IgG crosses the placenta and provides a high level of passive immunity at birth.

The antigen-independent differentiation within primary lymphoid organs and antigen-driven maturation in secondary lymphoid organs are summarized in figure 12.20.

## The evolution of the immune response

• Recognition of self is of fundamental importance for multicellular organisms, even lowly forms like sponges and earthworms.

• Invertebrates have defence mechanisms based on phagocytosis, killing by a multiplicity of microbicidal peptides and polyphenoloxidase metabolites, and

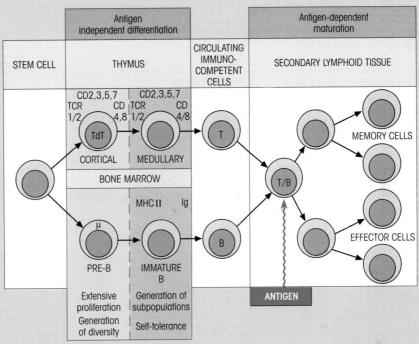

**Figure 12.20. Antigen-independent differentiation and antigen-dependent maturation of T- and B-cells.** Cortical thymocytes are also positively selected to recognize self-MHC haplotype. TCR1 = γδ T-cell receptor; TCR2 = αβ T-cell receptor; TdT = terminal deoxynucleotidyl transferase.

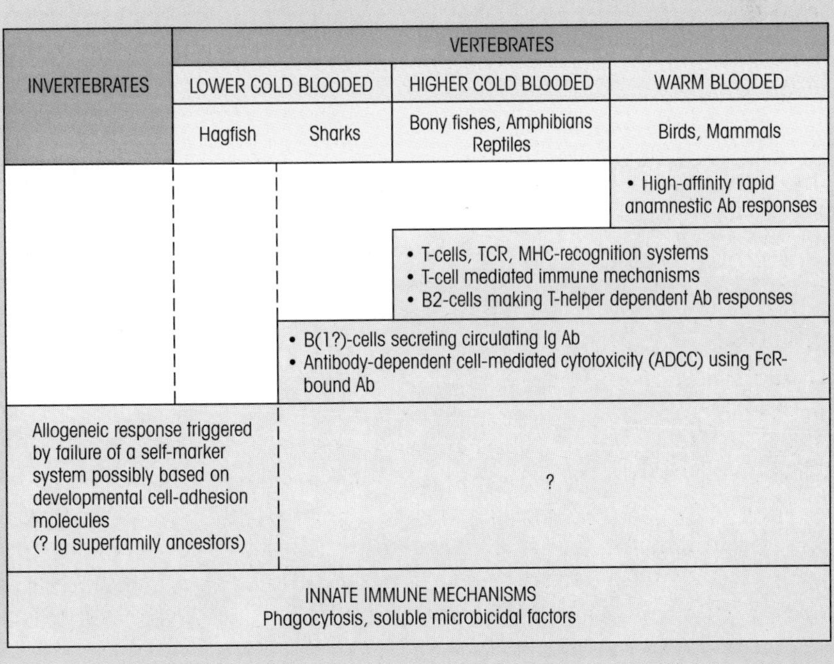

**Figure 12.21. The phylogeny of immune responses.** (Based partly on an article by Smith L.C. & Davidson E.H. (1992) *Immunology Today* **13**, 356, in which they argue that the allogeneic response in the lower orders is not a direct evolutionary antecedent of the mammalian homograft reaction.)

| INVERTEBRATES | VERTEBRATES | | | |
|---|---|---|---|---|
| | LOWER COLD BLOODED | | HIGHER COLD BLOODED | WARM BLOODED |
| | Hagfish | Sharks | Bony fishes, Amphibians Reptiles | Birds, Mammals |
| | | | | • High-affinity rapid anamnestic Ab responses |
| | | | • T-cells, TCR, MHC-recognition systems<br>• T-cell mediated immune mechanisms<br>• B2-cells making T-helper dependent Ab responses | |
| | | • B(1?)-cells secreting circulating Ig Ab<br>• Antibody-dependent cell-mediated cytotoxicity (ADCC) using FcR-bound Ab | | |
| Allogeneic response triggered by failure of a self-marker system possibly based on developmental cell-adhesion molecules (? Ig superfamily ancestors) | | | ? | |
| INNATE IMMUNE MECHANISMS Phagocytosis, soluble microbicidal factors | | | | |

(Continued on p. 250)

imprisonment of the invader by coagulation of the hemolymph or synthesis of a melanin.

• Higher plants can establish a persisting state of systemic acquired resistance.

• B- and T-cell responses are well defined in the vertebrates and the evolution of these distinct lineages was accompanied by the development of separate sites for differentiation.

• The success of the immunoglobulin domain structure, possibly through its ability to give noncovalent mutual binding, has been exploited by evolution to produce the very large Ig gene superfamily of recognition molecules including Ig, TCRs, MHC class I and II, $\beta_2$-microglobulin, CD4, CD8, the poly-Ig receptor and Thy 1. Another superfamily, the integrins, which include LFA-1 and the VLA molecules, are concerned with leukocyte binding to endothelial cells and extracellular matrix proteins.

A synthesis of the major emerging features of the immune response at different stages in phylogeny is outlined in figure 12.21.

## FURTHER READING

Arnold B., Schönrich G. & Hammerling G.J. (1993) Multiple levels of peripheral (T-cell) tolerance. *Immunology Today* **14**, 12.

Chothia C. (1992) One thousand families for the molecular biologist. *Nature* **357**, 543.

Hartley S.B., Crosbie J., Brink R., Kantor A.A., Basten A. & Goodnow C.C. (1991) Elimination from peripheral lymphoid tissues of self-reactive B-lymphocytes recognizing membrane-bound antigens. *Nature* **353**, 765.

Horton J. & Ratcliffe N. (1996) Evolution of immunity. In Roitt I.M., Brostoff J. & Male D.K. (eds) *Immunology*, 4th edn, p.15.1. Mosby, London.

Kruisbeek A.M. & Storb U. (eds) (1996) Lymphocyte development. *Current Opinion in Immunology* **8**, 257.

Liu Y-J. & Banchereau J. (1996) The paths and molecular controls of peripheral B-cell development. *The Immunologist* **4**(2), 55.

Miller J.F.A.P. (1994) The thymus: maestro of the immune system. *Bioessays* **16**, 509. (An intriguing historical account of the unravelling of the role of the thymus.)

Stall A.M. & Wells S.M. (eds) (1996) B-1 cells: origins and functions. *Seminars in Immunology* **8**, No. 1.

Turner R.J. (ed.) (1994) *Immunology: A Comparative Approach*. John Wiley & Sons Ltd, Chichester.

# P A R T 5

# IMMUNITY TO INFECTION

Immunology at this stage in evolution has been fashioned by the fight for survival against an incredible variety of infectious agents deploying a powerful range of aggressive strategies. Our existence testifies to the successful nature of the defenses that have been established. Chapter 13 takes us right into that never-ending battle. We take a deeper look at the vital defense mechanism of **inflammation** than was possible in the first two introductory chapters and then we describe the attack and counter-attack characterizing infections by **extra-** and **intra-cellular bacteria**, **viruses** and **parasites**, the latter having to achieve a balance of 'live and let live' with the host if they are to survive without eradicating the species which are to maintain them.

By and large, vaccination represents one of the really important public health measures and in Chapter 14 we discuss the advances that have been made using newer technologies, the influence of current immunological knowledge on the design of our strategies and the daunting problems that still beset us particularly with respect to parasitic infections.

# ADVERSARIAL STRATEGIES DURING INFECTION

We are engaged in constant warfare with the microbes which surround us and the processes of mutation and evolution have tried to select microorganisms which have evolved means of evading our defense mechanisms. In this chapter, we look at the varied, often ingenious, adversarial strategies which we and our enemies have developed over very long periods of time.

## INFLAMMATION REVISITED

The acute inflammatory process involves a protective influx of white cells, complement, antibody and other plasma proteins into a site of infection or injury and was discussed in broad outline in the introductory chapters. Now that we are ready to look in more detail at the aggressive gambits and wily counter-attacks which characterize the conflict between microbe and host, it is appropriate to re-examine the mechanisms of inflammation in greater depth. The reader may find it helpful to have another look at the relevant sections in Chapters 1 and 2, particularly those relating to figures 1.15/16/17 and 2.18.

## Mediators of inflammation

A complex variety of mediators is involved in acute inflammatory responses (figure 13.1). Some act directly on the smooth muscle wall surrounding the arterioles to alter blood flow. Others act on the venules to cause contraction of the endothelial cells with transient opening of the interendothelial junctions and consequent transudation of plasma. The migration of leukocytes from the bloodstream is facilitated by mediators which upregulate the expression of adherence molecules on both endothelial and white cells and others which lead the leukocytes to the inflamed site through chemotaxis.

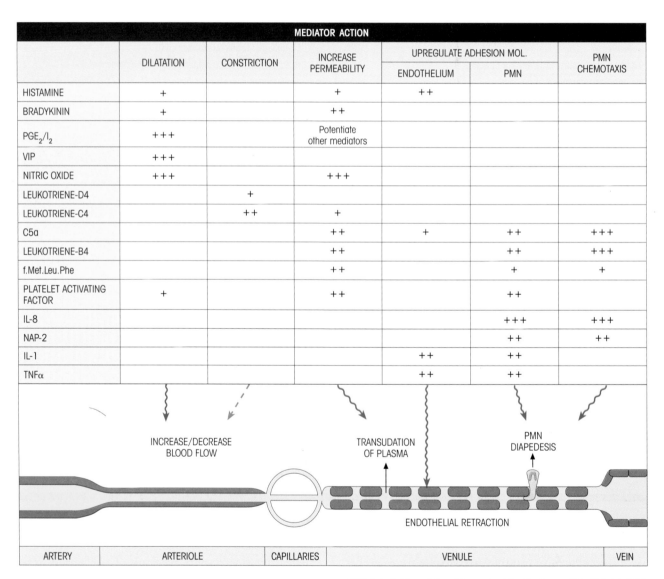

| | DILATATION | CONSTRICTION | INCREASE PERMEABILITY | UPREGULATE ADHESION MOL. | | PMN CHEMOTAXIS |
|---|---|---|---|---|---|---|
| **MEDIATOR ACTION** | | | | ENDOTHELIUM | PMN | |
| HISTAMINE | + | | + | + + | | |
| BRADYKININ | + | | + + | | | |
| PGE$_2$/I$_2$ | + + + | | Potentiate other mediators | | | |
| VIP | + + + | | | | | |
| NITRIC OXIDE | + + + | | + + + | | | |
| LEUKOTRIENE-D4 | | + | | | | |
| LEUKOTRIENE-C4 | | + + | + | | | |
| C5a | | | + + | + | + + | + + + |
| LEUKOTRIENE-B4 | | | + + | | + + | + + + |
| f.Met.Leu.Phe | | | + + | | + | + |
| PLATELET ACTIVATING FACTOR | + | | + + | | + + | |
| IL-8 | | | | | + + + | + + + |
| NAP-2 | | | | | + + | + + |
| IL-1 | | | | + + | + + | |
| TNFα | | | | + + | + + | |

INCREASE/DECREASE BLOOD FLOW          TRANSUDATION OF PLASMA          PMN DIAPEDESIS

ENDOTHELIAL RETRACTION

| ARTERY | ARTERIOLE | CAPILLARIES | VENULE | VEIN |

**Figure 13.1. The principal mediators of acute inflammation.** The readers should refer back to figure 1.15 to recall the range of products generated by the mast cell. The later-acting cytokines such as interleukin-1 (IL-1) are largely macrophage-derived and these cells also secrete prostaglandin E$_2$ (PGE$_2$), leukotriene-B4 and the neutrophil activating peptide (NAP-2.). PMN, polymorphonuclear neutrophil; VIP, vasoactive intestinal peptide; TNFα, α-tumor necrosis factor.

## Leukocytes bind to endothelial cells through paired adhesion molecules

Redirecting the leukocytes charging along the blood into the site of inflammation is somewhat like having to encourage bulls stampeding down the Pamplona main street to move quietly into the side roads. We have had occasion to confront this problem when discussing lymphocyte homing (cf. p. 155, figure 8.6) and, in the present context, the adherence of leukocytes to the endothelial vessel wall through the interaction of complementary binding of cell surface molecules is an absolutely crucial step. Several classes of molecule subserve this function (cf. p. 157, figure 8.7), some acting as lectins to bind a carbohydrate ligand on the complementary partner.

## Initiation of the acute inflammatory response

A very early event is the upregulation of P-selectin and platelet activating factor (PAF) on the endothelial cells lining the venules by histamine or thrombin released by the original inflammatory stimulus. Recruitment of the adhesion molecules from intracellular storage vesicles ensures that they appear very promptly on the cell surface. Engagement of the lectin-like domain on the tip of the long P-selectin molecule with sialyl Lewis$^x$ carbohydrate ligands on the polymorphonuclear neutrophil (PMN) surface mucins (possibly leukosialin) causes the neutrophil to **roll** along the endothelial wall and helps PAF to dock onto its corresponding receptor. This, in turn, increases surface expression of the integrins lymphocyte function-associated molecule-1 (LFA-1) and membrane attack complex-1 (MAC-1) which now bind the neutrophil very firmly to the endothelial surface (figure 13.2).

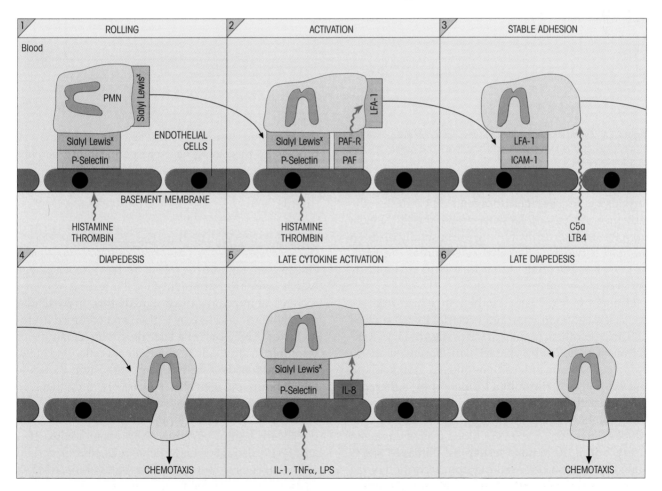

**Figure 13.2. Early events in inflammation affecting neutrophil margination and diapedesis.** Recognition of extracellular gradients of the chemotactic mediators by receptors on the polymorphonuclear neutrophil (PMN) surface triggers intracellular signals which generate motion. The neutrophils crawl rather than swim and migration along the extracellular matrix vitronectin is dependent upon very rapid cycles of integrin-dependent adhesion and detachment regulated by calcineurin. (Compare events involved in homing and transmigration of lymphocytes, figure 8.6.)

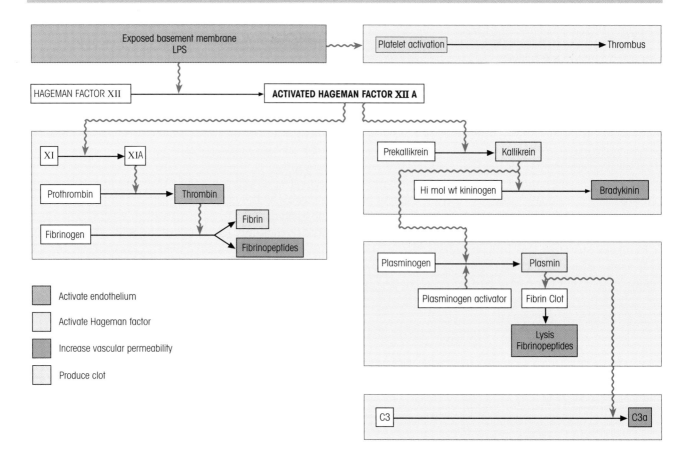

**Figure 13.3. Events initiated by damaged vascular endothelium.** Note that thrombin can also release platelet activating factor (PAF) which induces thrombus formation.

Activation of the neutrophils also makes them more responsive to chemotactic agents and, under the influence of C5a and leukotriene-B4, the PMN exits from the circulation by moving purposefully through the gap between endothelial cells, across the basement membrane (**diapedesis**) and up the chemotactic gradient to the inflammation site.

Damage to vascular endothelium which exposes the basement membrane and bacterial toxins such as LPS, trigger other complex systems (figure 13.3). Activation of platelets by contact with basement membrane collagen or induced endothelial PAF leads to aggregation and **thrombus** formation by adherence through platelet glycoprotein Ib to von Willebrand factor on the vascular surface. Such platelet plugs are adept at stemming the loss of blood from a damaged artery, but in the venous system the damaged site is sealed by a **fibrin clot** resulting from activation of the intrinsic clotting system via contact of Hageman factor (factor XII) with the exposed surface of the basement membrane. Activated Hageman factor also triggers the kinin and plasmin systems and several of

the resulting products influence the inflammatory process by increasing vascular permeability, activating endothelium, autocatalytically amplifying production of Hageman factor XII and cleaving C3 (figure 13.3).

## The ongoing inflammatory process

One must not ignore the role of the tissue macrophage which, under the stimulus of local infection or injury, secretes an imposing array of mediators. In particular the cytokines interleukin-1 (IL-1) and α-tumor necrosis factor (TNFα) act at a later time than histamine or thrombin to stimulate the endothelial cells. One of the late products is E-selectin, an adhesion molecule which binds and activates neutrophils, and others are the **chemokines** (*chemo*tactic cyto*kines*) IL-8 and epithelial derived neutrophil attractant-78 (ENA-78) which are highly effective PMN chemotaxins. IL-1 and TNFα also act on endothelial cells, fibroblasts and epithelial cells to secrete another chemokine, MCP-1, a potent monocyte chemotactic protein which attracts mononuclear phagocytes to the inflammatory site to strengthen and maintain the defensive reaction to infection.

**Table 13.1. Chemokines: leukocyte chemoattractant specificities.**

| Chemokine | Type | Chemoattractant specificity | | | | | |
|---|---|---|---|---|---|---|---|
| | | Neutrophils | Basophils | Eosinophils | NK cells | Monocytes | Lymphocytes |
| IL-8 | CXC | +++ | | | | | +++ |
| ENA-78 | CXC | +++ | | | | | |
| NAP-2 | CXC | ++ | | | | | |
| IP-10 | CXC | | | | | | +++ |
| Eotaxin | CC | | | +++ | | | |
| RANTES | CC | | +++ | ++ | + | +++ | |
| MCP-1 | CC | | ++ | | +++ | ++ | + |
| MCP-2 | CC | | | | | + | |
| MCP-3 | CC | | ++ | ++ | | ++ | |
| MIP-1α | CC | | | ++ | +++ | +++ | |
| MIP-1β | CC | | | | +++ | +++ | |
| Lymphotactin | C | | | | | | +++ |

CXC = chemokine with any amino acid X intervening between the first + second conserved cysteines of the four which characterize the chemokine structural motif; CC = no intervening residue; C = lacks first and third cysteines of the motif; except for IP-10, the CXC motif is preceded by the amino acids E-L-R; ENA-78 = epithelial derived neutrophil attractant-78; NAP-2 = neutrophil activating protein-2; IP-10 = interferon-inducible protein-10; RANTES = regulated upon activation normal T-cell expressed and secreted; MCP = monocyte chemotactic proteins; MIP = macrophage inflammatory protein. (Data summarized from Schall T.J. & Bacon K.B. (1994) *Current Opinion in Immunology* **6**, 865.)

Perhaps this is a good time to note the ongoing active interest in the chemokines which are a large family of secreted 8–10 kDa proteins that selectively attract multiple types of leukocytes to inflammatory foci (table 13.1). This pleiotropy results from the expression of multiple chemokine receptors on a given leukocyte and the ability of a given receptor to bind multiple ligands. In general, chemokines of the C-X-C subfamily such as IL-8 (table 13.1; cf. figure 10.8) are specific for neutrophils and, to varying extents, lymphocytes, whereas chemokines with the C-C motif are chemotactic for monocytes and variably for natural killer (NK) cells, basophils and eosinophils. Eotaxin is highly specific for eosinophils and the presence of significant concentrations of this mediator together with RANTES (regulated upon activation normal T-cell expressed and secreted) in mucosal surfaces could account for the enhanced population of eosinophils in those tissues. The different chemokines bind to particular heparin and heparan sulfate glycosaminoglycans so that, after secretion, the chemotactic gradient can be maintained by attachment to the extracellular matrix as a form of scaffolding.

Clearly this whole operation serves to focus the immune defenses around the invading microorganisms. These become coated with antibody, C3b and certain acute phase proteins and are ripe for phagocytosis by the granulocytes and macrophages; under the influence of the inflammatory mediators these have upregulated C3 and Ig receptors, enhanced phagocytic responses and hyped-up killing powers, adding up to bad news for the bugs.

Of course it is beneficial to recruit lymphocytes to sites of infection and we should remember that endothelial cells in these areas express VCAM-1 (cf. p. 155) which acts as a homing receptor for VLA-4 positive activated memory T-cells, while the chemokines, IL-8 and lymphotactin are chemotactic for lymphocytes.

## Regulation and resolution of inflammation

With its customary prudence, evolution has established regulatory mechanisms to prevent inflammation from getting out of hand. At the humoral level we have a series of complement regulatory proteins: C1 inhibitor, C4 binding protein, the C3 control proteins factors H and I, complement receptor CR1, decay accelerating factor (DAF), membrane cofactor protein (MCP) and immunoconglutinin, and finally the proteins which block the membrane attack complex, homologous restriction factor and CD59 (discussed further on p. 313). Some of the acute-phase proteins derived from the plasma transudate would be expected to act as protease inhibitors.

At the cellular level, PGE$_2$, transforming growth factor-β (TGFβ) and glucocorticoids are powerful regulators. PGE$_2$ is a potent inhibitor of lymphocyte proliferation and cytokine production by T-cells and macrophages. TGFβ deactivates macrophages by inhibiting the production of reactive oxygen intermediates and downregulating MHC class II expression; it also quells the cytotoxic enthusiasm of both macrophages and γ-interferon (IFNγ)-activated NK cells. Endogenous glucocorticoids produced via the hypothalamic–pituitary–adrenal axis probably exert their anti-inflammatory effects through control of lipocortin-1 which binds to the surface proteins on monocytes and neutrophils. IL-10 inhibits antigen presentation, cytokine production and nitric oxide (NO) killing by macrophages, the latter being greatly enhanced by synergistic action with IL-4 and TGFβ. Another control protein is the IL-1β receptor antagonist whose synthesis is promoted in macrophages activated by lipopolysaccharide (LPS) or IgG.

Once the inflammatory agent has been cleared, these regulatory processes will normalize the site. When the inflammation traumatizes tissues through its intensity and extent, TGFβ plays a major role in the subsequent wound healing by stimulating fibroblast division and the laying down of new extracellular matrix elements.

### Chronic inflammation

If an inflammatory agent persists, either because of its resistance to metabolic breakdown or through the inability of a deficient immune system to clear an infectious microbe, the character of the cellular response changes. The site becomes dominated by macrophages with varying morphology: many have an activated appearance, some form arrays of what are termed 'epithelioid' cells and others fuse to form giant cells. If an adaptive immune response is involved, lymphocytes in various guises will also be present. This characteristic **granuloma** walls off the persisting agent from the remainder of the body (see section on Type IV hypersensitivity in Chapter 16, p. 347 and examples in figure 16.8).

## EXTRACELLULAR BACTERIA SUSCEPTIBLE TO KILLING BY PHAGOCYTOSIS AND COMPLEMENT

### Bacterial survival strategies

The variety and ingenuity of these escape mechanisms are most intriguing and, as with virtually all infectious agents, if you can think of a possible avoidance strategy, some microbe will already have used it.

*Evading phagocytosis*

The cell walls of bacteria are multifarious (figure 13.4) and in some cases are inherently resistant to a number of microbicidal agents, but a common mechanism by which virulent forms escape phagocytosis is by synthesis of an outer **capsule**, which does not adhere readily to phagocytic cells and covers carbohydrate

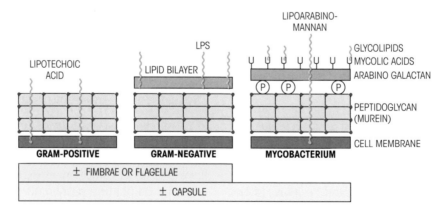

**Figure 13.4. The structure of bacterial cell walls.** All types have an inner cell membrane and a peptidoglycan wall which can be cleaved by lysozyme and lysozomal enzymes. The outer lipid bilayer of Gram-negative bacteria which is susceptible to the action of complement or cationic proteins, sometimes contains lipopolysaccharide (LPS; also known as endotoxin; composed of O-specific oligosaccharide side-chains attached to a basal core polysaccharide, itself linked to the mitogenic moiety, lipid A; 148 O antigen variants of *Escherichia coli* are known). The mycobacterial cell wall is highly resistant to breakdown. When present, outer capsules may protect the bacteria from phagocytosis.

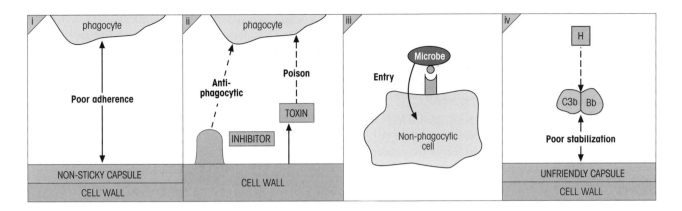

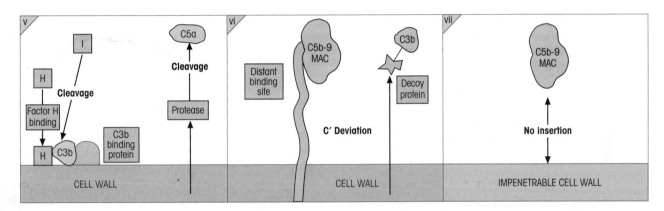

**Figure 13.5. Avoidance strategies by extracellular bacteria.** (i) Capsule gives poor phagocyte adherence. (ii) Exotoxin poisons phagocyte. (iii) Microbe attaches to surface component to enter nonphagocytic cell. (iv) Capsule provides nonstabilizing surface for alternative pathway convertase. (v) Accelerating breakdown complement by action of microbial products. (vi) Complement effectors are deviated from the microbial cell wall. (vii) Cell wall impervious to complement membrane attack complex (MAC).

molecules on the bacterial surface which could otherwise be recognized by phagocyte receptors (figure 13.5i). For example, as few as ten encapsulated pneumococci can kill a mouse, but if the capsule is removed by treatment with hyaluronidase, 10 000 bacteria are required for the job. Many pathogens evolve capsules which physically prevent access of phagocytes to C3b deposited on the bacterial cell wall.

Other organisms have actively **antiphagocytic** cell surface molecules and some go so far as to secrete **exotoxins**, which actually poison the leukocytes (figure 13.5ii). Yet another devious ruse is to exploit binding to the surface of a nonphagocytic cell so gaining entry into a shelter from the depradations of the professional phagocyte (figure 13.5iii). Presumably some

organisms try to avoid undue provocation of phagocytic cells by adhering to and *colonizing the external mucosal surfaces* of the intestine.

### Challenging the complement system

*Poor activation of complement.* Normal mammalian cells are protected from complement destruction by regulatory proteins such as complement receptor CR1, MCP and DAF, which cause C3 convertase breakdown (see p. 313 for further discussion). Microorganisms lack these regulatory proteins so that even in the absence of antibody, most of them would activate the alternative C pathway by stabilization of the C$\overline{\mathrm{3bBb}}$ convertase on their surfaces. However, bacterial capsules in general tend to be poor activators of the alternative complement pathway and selective pressures have obviously favored the synthesis of capsules whose surface components do not favor stable binding of the convertase complex (figure 13.5iv).

*Acceleration of complement breakdown.* Certain bacterial surface molecules, notably those rich in sialic acid, are grossly unsporting in their ability to bind factor H (figure 13.5v), which acts as a focus for the degradation of C3b by factor I (cf. p. 11). Several bacteria have developed molecules which can themselves act as cofactors for factor I cleavage: thus some have short consensus repeat motifs that resemble C4 binding protein, complement receptor CR1 and DAF and another has the impudence to display an integrin-like motif resembling CR3. Other bacteria may secrete enzymes which degrade peptides such as C5a, which play an essential role in the acute inflammatory response (figure 13.5v).

*Complement deviation.* Some species manage to avoid lysis by deviating the complement activation site either to a secreted decoy protein or to a position on the bacterial surface distant from the cell membrane (figure 13.5vi).

*Resistance to insertion of terminal complement components.* Gram-positive organisms (cf. figure 13.1) have evolved thick peptidoglycan layers which prevent the insertion of the lytic C5b–9 membrane attack complex into the bacterial cell membrane (figure 13.5vii). Many capsules do the same.

### Antigenic variation

Although the strategy of varying their antigens in the face of a determined host antibody response is more usually associated with viruses and parasites, there are a few well-defined examples in bacteria.

## The host counter-attack

The defense mechanisms exploit the specificity and variability of the antibody molecule. Antibodies can defeat these devious attempts to avoid engulfment by neutralizing the antiphagocytic molecules and by binding to the surface of the organisms to focus the site for fixation of complement, so 'opsonizing' them for ingestion by polymorphs and macrophages or preparing them for the terminal membrane attack complex (Milestone 13.1).

## Milestone 13.1—The Protective Effects of Antibody

The pioneering research which led to the recognition of the antibacterial protection afforded by antibody clustered in the last years of the 19th century. A good place to start the story is the discovery by Roux and Yersin in 1888 at the still famous Pasteur Institute in Paris, that the exotoxin of diphtheria bacillus could be isolated from a bacterium-free filtrate of the medium used to culture the organism. von Behring and Kitasato at Koch's Institute in Berlin in 1890 then went on to show that animals could develop an immunity to such toxins which was due to the development of specific neutralizing antidotes referred to generally as **antibodies**. They further succeeded in passively transferring immunity to another animal with serum containing the antitoxin. The dawning of an era of serotherapy came in 1894 with Roux's successful treatment of patients with diphtheria by injection of immune horse serum.

The immunological community then got its intellectual underwear in something of a twist over the next few years, first by advocates of the view that all bacterial immunity was due to antitoxins, and second by Metchnikoff's rigid espousal of phagocytosis itself as the main, if not the only, real bulwark of defense against infection. The situation was resolved by our shining knight Sir

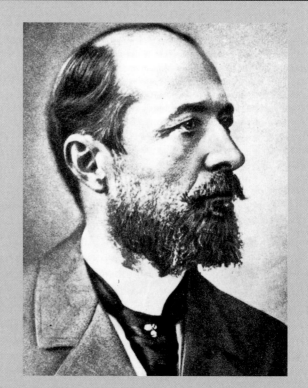

**Figure M13.1.1.** Emil von Behring (1854–1917). (Slide kindly supplied by The Wellcome Centre Medical Photographic Library, London.)

*(Continued)*

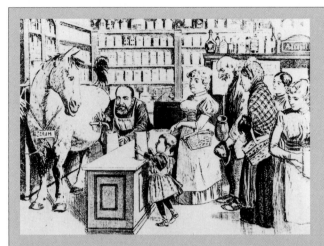

**Figure M13.1.2.** von Behring extracting serum using a tap. Caricature by Lustigen Blättern, 1894. (Legend: 'Serum direct from the horse! Freshly drawn.') (Slide kindly supplied by The Wellcome Centre Medical Photographic Library, London.)

Almroth Wright in London in 1903 who proposed that the main action of the increased antibody produced after infection was to reinforce killing by the phagocytes. He called the antibodies **opsonins** (Gk. *opson*, a dressing or relish) because they prepared the bacteria as food for the phagocytic cells, and amply verified his predictions by showing that antibodies dramatically increased the phagocytosis of bacteria *in vitro* thereby cleverly linking *innate* to *adaptive* immunity.

It was a feature of the time that major controversies were slugged out in pamphlets, books and plays and it was impressive that Bernard Shaw should enter the fray on the side of Almroth Wright in his play *The Doctor's Dilemma*. In the preface he gave an evocative description of the function of opsonins: 'Sir Almroth Wright, following up one of Metchnikoff's most suggestive biological

romances, discovered that the white corpuscles or phagocytes which attack and devour disease germs for us do their work only when we butter the disease germs appetizingly for them with a natural sauce which Sir Almroth named opsonins....' (More extended and very readable accounts of immunology at the turn of the 19th century may be found in Humphrey J.H. & White R.G. (1970) *Immunology for Students of Medicine*, 3rd edn, Ch. 1. Blackwell Scientific Publications, Oxford, and Craps L. (1993) *The Birth of Immunology*. Sandoz, Basel.)

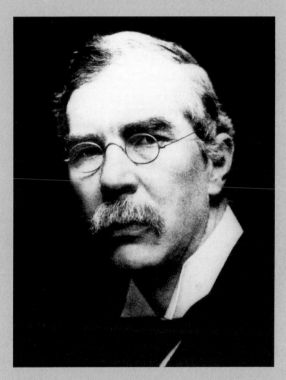

**Figure M13.1.3.** Sir Almroth Wright. (Slide kindly supplied by The Wellcome Centre Medical Photographic Library, London.)

## Toxin neutralization

Circulating antibodies act to neutralize the soluble antiphagocytic molecules and other exotoxins (e.g. phospholipase C of *Clostridium welchii*) released by bacteria. Combination near the biologically active site of the toxin would stereochemically block reaction with the substrate, particularly if it were macromolecular; combination distant from the active site may also cause inhibition through allosteric conformational changes. In its complex with antibody, the toxin may be unable to diffuse away rapidly and will be susceptible to phagocytosis, especially if the complex can be increased in size by the action of naturally

occurring autoantibodies to complexed IgG (antiglobulin factors) and C3b (immunoconglutinin, not to be confused with bovine *conglutinin*, a nonantibody molecule which combines with the carbohydrate portion of C3b).

## Opsonization of bacteria

*Independently of antibody.* Differences between the carbohydrate structures on bacteria and self are exploited by the **collectins**, a series of molecules with similar ultrastructure to C1q and which bear C-terminal lectin domains. These include mannose binding protein, lung surfactant proteins SP-A and

SP-D and conglutinin, which all recognize carbohydrate ligands. Mannose binding protein can bind to terminal mannose on the bacterial surface and then interacts with a serine proteinase MASP which is homologous in structure to C1r and C1s. Thus the interaction is closely similar to that of C1q with C1r and s (cf. p. 23) and in this way leads to the antibody-independent activation of the classical pathway. SP-A, SP-D and conglutinin can all act as opsonins (see Milestone 13.1) and mediate phagocytosis by virtue of their binding to the C1q receptor.

The all-important lipopolysaccharide endotoxin of Gram-negative bacteria, LPS, is recognized by three classes of receptor molecules (figure 13.6). Whole bacteria bind to and are taken into macrophages by CD18 without causing cell activation. Extracellular dispersions of LPS are recognized by a so-called 'scavenger' receptor, abundant in liver. This receptor binds to a wide range of anionic ligands, which it transports without much ado to the lysosomal compartment. Serum contains an acute phase LPS-binding protein which binds with high affinity to the chemically conserved region of LPS, lipid A. The resulting complexes attach to macrophage CD14 at very low levels, thereby inducing phagocytosis of the bacteria and TNF secretion.

*Augmented by antibody.* Encapsulated bacteria which resist phagocytosis become extremely attractive to polymorphs and macrophages when coated with

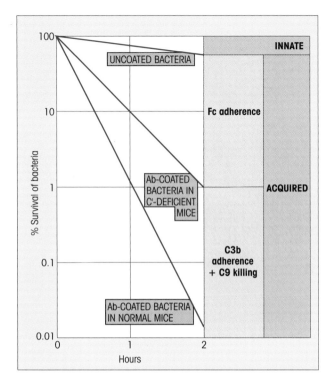

**Figure 13.7. Effect of opsonizing antibody and complement on rate of clearance of virulent bacteria from the blood.** The uncoated bacteria are phagocytosed rather slowly (*innate immunity*) but, on coating with antibody, adherence to phagocytes is increased many-fold (*acquired immunity*). The adherence is less effective in animals temporarily depleted of complement. This is a hypothetical but realistic situation; the natural proliferation of the bacteria has been ignored.

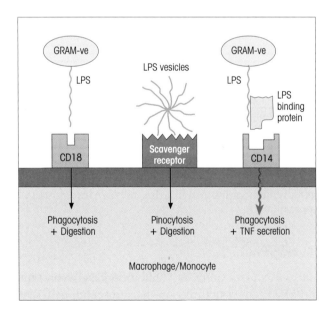

**Figure 13.6. Macrophage receptors for lipopolysaccharide (LPS) endotoxin.** The LPS-binding protein has considerable homology with the bactericidal/permeability increasing protein (BPI; figure 1.3). BPI also binds to lipid A and is directly bactericidal.

antibody and their rate of clearance from the bloodstream is strikingly enhanced (figure 13.7). The less effective removal of coated bacteria in complement-depleted animals emphasizes the synergism between antibody and complement for opsonization which is mediated through specific high affinity receptors for IgG and C3b on the phagocyte surface (figure 13.8). It is clearly advantageous that the subclasses which bind strongly to these Fc receptors (e.g. IgG$_1$ and IgG$_3$ in the human) also fix complement well, it being appreciated that the heterodimer of C3b bound to IgG Fd is a very efficient opsonin because it engages two receptors simultaneously. Complexes containing C3b may show immune adherence to the CR1 complement receptors on primate red cells and rabbit platelets to provide aggregates which are transported to the liver for phagocytosis.

Some elaboration on **complement receptors** may be pertinent at this stage. The CR1 receptors for C3b are also present on neutrophils, macrophages, B-cells and follicular dendritic cells in lymph nodes. Together with the CR3 receptor, they have the main responsibility for clearance of complexes containing

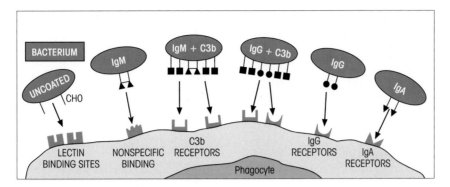

**Figure 13.8. Immunoglobulin and complement coats greatly increase the adherence of bacteria (and other antigens) to macrophages and polymorphs.** Uncoated bacteria adhere to lectin-like sites, including the mannose-binding receptor. There are no specific binding sites for IgM ( ▲ ▲ ) but there are high-affinity receptors for IgG (Fc) ( ● ) and iC3b ( ■ ; CR1 and CR3 types) on the macrophage surface which considerably enhance the strength of binding. The augmenting effect of complement is due to the fact that two adjacent IgG molecules can fix many C3b molecules, thereby increasing the number of links to the macrophage (cf. 'bonus' effect of multivalency; p. 88). Although IgM does not bind specifically to the macrophage, it promotes adherence through complement fixation. Specific receptors for the Fcα domains of IgA have also been defined.

C3. The *CR1* gene is linked in a cluster with C4b-binding protein and factor H, all of which subserve a regulatory function by binding to C3b or C4b to disassemble the C3/C5 convertases and act as cofactors for the proteolytic inactivation of C3b and C4b by factor I.

CR2 receptors for C3d, C3dg and iC3b are present on B-cells and follicular dendritic cells and transduce accessory signals for B-cell activation especially in the germinal centers (cf. p. 190). Their affinity for the Epstein–Barr virus (EBV) provides the means for entry of the virus into the B-cell.

CR3 receptors on polymorphs, macrophages and NK cells all bind the inactivated form C3bi. They are related to LFA-1 and CR4 (whose function is uncertain) in being members of the β₂ integrin subfamily (cf. table 8.1).

### Some further effects of complement

Some strains of Gram-negative bacteria which have a lipoprotein outer wall resembling mammalian surface membranes in structure are susceptible to the bactericidal action of fresh serum containing antibody. The antibody initiates the development of a complement-mediated lesion which is said to allow access of serum lysozyme to the inner peptidoglycan wall of the bacterium to cause eventual cell death. Activation of complement through union of antibody and bacterium will also generate the C3a and C5a anaphylatoxins leading to extensive transudation of serum components, including more antibody, and to the chemotactic attraction of polymorphs to aid in phagocytosis as described earlier under the acute inflammation umbrella (cf. figures 2.18 and 13.2).

### The secretory immune system protects the external mucosal surfaces

We have earlier emphasized the critical nature of the mucosal barriers, particularly in the gut where there is a potentially hostile interface with the microbial hordes. With an area of around 400 square meters, give or take a tennis court or two, the epithelium of the adult mucosae represents the most frequent portal of entry for common infectious agents, allergens and carcinogens. The need for well-marshalled, highly effective mucosal immunity is glaringly obvious. Awareness of such a need was evident even in byegone days. Per Brandtzaeg relates an amusing historical example:

In ancient times, kings were perpetually worried that they would be poisoned by their enemies. (I heard tell that the habit of clinking glasses together in a toast has its origin in the custom of pouring some of one's wine into the glass of the next person and so on until the operation had come full circle.) Anyway, Mithridates VI Eupator, King of Pontus (now part of Turkey) in the 1st century BC was so frightened of being poisoned that he attempted to increase his intestinal defenses by drinking the blood of ducks which had been fed poisonous weeds. After defeat by the Romans and mutiny in his army he tried unsuccessfully to poison himself, testimony to the effectiveness of oral immunization. As a grisly negative control, his two daughters had no difficulty in committing suicide using the same poison, whereupon the desperate king was forced to order his bodyguard to kill him with a more conventional weapon.

The mucosal surfaces are mainly defended by secretory IgA and IgM, with IgA1 predominating in the

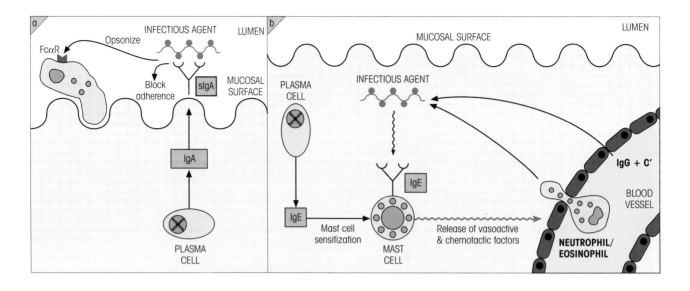

**Figure 13.9. Defense of the mucosal surfaces.** IgA opsonizes organisms and prevents adherence to the mucosa. IgE recruits agents of the immune response by firing the release of mediators from mast cells.

upper areas and IgA2 in the large bowel. The size of the task is highlighted by the fact that 80% of the Ig-producing B-cells in the body are present in the secretory mucosae and exocrine glands. IgA antibodies afford protection in the external body fluids, tears, saliva, nasal secretions and those bathing the surfaces of the intestine (so-called 'coproantibodies') and lung, by coating bacteria and viruses and preventing their adherence to the epithelial cells of the mucous membranes, which is essential for viral infection and bacterial colonization. It might be anticipated that in order to fulfil this function, secretory IgA molecules would themselves have very little innate adhesiveness for epithelial cells, but it is satisfying to read that high affinity Fc receptors for this Ig class have been identified on macrophages and polymorphs and can mediate phagocytosis (figure 13.9a). Two recent snippets: secretory IgA complexed with microbial products on the basolateral surface of the epithelial cells can be transcytosed to the lumen, whilst IgA being transported through epithelial cells can neutralize viruses within them. Those of a thrifty disposition will be uplifted by the knowledge that high affinity Fabγ fragments resulting from the normal catabolism of serum IgG, are carried via hepatobiliary secretions into the lumen of the digestive tract where they provide yet another blocking agent.

If an infectious agent succeeds in penetrating the IgA barrier, it comes up against the next line of defense of the secretory system (see p. 161) which is manned by IgE. There are obvious parallels between the ways in which complement-derived anaphylatoxins and IgE utilize the mast cell to cause local amplification of the immune defenses. It is worth noting that most serum IgE arises from plasma cells in mucosal tissues and in the lymph nodes that drain them. Although present in low concentration, IgE is bound very firmly to the Fc receptors of the mast cell (see p. 56) and contact with antigen leads to the release of mediators which effectively recruit agents of the immune response and generate a local acute inflammatory reaction. Thus histamine, by increasing vascular permeability, causes the transudation of IgG and complement into the area, while chemotactic factors for neutrophils and eosinophils attract the effector cells needed to dispose of the infectious organism coated with specific IgG and C3b (figure 13.9b). Engagement of the Fcγ and C3b receptors on local macrophages by such complexes will lead to secretion of peptides which further reinforce these vascular permeability and chemotactic events. Broadly one would say that immune exclusion in the gut is non-inflammatory but immune elimination of organisms which penetrate the mucosa is proinflammatory.

Where the opsonized organism is too large for phagocytosis, these cells can kill by an extracellular mechanism after attachment by their Fcγ receptors. This phenomenon, termed antibody-dependent cell-mediated cytotoxicity (ADCC), has been discussed earlier (see p. 34) and there is evidence for its involvement in parasitic infections (see p. 275). Yet another string to the bow is provided by dietary nitrates which, although vilified for their potential to form carcinogenic nitrosamines, can also be converted by nitrate-reducing bacteria on the tongue to nitrites; upon acidification in the stomach, these generate sufficient NO· to provide some protection from swallowed pathogens. NO· is also produced by epithelial cells in the paranasal sinuses and is present in sinus air in very high concentrations.

The mucosal tissues contain a variety of T-lymphocyte species, but their role and that of the mucosal epithelial cells other than in a helper function for local antibody production is of less relevance for the defense against extracellular bacteria.

## Some specific bacterial infections

First let us see how these considerations apply to the defense against infection by common organisms such as streptococci and staphylococci. β-Hemolytic **streptococci** were classified by Lancefield according to their carbohydrate antigen and the most important from the standpoint of human disease are those belonging to group A. *Streptococcus pyogenes* posed a major worldwide health threat; in 1981 more than six million children suffered from associated rheumatic disease in India alone and resurgence of a highly virulent strain causing rheumatic fever and toxic shock syndrome has occurred in the USA.

The most important virulence factor is the surface M-protein (variants of which form the basis of the Griffith typing). This protein is an acceptor for factor H which facilitates C3b breakdown, and binds fibrinogen and its fragments which cover sites that may act as complement activators (figure 13.10). It thereby inhibits opsonization and the protection afforded by antibodies to the M-component is attributable to the striking increase in phagocytosis which they induce. Their ability to elicit cross-reactive autoantibodies is thought to be involved in poststreptococcal autoimmune disease. High titer antibodies to the streptolysin O exotoxin (ASO), which damages membranes, are indicators of recent streptococcal infection. The pyrogenic exotoxins SPE A, B and C are superantigens associated with scarlet fever and streptococcal toxic shock syndrome. The toxins are neutralized by antibody and the erythematous intradermal reaction to injected toxin is only seen in individuals lacking antibody (Dick reaction). Antibody also neutralizes bacterial enzymes like hyaluronidase which act to spread the infection.

A growing body of evidence is tending to incriminate *Streptococcus mutans* as an important cause of **dental caries**. The organism has a constitutive enzyme, glucosyltransferase, able to convert sucrose to dextran which is utilized for adhesion to the tooth

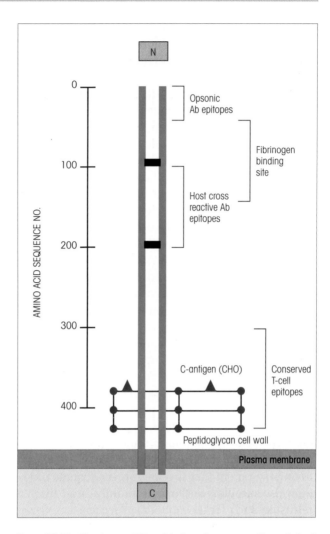

**Figure 13.10. Streptococcal M-protein from *S. pyogenes*.** The coiled-coil dimers are approximately 50 nm long. (Based on Robinson J.H. & Kehoe M.A. (1992) *Immunology Today* **13**, 362–367.)

surface. Passive transfer of IgG, but not IgA or IgM, antibodies to *S. mutans* in monkeys conferred protection against caries. It is thought that IgG antibody and complement in the gingival crevicular fluid bathing the tooth opsonize the bacteria to facilitate phagocytosis and killing by polymorphonuclear leukocytes. Curiously, a single treatment with a monoclonal anti-*S. mutans* kept teeth free of the microorganism for 1 year, perhaps due to a shift in bacterial ecology, with the place vacated by *S. mutans* being filled with another organism from the oral flora.

Virulent forms of **staphylococci**, of which *Staphylococcus aureus* is perhaps the most common, resist phagocytosis. This may be due partly to capsule formation *in vivo* and partly to the elaboration of factors such as a coagulase enzyme which could protect the bacterium by a barrier of fibrin. It has been suggested that the ability of a cell wall component, protein A, to combine with the Fc portion of IgG (other than subclass IgG3) is responsible for inhibition of phagocytosis by virulent strains, but IgG–protein A complexes fix complement and one study reports that protein A actually increases complement-mediated phagocytosis. We must return an open verdict on that issue. It seems to be accepted that *S. aureus* is readily phagocytosed in the presence of *adequate* amounts of antibody but a small proportion of the ingested bacteria survives and they are difficult organisms to eliminate completely. Where the infection is inadequately controlled, severe lesions may occur in the immunized host as a consequence of type IV delayed hypersensitivity reactions. Thus, staphylococci were found to be avirulent when injected into mice passively immunized with antibody but caused extensive tissue damage in animals previously given sensitized T-cells.

Other examples where antibodies are required to overcome the inherently antiphagocytic properties of **bacterial capsules** are seen in immunity to infection by pneumococci, meningococci and *Haemophilus influenzae*. *Bacillus anthrax* possesses an antiphagocytic capsule composed of a γ polypeptide of D-glutamic acid but although anticapsular antibodies effectively promote uptake by polymorphs, the exotoxin is so potent that vaccines are inadequate unless they also stimulate antitoxin immunity. In addition to releasing such lethal exotoxins, *Pseudomonas aeruginosa* also produces an elastase that inactivates C3a and C5a; as a result only minimal inflammatory responses are made in the absence of neutralizing antibodies.

The ploy of **diverting complement activation** to insensitive sites is seen rather well with different strains of Gram-negative *Salmonella* and *Escherichia coli* organisms which vary in the number of O-specific oligosaccharide side-chains attached to the lipid-A-linked core polysaccharide of the endotoxin (cf. figure 13.4). Variants with long side-chains are relatively insensitive to killing by serum through the alternative complement pathway (see p. 24); as the side-chains become shorter and shorter, the serum sensitivity increases. Although all variants activate the alternative pathway, only those with short or no side-chains allow the cytotoxic membrane attack complex to be inserted near to the outer lipid bilayer (figure 13.5vi). On the other hand, antibodies focus the complex to a more vulnerable site.

The destruction of gonococci by serum containing antibody is dependent upon the formation of the membrane attack complex and rare individuals lacking C8 or C9 are susceptible to *Neisseria* infection. *N. gonorrhoeae* specifically binds complement proteins and prevents their insertion in the outer membranes, but antibody, like a ubiquitous 'Mr Fixit', corrects this situation, at least so far as the host is concerned. With respect to the infective process itself, IgA produced in the genital tract in response to these organisms inhibits the attachment of the bacteria, through their pili, to mucosal cells, but seems unable to afford adequate protection against reinfection. This seems to be due to a very effective antigenic shift mechanism which alters the sequence of the expressed pilin by gene conversion. Failure to achieve good protection might also be a reflection of the ability of gonococcal protease to split $IgA_1$ dimers. Meningococci which frequently infect the nasopharynx, *H. influenzae* and *S. pneumoniae* have similar unfair proteases.

**Cholera** is caused by the colonization of the small intestine by *Vibrio cholerae* and the subsequent action of its enterotoxin. The B subunits of the toxin bind to specific GM1 monosialoganglioside receptors and translocate the A subunit across the membrane where it activates adenyl cyclase. The increased cAMP then causes fluid loss by inhibiting uptake of sodium chloride and stimulating active Cl⁻ secretion by intestinal epithelial cells. Locally synthesized IgA antibodies against *V. cholerae* lipopolysaccharide and the toxin provide independent protection against cholera, the first by inhibiting bacterial adherence to the intestinal wall, the second by blocking attachment of the toxin to its receptor. In accord with this analysis is the epidemiological data showing that children who drink milk with high titers of IgA antibodies specific for either of these antigens are less likely to develop clinical cholera.

*Yersiniae* and *Salmonellae* are among the select number of bacterial pathogens which have evolved special mechanisms to enter, survive and replicate within normally **nonphagocytic host cells**. The former gain entry through binding of their outer membrane protein, invasin, to multiple $\beta_1$ integrin receptors on the host cell. *Salmonellae*, on the other hand, induce membrane ruffling on the target cell, linked in some way to signaling events which lead to bacterial uptake.

I thought it might be helpful to summarize the ways in which antibody can parry the different facets of bacterial invasion in figure 13.11.

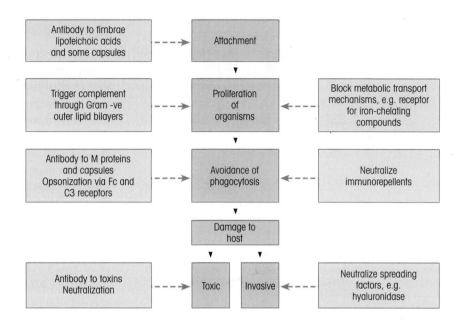

Figure 13.11. Antibody defenses against bacterial invasion.

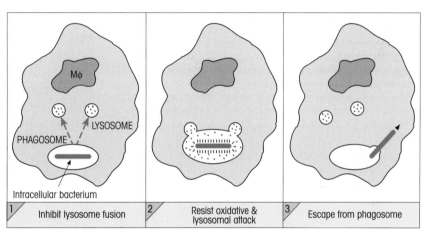

Figure 13.12. Evasion of phagocytic death by intracellular bacteria.

## BACTERIA WHICH GROW IN AN INTRACELLULAR HABITAT

### Bacterial gambits

Some strains of bacteria, such as the tubercle and leprosy bacilli and *Listeria* and *Brucella* organisms, escape the wrath of the immune system by cheekily fashioning an intracellular life within one of its strongholds, the macrophage no less. Mononuclear phagocytes are a good target for such organisms in the sense that they are very mobile and allow wide dissemination throughout the body. Entry of opsonized bacteria is facilitated by phagocytic uptake after attachment to Fcγ and C3b receptors but once inside many of them defy the mighty macrophage by subverting the innate killing mechanisms in a variety

of ways. Organisms such as *Mycobacterium tuberculosis* inhibit fusion of the lysosomes with the phagocytic vacuole containing the ingested bacterium (figure 13.12). Mycobacterial lipids such as lipoarabinomannan obstruct priming and activation of the macrophage and also protect the bacteria from attack by scavenging reactive oxygen intermediates such as superoxide anion, hydroxyl radicals and hydrogen peroxide (cf. p. 9). Organisms such as *Listeria monocytogenes* use a special lysin to escape from their phagosomal prison to lie happily free within the cytoplasm; some rickettsias and the protozoon *Trypanosoma cruzi* can do the same. Legionella are said to inhibit the respiratory burst, further confirming the view that if there is a mechanism available to inhibit, some microorganisms will eventually find a way to do it.

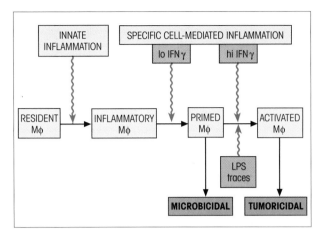

**Figure 13.13. Stages in the activation of macrophages (Mφ) for microbicidal and tumoricidal function.** Macrophages taken from sites of inflammation induced by complement or nonimmunological stimuli, such as thioglycollate, are considerably increased in size, acid hydrolase content, secretion of neutral proteinases and phagocytic function. If I may give one example, the C3b receptors on resident Mφ are not freely mobile in the membrane so cannot permit the 'zippering' process required for phagocytosis (see p. 8); consequently, they bind but do not ingest C3b-coated red cells. Inflammatory Mφ, on the other hand, have C3 receptors which display considerable lateral mobility and the C3 opsonized erythrocytes are readily phagocytosed. In addition to the dramatic upregulation of intracellular killing mechanisms, striking changes in surface components accompany activation. In mouse macrophages there is an increase in class II MHC (dramatic), Fc receptors for IgG2b and binding sites for tumor cells; in contrast, the mannose receptor, the F4/80 marker and IgG2a receptors all decline, while the Mac-I component associated with the CR3 iC3b receptor remains unchanged.

## Defense is by T-cell-mediated immunity (CMI)

In an elegant series of experiments, Mackaness demonstrated the importance of CMI reactions for the killing of these intracellular parasites and the establishment of an immune state. Animals infected with moderate doses of *M. tuberculosis* overcome the infection and are immune to subsequent challenge with the bacillus. The immunity can be transferred to a normal recipient with T-lymphocytes but not macrophages or serum from an immune animal. Supporting this view, that specific immunity is mediated by T-cells, is the greater susceptibility to infection with tubercle and leprosy bacilli of mice in which the T-lymphocytes have been depressed by thymectomy plus anti-T-cell monoclonals, or in which the TCR genes have been disrupted by homologous gene recombination (knockout mice).

## Activated macrophages kill intracellular parasites

When monocytes first settle down in the tissue to become 'resident' macrophages they are essentially downregulated with respect to expression of surface receptors and function. They can be activated in several stages (figure 13.13), but the ability to kill obligate intracellular microbes only comes after stimulation by macrophage activating factor(s)

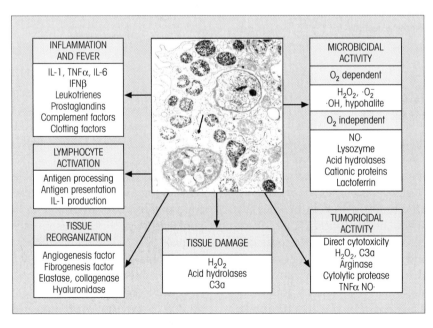

**Figure 13.14. The role of the activated macrophage in the initiation and mediation of chronic inflammation** with concomitant tissue repair, and in the killing of microbes and tumor cells. It is possible that macrophages differentiate along distinct pathways to subserve these different functions. The electron micrograph shows a highly activated macrophage with many lysozomal structures which have been highlighted by the uptake of thorotrast; one (arrowed) is seen fusing with a phagosome containing the protozoon *Toxoplasma gondii*. (Courtesy of Professor C. Jones.)

such as IFNγ released from stimulated lymphokine-producing T-cells. Foremost amongst the killing mechanisms which are upregulated are those mediated by reactive oxygen intermediates and NO·. The activated macrophage is undeniably a remarkable and formidable cell, capable of secreting the 60-odd substances which are concerned in chronic inflammatory reactions (figure 13.14)—not the sort to meet in an alley on a dark night!

The mechanism of T-cell-mediated immunity in the Mackaness experiments now becomes clear. Specifically primed T-cells react with processed antigen derived from the intracellular bacteria present on the surface of the infected macrophage in association with MHC II; the subsequent release of lymphokines activates the macrophage and endows it with the ability to kill the organisms it has phagocytosed (figure 13.15).

## Examples of intracellular bacterial infections

### Listeria

Undoubtedly, T-helper-1 (TH1)-activated macrophages are crucially important for the ultimate elimination of intracellular *Listeria* but the complex role of innate mechanisms early in infection must be considered. These are outlined in figure 13.16 where attention should be drawn to the bactericidal action of polymorphs and the central action of IL-12 which generates the macrophage-activator IFNγ through its stimulation of NK cells and recruitment of TH1 helpers. Mutant mice lacking αβ and/or γδT-cells reveal that TCR1 and TCR2 cells make comparable contributions to resistance against primary *Listeria* infection but that the TCR2 (αβ) set bears the major responsibility for conferring protective immunity. TCR1 (γδ) cells control the local tissue response at the site of microbial replication and γδ knockout mutants develop huge abscesses when infected with *Listeria*.

### Tuberculosis

Tuberculosis (TB) is beginning to rampage. Some 90 million new cases and 30 million deaths are forecast for the nineties if control measures do not improve. Newly emerging multi-drug-resistant strains are emerging and human immunodeficiency virus (HIV)-infected individuals with low CD4 counts have increased susceptibility.

With respect to host defense mechanisms, as seen with *Listeria* infection, murine macrophages activated by IFNγ can destroy intracellular mycobacteria with

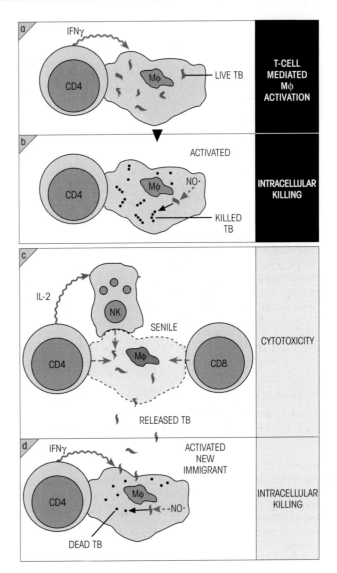

**Figure 13.15. The 'cytokine connection': nonspecific murine macrophage killing of intracellular bacteria triggered by a specific T-cell mediated immunity reaction.** (a) Specific CD4 TH1 cell recognizes mycobacterial peptide associated with MHC class II and releases Mϕ activating IFNγ. (b) The activated Mϕ kills the intracellular TB, mainly through generation of toxic NO·. (c) A 'senile' Mϕ, unable to destroy the intracellular bacteria, is killed by CD8 and CD4 cytotoxic cells and possibly by IL-2 activated NK cells. The Mϕ then releases live tubercle bacilli which are taken up and killed by newly recruited Mϕ susceptible to IFNγ activation. Human monocytes require activation by both IFNγ and IL-4 plus a CD23-mediated signal for induction of iNO synthase and production of NO·.

magisterial ease, largely through generation of toxic NO·. Some parasitized macrophages reach a stage at which they are too incapacitated to be stirred into action by T-cell messages and here a somewhat ruthless strategy has evolved in which the host deploys cytotoxic CD8, and possibly CD4 and NK cells, to execute the helpless macrophage and release the live *Mycobacteria*; these should now be taken up by newly

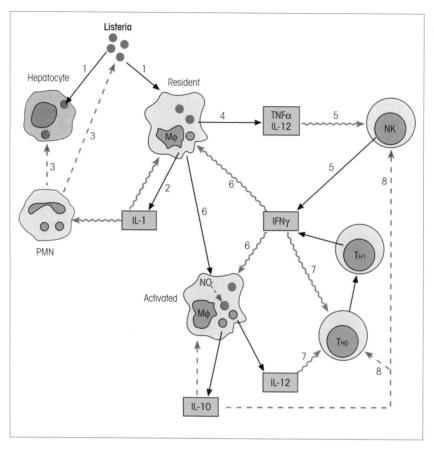

**Figure 13.16. Immune response to *Listeria* infection.** (1) *Listeria* infects resident macrophages and hepatocytes; (2) the Mϕ release IL-1 which activates polymorphs; (3) the activated PMN destroy *Listeria* bacilli by direct contact and are cytotoxic for infected hepatocytes; (4) the infected Mϕ release TNFα and IL-12 which stimulate NK cells; (5) NK cells secrete IFNγ, which (6) activates the macrophage to produce NO· and kill intracellular *Lis-* *teria*; (7) IFNγ plus Mϕ-derived IL-12 recruit TH1 cells which reinforce Mϕ activation through production of IFNγ. (8) Eventual synthesis of IL-10, encouraged by the action of immune complexes, downregulates Mϕ, NK and TH1 activity. (Based on an article by Rogers H.W., Tripps C.S. & Unanue E.R. (1995) *The Immunologist* **3**, 152.)

immigrant phagocytic cells susceptible to activation by IFNγ and summarily disposed of (figure 13.15).

The position is more complicated in the human. IFNγ-stimulated human monocytes cannot eliminate intracellular TB, although there is some stasis and IFNγ does upregulate expression of the 1-hydroxylase which converts vitamin D$_3$ into the 1,25-dihydroxy form, a potent activator of antimycobacterial mechanisms. However, there is no induction of NO· synthase (iNOS type II) unless IL-4 is also added to the system, whereupon there is copious production of NO· in a CD23-dependent reaction.

A further plethora of potential defensive mechanisms is emerging. The TB products Ag85B (a mycolyl transferase) and ESAT-6 are potent inducers of IFNγ from CD4 cells. CD4–8–αβ T-cells proliferate in response to mycolic acid and lyse cells presenting the acid in the context of CD1b, while human Vγ$_2$Vδ$_2$ T-cells recognize protein antigens, isopentenyl pyrophosphates and prenyl pyrophosphates from *M. tuberculosis*. The TCR1 T-cells bearing γδ-receptors have an eerie, almost compelling, relationship to mycobacterial antigens. Limiting dilution analysis indicates that almost every γδ-T-cell in the peripheral blood of normal individuals is stimulated by mycobacterial lysates. They can lyse target cells presenting mycobacterial antigens and, in the mouse, a high percentage react to the 65 kDa heat-shock protein. A vital role for these cells in murine TB is indicated by the death of TCR1-deletion mutants after an infection with *M. tuberculosis* which was still tolerated by immunocompetent animals.

Given these potential CMI defenses, why do some individuals fail to eradicate their infections with mycobacteria and other intracellular facultative bacteria and so suffer from diseases such as TB and leprosy even though they have established TH1 responses? One important clue is provided by the demonstration that inbred strains of mice differ dramatically in their susceptibility to infection by various mycobacteria, *Salmonella typhimurium* and *Leishmania donovani*. Control of the resistance/susceptibility phenotype is by two alleles of a single autosomal dominant gene, *Bcg*, and resistance is linked to a T-cell-independent enhanced state of macrophage priming for bactericidal activity involving oxygen and nitrogen radicals. Moreover, macrophages from resistant strains had increased MHC class II expression and a higher respiratory burst, were more readily activated by IFNγ, and induced better stimulation of T-cells, whereas macrophages from susceptible strains tended to have suppressor effects on T-cell proliferation to mycobacterial antigens. The likely candidate gene is *Nramp-1*, probably concerned with the transport or metabolism of NO·. The human homolog has been cloned and obviously there will be a search for alleles linked with susceptibility to mycobacterial infection.

Where the host has difficulty in effectively eliminating these organisms, the chronic CMI response to local antigen leads to the accumulation of densely packed macrophages which release angiogenic and fibrogenic factors and stimulate the formation of granulation tissue and ultimately fibrosis. The activated macrophages, perhaps under the stimulus of IL-4, transform to epithelioid cells and fuse to become giant cells. As suggested earlier, the resulting granuloma represents an attempt by the body to isolate a site of persistent infection.

*Leprosy*

In human leprosy, the disease presents as a spectrum ranging from the **tuberculoid** form with lesions containing small numbers of viable organisms, to the **lepromatous** form characterized by an abundance of *M. leprae* within the macrophages. The tuberculoid state is associated with good cell-mediated dermal hypersensitivity reactions and a bias towards TH1 type responses, although these are still not good enough completely to eradicate the bacilli. In the lepromatous form, there is poor T-cell reactivity to whole bacilli and poor lepromin dermal responses, although there are numerous plasma cells which contribute to a high level of circulating antibody and indicate a more prominent TH2 activity. Clearly CMI rather than humoral immunity is important for the control of the leprosy bacillus but reasons for the inadequate responses of the lepromatous patients are still uncertain.

## IMMUNITY TO VIRAL INFECTION

Genetically controlled constitutional factors which render a host or certain of their cells nonpermissive (i.e. resistant to takeover of their replicative machinery by virus) play a dominant role in influencing the vulnerability of a given individual to infection. Macrophages may readily take up viruses nonspecifically and kill them. However, in some instances the macrophages allow replication and, if the virus is capable of producing cytopathic effects in various organs, the infection may be lethal; with noncytopathic agents such as lymphocytic choriomeningitis, Aleutian mink disease and equine infectious anemia viruses, a persistent infection may result. Viruses can avoid recognition by the host's immune system by latency or by sheltering in privileged sites but they have also evolved a maliciously cunning series of evasive strategies.

### Immunity can be evaded by antigen changes

*Changing antigens by drift and shift*

In the course of their constant duel with the immune system, viruses are continually changing the structure of their surface antigens. They do so by processes termed 'antigenic drift' and 'antigenic shift', the nature of which may be made more apparent by consideration of different influenza strains. The surface of the influenza virus contains a hemagglutinin, by which it adheres to cells prior to infection, and a neuraminidase, which releases newly formed virus from the surface sialic acid of the infected cell; of these the hemagglutinin is the more important for the establishment of protective immunity. Minor changes in antigenicity of the hemagglutinin occur through point mutations in the viral genome (**drift**) but major changes arise through wholesale swapping of genetic material with reservoirs of different viruses in other animal hosts (**shift**) (figure 13.17). When alterations in the hemagglutinin are sufficient to render previous immunity ineffective, new influenza epidemics break out.

Mutant forms can be favored by selection pressure from antibody. In fact one current strategy for generating mutants in a given epitope is to grow the virus in tissue culture in the presence of a monoclonal antibody which reacts with that epitope; only mutants which do not bind the monoclonal will escape and grow out. This principle underlies the antigenic variation characteristic of the common cold rhinoviruses. The site for attachment and penetration of mucosal

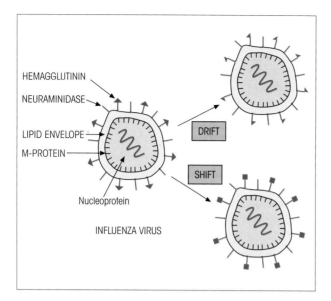

**Figure 13.17. Antigenic drift and shift in influenza virus.** The changes in hemagglutinin structure caused by drift may be small enough to allow protection by immunity to earlier strains. This may not happen with radical changes in the antigen associated with antigenic shift and so new virus epidemics break out. Over the last 50 years epidemics have been associated with the emergence by antigenic shift of the A/PR8 strain in 1933 with the structure $H_0N_1$ (the official nomenclature assigns numbers to each hemagglutinin and neuraminidase major variant), A/FM1 in 1947 ($H_1N_1$), A/Singapore in 1957 ($H_2N_2$) and A/Hong Kong in 1968 ($H_3N_2$); note that each new epidemic was associated with a fundamental change in the hemagglutinin.

cells bearing ICAM-1 is a hydrophobic pocket lying on the floor of a canyon which antibodies were thought to be too large to penetrate. Antibodies react with the rim of the viral canyon and mutations in the rim would thus enable the virus to escape from the host immune response without affecting the conserved site for binding to the target cell. This cosy picture has been challenged by a recent structural study which revealed that a neutralizing antibody Fab could modify its shape to penetrate deeply within the canyon. Hydrophobic drugs have been synthesized which fit the rhinovirus canyon and cause a change in conformation which prevents binding to cells and, since host proteins have very different folds to those of the viral capsid molecule, the drugs have limited cytotoxicity. A more recent drug has been designed to slot into the substrate binding site of the neuraminidase, so inhibiting its biological activity.

### Mutation can produce antagonistic T-cell epitopes

Hepatitis B virus isolates from chronically infected patients can present variant epitopes which act as TCR antagonists capable of inhibiting naturally occurring antiviral cytotoxic T-cells. Mutations which modify residues critical for recognition by MHC or TCR may generate partial agonists that can induce a profound and long-lasting state of T-cell anergy (cf. p. 235 and figure 9.6). Either strategy can lead to persistent infection.

### Some viruses can affect antigen processing

The Tap-mediated translocation of peptides from the cytosol to the endoplasmic reticulum can be adversely affected by adenovirus 12 infection or by the immediate early protein ICP-47 of herpes simplex virus. EBNA-1, the Epstein–Barr virus (EBV) nuclear antigen-1, contains Gly.Ala repeats which behave as *cis*-acting elements that repress class I antigen presentation, probably by influencing protein degradation. The net effect is a lack of surface target for cytotoxic T-cells.

## Viruses can interfere with immune effector mechanisms

### Playing games with the complement system

Blocking of complement-mediated induction of the inflammatory response and viral killing is achieved by an abundant vaccinia virus product structurally related to C4b binding protein. For its part, Herpes simplex type I subverts the complement cascade by producing a C3-binding molecule which augments decay of the alternative pathway $\overline{C3bBb}$ convertase.

Several viruses utilize complement receptors to gain entry into cells, especially since engagement of the complement receptor alone on a macrophage is a feeble activator of the respiratory burst. Flavivirus coated with iC3b enters through the CR3 receptors. As noted previously, EBV infects B-cells by binding to the CR2 surface receptors. Ominously, HIV coated with antibody and complement is more virulent than unopsonized virus.

### Sabotaging cell-mediated immunity

Para-influenza virus type 2 strongly inhibits Tc cells by downregulating granzyme B expression (cf. p. 19). Numerous viral open-reading frames encode proteins homologous to host cytokines and their receptors. For example, one EBV product with 84% identity to human IL-10 helps the virus to escape the antiviral effects of IFNγ. Others produce soluble proteins which bind and therefore subvert cytokines such as RANTES and IL-6.

## Protection by serum antibody

The antibody molecule can neutralize viruses by a variety of means. It may stereochemically inhibit combination with the receptor site on cells, thereby preventing penetration and subsequent intracellular multiplication, the protective effect of antibodies to influenza viral hemagglutinin providing a good example. Similarly, antibodies to the measles hemagglutinin prevent entry into the cell but spread of virus from cell to cell is stopped by antibodies to the fusion antigen. Antibody may destroy a free virus particle directly through activation of the classical complement pathway or produce aggregation, enhanced phagocytosis and intracellular death by mechanisms already discussed.

Relatively low concentrations of circulating antibody can be effective and one is familiar with the protection afforded by poliomyelitis antibodies, and by human γ-globulin given prophylactically to individuals exposed to measles. The most clear-cut protection is seen in diseases with long incubation times where the virus has to travel through the bloodstream before it reaches the tissue which it finally infects. For example, in poliomyelitis the virus gains access to the body via the gastrointestinal tract and eventually passes through the circulation to reach the brain cells which become infected. Within the blood, the virus is neutralized by quite low levels of specific antibody while the prolonged period before the virus infects the brain allows time for a secondary immune response in a primed host.

## Local factors

With other viral diseases, such as influenza and the common cold, there is a short incubation time related to the fact that the final target organ for the virus is the same as the portal of entry and no intermediate stage involving passage through the body occurs. There is little time for a primary antibody response to be mounted and in all likelihood the **rapid production of interferon** is the most significant mechanism used to counter the viral infection. Experimental studies certainly indicate that after an early peak of interferon production, there is a rapid fall in the titer of live virus in the lungs of mice infected with influenza (figure 13.18). Antibody, as assessed by the serum titer, seems to arrive on the scene much too late to be of value in aiding recovery. However, recent investigations have shown that antibody levels may be elevated in the local fluids bathing the infected surfaces, e.g. nasal mucosa and lung, despite low serum titers and it is

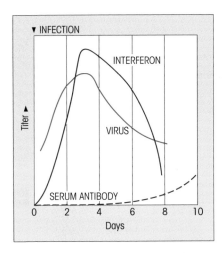

**Figure 13.18. Appearance of interferon and serum antibody in relation to recovery from influenza virus infection of the lungs of mice.** (From Isaacs A. (1961) *New Scientist* **11**, 81.)

the production of **antiviral antibody** (most prominently IgA) by locally deployed immunologically primed cells which is of major importance for the **prevention of subsequent infection**. Unfortunately, in so far as the common cold is concerned, a subsequent infection is likely to involve an antigenically unrelated virus so that general immunity to colds is difficult to achieve.

## Cell-mediated immunity gets to the intracellular virus

In Chapter 2 we emphasized the general point that to a first approximation, antibody dealt with extracellular infective agents and CMI with intracellular ones. The same holds true for viruses which try to shelter from antibody in an intracellular habitat. Local or systemic antibodies can block the spread of cytolytic viruses which are released from the host cell they have just killed, but alone they are usually inadequate to control those viruses which bud off from the surface as infectious particles because they are also capable of spreading to adjacent cells without becoming exposed to antibody (figure 13.19). The importance of CMI for recovery from infection with these agents is underlined by the inability of children with primary T-cell immunodeficiency to cope with such viruses, whereas patients with Ig deficiency but intact CMI are not troubled in this way.

### NK cells can kill virally infected targets

In earlier chapters we have explained how early recognition and killing of a virally infected cell before

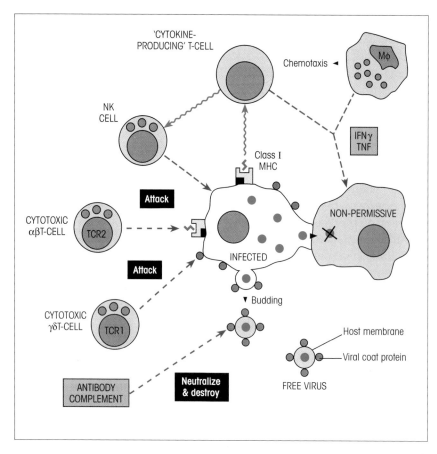

**Figure 13.19. Control of infection by 'budding' viruses.** Free virus released by budding from the cell surface is neutralized by antibody. Specific cytotoxic T-cells kill virally infected targets directly. Interaction with a (separate?) sub-population of T-cells releases lymphokines which attract macrophages, prime contiguous cells with IFNγ and TNF to make them resistant to viral infection and activate cytotoxic NK cells. NK cells are large granular lymphocytes, CD3−, majority CD16+ (FcγRIIIa) and CD56+ (NCAM) in humans; powerful producers of IFNγ and GM-CSF. They recognize neocarbohydrates (?) on the infected cell membrane and antibody coating viral envelope protein (ADCC). Included in this group of budding viruses are: oncorna (= oncogenic RNA virus, e.g. murine leukemogenic), orthomyxo (influenza), paramyxo (mumps, measles), toga (dengue), rhabdo (rabies), arena (lymphocytic choriomeningitis), adeno, herpes (simplex, varicella zoster, cytomegalo, Epstein–Barr, Marek's disease), pox (vaccinia), papova (SV40, polyoma) and rubella viruses.

replication occurs is of obvious benefit to the host. The importance of the NK cell in this role as an agent of preformed innate immunity can be gauged from observations on the exceedingly rare patients with complete absence of these cells who suffer recurrent life-threatening viral infections including EBV, varicella and cytomegaloviruses (CMV). The surface of a virally infected cell undergoes modification, probably in its surface carbohydrate structures, making it an attractive target for NK cells which can be shown to be cytotoxic *in vitro* to cells infected with a number of different viruses. The NK cell possesses two families of surface receptors. One, lectin-like, binds to the novel structures expressed by the infected cell, the other, a newly cloned class of p58/NKAT receptors, recognizes supertypic or public specificities common to several MHC class I alleles. The first activates killing but the recognition of class I delivers an inhibitory signal. Thus, the sensitivity of the target cell is closely related to self-MHC class I expression; sensitive targets have low class I but transfection with the self-MHC molecule will generally protect them. Karrer has suggested that, whereas T-cells search for the presence of foreign shapes, NK cells survey tissues for the absence of self as indicated by aberrant or absent expression of MHC class I which might occur in tumorigenesis or certain viral infections. The ability of EBV to downregulate class I would explain the drastic nature of this infection in NK-deficient patients mentioned above. The production of IFNα during viral infection not only protects surrounding cells but also activates NK cells and upregulates MHC expression on the adjacent cells, making them more resistant to cytotoxicity.

## Cytotoxic T-cells (Tc) are crucial elements in immunity to infection by budding viruses

T-lymphocytes from a sensitized host are directly cytotoxic to cells infected with viruses, the new MHC-associated peptide antigens on the target cell surface being recognized by specific αβ receptors on the aggressor lymphocytes. The need for CD4 T-cell help in the generation of Tc is still equivocal in the light of studies showing the production of influenza and lymphocytic choriomeningitis virus (LCMV)-specific Tc cells in class II knockout mice. Tc are less strain-specific in that they show broader cross-reaction than antibody, presumably reflecting a greater conservation of the T- as distinct from the B-cell epitopes. There is a quite surprising frequency of dual specificities in target cell recognition by virus-specific Tc clones, which can lyse uninfected allogeneic cells or targets expressing peptides with little homology from different regions of the same viral protein, from different proteins of the same virus, or even from different unrelated viruses. Thus activation by a second virus may help to maintain memory and there may be a spontaneous immunity to an unrelated virus after initial infection with a cross-reacting strain. Could the dual specificity be related to expression of two TCR α-chain genes due to lack of allelic exclusion (cf. p. 229)? Downregulation of MHC class I poses no problems for **TCR1 γδ Tc** which recognize native viral coat protein (e.g. herpes simplex virus glycoprotein) on the cell surface (figure 13.19).

Tc cells can usually be detected in the peripheral blood lymphocytes of individuals who have recovered from infection with influenza, CMV or EBV by re-exposure *in vitro* to appropriately infected cells. In the case of CMV, for example, the targets are cells with the 'early antigen' on their surface expressed within 6 hours of infection. As discussed above, it is clearly advantageous for the cytotoxic cell to strike so soon after infection. Studies on volunteers, showing that high levels of cytotoxic activity before challenge with live influenza correlated with low or absent shedding of virus, speak in favour of the importance of Tc in human viral infection.

After a natural infection, both antibody and Tc cells are generated; subsequent protection is long lived without reinfection, possibly being reinforced by bystander activation through cytokines released from other stimulated T-cells or perhaps by random triggering with unrelated viruses based on the dual specificity described earlier. By contrast, injection of killed influenza produces antibodies but no Tc and protection is only short term.

## Cytokines recruit effectors and provide a 'cordon sanitaire'

A number of studies on transfer of protection to influenza, lymphocytic choriomeningitis, vaccinia, ectromelia and CMV infections focus on CD8 rather than CD4 T-cells as the major defensive force. The knee-jerk response would be to implicate cytotoxicity but it is becoming increasingly clear that CD8 cells also produce cytokines. This may well be crucial when viruses escape the cytotoxic mechanism and manage to sidle laterally into an adjacent cell. CMI can now play some new cards: if T-cells (CD8?) stimulated by viral antigen release lymphokines such as IFNγ and macrophage or monocyte chemotaxin, the mononuclear phagocytes attracted to the site will be activated to secrete TNF, which will synergize with the IFNγ to render the contiguous cells nonpermissive for the replication of any virus acquired by intercellular transfer (figure 13.19). In this way the site of infection can be surrounded by a cordon of resistant cells. Like IFNα, IFNγ may also increase the nonspecific cytotoxicity of NK cells (see p. 19) for infected cells. This generation of 'immune interferon' (IFNγ) and TNF in response to non-nucleic acid viral components provides a valuable back-up mechanism when dealing with viruses which are intrinsically poor stimulators of interferon synthesis.

### Antibody has a part too

The neutralization of free virus particles by antibody is relatively straightforward but the interaction with infected cells is rather more complex. Access to the surface antigens by αβ-T-cells cannot be blocked by antibody since they recognize processed, and antibody, native antigen molecules. Antibodies can however block γδ Tc by reacting with surface antigen on incipiently budding virions but should be able to initiate ADCC (p. 34) as has been reported with herpes, vaccinia and mumps-infected target cells.

Do not forget the importance of antibody in **preventing reinfection** with most viruses.

## IMMUNITY TO FUNGI

Not too much is known about this subject. Many fungal infections become established in immunocompromised hosts or when the normal commensal flora are upset by prolonged administration of broad-spectrum antibiotics. T-cells are important in defense and can interact directly with the surface of organisms such as *Cryptococcus neoformans* and *Candida albicans*, killing them by the granzyme system. NK cells can also lyse *C. neoformans*.

## IMMUNITY TO PARASITIC INFECTIONS

The diverse organisms responsible for the major parasitic diseases are listed in figure 13.20. The numbers affected are truly horrifying and the sum of misery they engender is too large to comprehend. The consequences of parasitism could be at one extreme a lack of immune response leading to overwhelming superinfection, and at the other an exaggerated life-threatening immunopathologic response. To be successful, a parasite must steer a course *between* these extremes, avoiding wholesale killing of the human host and yet at the same time escaping destruction by the immune system. In practice, each type of parasite is virtually a world unto itself in the complexity of the mechanisms by which this is achieved.

### The host responses

A wide variety of defensive mechanisms are deployed by the host but the rough generalization may be made that a humoral response develops when the organisms invade the bloodstream (malaria, trypanosomiasis), whereas parasites which grow within the tissues (e.g. cutaneous leishmaniasis) usually elicit CMI (table 13.2). Often, a chronically infected host will be resistant to reinfection with fresh organisms, a situation termed **concomitant immunity**. This is seen particularly in schistosomiasis but also in

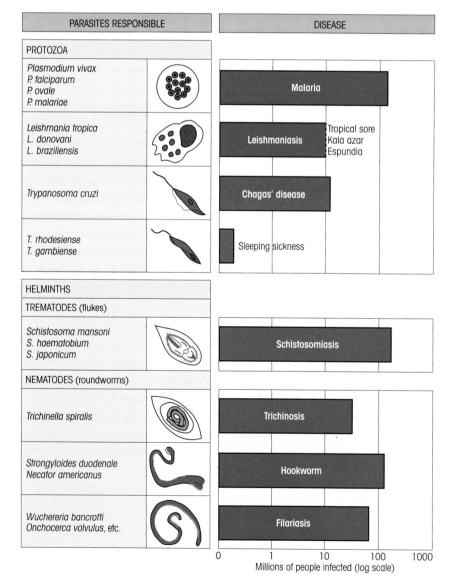

**Figure 13.20.  The major parasites in man** and the sheer enormity of the numbers of people infected. (Data from World Health Organization, 1990.)

**Table 13.2.** The relative importance of antibody and cell-mediated responses in protozoal infections.

| PARASITE | TRYPANOSOMA BRUCEI | PLASMODIUM | TRYPANOSOMA CRUZI | LEISHMANIA |
|---|---|---|---|---|
| HABITAT | Free in blood | Inside red cell | Inside macrophage | Inside macrophage |
| **ANTIBODY** | | | | |
| Importance | + + + + | + + + | + + | + |
| Mechanism | Lysis with complement Opsonizes for phagocytosis | Blocks invasion Opsonizes for phagocytosis | Limits spread in acute infection | Limits spread |
| Means of evasion | Antigenic variation | Intracellular habitat Antigenic variation | Intracellular habitat | Intracellular habitat |
| **CELL-MEDIATED** | | | | |
| Importance | – | + | + + + (Chronic phase) | + + + + |
| Mechanism | – | | Lymphokine-mediated activation of macrophages and NK cells | Macrophage activation by lymphokines and killing by TNF, metabolites of O$_2$ and NO· Role for cytotoxic T-cells |

malaria, where historically the phenomenon was called 'premunition'. The resident and the infective forms must differ in some way yet to be pinpointed.

*Humoral immunity*

Antibodies of the right specificity present in adequate concentrations and affinity are reasonably effective in providing protection against blood-borne parasites such as *Trypanosoma brucei* and the sporozoite and merozoite stages of malaria. Thus individuals receiving IgG from solidly immune adults in malaria endemic areas are themselves temporarily protected against infection, the effector mechanisms being opsonization and phagocytosis, and complement-dependent lysis.

A marked feature of the immune reaction to helminthic infections such as *Trichinella spiralis* in man and *Nippostrongylus brasiliensis* in the rat is the eosinophilia and the high level of IgE antibody produced. In man, serum levels of IgE can rise from normal values of around 100 ng/ml to as high as 10 000 ng/ml. These changes have all the hallmarks of response to TH2-type lymphokines (cf. p. 184) and it is notable that in animals infected with helminths, injection of anti-IL-4 greatly reduces IgE production and anti-IL-5 suppresses the eosinophilia. This exceptional increase in IgE has encouraged the view that it represents an important line of defense. One can see

that antigen-specific triggering of IgE-coated mast cells would lead to exudation of serum proteins containing high concentrations of protective antibodies in all the major Ig classes and the release of eosinophil chemotactic factor. It is relevant to note that schistosomules, the early immature form of the schistosome, have been killed in cultures containing both specific IgG and eosinophils, which induce a form of ADCC by binding through their FcγRII receptors to the IgG-coated organism (figure 13.21); after 12 hours or so, the major basic protein forming the electron-dense core of the eosinophilic granules is released onto the parasite and brings about its destruction. A contribution to this process from CMI is emerging, since eosinophils can express class II MHC and their IgG-mediated ADCC is strongly enhanced by granulocyte–macrophage colony-stimulating factor (GM-CSF) and TNF. Further evidence for an involvement of this cell comes from the experiment in which the protection afforded by passive transfer of antiserum *in vivo* was blocked by pretreatment of the recipient with an antieosinophil serum. It has recently been found that eosinophils can also kill IgE-coated schistosomules but the mechanism is different because activation of the IgE (FcεRI) receptors now triggers release of platelet activating factors and the eosinophil peroxidase. This dichotomy in Fcγ and Fcε receptor pathways is also evident from reports that IgE but not IgG can mediate schistosome killing by

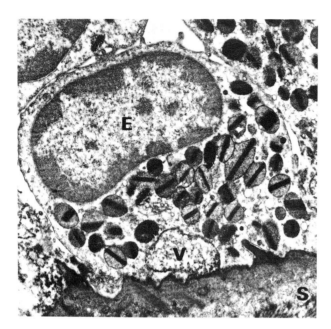

**Figure 13.21.** Electron micrograph showing an eosinophil (E) attached to the surface of a schistosomulum (S) in the presence of specific antibody. The cell develops large vacuoles (V) which appear to release their contents on to the parasite (×16 500). (Courtesy of Drs D.J. McLaren & C.D. Mackenzie.)

macrophages or platelets. There is a further complication: engagement of the eosinophil receptor for secretory IgA releases the peroxidase plus a neurotoxic protein derived from the granules. There is no telling what will happen next.

Two further points are in order. The IgE-mediated reactions may be vital for recovery from infection, whereas the resistance in vaccinated hosts may be more dependent upon preformed IgG and IgA antibodies.

### Cell-mediated immunity

Just like mycobacteria, many parasites have adapted to life within the macrophage despite the possession by that cell of potent microbicidal mechanisms recently shown to include NO· (figure 13.22). Intracellular organisms such as *Toxoplasma gondii*, *Trypanosoma cruzi* and *Leishmania* spp. use a variety of ploys to subvert the macrophage killing systems (see below) but again, as with mycobacterial infections, cytokine-producing T-cells are crucially important for the stimulation of macrophages to release their killing power and dispose of the unwanted intruders. The whole effect can be witnessed *in vitro* when IFNγ, preferably amplified by TNFα, is added to cultures of macrophages supporting the intracellular growth of *Leishmania donovani* and *T. cruzi*.

*In vivo*, the balance of cytokines produced may be of

the utmost importance. Infection of mice with *Leishmania major* is instructive in this respect; the organism produces fatal disease in susceptible mice but other strains are resistant. This is partly controlled by alleles of the *Nramp-1* gene (cf. p. 271) but as discussed earlier in Chapter 10, in susceptible mice there is excessive stimulation of TH2-like cells producing IL-4 which do not help to eliminate the infection, whereas resistant strains are characterized by the expansion of TH1-type cells which secrete IFNγ in response to antigen presented by macrophages harboring *living* protozoa. Combined therapy of susceptible strains with the leishmanicidal drug, Pentostam, plus IL-12 which recruits TH1 cells, provides promise that TH2 activities which exacerbate disease can be switched to protective TH1 responses. CD4 clones which recognize only *lysates* of the organism do not confer protection even though they produce IFNγ, a point to be borne in mind in designing vaccines. As for CD8 cells, little ripples here and there betoken an important contribution yet to be revealed. For example, susceptible strains of mice immunized with killed *L. major* lose their resistance to infection with live parasites if depleted of their CD8 cells. Further, β2-microglobulin 'knockout' mice which cannot express MHC class I, are readily infected with *T. cruzi*; there are no inflammatory cells around the parasites which raises a question regarding the role of CD8 lymphocytes in recruiting inflammatory cells into the lesion.

Organisms such as malarial plasmodia, and incidentally rickettsiae and chlamydiae, that live in cells which are not professional phagocytes, may be elimi-

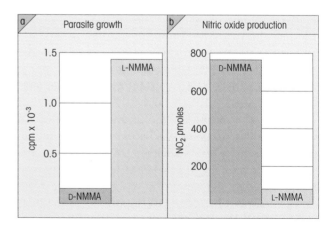

**Figure 13.22. Role of NO· in macrophage leishmanicidal activity.** The NO· synthase inhibitor L-NMMA (50 mM) inhibits the ability of macrophages to kill intracellular *Leishmania* (a) where growth is monitored by [3H]thymidine incorporation and also blocks NO production (b) measured by accumulation of $NO_2^-$ in the culture supernatant at 72 hours. The D-isomer, D-NMMA, used as a control does not inhibit the enzyme. (Data taken from Liew F.Y. & Cox F.E.G. (1991) *Immunology Today* **12**, A17–21.)

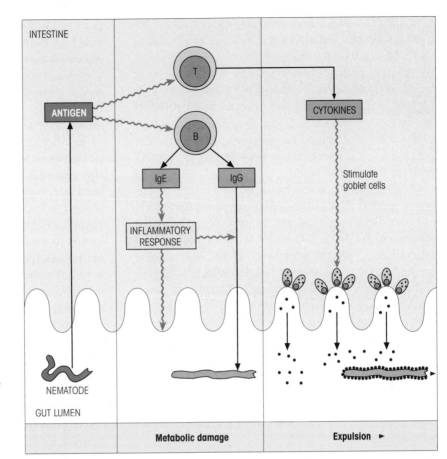

**Figure 13.23. The expulsion of nematode worms from the gut.** The parasite is first damaged by IgG antibody passing into the gut lumen, perhaps as a consequence of IgE-mediated inflammation and possibly aided by accessory ADCC cells. Cytokines released by antigen-specific triggering of T-cells stimulate proliferation of goblet cells and secretion of mucous materials, which coat the damaged worm and facilitate its expulsion from the body by increased gut motility induced by mast cell mediators such as leukotriene-D4 and diarrhea resulting from inhibition of glucose-dependent sodium absorption by mast cell-derived histamine and $PGE_2$.

nated through activation of intracellular defense mechanisms by IFNγ released from CD8-positive T-cells or even by direct cytotoxicity. This is very much the case in hepatic cells harboring malarial sporozoites, and it is pertinent to note that, following the recognition of an association between HLA-Bw53 and protection against severe malaria, Bw53-restricted Tc reacting with a conserved nonamer from a liver stage-specific antigen have been demonstrated in the peripheral blood of such resistant individuals. A large case control study of malaria in Gambian children showed that the protective Bw53 class I antigen is common in West Africa but rare in other racial groups, lending further credence to the hypothesis that MHC polymorphism has evolved primarily through natural selection by infectious pathogens.

Eliminating worm infestations of the gut is a more tricky operation and the combined forces of cellular and humoral immunity are required to expel the unwanted guest. One of the models studied is the response to *Nippostrongylus brasiliensis*; transfer studies in rats (Ogilvie) have shown that, although antibody produces some damage to the worms, T-cells from *immune* donors are also required for vigor-

ous expulsion which is probably achieved through a combination of mast cell-mediated stimulation of intestinal motility and cytokine activation of the innumerable intestinal goblet cells. These secrete a complex mixture of densely glycosylated high molecular weight molecules which form a viscoelastic gel around the worm, so protecting the colonic and intestinal surfaces from invasion (figure 13.23). Another model, this time of *Trichinella spiralis* infection in mice, again hints at a duality of T-subset cytokine responses. One strain, which expels adult worms rapidly, makes large amounts of IFNγ and IgG2a antibody, while in contrast, more susceptible mice made miserly amounts of IFNγ and favored IgG1, IgA and IgE antibody classes. Clearly the protective strategy varies with the infection.

## Evasive strategies by the parasite

### Resistance to effector mechanisms

Two tricks to pre-empt the complement defenses are of interest. *T. cruzi* has elegantly created a DAF-like molecule (cf. p. 313) which accelerates the decay of

C3b. The cercarii of *Schistosoma mansoni* activate complement directly but eject the bound C3 by shedding their glycocalyx. In a similar fashion, malarial sporozoites shed their circumsporozoite antigen when it binds antibody and *Trypanosoma brucei* releases its surface antigens into solution to act as decoy proteins (p. 260). In each case, these shedding and decoy systems are well suited to parasites or stages in the parasite life cycle which are only briefly in contact with the immune system.

We have already mentioned the way in which different protozoal parasites hide away from the effects of antibody by using the interior of a macrophage as a sanctuary. To do this they must block the normal microbicidal mechanisms and they use similar methods to those deployed by intracellular obligate and facultative bacteria (cf. p. 267). *Toxoplasma gondii* inhibits phagosome–lysosome fusion by lining up host cell mitochondria along the phagosome membrane. *Trypanosoma cruzi* escapes from the confines of the phagosome into the cytoplasm, while *Leishmania* parasites are surrounded by a lipophosphoglycan which protects them from the oxidative burst by scavenging oxygen radicals. They also downregulate expression of MHC and B7 so diminishing T-cell stimulation.

### Avoiding antigen recognition by the host

Some parasites **disguise** themselves to look like the host. This can be achieved by molecular mimicry as instanced by cross-reactivity between *Ascaris* antigens and human collagen. Another way is to cover the surface with host protein. Schistosomes are very good at that; the adult worm takes up host red-cell glycoproteins, MHC molecules and IgG and lives happily in the mesenteric vessels of the host, despite the fact that the blood which bathes it contains antibodies which can prevent reinfection.

Another very crafty ruse, rather akin to moving the goalposts in football, is **antigenic variation**, in which the parasites escape from the cytocidal action of humoral antibody on their cycling blood forms by the ingenious trick of altering their antigenic constitution. Figure 13.24 illustrates how the trypanosome continues to infect the host, even after fully protective antibodies appear, by switching to the expression of a new antigenic variant which these antibodies cannot inactivate; as antibodies to the new antigens are synthesized, the parasite escapes again by changing to yet a further variant and so on. In this way the parasite can remain in the bloodstream long enough to allow an opportunity for transmission by blood-sucking insects or blood-to-blood contact. The same phenomenon has been observed with *Plasmodium* spp. and this may explain why, in hyperendemic areas, children are subjected to repeated attacks of malaria for their first few years and are then solidly immune to further infection. Immunity must presumably be developed against all the antigenic variants before full protection can be attained, and indeed it is known that IgG from individuals with solid immunity can effectively terminate malaria infections in young children.

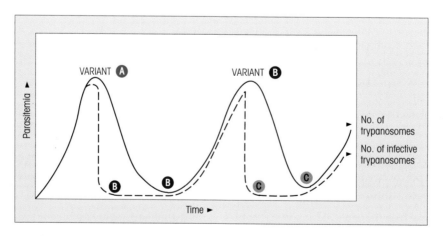

**Figure 13.24. Antigenic variation during chronic trypanosome infection.** As antibody to the initial variant A is formed, the blood trypanosomes become complexed prior to phagocytosis and are no longer infective, leaving a small number of viable parasites which have acquired a new antigenic constitution. This new variant (B) now multiplies until it, too, is neutralized by the primary antibody response and is succeeded by variant C (after A.R. Gray, see Further Reading). At any time, only one of the variant surface glycoproteins (VSG) is expressed and covers the surface of the protozoon to the exclusion of all other antigens. Nearly 9% of the genome (approx. 1000 genes) is devoted to generation of VSGs. Switching occurs by insertion of a duplicate gene into a new genomic location in proximity to the promoter.

## Deviation of the host immune response

Immunosuppression has been found in most of the parasite infections studied. During infection by *T. brucei*, for example, antibody and CMI is only 5–10% of the normal value while T-suppressor activity is prominent, presumably related to an excessive load of antigen. *Schistosoma mansoni* possesses a gene with homology for proopiomelanocortin which in the human is a prohormone that is cleaved to generate adrenocorticotropic hormone (ACTH), melanocyte stimulating hormones (MSH) and the opioid, β-endorphin. All have immunomodulatory properties and both ACTH and β-endorphin have been demonstrated in the culture medium when adult worms were incubated at 37°C in minimum essential medium; if neutrophils are added to the system, α-melanocyte stimulating hormone derived from ACTH by the PMN endopeptidase (CD10; CALLA, p. 387) is also formed.

Parasites may also manipulate T-cell subsets to their own advantage. Filiariasis provides a case in point: it has been suggested that individuals with persistent microfilariae fail to mount presumably protective immediate hypersensitivity responses including IgE and eosinophilia as a result of active suppression of T$_{H2}$ type lymphocytes.

Epidemiological surveys accord with a protective role for IgE antibodies in schistosomiasis but they also reveal a susceptible population producing IgM and IgG4 antibodies which can block ADDC dependent upon IgE. The ability of certain helminths to activate IgE producing B-cells polyclonally is good for the parasite and correspondingly not so good for the host, since a high concentration of irrelevant IgE binding to a mast cell will crowd out the parasite-specific IgE molecules and diminish the possibility of triggering the mast cell by specific antigen to initiate a protective defensive reaction.

## Immunopathology

Where parasites persist chronically in the face of an immune response, the interaction with foreign antigen frequently produces tissue damaging reactions. One example is the immune-complex induced-nephrotic syndrome of Nigerian children associated with quartan malaria. Increased levels of TNF are responsible for pulmonary changes in acute malaria, cerebral malaria in mice and severe wasting of cattle with trypanosomiasis. Another example is the liver damage resulting from IL-4-mediated granuloma formation around schistosome eggs (cf. figure 16.8o); one of the egg antigens directly induces IL-10 production in B-cells thereby contributing to T$_{H2}$ dominance. Remarkably, the hypersensitivity reaction helps the eggs to escape from the intestinal blood capillaries into the gut lumen to continue the cycle outside the body, an effect mediated by TNFα.

Cross-reaction between parasite and self may give rise to autoimmunity and this has been proposed as the basis for the cardiomyopathy in Chagas' disease. It is also pertinent that the nonspecific immunosuppression which is so widespread in parasitic diseases tends to increase susceptibility to bacterial and viral infections and, in this context, the association between Burkitt's lymphoma and malaria has been ascribed to an inadequate host response to the Epstein–Barr virus.

## SUMMARY

Immunity to infection involves a constant battle between the host defenses and the mutant microbes trying to evolve evasive strategies.

### Inflammation revisited

• Inflammation is a major defensive reaction initiated by infection or tissue injury.
• The mediators released upregulate adhesion molecules on endothelial cells and leukocytes, which pair together causing first rolling of leukocytes along the vessel wall and then passage across the blood vessel up the chemotactic gradient to the site of inflammation.

• IL-1, TNFα and chemokines such as IL-8 are involved in maintaining the inflammatory process.
• Inflammation is controlled by complement regulatory proteins, PGE$_2$, TGFβ, glucocorticoids and IL-10. LPS is scavenged by specific receptors.
• Inability to eliminate the initiating agent leads to a chronic inflammatory response dominated by macrophages often forming granulomata.

### Extracellular bacteria susceptible to killing by phagocytosis and complement

• Bacteria try to avoid phagocytosis by surrounding

*(Continued on p. 282)*

themselves with capsules, secreting exotoxins which kill phagocytes or impede inflammatory reactions, deviating complement to inoffensive sites or by colonizing relatively inaccessible locations.

• Antibody combats these tricks by neutralizing the toxins, making complement deposition more even on the bacterial surface, overcoming the antiphagocytic nature of the capsules by opsonizing them with Ig and C3b.

• The secretory immune system protects the external mucosal surfaces. IgA inhibits adherence of bacteria and can opsonize them. IgE bound to mast cells can initiate the influx of protective IgG, complement and polymorphs to the site by a miniature acute inflammatory response.

## Bacteria which grow in an intracellular habitat

• Intracellular bacteria such as tubercle and leprosy bacilli grow within macrophages. They defy killing mechanisms by blocking macrophage activation, scavenging oxygen radicals, inhibiting lysosome fusion, having strong outer coats and by escaping from the phagosome into the cytoplasm.

• They are killed by CMI: specifically sensitized T-helpers release lymphokines on contact with infected macrophages which powerfully activate the formation of nitric oxide (NO·), reactive oxygen intermediates (ROI) and other microbicidal mechanisms.

## Immunity to viral infection

• Viruses try to avoid the immune system by changes in the antigenicity of their surface antigens. Point mutations bring about minor changes (antigenic drift) but radical changes leading to endemics can result from wholesale swapping of genetic material with different viruses in other animal hosts (antigenic shift).

• Some viruses subvert the function of the complement system to their own advantage.

• Antibody neutralizes free virus and is particularly effective when the virus has to travel through the bloodstream before reaching its final target.

• Where the target is the same as the portal of entry, e.g. the lungs, interferon is dominant in recovery from infection.

• Antibody is important in preventing reinfection.

• 'Budding' viruses which can invade lateral cells without becoming exposed to antibody are combated by CMI. Infected cells express a processed viral antigen peptide on their surface in association with MHC class I a short time after entry of the virus, and rapid killing of the cell by cytotoxic αβ-T-cells prevents viral multiplication which depends upon the replicative machinery of the intact host cell. γδ-Tc recognize native viral coat protein on the target cell surface. NK cells are also cytotoxic.

• T-cells and macrophages producing γ-interferon and TNF bathe the contiguous cells and prevent them from becoming infected by lateral spread of virus.

## Immunity to parasitic infections

• Diseases involving *protozoal parasites* and *helminths* affect hundreds of millions of people. Antibodies are usually effective against the blood-borne forms. IgE production is notoriously increased in worm infestations and can lead to mast-cell-mediated influx of Ig and eosinophils; schistosomes coated with IgG or IgE are killed by adherent eosinophils through extracellular mechanisms involving release of cationic proteins and peroxidase.

• Organisms such as *Leishmania* spp., *Trypanosoma cruzi* and *Toxoplasma gondii* hide from antibodies inside macrophages and use the same strategies as intracellular parasitic bacteria to survive, and like them are killed when the macrophages are activated by TH1 cytokines produced during cell-mediated immune responses. NO· is an important killing agent.

• CD8 cells also have a protective role.

• Expulsion of intestinal worms usually depends heavily on TH2 responses and requires the coordinated action of antibody, the release of mucin by cytokine-stimulated goblet cells and the production of intestinal contraction and diarrhea by mast cell mediators.

• Some parasites avoid recognition by disguising themselves as the host, either through molecular mimicry or by absorbing host proteins to their surface.

• Other organisms such as *Trypanosoma brucei* and various malarial species have the extraordinary ability to cover their surface with a dominant antigen which is changed by genetic switch mechanisms to a different molecule as antibody is formed to the first variant.

• Most parasites also tend to produce nonspecific suppression of host responses.

• Chronic persistence of parasite antigen in the face of an immune response often produces tissue-damaging immunopathological reactions such as immune complex nephrotic syndrome, liver granulomata and autoimmune lesions of the heart. Generalized immunosuppression increases susceptibility to bacterial and viral infections.

• As the features of the response to infection are analysed, we see more clearly how the specific acquired response operates to amplify and enhance innate immune mechanisms; the interactions are summarized in figure 13.25.

(Continued)

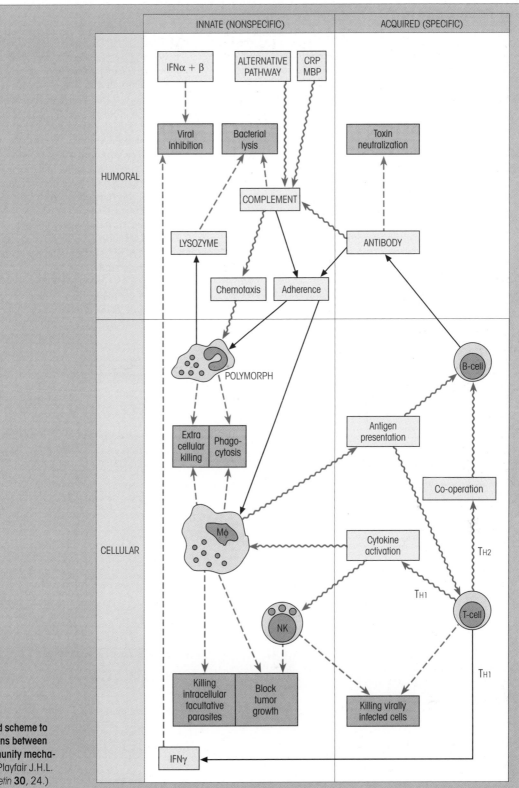

**Figure 13.25. Simplified scheme to emphasize the interactions between innate and acquired immunity mechanisms.** (Developed from Playfair J.H.L. (1974) *British Medical Bulletin* **30**, 24.)

# FURTHER READING

Adamson J.W. (ed.) (1993) *Current Opinion in Hematology*. Current Science, London. (Articles on 'Cytokines in acute inflammation', pp. 26–32, and series on 'Functions and disorders of leukocytes', pp. 91–166.)

Blackwell J.M. (1996) Structure and function of the natural-resistance-associated macrophage (Nramp 1), a candidate protein for infectious disease susceptibility. *Molecular Medicine Today* **2**, 205.

Bloom B.R. (ed.) (1994) *Tuberculosis: Pathogenesis, Protection and Control*. American Society Press, Washington, DC. (Reviewed by Rom W. (1996) in *Nature Medicine* **2**, 244, who suggests that this is a terrific book on the basic nature of the immune response to tuberculosis in animal research but is critical that not enough support goes to what he calls 'patient-oriented research' in which greater study is made of the phenomena which occur in the interaction between the parasite and host in the infected patient where there are many phenomena which do not occur in the experimental models.)

Bloom B. & Zinkernagel R. (eds) (1996) Immunity to infection. *Current Opinion in Immunology* **8**, 465.

Brandtzaeg P. (1995) Basic mechanisms of mucosal immunity: a major adaptive defense system. *The Immunologist* **3**, 89–96.

Cotran R.S., Kumar V. & Robbins S.L. (1989) *Pathologic Basis of Disease* Chs 1, 2. W.B. Saunders, Philadelphia.

Gazzinelli R.T. (1996) Molecular and cellular basis of interleukin 12 activity in prophylaxis and therapy against infectious diseases. *Molecular Medicine Today* **2**, 258.

Gray A.R. (1969) Antigenic variation in trypanosomes. *Bulletin of the World Health Organization* **41**, 805.

Hill A.V.S. (1992) Molecular analysis of the association of HLA-53 and resistance to severe malaria. *Nature* **360**, 434–439.

Mims C.A., Playfair J.H.L., Roitt I.M., Wakelin D. & Williams R. (1993) *Medical Microbiology*. C.V.Mosby, London. (Based on conflict of host vs microbe; systems treatment of infections; reference tables of organisms.)

Ogra P.E. *et al.* (eds) (1994) *Handbook of Mucosal Immunology*. Academic Press, Orlando.

Rollins B.J. (1996) Monocyte chemoattractant protein 1: a potential regulator of monocyte recruitment in inflammatory disease. *Molecular Medicine Today* **2**, 198.

# PROPHYLAXIS

## CONTENTS

The control of infection is approached from several directions. One method of breaking the chain of infection has been achieved in the UK with rabies and psittacosis by controlling the importation of dogs and parrots respectively. Improvements in public health—water supply, sewage systems, education in personal hygiene — prevent the spread of cholera and many other diseases; and of course when other measures fail we can fall back on the induction of immunity (Milestone 14.1).

## PASSIVELY ACQUIRED IMMUNITY

Temporary protection against infection can be established by giving preformed antibody from another individual of the same or a different species (table 14.1). As the acquired antibodies are utilized by combination with antigen or catabolized in the normal way, this protection is gradually lost.

Horse globulins containing antitetanus and antidiphtheria toxins have been extensively employed

# Milestone 14.1—Vaccination

The notion that survivors of serious infectious disease seldom contract that infection again has been embedded in folklore for centuries. In an account of the terrible plague which afflicted Athens, Thucydides noted that, in the main, those nursing the sick were individuals who had already been infected and yet recovered from the plague. Deliberate attempts to ward off infections by inducing a minor form of the disease in otherwise healthy subjects were common in China in the Middle Ages. There, they developed the practice of inhaling a powder made from **smallpox** scabs as protection against any future infection. The Indians inoculated the scab material into small skin wounds and this practice of **variolation** (Latin *varus*, a pustular facial disease) was introduced into Turkey where the inhabitants of Circassia were determined to prevent the ravages of smallpox epidemics interfering with the lucrative sale of their gorgeous daughters to the harems of the wealthy.

Voltaire, in 1773, tells us that the credit for spreading the practice of variolation to Western Europe should be attributed to Lady Wortley Montague, a remarkably enterprising woman who was the wife of the English Ambassador to Constantinople in the time of George I. With little scruple, she inoculated her daughter with smallpox in the face of the protestations of her Chaplain who felt that it could only succeed with infidels, not Christians. All went well however and the practice was taken up in England despite the hazardous nature of the procedure which had a case fatality of 0.5–2%. These dreadful risks were taken because at that time, as Voltaire recorded '… three score persons in every hundred have the smallpox. Of these three score, twenty die of it in the most favourable season of life, and as many more wear the disagreeable remains of it on their faces so long as they live.'

Edward Jenner (1749–1823), a country physician in Gloucestershire, suggested to one of his patients that she might have smallpox but she assured him that his diagnosis was impossible since she had already contracted cowpox through her chores as a milkmaid (folklore again!). This led Jenner to the series of experiments in which he showed that prior inoculation with cowpox, which was nonvirulent (i.e. nonpathogenic) in the human, protected against subsequent challenge with smallpox (cf. p. 33). His ideas initially met with violent opposition but were eventually accepted and he achieved world fame; learned societies everywhere elected him to membership, although it is intriguing to note that the College of Physicians in London required him to pass an examination in classics and the Royal Society honored him with a Fellowship on the basis of his work on the nesting behavior of the cuckoo. In the end he inoculated thousands in the shed in the garden of his house in Berkeley, Gloucestershire which now functions as a museum and venue for small symposia organized by the British Society of Immunology (rather fun to visit if you get the chance).

The next seminal development in vaccines came through the research of Louis Pasteur who had developed the germ theory of disease. A culture of chicken cholera bacillus which had accidently been left on a bench during the warm summer months lost much of its ability to cause disease; nonetheless, birds which had been inoculated with this old culture were resistant to fresh virulent cultures of the bacillus. This **attenuation** of **virulent** organisms was reproduced by Pasteur for anthrax and rabies using abnormal culture and passage conditions. Recognizing the relevance of Jenner's research for his own experiments, Pasteur called his treatment **vaccination**, a term which has stood the test of time.

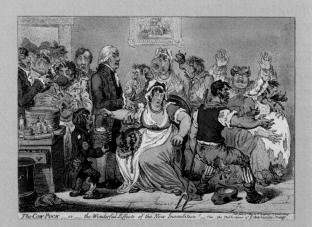

**Figure M14.1.1.** Edward Jenner among patients in the Smallpox and Inoculation Hospital at St Pancras. Etching after J. Gillray, 1802. (Kindly supplied by The Wellcome Centre Medical Photographic Library, London.)

**Table 14.1. Passive immunotherapy with antibody.**

| INFECTION | SOURCE OF ANTIBODY | | USE |
|---|---|---|---|
| | HORSE | HUMAN | |
| Tetanus Diphtheria | √ | √ | Prophylaxis Treatment |
| Botulism Gas gangrene Snake or scorpion bite | √ | – | Treatment |
| Varicella zoster | – | √ | Treatment immunodeficiency |
| Rabies | – | √ | Post-exposure to vaccine |
| Hepatitis B | – | √ | Treatment |
| Hepatitis A Measles | – | Pooled Ig | Prophylaxis (Travel) Treatment |

prophylactically, but at the present time the practice is more restricted because of the complication of serum sickness developing in response to the foreign protein. This is more likely to occur in subjects already sensitized by previous contact with horse globulin; thus individuals who have been given horse antitetanus (e.g. for immediate protection after receiving a wound out in the open) are later advised to undergo a course of active immunization to obviate the need for further injections of horse protein in any subsequent emergency.

## Maternally acquired antibody

In the first few months of life while the baby's own lymphoid system is slowly getting under way, protection is afforded by maternally derived antibodies acquired by placental transfer and by intestinal absorption of colostral immunoglobulins. The major immunoglobulin in milk is secretory IgA and this is not absorbed by the baby but remains in the intestine to protect the mucosal surfaces. In this respect it is quite striking that the sIgA antibodies are directed against bacterial and viral antigens often present in the intestine, and it is presumed that IgA-producing cells, responding to gut antigens, migrate and colonize breast tissue (as part of the MALT immune system; see p. 161), where the antibodies they produce appear in the milk. The case for mucosal vaccination of future mothers against selected infections is inescapable.

## Pooled human γ-globulin

Regular injection of pooled human adult γ-globulin is an essential treatment for patients with long-standing immunodeficiency. The preparations are also of value to modify the effects of chicken pox or measles in other individuals with defective immune responses, such as premature infants, children with protein malnutrition or patients on steroid treatment. Contacts with cases of infectious hepatitis and smallpox may also be afforded protection by γ-globulin, especially when in the latter case the material is derived from the serum of individuals vaccinated some weeks previously. Human antitetanus immunoglobulin is preferable to horse antitoxin serum, which may cause hypersensitivity reactions. Curiously, pooled γ-globulin is being increasingly used as a treatment for autoimmune diseases such as idiopathic thrombocytopenic purpura, possibly acting through anti-idiotypic mechanisms.

Isolated γ-globulin preparations tend to form small aggregates spontaneously and these can lead to severe anaphylactic reactions when administered intravenously, on account of their ability to aggregate platelets and to activate complement and generate C3a and C5a anaphylatoxins. For this reason the material is always injected intramuscularly. Preparations free of aggregates are available and separate pools with raised antibody titers to selected organisms such as vaccinia, Herpes zoster, tetanus and perhaps rubella would be welcome. This need may ultimately be satisfied as it becomes possible to produce human monoclonal antibodies on demand.

## Cultured antibodies made to order

The techniques for producing human monoclonal antibodies to predetermined specificities still leave something to be desired but they are improving steadily. Restlessly we look to recombinant DNA technology to engineer antibodies of very high affinity. We have described different approaches to the production of antibodies which circumvent the need for intervention by a host immune system such as the single chain Fv ($V_H$-$V_L$) construct (cf. p. 124) and the single $V_H$ domain antibodies. The latter, being so small, may well be capable of reaching cell receptors on viruses which are tucked away at the bottom of protein canyons where they might be inaccessible to the Fv of an intact antibody but the sticky nature of these $V_H$ domains could be a serious impediment to their use. Expression of **antibody genes in plants** is going to be big business. If it were feasible to produce IgA antibodies coupled to secretory piece in this way, they should provide an invaluable supplement to dried cows' milk baby food in cases where the mother's milk was of poor quality.

Never neglect innate immune mechanisms. Defensins, the broad range antimicrobial peptides present in polymorphonuclear neutrophil (PMN) granules (cf. p. 10), are now being engineered in tobacco plants and it is planned to use them for fungal and bacterial infections which become refactory to conventional antibiotics. A good example of lateral thinking by the project leaders.

## Adoptive transfer of cytotoxic T-cells

This is a labor-intensive operation and will be restricted to instances where the donor shares an MHC class I allele. To give one example, up to 30% of recipients of bone marrow allografts from mismatched family members or matched unrelated donors develop Epstein–Barr virus (EBV) lymphoma. Pilot studies aimed at potential prophylaxis showed that EBV-induced cytotoxic T-cell (Tc) lines transferred to the bone marrow recipients reconstituted the patients' immune responses to EBV for at least 18 months.

# VACCINATION

## Herd immunity

In the case of tetanus, active immunization is of benefit to the individual but not to the community since it will not eliminate the organism which is formed in the faeces of domestic animals and persists in the soil as highly resistant spores. Where a disease depends on human transmission, immunity in just a proportion of the population can help the whole community if it leads to a fall in the reproduction rate (i.e. the number of further cases produced by each

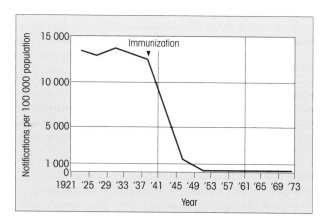

**Figure 14.1.  Notification of diphtheria in England and Wales per 100 000 population** showing dramatic fall after immunization. (Reproduced from Dick G. (1978) *Immunisation.* Update Books; with kind permission of the author and publishers.)

infected individual) to less than one; under these circumstances the disease will die out, witness for example the disappearance of diphtheria from communities in which around 75% of the children have been immunized (figure 14.1). But this figure must be maintained; there is no room for complacency. In contrast, focal outbreaks of poliomyelitis have occurred in communities which object to immunization on religious grounds, raising an important point for parents in general.

## Strategic considerations

The objective of vaccination is to provide effective immunity by establishing adequate levels of antibody and a primed population of memory cells which can rapidly expand on renewed contact with antigen and so provide protection against infection. Sometimes, as with polio infection, a high blood titer of antibody is required; in mycobacterial diseases such as tuberculosis (TB), a macrophage-activating cell-mediated immunity (CMI) is most effective, whereas with influenza virus infection, cytotoxic T-cells probably play a significant role. The site of the immune response evoked by vaccination may also be most important. For example in cholera, antibodies need to be in the gut lumen to inhibit adherence to and colonization of the intestinal wall.

Eradication of the infectious agent is not always the most practical goal. To take the example of malaria, the blood-borne form releases molecules which trigger tumor necrosis factor (TNF) and other cytokines from monocytes and the secretion of these mediators is responsible for the unpleasant effects of the disease. Accordingly, an antibody response targeted to these released antigens with structurally conserved epitopes may be a more realistic strategy than running after the more elusive antigen-swapping parasite itself. Under these circumstances life with the parasite might be acceptable.

In addition to an ability to engender effective immunity, a number of mundane but nonetheless crucial conditions must be satisfied for a vaccine to be considered successful (table 14.2). The antigens must be readily available, the preparation should be stable, it should be cheap and, certainly, safe. Clearly the first contact with antigen during vaccination should not be injurious and the maneuver is to avoid the pathogenic effects of infection, while maintaining protective immunogens.

## KILLED ORGANISMS AS VACCINES

The simplest way to destroy the ability of microbes to

Table 14.2. Factors required for a successful vaccine.

| FACTOR | REQUIREMENTS |
|---|---|
| Effectiveness | Must evoke protective levels of immunity: at the appropriate site of relevant nature (Ab, Tc, $T_{H1}$, $T_{H2}$) of adequate duration |
| Availability | Readily cultured in bulk or accessible source of subunit |
| Stability | Stable under extreme climatic conditions, preferably not requiring refrigeration |
| Cheapness | What is cheap in the West may be expensive in developing countries but WHO tries to help |
| Safety | Eliminate any pathogenicity |

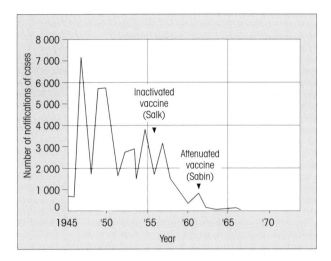

**Figure 14.2. Notifications of paralytic poliomyelitis in England and Wales** showing the beneficial effects of community immunization with killed and live vaccines. (Reproduced from Dick G. (1978) *Immunisation*. Update Books; with kind permission of the author and publishers.)

cause disease yet maintain their antigenic constitution is to prevent their replication by killing in an appropriate manner. Parasitic worms and, to a lesser extent, protozoa are extremely difficult to grow up in bulk to manufacture killed vaccines. This problem does not arise for many bacteria and viruses and, in these cases, the inactivated microorganisms have generally provided safe antigens for immunization. Examples are typhoid (in combination with the relatively ineffective paratyphoid A and B), cholera and killed poliomyelitis (Salk) vaccines. The success of the Salk vaccine was slightly marred by a small rise in the incidence of deaths from poliomyelitis in 1960–61 (figure 14.2), but this has now been attributed to poor antigenicity of one of the three different strains of virus used and present-day vaccines are far more potent. Care has to be taken to ensure that important protective antigens are not destroyed in the inactivation process. During the production of an early killed measles vaccine, the fusion antigen, which permits cellular spread of virus, was inactivated; as a result, incomplete immunity was produced and this left the individual susceptible to the development of immunopathological complications on subsequent natural infection. The dangers of incomplete immunity are especially worrying in areas where measles is endemic and the immune response is relatively enfeebled due to protein malnutrition. Since the widespread correction of this dietary deficiency is unlikely in the near future, it is worth considering whether nonspecific stimulation by immunopotentiating drugs or thymus hormones at the time of vaccination might provide a feasible solution.

This idea of supplementing a deficient adaptive immune response with some synergistic treatment has surfaced in other contexts. Thus, the antibiotic polymyxin B is too toxic for normal use; however, if certain end groups are removed, the molecule loses its

toxicity but still retains its ability to disturb the outer wall of Gram-negative bacteria, thereby allowing potentially lytic antibodies and complement to reach previously inaccessible bacterial inner membranes. Another curious phenomenon which might be exploited is the finding that the amoeba *Entamoeba histolytica*, which is resistant to lysis by antibody and complement, shows greatly increased susceptibility if treated with an otherwise nontoxic protein inhibitor.

## LIVE ATTENUATED ORGANISMS HAVE MANY ADVANTAGES AS VACCINES

The objective of attenuation is to produce a modified organism which mimics the natural behavior of the original microbe without causing significant disease. In many instances the immunity conferred by killed vaccines, even when given with adjuvant (see below), is often inferior to that resulting from infection with live organisms. This must be partly because the replication of the living microbes confronts the host with a **larger and more sustained dose of antigen** and that, with budding viruses, infected cells are required for the establishment of good **cytotoxic T-cell memory**. Another significant advantage of using live organisms is that the immune **response takes place largely at the site of the natural infection**. This is well illustrated by the nasopharyngeal IgA response to immunization with polio vaccine: In contrast with the ineffectiveness of parenteral injection of killed vaccine, intranasal administration evoked a good local antibody response; however, whereas this declined over a period of 2 months or so, per oral

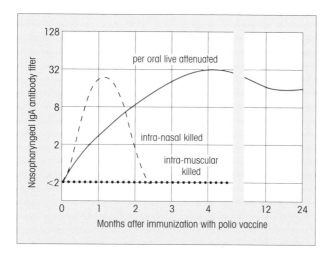

**Figure 14.3. Local IgA response to polio vaccine.** Local secretory antibody synthesis is confined to the specific anatomical sites which have been directly stimulated by contact with antigen. (Data from Ogra P.L. *et al.* (1975) In: Notkins A.L. (ed.) *Viral Immunology and Immunopathology*, p. 67. Academic Press, New York.)

immunization with *live attenuated* virus established a persistently high IgA antibody level (figure 14.3).

There is in fact a strong upsurge of interest in strategies for mucosal immunization. Remember, the MALT system involves mucous membranes covering the aerodigestive and urogenital tracts as well as the conjunctiva, the ear and the ducts of all exocrine glands which are essentially protected by sIgA antibodies. Resident T-cells in these tissues produce large amounts of transforming growth factor-β (TGFβ), and the interleukins IL-10 and IL-4, which promote the B-cell switch to IgA, and note also that human intestinal epithelial cells themselves are major sources of TGFβ and IL-10. Site-specific vaccination can lead to a degree of compartmentalization within the MALT system. After oral immunization there is antibody production in the small intestine and some exocrine glands including mammary and salivary glands, but little in the large intestine, tonsil or female genital tract. Intranasal immunization, on the other hand, gives rise to antibody production in the mucosa of the upper airways and in salivary glands without evoking an immune response in the gut.

## Classical methods of attenuation

The objective of attenuation, that of producing an organism which causes only a very mild form of the natural disease, can be equally well attained if one can identify heterologous strains which are virulent for another species, but avirulent in man. The best example of this was Jenner's seminal demonstration that cowpox would protect against smallpox. Since

then, a truly remarkable global effort by the World Health Organization, combining extensive vaccination and selective epidemiological control methods, **has completely eradicated the human disease** — a wonderful achievement.

Attenuation itself can be achieved by modifying the conditions under which an organism grows. Pasteur first achieved the production of live but nonvirulent forms of chicken cholera bacillus and anthrax (cf. Milestone 14.1) by such artifices as culture at higher temperatures and under anaerobic conditions, and was able to confer immunity by infection with the attenuated organisms. A virulent strain of *Mycobacterium tuberculosis* became attenuated by chance in 1908 when Calmette and Guérin at the Institut Pasteur, Lille, added bile to the culture medium in an attempt to achieve dispersed growth. After 13 years of culture in bile-containing medium, the strain remained attenuated and was used successfully to vaccinate children against tuberculosis. The same organism, BCG (bacille Calmette–Guérin), is widely used today for immunization of tuberculin-negative individuals. Attenuation by cold adaptation of influenza and other respiratory viruses seems hopeful; the organism can grow at the lower temperatures (32–34°C) of the upper respiratory tract, but fails to produce clinical disease because of its inability to replicate in the lower respiratory tract (37°C).

## Attenuation by recombinant DNA technology

Genetic recombination is being used to develop various attenuated strains of viruses such as influenza with lower virulence for man and some with an increased multiplication rate in eggs (enabling newly endemic strains of influenza to be adapted for rapid vaccine production). The potential is clearly quite enormous.

The **tropism** of attenuated organisms for **the site** at which **natural infection** occurs is likely to be exploited dramatically in the near future to establish gut immunity to typhoid and cholera using attenuated forms of *Salmonella* strains and *Vibrio cholerae* in which the virulence genes have been identified and modified by genetic engineering.

## Microbial vectors for other genes

An ingenious trick is to use a virus as a 'piggyback' for genes from another virus, particularly one that cannot be grown successfully, or which is inherently dangerous. Large DNA viruses, such as vaccinia, can act as carriers for one or many foreign genes while retaining infectivity for animals and cultured cells. The proteins encoded by these genes are appropriately expressed *in vivo* with respect to glycosylation and secretion, and are processed for major histocompatibility complex (MHC) presentation by the infected cells, thus effectively endowing the host with both humoral and CMI. Proteins placed under the control of promoters for early gene expression tend to favor the generation of cytotoxic T-cells, whereas both early and late promoters engender good antibody production. An example of a construct in which vaccinia is a vector for an inserted foreign gene is described in figure 14.4.

A wide variety of genes has been expressed by vaccinia virus vectors and it has been demonstrated that the products of genes coding for viral envelope proteins such as influenza virus hemagglutinin, vesicular stomatis virus glycoprotein, human immunodeficiency virus (HIV)-1 gp120 and herpes simplex virus glycoprotein D, could be correctly processed and inserted into the plasma membrane of infected cells. Hepatitis surface antigen (HBsAg) was secreted from recombinant vaccinia virus infected cells as the characteristic 22 nm particles. It is an impressive approach and chimpanzees have been protected against the

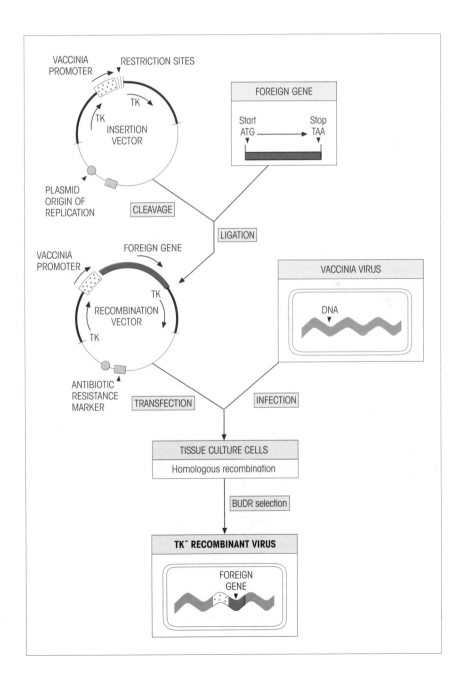

**Figure 14.4. Construction of vaccinia virus recombinants that express a foreign gene.** The gene in question, say encoding hepatitis surface antigen (HBsAg), is first inserted into an appropriate vector so that it is adjacent to a vaccinia promoter and flanking vaccinia DNA sequences (in this case thymidine kinase—TK) which determines the site of recombination with the virus. The plasmid is replicated and then used to transfect cells that are simultaneously infected with vaccinia. Homologous recombination inserts the promoter plus foreign gene into the viral genome and the resulting TK recombinant is selected by picking viral plaques resistant to 5-bromodeoxyuridine (BUDR). TK is not essential for viral growth. (Reproduced from Moss B. (1985) *Immunology Today* **6**, 243, with permission.)

clinical effects of hepatitis B virus, while mice inoculated with recombinant influenza hemagglutinin generated cytotoxic T-cells and were protected against influenza infection. Spectacular neutralizing antibody titers were produced by a construct with the gene encoding rabies virus glycoprotein and protected animals against a severe intracerebral challenge. It is even possible to make a vector with two inserts.

No system is trouble free and some recombinants grow poorly *in vivo*. Furthermore, immunodeficient individuals have difficulty in clearing the virus, although the resistance of nude mice lacking T-cells to $10^8$ plaque-forming units of recombinant vaccinia expressing the IL-2 gene suggests a way around this problem. There is also the objection that a viral vaccine which produces occasional but serious side-effects should not be used in a world free of smallpox. The attenuated strains so far employed have unacceptably high levels of complications, ranging from 1 in 300 000 for severe neurological effects to 1 in 1000 for serious complications such as disseminated vaccinia and vaccinia gangrenosum. The classic Copenhagen strain has now been subject to precise deletions in 18 open-reading frames and should therefore be highly attenuated. Avipoxes such as canary pox virus produce abortive infections in mammalian cells and look to have a future. Although based on the same principles as those used for vaccinia virus, there may be a more favorable climate regarding the acceptance of hybrid polio viruses as potential vaccines in the human, and HIV and hepatitis A genes have all been inserted into the polio genome and shown to produce neutralizing antibodies.

The real issue, as ever, is whether the recombinant vaccine causes more problems than the disease for which a vaccine is sought. For veterinary use, of course, there is no problem and excellent results have been obtained using existing vaccinia strains with rinderpest in cattle and rabies in foxes for example. In the latter case, a recombinant vaccinia virus vaccine expressing the rabies surface glycoprotein was distributed with bait from the air and immunized approximately 80% of the foxes in that area. No cases of rabies have since been seen but epidemiological considerations indicate that with the higher fox density that this leads to, the higher the percentage which have to be made immune; thus, either one has to increase the efficacy of the vaccine, or culling of the animals must continue — an interesting consequence of interference with ecosystems. Less complicated is the use of such immunization to control local outbreaks of rabies in rare mammalian species such as

the African wild dog in certain game reserves which are threatened with extinction by the virus.

For humans, there is more safety in switching to plants, using viruses such as cowpea mosaic virus and potato virus X, which cannot infect mammalian cells, to express recombinant proteins. Their robustness and resistance to acid and proteolysis makes them attractive vehicles for oral immunization.

Attention has turned to BCG as a vehicle for antigens required to evoke CD4-mediated T-cell immunity. The organism is avirulent, has a low frequency of serious complications, can be administered any time after birth, has strong adjuvant properties, gives long-lasting CMI after a single injection and is a bargain at around US $0.05 a shot. The development of shuttle vectors which can replicate in *E. coli* as plasmids and in mycobacteria as phages has allowed foreign DNA to be introduced into *M. smegmatis* and BCC vaccine strains. We can expect many advances on this front: thus incorporation of a gene for kanamycin resistance into the plasmid provides a selectable marker for transformed bacteria, while inclusion of a signal sequence permits secretion of the recombinant protein. Recombinant BCG, engineered to express the outer surface protein A (OspA) of *Borrelia* in its cell membrane, induced excellent antibody titres. For those interested, *Borrelia burgdorferi* is the cause of Lyme disease associated with an arthritic condition.

The ability of *Salmonella* to elicit **mucosal responses by oral immunization**, has been exploited by the design of vectors which allow the expression of any protein antigen linked to *E. coli* enterotoxin, a powerful mucosal immunostimulant. There is an attractive possibility that the oral route of vaccination may be applicable not only for the establishment of gut mucosal immunity but also for providing systemic protection. For example, *Salmonella typhimurium* not only invades the mucosal lining of the gut, but also infects cells of the mononuclear phagocyte system throughout the body, thereby stimulating the production of humoral and secretory antibodies as well as CD4 and CD8 cell-mediated immunity. Since attenuated *Salmonella* can be made to express proteins from *Shigella*, cholera, malaria-sporozoites and so on, it is entirely feasible to consider these as potential oral vaccines. Quite strikingly, these attenuated organisms are very effective when inhaled; for example, intranasal immunization with recombinant BCG expressing the OspA lipoprotein (*vide supra*) elicited substantive mucosal and systemic immune responses comparable to those obtained by the parenteral route. Vaccinologists are confidently predicting **'the age of the nose'**.

## Constraints on the use of attenuated vaccines

Attenuated vaccines for poliomyelitis (Sabin), measles and rubella have gained general acceptance. However, with live viral vaccines there is a possibility that the nucleic acid might be incorporated into the host's genome or that there may be reversion to a virulent form, although this will be unlikely if the attenuated strains contain several mutations. Another disadvantage of attenuated strains is the difficulty and expense of maintaining appropriate cold-storage facilities, especially in out-of-the-way places. In diseases such as viral hepatitis, AIDS and cancer, the dangers associated with live vaccines would make their use virtually unthinkable. As discussed above, with certain vaccines there is a very small, but still real, risk of developing complications and it cannot be emphasized too often that this risk must be balanced against the expected chance of contracting the disease with its own complications. Where this is minimal some may prefer to avoid general vaccination and to rely upon a crash course backed up if necessary by passive immunization in the localities around isolated outbreaks of infectious disease.

It is important to recognize those children with immunodeficiency before injection of live organisms; a child with impaired T-cell reactivity can become overwhelmed by BCG and die. Perhaps this is only a sick story, but it is said that in one particular country at a certain time there were no adults with T-cell deficiency. The reason? All children had been immunized with live BCG as part of a community health program(!). The extent to which children with partial deficiencies are at risk has yet to be assessed. It is also inadvisable to give live vaccines to patients being treated with steroids, immunosuppressive drugs or radiotherapy or who have malignant conditions such as lymphoma and leukemia; pregnant mothers must also be included here because of the vulnerability of the fetus.

## SUBUNIT VACCINES CONTAINING INDIVIDUAL PROTECTIVE ANTIGENS

A whole parasite or bacterium usually contains many antigens which are not concerned in the protective response of the host but may give rise to problems by suppressing the response to protective antigens or by provoking hypersensitivity, as we saw in the last chapter. Vaccination with the isolated protective antigens may avoid these complications and identification of these antigens then opens up the possibility of producing them synthetically in circumstances where bulk growth of the organism is impractical or isolation of the individual components too expensive.

Identification of protective antigens is greatly facilitated if one has an experimental model. If protection is antibody-mediated, one can try out different monoclonal antibodies and use the successful ones to pull out the antigen. Where antigenic variation is a major factor, desperate attempts are being made to identify some element of constancy which could provide a basis for vaccination, again using monoclonal antibodies with their ability to recognize a single specificity in a highly complex mixture. If protection is based primarily on T-cell activity, the approach would then be through the identification of individual T-cell clones capable of passively transferring protection. Switching back to humans, one seeks encouragement that the experimental models have kept the focus on the right target by confirming that the immune response to the antigen identified in the models correlates with protection in naturally infected individuals.

## The use of purified components

Bacterial exotoxins such as those produced by diphtheria and tetanus bacilli have long been used as immunogens. First, they must of course be detoxified and this is achieved by formaldehyde treatment, which fortunately does not destroy the major immunogenic determinants (figure 14.5). Immunization with the **toxoid** will therefore provoke the formation of protective antibodies, which neutralize the toxin by stereochemically blocking the active site, and encourage removal by phagocytic cells. The toxoid is generally given after adsorption to aluminum hydroxide which acts as an adjuvant and produces higher antibody titers. Coupling a protein antigen to cholera toxin B subunit targets the vaccine to the epithelial cells of the intestinal tract and usually produces good IgG and IgA antibodies which appear also in the saliva, tears and milk, indicating that the

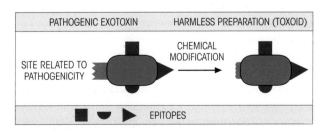

**Figure 14.5. Modification of toxin to harmless toxoid** without losing many of the antigenic determinants. Thus antibodies to the toxoid will react well with the original toxin.

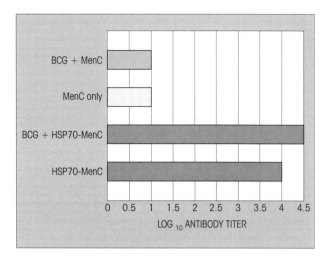

**Figure 14.6. The carrier effect of mycobacterial heat-shock protein (hsp70) without adjuvant.** Antibody responses to group C meningococcal polysaccharide (MenC) conjugated to hsp70 injected into mice with and without priming to the attenuated *Mycobacterium* BCG. (From Lambert P.-H., Louis J.A. and del Giudice G. (1992) In Gergely *et al.* (eds) *Progress in Immunology* VIII, pp. 683–689. Springer-Verlag, Budapest.)

antigen-specific IgA precursor cells become disseminated throughout the MALT system. Whether the immune response to the cholera precludes its use as a carrier for immunization with further antigens, remains an open question.

The emphasis now is to move towards gene cloning of individual proteins once they have been identified immunologically and biochemically. In general a protein subunit used in a vaccine should contain a sufficient number of T-cell epitopes to avoid human leukocyte antigen (HLA)-related unresponsiveness within the immunized population. In order to maintain a pool of memory cells over a reasonable period of time, persistence of antigen on the follicular dendritic cells in a form resistant to proteolytic degradation with retention of the native three-dimensional configuration is needed. Glycosylation of the protein contributes to this stability but by the same token might not give a good T-cell response so that the vaccine may need to be supplemented with a separate denatured source of T-cell epitopes. Purified polysaccharide vaccines are in a different category in that they normally require coupling to some immunogenic carrier protein such as tetanus toxoid or mycobacterial heat-shock protein (figure 14.6), since they fail to stimulate T-helpers or induce adequate memory. This maneuver can give respectable antibody titers but these will only be boosted by a natural infection if the carrier is derived from or related to the infecting agent itself.

## Antigens can be synthesized through gene cloning

Recombinant DNA technology enables us to make genes encoding part or the whole of a protein peptide chain almost at will, and express them in an appropriate vector. We have already ruminated upon vaccinia virus and other recombinant vectors. Another strategy is to fuse the gene with the Ty element of yeast which self-assembles into a highly immunogenic virus-like particle. In a similar fashion, peptides can be fused with the core antigen of hepatitis B virus, which spontaneously polymerizes into 27 nm particles capable of eliciting strong T-cell help. However, we often wish to develop vaccines which utilize the gene product on its own, incorporated in an adjuvant. Baculovirus vectors in moth cell lines produce large amounts of glycosylated recombinant protein, while the product secreted by yeast cells expressing the HBsAg gene is available as a commercial vaccine. Stably transformed transgenic bananas are now being developed to express protein vaccines. Bananas are cheap and easy to grow in the developing world and children like to eat them raw so avoiding inactivation by cooking. It is a sobering thought that a few hectares of the fruit could satisfy the annual global requirement for a single dose of oral immunogen.

The potential of gene cloning is clearly vast and, in principle, economical, but there are sometimes difficulties in identifying a good expression vector, in obtaining correct folding of the peptide chain to produce an active protein, and in separating the required product from the culture melange in an undenatured state. It could be instructive to follow one particular study on production of a vaccine against ovine cysticercosis. This disease in sheep is caused by larval tapeworms (*Taenia ovis*) and an extract of the early larval oncosphere stage will immunize completely against reinfection. Immune sera reacted strongly on Western immunoblots with oncosphere antigens of molecular weight 47–52 kDa (figure 14.7), and when cut out of the gel this fraction gave good protection. Antibodies affinity-purified from the 47 to 52 kDa immunoblots were used to screen a cDNA expression library to identify two clones producing antigen linked to β-galactosidase. Although one of the fusion proteins generated antibodies, it could not protect against infection, suggesting that the antigen may have been denatured. When glutathione-*S*-transferase from *Schistosoma japonicum* was used as the fusion partner, the antigen could be isolated under nondenaturing conditions and now gave almost complete protection when administered

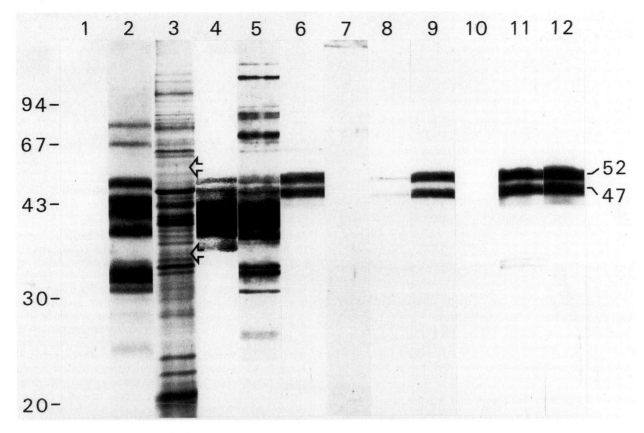

**Figure 14.7.** *T. ovis* **oncosphere antigens separated by SDS–PAGE** (cf. figure 6.18). Lanes were immunoblotted with: (1) preimmune sheep sera; (2) sera from sheep immunized with oncosphere extract; (4) sheep immunized with gel cut-out fraction in lane 3; (5) rabbit hyperimmune to extract; (6) rabbit affinity-purified antibodies eluted from blots of 47–52 kDa antigens; (7) sheep immunized with β-galactosidase (β-gal); (8) sheep immunized with clone β-gal-45S, a fusion protein of antigen linked to β-galactosidase (see text); (9) same using clone β-gal-45W; (10) same using glutathione-*S*-transferase (GST); (11) same using clone GST-45S; (12) same using clone GST-45W. The 45S antigen fused with GST but not with β-gal folded to generate epitopes reacting with antibody (lane 11 vs 8). (Reproduced from Johnson K.S. *et al.* (1989) *Nature* **338**, 585, with permission.)

to sheep in the adjuvant saponin. A valuable vaccine is on its way.

One restriction to gene cloning is that carbohydrate antigens cannot be synthesized directly by recombinant DNA technology, although preliminary attempts to clone the cohort of genes which encode the cascade of synthetic enzymes needed to produce complex carbohydrates are under way.

## The naked gene itself acts as a vaccine

Teams working with J. Wolff and P. Felgner experimented with a new strategy for gene therapy which involved binding the negatively charged DNA to cationic lipids which would themselves attach to the negatively charged surface of living cells and then presumably gain entry. The surprise was that controls injected with DNA without the lipids actually showed an *even higher uptake of DNA* and expression of the protein it encoded, so giving rise to the whole

new technology of **naked DNA therapy**. As Wolff put it: 'We tried it again and it worked. By the fourth or fifth time we knew we were onto something big. Even now I get a chill down my spine when I see it working.' Well, there is the real excitement of a blockbuster finding, even if, as usually happens to be the case, it arises from serendipity. It was quickly appreciated that the injected DNA functions as a source of immunogen *in situ* and can induce strong immune responses. So now, vaccinologists everywhere are scurrying around trying to adapt the new technology.

The gene is stitched in place in a DNA plasmid with appropriate promoters and enhancers and injected into muscle where it can give prolonged expression of protein. Broad immune responses are observed but naked DNA is also rather good at inducing Tc cells, presumably reflecting the cytosolic expression of the protein and its processing with MHC class I. Let's look at an example. It will be recalled that frequent point mutations (drift; p. 259) in antigenically important regions of influenza surface hemagglutinin give rise to substantial antigenic variation, whereas the major internal proteins which elicit T-cell-mediated immunity responses have been relatively conserved over the last 60 years. On this line of reasoning, nucleoprotein DNA should give broad protection against other influenza strains and indeed it does (figure 14.8). A combination of DNAs encoding the hemagglutinin (included only for statutory reasons) and nucleoprotein genes gave nonhuman primates and ferrets good protection against infection and protected ferrets against challenge with an antigenically distinct epidemic human virus strain more effectively than the contemporary clinically licensed vaccine. Excellent antibody responses to the viral hemagglutinin were also readily obtained in monkeys (figure 14.9).

DNA for this procedure can be obtained directly from current clinical material without having to select specific mutant strains. Altogether, the speed and simplicity mean that the 2 years previously needed to make a recombinant vaccine can be reduced to months. DNA vaccines do not need the cumbersome and costly protein synthesis and purification procedures that subunit formulations require; almost identical production facilities can be used for totally different vaccine candidates; they can be prepared in a highly stable powder form which does not depend on the cold complex chain logistically needed for heat-sensitive vaccines such as the oral polio vaccine in tropical countries. But, above all, they are incredi-

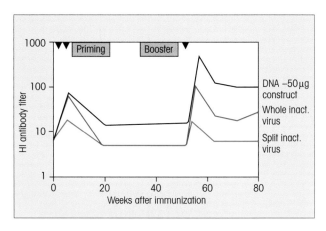

**Figure 14.9. Immunization of primates with influenza hemagglutinin (HA)-DNA.** Groups of three young adult African green monkeys were immunized twice with a DNA vaccine consisting of 50 µg each of plasmids encoding HA from A/Georgia/03/93, A/Texas/36/91 (H1N1), and B/Panama/45/90. Control groups received commercially inactivated vaccine or split inacti-vated vaccine (15 µg HA strain, the full human dose), 1993–1994 formulation, containing A/Beijing/32/92 (H3N2), A/Texas/36/91 and B/Panama/45/95). At week 48 a single booster immunization was given with the same vaccine at the same dose as was given for the primary immunization. Geometric mean hemagglutination inhibition antibody titers against the homologous strain (A/Georgia/03/93 for the DNA immunized monkeys and A/Beijing/32/92 for inactivated virus immunized animals) are shown. (Unpublished data kindly provided by Dr Margaret A. Liu and colleagues; to be published in *Vaccines*.)

bly cheap. The $3 required for an injection of recombinant hepatitis B represents the whole health budget for a single individual in some countries, whereas the single shot of DNA vaccine would be a tiny fraction of that. Before there is widespread use in humans, a number of safety considerations, such as the possibility of permanent incorporation of a plasmid into the host genome, need to be addressed.

## EPITOPE-SPECIFIC VACCINES MAY BE NEEDED

Most immunogens, especially proteins, present a variety of B- and T-cell epitopes to the immune system. Most, if not all, will elicit protective responses but some may have undesirable characteristics. For example, if there is cross-reaction with a self-epitope as between *Trypanosoma cruzi* and heart muscle, potentially pathogenic autoimmune reactions may result. Sometimes an immunodominant region such as the V3 loop in HIV gp120, hogs the antibody response at the expense of the more weakly immunogenic conserved regions, but continually escapes from capture by a high mutation rate. Similar escape mutants crop up in the Tc response to highly mutating dominant T-cell epitopes in malaria and various

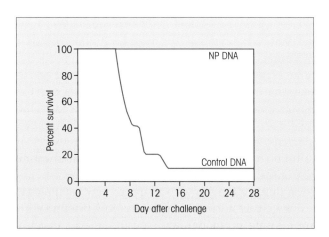

**Figure 14.8. Protection from cross-strain influenza challenge after vaccination with nucleoprotein DNA.** Mice were immunized three times at 3-week intervals with 200 µg of nucleoprotein (NP) or vector (control) DNA and lethally challenged with a heterologous influenza strain 3 weeks after the last immunization. Survival of mice given NP-DNA was significantly higher than in mice receiving vector (p = 0.0005). (Data kindly provided by Dr Margaret A. Liu and colleagues from *DNA and Cell Biology* (1993) **12**(9), and reproduced by permission of Mary Ann Liebert Inc..)

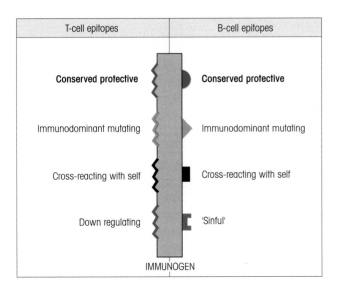

| T-cell epitopes | B-cell epitopes |
|---|---|
| **Conserved protective** | **Conserved protective** |
| Immunodominant mutating | Immunodominant mutating |
| Cross-reacting with self | Cross-reacting with self |
| Down regulating | 'Sinful' |

IMMUNOGEN

**Figure 14.10. Desirable (green) and unwanted (red) epitopes on a protein immunogen.** Conserved epitopes give broader protection against mutant variant strains. Epitopes may be unwanted because (i) they are immunodominant and attract the main immune response but continually escape by mutation; (ii) they cross-react with self-epitopes and can trigger autoimmunity; (iii) they are responsible for 'original antigenic sin' (see text); or (iv) they downregulate or antagonize T-cell-mediated immunity.

viral protein antigens. Unwanted epitope effects are seen in the phenomenon of **'original antigen sin'**, in which a second infection with influenza virus involving an antigenically related but not identical strain generates antibodies with a higher titer for the strain which produced the first infection. It is conceivable also that certain epitopes may bias T-helpers towards an inappropriate subset or may engender a predominantly suppressive, antagonistic or anergic response which could downregulate T-cell reactivity to linked epitopes on the same immunogen (figure 14.10). For such reasons, the requirement may arise for a vaccine in which the good protective epitopes can be dissociated from the 'bad guys' which compromise the protective responses; in other words, we need to construct **epitope-specific vaccines**, preferably based on conserved regions which provide broad defense. Several approaches are possible.

## Epitopes can be mimicked by synthetic peptides

### B-cell epitopes

Small peptide sequences corresponding with important epitopes on a microbial antigen can be synthesized readily and economically; long ones are rather expensive to manufacture. One might predict that, although the synthetic peptide has the correct linear *sequence* of amino acids, its random structure would

make it a poor model for the *conformation* of the parent antigen and hence a poor vaccine for evoking humoral immunity. Curiously this does not always seem to be a serious drawback. The 20 amino acid peptide derived from the foot and mouth virus-specific protein (VP1) evokes a good neutralizing response. The explanation has been forthcoming from X-ray structural analysis which shows the peptide sequence to be in a 'loop' region with blurred electron density indicative of dramatic disorder. In this case, the epitope is linear and evidently the flexibility of the loop structure may approach that of the free peptide which can thus mimic the epitope on the native VP1 molecule and stimulate a protective antibody response when used as a vaccine (figure 14.11a and b). Where the epitope is linear but is restricted in conformation by adjacent structures in the intact protein, immunization with free peptide tends to produce antibodies of disappointing affinity for the protein itself for reasons outlined in figure 14.11c.

### T-cell epitopes

Although short peptides may not have the conformation to stimulate adequate B-cell responses, they can prime antigen-specific T-cells which recognize the primary sequence rather than the tertiary configuration of the protein. If the primed T-cells mediate CMI and possibly act to help B-cells make antibody, they could enable the host to mount an effective response on subsequent exposure to natural infection and this would prove to be a useful prophylactic strategy. This seems to have been the case when a peptide sequence from polio virus VP1 induced poor neutralizing antibody but did prime the recipient for a good response to infection.

We have already alluded to T-cell epitopes, often dominant and subject to high mutation rates, which can downregulate or subvert protective CMI responses. Under these circumstances, conserved peptide sequences which form **subdominant or cryptic epitopes (cf. p. 202) can function as effective vaccines**. The ineffectiveness of these sequences in providing adequate MHC/peptide levels to *prime* resting T-cells when the whole protein is processed by antigen-presenting cells, can be side-stepped by immunizing with adequate doses of the preformed synthetic peptide. Because **primed**, as compared with **resting**, T-cells can be stimulated by much lower concentrations of MHC/peptide and do not necessarily require major costimulatory signals, they will react with infected cells which have processed and presented the cryptic epitopes; furthermore, because the

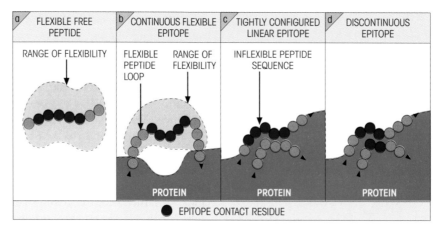

**Figure 14.11. Structural basis for peptide mimicry of protein epitopes.** (a) The free peptide is very flexible and can adopt a large number of structures in solution. (b) If the peptide sequence is present as a linear epitope on a part of a protein which is a flexible loop or chain, this will also exist in a variety of structures resembling the free peptide to a fair extent and will behave comparably as an antigen and as an immunogen (vaccine) so that the peptide will raise antibodies which react well with the native protein. (c) If the linear epitope on the protein is structurally constrained (i.e. inflexible), it represents only one of the many structures adopted by the free peptide; thus if this peptide is used for immunization, only a minority of the B-cells stimulated will be complementary in shape to the native protein, so the peptide would be a poor vaccine for humoral immunity to microbes containing the protein antigen. (Note, however, the antibodies produced would be good for Western immunoblots where the protein has been denatured after sodium dodecyl sulfate (SDS) treatment and the peptide structure is relatively free.) Preformed antibodies to the protein would react with the peptide, albeit with lower affinity because energy must be used to constrain the peptide to the one structure which fits the antibody—just like the force used to restrain a madman in a strait-jacket. Where the sequence has a comparable degree of constraint in both peptide and protein, as in the disulfide-bonded loops in diphtheria toxin and hepatitis B surface antigen, antipeptide sera react reasonably well with the native protein. (d) Most commonly, the epitopes are discontinuous and, even if with difficulty, we can predict the contact residues, the techniques for designing a peptide with appropriate structure are not robust although some progress is being made using antibody to select from a random bacteriophage library in which the peptides are constrained on a structural scaffold such as that supporting the Ig CDR3 loop.

primed T-cells will be directed against conserved sequences, they will therefore provide broad CMI protection against mutated strains.

A major worry about peptides as T-cell vaccines is the variation in ability to associate with the different polymorphic forms of MHC molecules present in an outbred population, which contributes to the immune response (*Ir*) gene effect described earlier (see p. 214). One either has to use a cocktail of peptides in a general vaccine to cover HLA variation, or if that is too difficult, go back to a gene-cloned version of the whole protein antigen. Residues 378–398 of the malaria circumsporozoite protein provide an exception in being virtually a universal T-cell epitope recognizable by all individuals so far tested. Other examples are residues 307–319 in influenza hemagglutinin and both 830–843 and 947–967 in tetanus toxin. These sequences, and possibly the highly conserved heat-shock proteins, can provide promiscuous (i.e. HLA independent) T-cell epitopes to conjugate with peptide vaccines.

*Making the peptides immunogenic*

Immunogenicity of peptides for B-cells is invariably bound up with a dependence on T-cell help and failure to provide linked T-cell epitopes is thought to be responsible for poor antibody responses to the foot and mouth disease VP1 loop peptide in cattle and pigs, and to polymers of the tetrapeptide asparagyl-alanylasparagylproline (NANP) of malarial circumsporozoite antigens in man (cf. p. 301). When the general T-cell carrier, peptide 378–398 (see above), was coupled to (NANP)$_3$ tetramer repeat, good antibody responses were obtained in all strains of mice tested. Furthermore, after priming with this synthetic peptide, whole sporozoites would boost antibody titers. This brings up two points: first, as we have already noted, in order for the natural infection to boost, the T- and B-cell epitopes must both be present and, second, they must be linked so that the T-cell epitope is taken up for processing by the lymphocyte which recognizes the B-cell epitope (figure 9.9). This does not always imply that the link in the infectious agent must be covalent, since mice primed with the core antigen of hepatitis B virus gave excellent responses to the surface antigen when challenged with whole virions, i.e. an interstructural relationship may function in this regard as well as an intramolecular one. In contrast, animals immunized with an HBs B-cell peptide coupled with a streptococcal peptide T-cell carrier require boosting with the original vaccine but do not receive a boost from natural infection. Mycobacterial heat-shock proteins are excellent carriers for peptides even in the absence of adjuvants and irrespective of BCG priming (figure 14.6), possibly due to the preprogramming of responses to cross-reacting self heat-shock proteins in the 'immunological homunculus' (cf. p. 209). It has been suggested that in some cases, antibodies induced by protein carriers might suppress a boosting injection of vaccine and in this respect, peptides providing the carrier T-cell epitope have an advantage. It is worth noting that the presentation of a peptide such as the foot and mouth disease virus VP1 loop in the form of an octamer coupled to a poly-L-lysine backbone produces responses of far greater magnitude than the monomer, a strategy which has proved successful when multiple clusters of peptides are linked to a small central oligolysine core in what has been labeled 'the multiple antigen peptide (MAP) system'. Are not the multiple peptide units acting as carriers for each other?

Notwithstanding these considerations, the evidence is mounting that the majority of protein determinants are discontinuous, i.e. involve amino acid residues far apart in the primary sequence but brought close to each other by peptide folding (figure 14.11d; cf. p. 81). In such cases, peptides which represent linear sequences of the primary structure will, at best, only mimic part of a determinant and generate low affinity responses. Defining a discontinuous determinant by X-ray crystallography and site-related mutagenesis takes a long time and by computer analysis, perhaps even longer. Even when armed with this information, synthesis of a configured peptide which will topographically mimic the contact residues which constitute such an epitope still remains a serious challenge. Progress might be anticipated from attempts to use antibodies to select peptide epitopes binding with higher affinity from bacteriophage libraries of random hexa- or heptapeptides which are constrained on a structural scaffold such as that holding the CDR3 loop in the immunoglobulin variable region.

## Idiotypes can be exploited as epitope-specific vaccines

In principle, internal image anti-idiotypes provide surrogates for discontinuous B-cell epitopes through possession of an innate structure capable of binding with the antigen-combining site of the idiotype antibody. If the reader trundles back to figure 11.9, it will be seen that there are two main categories of anti-idiotype: Ab2α, which recognize cross-reacting, presumably regulatory, idiotypes and Ab2β, which are thought to behave as internal images of the antigenic determinant. In those instances where the major Id is mostly associated with a given specificity (e.g. murine T15 Id is largely present on antibodies to phosphoryl choline), then Ab2α anti-Ids could provide useful potential vaccines, particularly for carbohydrates which are notoriously poor immunogens in the very young. They might also be applicable to the expansion of specific antitumor clones with their own private idiotypes in cancer patients. In general, the Ab2β are capable of stimulating a wider range of lymphocytes. Although the internal image anti-idiotypes concerned with the majority of microbial antigens are probably rather poorly represented in the B-cell repertoire, they could be pulled out by monoclonal antibody technology or selected from bacteriophage scFv libraries by cross-reaction with polyclonal antisera specific for the original antigen. Regrettably, to date no serious idiotype vaccines have yet emerged.

## Unwanted epitope-loss mutants can correctly fold desired discontinuous B-cell epitopes

The most natural way to achieve a correctly configured discontinuous B-cell epitope is to allow the protein to fold spontaneously. If the gene encoding the protein antigen is mutated so that the unwanted epitope is eliminated by replacement of its amino acid side-chains without affecting the folding of the protein chain which generates the epitopes we wish to preserve, our object is achieved. Preservation of the desired epitopes and destruction of the 'bad' epitopes by 'genetic sandpapering' can obviously be monitored by following the reactivity of the mutants with the appropriate monoclonal antibody (figure 14.12). It will be apparent that 'bad' T-cell epitopes can also be eliminated by targeted mutations.

## CURRENT VACCINES

The established vaccines in current use and the schedules for their administration are set out in tables 14.3 and 14.4.

Because of the pyrogenic reactions and worries about possible hypersensitivity responses to the whole-cell component of the conventional pertussis vaccine, a new generation containing one or more purified components of *Bordetella pertussis* and therefore termed 'acellular' vaccines have been licensed in the USA. The combination with diphtheria and tetanus toxoids (DTaP) is recommended for the later

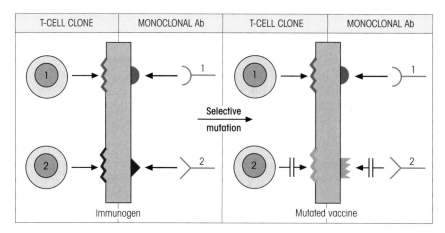

**Figure 14.12. Selective mutation of unwanted (purple) with retention of desirable (green) epitopes in a protein vaccine.** Success of the mutation strategy can be monitored by reactivity with monoclonal antibodies (B-epitopes) and T-cell clones (T-epitopes). Our immunoprotein engineering group at University College London have used this strategy to mutate human chorionic gonadotropin-β (βhCG) so that it still retains βhCG-specific epitopes but has lost those shared with human luteinizing hormone (hLH). βhCG has been investigated as a contraceptive vaccine to aid population control since antibodies to βhCG neutralize the hormone and prevent successful pregnancy. However, the production of antibodies to hLH is undesirable since this hormone is present all the time, not just during pregnancy as is essentially the case for hCG (cf. figure 17.20). The mutant epitopes (orange) avoid this unwanted LH cross-reactivity. The C-terminal end of the construct can be extended to encode suitable T-helper carrier epitopes. For simplicity the T-cell recognition of MHC/peptide has been ignored.

4th and 5th 'shots' and for children at increased risk for seizures. Children under 2 years of age make inadequate responses to the T-independent *H. influenzae* capsular polysaccharide, so they are now routinely immunized with the antigen conjugated with tetanus or diphtheria toxoids.

A resurgence of **measles** outbreaks in recent years has prompted recommendations for reimmunizing children, at the age of school entry or at the change to middle school, with measles. The considerable morbidity and mortality associated with hepatitis B infection, its complex epidemiology and the difficulty in identifying high risk individuals has led to recommendations for vaccination in the 6–18 month age group.

The deviating influence of maternally derived IgG antibody has been discussed in an earlier chapter. Preliminary results suggest that infants of 4–6 months can be seroconverted by inhaled aerosol measles vaccine which presumably evades the maternal antibody; this will have singular relevance in endemic measles areas, where almost split-second timing is required with conventional immunization as passively acquired antibody wanes. Naked DNA vaccines may also have a role to play here.

**Tuberculosis** is the largest cause of death in the world from a single infectious disease and, while it remains a truly major problem in developing countries, cases have increased by around one-third in Western countries. There is an alarmingly heightened susceptibility to TB of individuals with the HIV and worldwide multidrug-resistant strains are appearing. Thus, although BCG has been in use for 70 years and is reasonably efficacious and safe in healthy non-T-cell deficient subjects, there is certainly a vital need for the development of new drugs and vaccines. It remains to be seen whether the disappointing degree of protection against TB and *Mycobacterium leprae* found with BCG in field trials in certain parts of the globe is due to the use of high doses, deficient strains or subversion of the response to group i cross-reacting antigens by suppressive mycobacterial species in the local environment.

## EXPERIMENTAL VACCINES IN DEVELOPMENT

### Malaria

Don't sneer at low technology. The major advance in malaria control has been the finding that impregnation of bed nets with the insecticide pyrethroid reduces *Plasmodium falciparum* deaths by 40%. However, with the emergence of drug-resistant strains of mosquito, vaccines must be developed. The goal is achievable since, although children are very susceptible, adults resident in highly endemic areas acquire a protective but nonsterilizing immunity.

Antigen variation poses a big problem for vaccine development and a number of investigators in the malaria field have turned their attention to the invari-

**Table 14.3. Current and experimental vaccines.**

| Type | Established | Experimental |
|---|---|---|
| **BACTERIAL VACCINES** | | |
| Live attenuated | Mycobacterium tuberculosis (BCG) | ● Vibrio cholerae<br><br>● Salmonella typhi (Ty21a: Vi⁻ mutant)<br><br>● S. typhi (aroA: aromatic pathway mutant) |
| Inactivated | V. cholerae<br>B. pertussis<br>S. typhi | ● V. cholerae + toxin B subunit<br>M. leprae |
| Subunit | Haemophilus influenzae<br>Neisseria meningitidis<br>Streptococcus pneumoniae | S. typhi (capsular Vi⁻carrier)<br>H. Influenzae (dip/tet toxoid)<br>M. tuberculosis (naked DNA) |
| Toxoid | Tetanus, diphtheria | |
| **VIRAL VACCINES** | | |
| Live attenuated | Vaccinia<br>Measles<br>Mumps<br>Rubella<br>● Polio (Sabin)<br>Varicella zoster<br>● Adeno<br>Yellow fever | Cytomegalovirus<br>Hepatitis A<br>Influenza<br>Dengue<br>● Rota<br>Parainfluenza<br>Japanese encephalitis<br>● Polio |
| Inactivated | Polio (Salk)<br>Influenza<br>Rabies<br>Japanese encephalitis | Hepatitis A |
| Subunit | Hepatitis B, influenza | HIV, influenza, hepatitis B/C, herpes, cytomegalovirus, rabies (all naked DNA in experimental animals) |

● Given orally

**Table 14.4. Current vaccination practice.**

| VACCINE | | ADMINISTRATION | | |
|---|---|---|---|---|
| | | UK | USA | OTHER COUNTRIES |
| **CHILDREN** | | | | |
| Triple (DTP) vaccine: diphtheria, tetanus, pertussis | Primary | 2–6 mo (3x/4 weekly) | | Japan: 2 yr |
| | Boost | 3–5yr | 15 mo/4 yr DT every 10 yr | |
| Polio: live | Primary | Concomitant with DTP | | |
| | Boost | 4/6 yr | 15 mo, 4 yr high-risk adult | |
| killed | | Immunocompromised | | |
| MMR vaccine: measles, mumps rubella | Primary | 12–18 | | Africa: 6 mo |
| | Boost | 3–5yr 10–14 yr seronegative girls selectively with rubella | | |
| BCG (TB, leprosy) | | 10–14 yr | high risk only | Tropics: at birth |
| Haemophilus | | 18 mo | | |
| Varicella | | Neonates at risk, immunocompromised | | |
| **ELDERLY** | | | | |
| Pneumococcal polysaccharide serotypes | | Aged & high risk | | |
| Influenza | | Aged & high risk | | |
| **SPECIAL GROUPS** | | | | |
| Hepatitis B | | Travellers, high risk groups | | |
| Hepatitis A Meningitis (A+C) | | Travellers to endemic areas | | |
| Yellow fever Typhoid Cholera | | Travellers to endemic areas | | Tropics: infants Yellow fever: boost residents and frequent visitors every 10 yr |
| Rabies | | Prophylactically in high risk groups Post-exposure to contacts in endemic areas | | |

ant antigens of the sporozoite, which is the form with which the host is first infected; this rapidly reaches the liver to emerge later as merozoites which infect the red cells (figure 14.13). Because the sporozoite only takes 30 minutes to reach the liver, the antibody has to act fast so that inactivation is limited by diffusion events and hence dependent on the concentration of antibody molecules. The sporozoite has a characteristic antigen with multiple tetrapeptide repeats. *Plasmodium falciparum*, for example, has 37 repeats of NANP. Field trials of vaccines with polymers of NANP and similar tetrapeptides from other species have not so far been spectacularly successful but building in powerful T-cell help in the form of the promiscuous 378–398 epitope (see p. 298) or a

mycobacterial heat-shock protein hsp65 carrier (which obviates the need for adjuvant) should improve efficacy. Mice immunized with circumsporozoite protein linked to attenuated *Salmonella* were resistant to live challenge with sporozoites. No antibodies were detectable so T-cells can offer protection against the liver stage; additionally, the response of cytokines such as γ-interferon (IFNγ) is thought to stimulate the production of NO·, TNF and reactive oxygen intermediates which are active against the blood-stage merozoites.

Many laboratories have been targeting the various antigens associated with the blood stages and much publicity has been given to trials using the vaccine SPf66, which consists of three peptide epitopes from

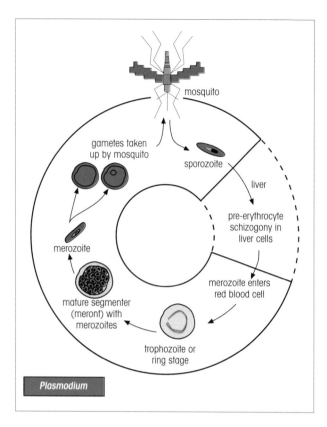

**Figure 14.13. The life cycle of the malaria parasite.**

three blood stage proteins intercalated with NANP sequences. Some clear protection was originally obtained in large scale trials in South America, but two further trials in other areas were unfortunately ineffective. One of the products of the infected erythrocytes is a glycophospholipid with features of the insulin second messenger. This may be responsible for many of the secondary features of malaria by acting as an excessive stimulator of TNF production. A strategy based on using the molecule as a vaccine would resemble the well-established approach to tetanus and diphtheria, where the toxin rather than the organism is attacked. Other groups are focusing on antigens which elicit antibodies able to block transmission (see legend figure 14.14); these would be altruistic vaccines in that they only help the next guy down the line and finally the community as a whole. A brief summary of the many different vaccine strategies being deployed to counter this complex parasite is presented in figure 14.14, and there may be a consensus that, ultimately, vaccines will contain antigens from all stages probably presented as a mixture of the naked DNA genes which encode them.

## Schistosomiasis

The morbidity in this chronic and debilitating disease is related to the remarkable fecundity of the female worm which lays hundred of eggs every day. These are deposited in numerous mucous membranes and tissues and the granulomas which form around them (cf. figure 16.8) lead to the development of severe fibrotic and often irreversible lesions. Specific IgE can

| STAGE | VACCINE | STRATEGY |
|---|---|---|
| 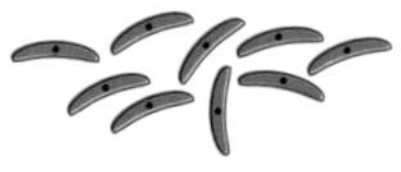 SPOROZOITES | CIRCUMSPOROZOITE (CS) PROTEIN OR PEPTIDES | Ab blocks infection of liver |
| 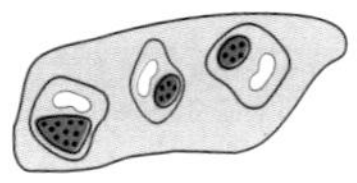 LIVER STAGE | CS PROTEIN OR PEPTIDES | T-cell mediated immunity destroys liver stage |
| 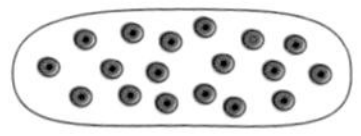 MEROZOITES | MEROZOITE ANTIGENS | Block infection of red cells |
| 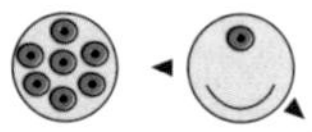 ASEXUAL ERYTHROCYTE STAGE / TOXIC ANTIGEN | ASEXUAL STAGE RBC | Destroy infected red cells |
| | TOXIC PRODUCT | Ab neutralizes toxin |
| 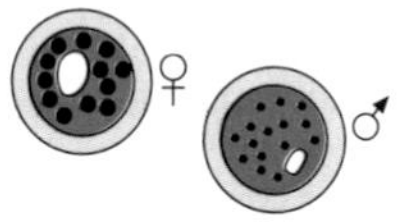 GAMETOCYTES / GAMETES | SEXUAL STAGES | Ab blocks transmission |
| 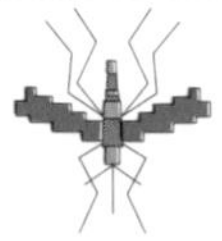 MOSQUITO | MOSQUITO TRYPSIN | |

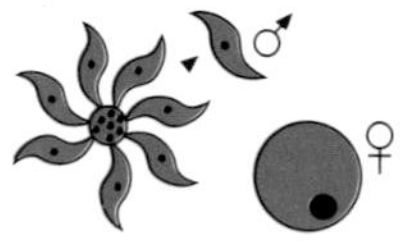

**Figure 14.14. Strategies for a malaria vaccine.** A vaccine incorporating a yeast-derived polypeptide representing the zygote-specific antigen Pfs25 which can induce transmission-blocking antibodies looks like the next candidate for big field trials of efficacy. If antibodies to the mosquito midgut trypsin are taken into the blood meal with the gametocytes, they block the trypsin-mediated activation of the parasite prochitinase enzyme required for penetration of the chitin layer lining the midgut by the ookinates (differentiated from the gametocyte stage).

produce worm damage through antibody-dependent cell-mediated cytotoxicity (ADCC) mechanisms (cf. p. 34 and figure 13.21) involving eosinophils and possibly mononuclear phagocytes as effector cells and may be regarded as a factor in recovery from infection together with TH1 CMI, schistosomes being susceptible to the lethal effects of NO· produced by activated macrophages. IgE, G and A antibodies correlate with resistance to reinfection in drug-cured patients, while IgA appears to control fecundity as shown by passive transfer experiments. Our abilities to stimulate IgE and, to a lesser extent, IgA antibodies at will are, to put it mildly, still somewhat underdeveloped but it is encouraging to note that a monoclonal antibody to the glutathione-S-transferase of *S. mansoni* inhibits the enzyme, protects against challenge and dramatically reduces laying and viability of eggs. Another protective monoclonal to a different epitope has no effect on enzymic activity or on the production and viability of eggs, but does reduce the worm burden. The recombinant enzyme, possibly in a cocktail with other schistosome antigens and cercerial proteases, could provide a promising future vaccine.

## Cholera

In the case of **cholera**, an oral vaccine which combines the B subunit of cholera toxin with killed vibrios is reported in a big field trial in Bangladesh to stimulate excellent gut mucosal antibody formation, the response being said to equal that seen after clinical cholera. The vaccine also afforded cross-protection against the enterotoxin of *E. coli*, responsible for travellers' diarrhea.

## Tuberculosis

Extensive field trials of the nonvirulent *Mycobacterium vaccae* are underway using the killed organisms which generate strong TH1 responses. To obviate potential adverse effects of live BCG vaccine in immunodeficient subjects (e.g. HIV-positive), auxotrophic strains which fail to grow in the absence of essential amino acids such as methionine and leucine, were created by insertional mutagenesis. The strains died out within 16–32 weeks in mice and severe combined immunodeficient (SCID) mice survived for at least 230 days compared with 8 weeks for a conventional BCG vaccine. These auxotrophic strains gave excellent protection against challenge with virulent bacilli and so offer a potentially safe vaccine against TB for populations at risk for HIV.

At the subunit level, as might now be anticipated, naked DNA vaccines for heat-shock and other common mycobacterial antigens are being developed and seem to be highly effective, in mice at least.

# ADJUVANTS

For practical and economic reasons, prophylactic immunization should involve the minimum number of injections and the least amount of antigen. We have referred to the undoubted advantages of replicating attenuated organisms in this respect but nonliving organisms, and especially purified products, frequently require an adjuvant which by definition is a substance incorporated into or injected simultaneously with antigen which potentiates the immune response (Latin *adjuvare*—to help). It is interesting that bacterial structures provide the major source of immunoadjuvants, presumably because they provide danger signals of infection. In a sense, the basis of adjuvanticity is often the recognition of these signals by phylogenetically ancient receptors on accessory cells. The mode of action of adjuvants may be considered under several headings.

## Depot effects

Free antigen usually disperses rapidly from the local tissues draining the injection site and an important function of the so-called repository adjuvants is to counteract this by providing a long-lived reservoir of antigen, either at an extracellular location or within macrophages. The most common adjuvants of this type used in man are **aluminum compounds** (phosphate and hydroxide). Freund's incomplete adjuvant (in which the antigen is incorporated in the aqueous phase of a stabilized water in paraffin oil emulsion) also increases the antibody response but the emulsions tend to produce higher and far more sustained antibody levels with a broadening of the response to include more of the epitopes in the antigen preparation. However, because of the lifelong persistence of oil in the tissues and the occasional production of sterile abscesses, and the unpalatable fact that paraffin oil produces tumors in mice, attention has been focused on the replacement of incomplete Freund's with different types of oils such as squalene or biodegradable peanut oil. It is reassuring that recent analysis of large-scale trials of vaccines containing emulsified mineral oils performed 30–40 years ago has shown that such procedures do not increase the incidence of neoplasms or autoimmune disease.

## Macrophage activation

Under the influence of the repository adjuvants, macrophages form granulomas which provide sites for interaction with antibody-forming cells. The maintenance by the depot of consistent antigen concentrations ensures that as antigen-sensitive cells divide within the granuloma, their progeny are highly likely to be further stimulated by antigen. Virtually all adjuvants stimulate macrophages which are thought to act by improving immunogenicity through an increase in the concentration of processed antigen on their surface and the efficiency of its presentation to lymphocytes, by the provision of accessory costimulatory signals to direct lymphocytes towards an immune response rather than tolerance, and by the secretion of soluble stimulatory factors (e.g. interleukin (IL)-1) which influence the proliferation of lymphocytes.

## Specific effects on lymphocytes

In mice, alum tends to stimulate helper cells of the T$_{H}$2 family, whereas complete Freund's adjuvant favors the T$_{H}$1 subset. It will be recalled that complete Freund's is made from the incomplete adjuvant by addition of killed mycobacteria (cf. p. 193), the active component being the water-soluble **muramyl dipeptide** (MDP; *N*-acetyl-muramyl-L-alanyl-D-isoglutamine). Hydrophilic MDP analogs with aqueous antigen preferentially stimulate antibody responses, but if administered in a hydrophobic microenvironment such as mineral oil or incorporation into liposomes, CMI is the major outcome. Lipophilic MDP derivatives enhance CMI without the need for the water-in-oil emulsion. The immunopathological effects of the mycobacterial component in complete Freund's are so striking that their use in man is not normally countenanced; undoubtedly hope lies in the exploration of suitable MDP analogs and a number of acceptable derivatives are now available.

Looking at other materials with adjuvant properties, BCG is a potent stimulator of T- and B-cells and macrophages and we have already noted the ability of mycobacterial hsp70 to act as a powerful carrier without the need for adjuvants (figure 14.6). Purified lipid A from bacterial lipopolysaccharide is a B-cell mitogen in mice with a preferential effect on Bμ cells. However, in general it is a very potent stimulator of macrophages but has many side-effects and interest is developing in its derivative, monophosphoryl lipid A (MLA), which is less toxic than lipopolysaccharide (LPS); it promotes IFNγ production by T-cells and TNF by macrophages, a combination which activates T$_{H}$1 and natural killer (NK) cells. The adjuvanticity of LPS derivatives is improved when combined with nonionic block copolymer surfactants which have a hydrophobic polyoxypropylene core linked to hydrophilic polymers of polyoxyethylene. Of course, no matter how cleverly these materials behave in mice, the acid test which destroys so many promising compounds is the long-term effect in the human.

The role of modulatory cytokines in these interactions is important and several experimental approaches are exploring the effect of cytokines administered simultaneously with antigen. In one study, a construct of the macrophage stimulator granulocyte–macrophage colony-stimulating factor (GM-CSF) linked to a monoclonal immunoglobulin, successfully induced anti-idiotypic responses relevant to the treatment of chronic lymphocytic leukemia. IL-2 has an adjuvant activity in unresponsive leprosy patients and a single injection in dialysis patients effectively induced their seroconversion to hepatitis B surface antigen. The potential of IL-12 to encourage T$_{H}$1 responses is yet to be realized.

## NEW APPROACHES TO THE PRESENTATION OF ANTIGEN

Recent interest has centered on the use of small lipid membrane vesicles (**liposomes**) as agents for the presentation of antigen to the immune system. It may be that the liposome acts as a storage vacuole within the macrophage or perhaps fuses with the macrophage membrane to provide a suitably immunogenic complex. The differing pathways for processing peptides within antigen-presenting cells can be turned to advantage by encapsulating antigen in acid-resistant liposomes so that they can only enter the MHC class I route and stimulate CD8 T-cells. Antigens within acid-sensitive liposomes become associated with both class I and class II molecules. Proteins anchored in the lipid membrane by hydrophobic means give augmented CMI. Short synthetic peptides coupled covalently to monophosphoryl lipid A or tripalmitoyl-S-glyceryl-cysteinyl-seryl-serine (P3CSS) have high priming efficiency.

One can readily envisage the possibility of a single-shot liposome vaccine with multiple potentialities which incorporate several antigens, different adjuvants and specialized targeting molecules (figure 14.15).

Another innovation is the **Iscom** (immunostimulating complex), a hydrophobic matrix of the adjuvant saponin, with antigen, cholesterol and phosphatidyl-

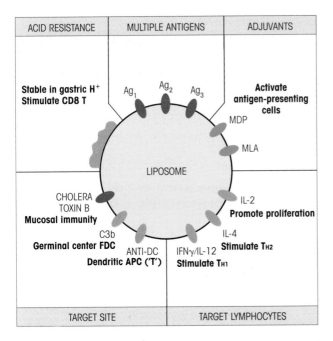

**Figure 14.15. The 'do-it-all-in-one' omnipotent liposome particle** illustrating some possible ways to build immunogenic flexibility into a single-shot liposome vaccine. The interior of the liposome may also contain depots of certain components. MDP = muramyl dipeptide; MLA = monophosphoryl lipid A.

choline. Antigens with a transmembrane hydrophobic region, such as surface molecules of lipid-containing viruses, are powerfully immunogenic in this vehicle and may engender cytotoxic T-cell responses. Iscoms are extremely resistant to acid and bile salts and are immunogenic by the oral route producing systemic immunity and good local secretory IgA. Intranasal exposure established protective immunity to influenza in mice.

It may be useful to focus on the notion floated earlier that polymeric antigens tend to be more immunogenic and to note a novel form of solid matrix of the Cowan strain of *S. aureus* which can bind several molecules of monoclonal antibody, which can, in turn, immobilize several molecules of antigen. Using a variety of monoclonals, one can purify onto

their binding sites appropriate antigens from a mixture to give a multivalent subunit vaccine. One could also incorporate cholera toxin to give good mucosal immunity.

We should not ignore the practicability of one-shot **biolistics** (cf. p. 144) to introduce gold microspheres coated with a construct of the gene encoding the vaccine antigen linked to a muscle promoter; muscle cells which are penetrated will then synthesize the antigen and export it if a leader sequence is provided.

There have been some very important advances in the design of controlled-release systems for antigen delivery *in vivo*. Polymers of polylactic-polyglycolic esters are nontoxic biodegradable vehicles which can be prepared in different formulations to provide **slow release** of an antigen (or any active drug or hormone) for periods up to several months. Figure 14.16 shows the principle of a one-shot controlled-release vaccine for tetanus designed to provide a priming dose and two boosting doses of toxoid to mimic the conventional immunization schedule.

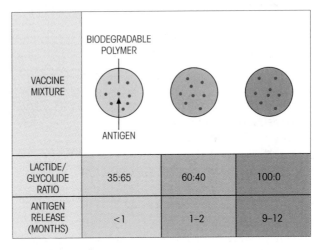

**Figure 14.16. One-shot controlled release vaccine.** The polymer is biodegraded at different times, depending upon the formulation. The net result is equivalent to a conventional schedule for tetanus toxoid immunization. (From Lambert P.H. (1993) New vaccines for the world — needs and prospects. *The Immunologist* **1**, 50–55.)

## SUMMARY

*Passively acquired immunity*

• Passive immunity can be acquired by maternal antibodies or from homologus pooled γ-globulin.

• Horse antisera are more restricted because of the danger of serum sickness.

• Antibodies are being constructed to order using recombinant DNA technology and can be produced in bulk in plants.

*(Continued on p. 306)*

## Vaccination

• Active immunization provides a protective state through contact with a harmless form of the disease organism.
• A good vaccine should be based on antigens which are easily available, cheap, stable under extreme climatic conditions and nonpathogenic.

## Killed organisms as vaccines

• Killed bacteria and viruses have been widely used.

## Live attenuated organisms

• The advantages are: replication gives a bigger dose, the immune response is produced at the site of the natural infection.
• Attenuated vaccinia or polio can provide a 'piggyback' carrier for genes from other organisms which are difficult to attenuate.
• BCG is a good vehicle for antigens requiring CD4 T-cell immunity and salmonella constructs may give oral and systemic immunity. Intranasal immunization is fast gaining popularity.
• Risks are reversion to the virulent form and danger to immunocompromised individuals.

## Subunit vaccines

• Whole organisms have a multiplicity of antigens, some of which are not protective, may induce hypersensitivity or might even be frankly immunosuppressive.
• It makes sense in these cases to use purified components.
• There is greatly increased use of recombinant DNA technology to produce these antigens. Expression in bananas provides a very cheap way of achieving oral immunization in the developing world.
• Naked DNA encoding the vaccine subunit can be injected directly into muscle, where it expresses the protein and produces immune responses. The advantages are stability, ease of production and cheapness.
• Epitope-specific vaccines based on conserved structures have the advantage that they can provide broad protection and may avoid the possible deleterious effects of other epitopes (autoimmunity, T-downregulation, original antigenic sin, escape by mutation of immunodominant epitopes) when certain whole antigens are used for immunization.

• Epitope-specific vaccines can be based on peptides, internal image anti-idiotypes or epitope-loss mutants.
• Peptides may only usefully mimic the native protein for vaccination to produce antibody if the epitope is linear and relatively unconstrained in structure. Carriers such as tetanus toxoid or mycobacterial heat shock proteins are needed to make the peptide immunogenic. Linear peptides can mimic T-cell epitopes in the whole protein.
• Epitope-loss mutants have undesirable epitopes replaced but still fold correctly to produce the wanted discontinuous B-cell epitope(s).

## Current vaccines

• Children in the USA and UK are routinely immunized with diphtheria and tetanus toxoids and pertussis (DTP triple vaccine) and attenuated strains of measles, mumps and rubella (MMR) and polio. BCG is given at 10–14 years.
• Subunit forms of pertussis lacking side-effects are being introduced.
• The capsular polysaccharide of *H. influenza* has to be linked to a carrier.
• The elderly receive vaccines of influenza and *Pneumococcus* polysaccharides.
• Vaccines for hepatitis A and B, meningitis, yellow fever, typhoid, cholera and rabies are available for travellers and high-risk groups.

## Vaccines in development

• In malaria the experimental vaccines are targeted at the *sporozoite and blood stages*, the *toxin* producing serious side-effects; the *gametes* and the insect gut trypsin.
• Recombinant glutathione-*S*-transferase is a promising candidate for a vaccine against schistosomiasis.
• An oral vaccine composed of cholera toxin B subunit and killed vibrios, induced good mucosal immunity to cholera.

## Adjuvants

• Adjuvants work by producing depots of antigen, and by activating macrophages; they sometimes have direct effects on lymphocytes.
• Adjuvants such as the muramyl dipeptide analogs derived from mycobacterial cell walls and the monophosphoryl lipid A derivative from Gram-negative LPS may soon be in general use.
• New methods of delivery include linking the antigen

*(Continued)*

to small lipid membrane vesicles (liposomes) or a special glycoside matrix (Iscom). These delivery particles can be furnished with many factors which improve their immunogenicity and flexibility. One can build in several antigens into the same particle, adjuvants such as MDP and MLA, cytokines to influence lymphocyte subset responses and molecules such as cholera toxin B to target particular sites in the body.

• Antigens built into biodegradable polymers of varying half-life can provide single-shot vaccines which mimic a conventional course of immunization requiring several injections.

The overall strategies for vaccination are summarized in figure 14.17.

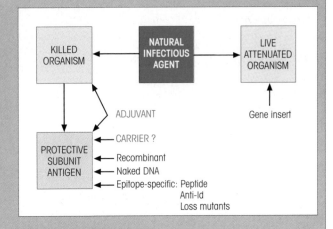

**Figure 14.17. Strategies for vaccination.**

# FURTHER READING

Featherstone C. (1996) Vaccines by agriculture. *Molecular Medicine Today* **2**, 278.

Harding C.V., Collins D.S., Kanagawa O. & Unanue E.R. (1991) Liposome-encapsulated antigens engender liposomal processing for class II MHC presentation and cytosolic processing for class I presentation. *Journal of Immunology* **147**, 2860–2863.

Kumar V. & Sercarz E. (1996) Genetic vaccination: The advantages of going naked. *Nature Medicine* **2**(8), 857–859.

Lambert P.H. (1993) New vaccines for the world — needs and prospects. *The Immunologist* **1**, 50–55.

Mims C.A., Playfair J.H.L., Roitt I.M., Wakelin D. & Williams R. (1993) *Medical Microbiology*. Mosby, London.

Nicholson B.H. (ed.) (1994) *Synthetic Vaccines*. Blackwell Science, Oxford.

Peter G. (1992) Current concepts: childhood immunizations. *New England Journal of Medicine* **327**, 1794–1800.

Powell M.F. & Newman M.J. (eds) (1995) *Vaccine Design*. Plenum Publishing, New York.

Sherwood J.K. *et al.* (1996) Controlled release of antibodies for long-term topical passive immunoprotection of female mice against genital herpes. *Nature Biotechnology* **14**(4), 468.

Whittum-Hudson J.A. *et al.* (1996) Oral immunisation with anti-idiotype to exoglycolipid antigen protects against *Chlamydia trachomatis* infection. *Nature Medicine* **2**, 1116–1121.

Yap P.L. (ed.) (1992) *Clinical Applications of Intravenous Immunoglobulin Therapy*. Churchill Livingstone, Edinburgh.

Zinkernagel R. & Lambert P.H. (1992) Immunity to infection. *Current Opinion in Immunology* **4**, 385–460 (also 1993, **5**, issue 4).

# CLINICAL IMMUNOLOGY

We are now ready to look at the clinical consequences of failure or abnormal operation of the body's immunological defenses. Not surprisingly, when the immune systems fail, the individual is susceptible to infection and Chapter 15 is concerned with the underlying mechanisms and infectious consequences of what are essentially **primary immunodeficiency** states and **immunodeficiency secondary** to some clearly defined cause such as the AIDS viruses.

Abnormally heightened immune responses or unusually excessive amounts of antigen can lead to tissue damage and Chapter 16 looks at a variety of these **hypersensitivity** reactions. Some disorders (e.g. allergy, Rhesus disease of the newborn) are caused by antibody and others (e.g. systemic lupus erythematosus (SLE)) by immune complexes; T-cell-mediated, delayed-type hypersensitivity often underlies severe reactions to infection while reactions to bacterial products such as lipopolysaccharide (LPS) can activate the innate system adversely.

The realization that **graft rejection** is an immunological phenomenon has spawned frenetic attempts to overcome this barrier and the achievements of matching histocompatibility tissue types and developing antigen-specific and nonspecific therapies are closely monitored in Chapter 17. We also discuss the allograft problem faced by the fetus as a result of the tremendous polymorphism of the major histocompatibility antigens and open the curtain on immunological contraception as one approach to population control.

Tumor immunology is becoming exciting again and increasing evidence that certain **tumors** may be susceptible to attack by both the innate and acquired arms of the immune response is debated in Chapter 18. We also give an account of the **lymphoproliferative diseases**, such as leukemia, which arise when there is dysregulated development of lymphoid cells.

It is inevitable that from time to time the body's fail-safe mechanisms which prevent self-reactivity from emerging within the lymphoid population are circumvented, and we are faced with the prospect of **autoimmune disease**. The surprising **range of disorders** encompassed by this pathogenic umbrella is introduced in Chapter 19, where possible **etiological scenarios** are entertained.

Finally, Chapter 20 updates our views on the **pathogenic mechanisms** which operate, the value of the **diagnostic tests** available in the clinical immunology laboratory and the efficacy of current and possible future **therapeutic modalities**.

# IMMUNODEFICIENCY

C O N T E N T S

## PRIMARY IMMUNODEFICIENCY STATES IN THE HUMAN

In accord with the dictum that 'most things that can go wrong, do so', a multiplicity of immunodeficiency states in man which are **not secondary** to environmental factors, have been recognized. We have earlier stressed the manner in which the interplay of complement, antibody and phagocytic cells constitutes the basis of a tripartite defense mechanism against pyogenic (pus-forming) infections with bacteria which require prior opsonization before phagocytosis. It is not surprising then, that deficiency in any one of these factors may predispose the individual to repeated infections of this type. Patients with T-cell deficiency of course present a markedly different pattern of infection, being susceptible to those viruses and moulds which are normally eradicated by cell-mediated immunity (CMI).

A relatively high incidence of malignancies, and of autoantibodies with or without autoimmune disease, has been documented in patients with immunodeficiency but the reason for this association is not yet clear, although failure of T-cell regulation or inability to control key viral infections are among the suggestions canvassed.

The following sections examine various forms of these primary immunodeficiencies.

## DEFICIENCIES OF INNATE IMMUNE MECHANISMS

### Phagocytic cell defects

In **chronic granulomatous disease** the monocytes and polymorphs fail to produce reactive oxygen intermediates (figure 15.1) due to a defect in the cytochrome $b_{-245}$ oxidase system (cf. p. 8) normally

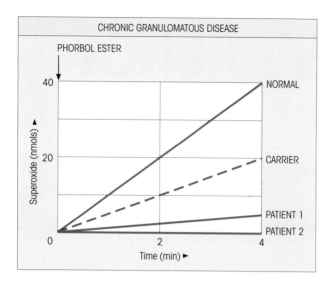

**Figure 15.1. Defective respiratory burst in neutrophils of patients with chronic granulomatous disease.** The activation of the NADP/cytochrome oxidase is measured by superoxide anion ($\cdot O_2^-$; cf. figure 1.9) production following stimulation with phorbol myristate acetate. Patient 2 has a p92*phox* mutation which prevents expression of the protein, whilst patient 1 has the variant p92*phox* mutation producing very low but measurable levels. Many carriers of the X-linked disease express intermediate levels, as in the individual shown who is the mother of patient 2. (Data from Smith R.M. & Curnutte J.T. (1991) *Blood* **77**, 673–686.)

activated by phagocytosis. The cytochrome has 92 and 22 kDa subunits and in the X-linked form of the disease there are mutations in the gene encoding the larger of these subunits. In the majority of cases, no cytochrome is produced but one variant gp92 mutation permits the synthesis of low levels of the protein (figure 15.1) and the condition can be improved by treatment with γ-interferon. The 30% of chronic granulomatous disease patients who inherit their disorder in an autosomal recessive pattern express a defective form of the oxidase resulting from mutations in the smaller p22*phox* cytochrome subunit and in the cytosolic p47*phox* and p67*phox* (*phox* = phagocyte oxidase) components of the total NADPH-oxidase system. Not unexpectedly, the knockout of gp92*phox* provides a handy mouse model (cf. figure 1.9).

Curiously, the range of infectious pathogens which trouble these patients is relatively restricted. The most common pathogen is *Staphylococcus aureus* but certain Gram-negative bacilli and fungi such as *Aspergillus fumigatus* and *Candida albicans* are frequently involved. The factors underlying this restriction are 2-fold. First, many bacteria help to bring about their own destruction by generating $H_2O_2$ through their own metabolic processes, but if they are catalase positive, the peroxide is destroyed and the bacteria will survive. Thus polymorphs from these patients readily take up catalase-positive staphylo-

cocci in the presence of antibody and complement but fail to kill them intracellularly. Second, the organisms which are most virulent tend to be those that are highly resistant to the oxygen-independent microbicidal mechanisms of the phagocyte.

In **Chediak–Higashi** disease, the lysosomes are deficient in elastase and cathepsin G and the patients suffer from pyogenic infections which can be fatal. Beige mice which represent a murine model of this disease have neutrophils which lack azurophilic granules. Among other rare conditions, **myeloperoxidase deficiency** is associated with susceptibility to systemic candidiasis, while a defective polymorph response to chemotactic stimuli characterizes the **lazy leukocyte syndrome**.

Lack of the CD18 β-subunit of the $β_2$-integrins produces a **leukocyte adhesion deficiency** causing impaired neutrophil chemotaxis and recurrent bacterial infection. Emigration of monocytes, eosinophils and lymphocytes is unaffected since these can fall back on the alternative VCAM-1/VLA-4 $β_1$-integrin system. Two cases (remember these primary immunodeficiencies tend to be pretty rare) of leukocyte adhesion deficiency associated with mental retardation and Bombay hh blood group phenotype had defective neutrophil motility due to a failure to produce sialyl Lewis[x], the ligand used to bind to the selectins on endothelial cells. The defect in the synthesis of blood group H antigen, which is also a fucosylated carbohydrate, suggests a defect in fucose metabolism. Allogeneic bone marrow grafts used to correct the CD18-linked disease are surprisingly well tolerated, possibly because of the LFA-1 defect. Seizing on this clue, one group has increased allogeneic bone marrow survival in general to 50% by treating recipients with monoclonal anti-LFA-1. In a totally different disorder, **congenital agranulocytosis**, it is encouraging to report that daily infusion of recombinant granulocyte colony-stimulating factor (G-CSF) (p. 181) raises the granulocyte counts in the majority of patients.

## Complement system deficiencies

### Defects in control proteins

The importance of complement in defense against infections is emphasized by the occurrence of repeated life-threatening infection with pyogenic bacteria in a patient lacking factor I, the C3b inactivator. Because of this inability to destroy C3b, there is continual activation of the alternative pathway through the feedback loop leading to very low C3 and factor B levels with normal C1, 4 and 2.

Each red blood cell is bombarded daily with 1000 molecules of C3b generated through the formation of fluid phase alternative pathway C3 convertase from the spontaneous hydrolysis of the internal thioester of C3. There are several regulatory components on the red cell surface to deal with this. The C3 convertase complex is dissociated by decay-accelerating factor (DAF) and by CR1 complement receptors (not forgetting factor H from the fluid phase, cf. p. 11), after which the C3b is dismembered by factor I in concert with CR1, membrane cofactor protein (MCP) or factor H (figure 15.2). There are also two inhibitors of the membrane attack complex, homologous restriction factor (HRF) and the abundant protectin molecule (CD59) which, by binding to C8, prevent the unfolding of the first C9 molecule needed for membrane insertion. DAF, HRF and CD59 bind to the membrane through glycosyl phosphatidylinositol anchors. In a condition known as **paroxysmal nocturnal hemoglobinuria (PNH)** there is a defect in the ability to synthesize these anchors and, in the absence of these complement regulators, serious lysis of the red cells occurs. In the less severe type II PNH, there is a defect in DAF, but in the type III form, associated also with deficiency of CD59, susceptibility to spontaneous complement-mediated lysis is greatly increased (figure 15.2). The erythrocytes can be normalized by adding back the deficient factors.

In **acute myocardial infarction**, the expression of the CD59 protectin decreases, perhaps due to the shedding of small membrane vesicles, and this sensitizes the injured myocardial cells to attack by the membrane attack complex (MAC) leading to a clear demarcation between nonviable and viable tissue areas.

An inhibitor of active C1 is grossly lacking in **hereditary angioedema** and this can lead to recurring episodes of acute circumscribed non-inflammatory edema mediated by a vasoactive C2 fragment (figure 15.3). The patients are heterozygotes and synthesize small amounts of the inhibitor which can be raised to useful levels by administration of the synthetic anabolic steroid danazol or, in critical cases, of the purified inhibitor itself. ε-Aminocaproic acid, which blocks the plasmin-induced liberation of the C2 kinin, provides an alternative treatment.

## Deficiency of components of the complement pathway

Failure to generate the classical C3-convertase through deficiencies in C1q, C1r, C4 and C2 has been reported in a small number of cases associated with

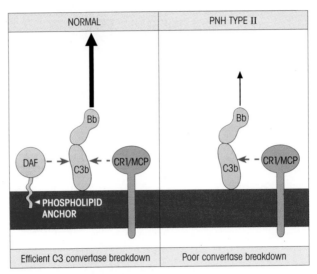

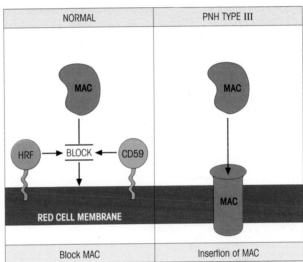

**Figure 15.2. Paroxysmal nocturnal hemoglobinuria (PNH).** A mutation in the *PIG-A* gene, which encodes α-1,6-*N*-acetylglucosaminyl-transferase, results in an inability to synthesize the glycosyl phosphatidylinositol anchors, deprives the red cell membrane of complement control proteins and renders the cell susceptible to complement-mediated lysis. Type II is associated with a DAF defect and the more severe type III with additional CD59 deficiency. (DAF = decay accelerating factor; CR1 = complement receptor type 1; MCP = membrane cofactor protein; HRF = homologous restriction factor; MAC = membrane attack complex.)

an unusually high incidence of SLE-like syndromes (cf. p. 429), perhaps due to a decreased ability to mount an adequate host response to infection with a putative etiologic agent or, more probably, to eliminate antigen–antibody complexes effectively (cf. p. 342). Permanent deficiencies in C5, C6, C7, C8 and C9 have all been described in man, yet in virtually every case the individuals are healthy and not particularly prone to infection apart from an increased susceptibility to disseminated *Neisseria gonorrhoeae* and *N. meningitidis*. Thus full operation of the terminal complement system does not appear to be essential

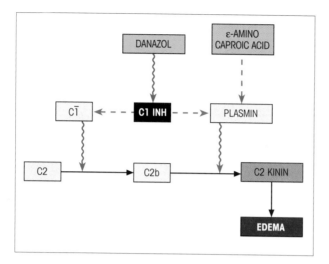

**Figure 15.3. C1 inhibitor deficiency and angioedema.** C1 inhibitor stoichiometrically inhibits C1, plasmin, kallikrein and activated Hageman factor and deficiency leads to formation of the vasoactive C2 kinin by the mechanism shown. The synthesis of C1 inhibitor can be boosted by methyltestosterone or preferably the less masculinizing synthetic steroid, danazol; alternatively, attacks can be controlled by giving ε-aminocaproic acid to inhibit the plasmin.

for survival and adequate protection must be largely afforded by opsonizing antibodies and the immune adherence mechanism.

## PRIMARY B-CELL DEFICIENCY

**Bruton's congenital a-γ-globulinemia** is one of several immunodeficient syndromes which have been mapped to the X-chromosome (figure 15.4). The defect occurs at the pre-B-cell stage and the production of immunoglobulin in affected males is grossly depressed, there being few lymphoid follicles or plasma cells in lymph node biopsies. Mutations occur in Bruton's tyrosine kinase (*BTK*) gene, which is also responsible for the *xid* defect in mice. The children are subject to repeated infection by pyogenic bacteria — *Staphylococcus aureus, Streptococcus pyogenes* and *pneumoniae, Neisseria meningitidis, Haemophilus influenzae* — and by a rare protozoon, *Pneumocystis carinii*, which produces a strange form of pneumonia. Cell-mediated immune responses are normal and viral infections such as measles and smallpox are readily brought under control. Therapy involves the repeated administration of human γ-globulin to maintain adequate concentrations of circulating immunoglobulin.

**IgA deficiency** due to a failure of IgA-bearing lymphocytes to differentiate into plasma cells, is encountered with relative frequency. Antibodies to IgA are often detectable but it is uncertain whether these anti-

bodies prevented development of the IgA system or whether lack of tolerance resulting from an absent IgA system allowed the body to make antibodies to exogenous determinants immunologically related to IgA.

The most common form of immunodeficiency, not surprisingly known as **common variable immunodeficiency**, is characterized by recurrent pyogenic infections and probably includes many entities. The marrow contains normal numbers of immature B-cells, but one-third of the patients lack circulating B-cells with surface Ig and, of the remainder, half have subnormal numbers. Where present they are unable to differentiate to plasma cells in some cases or to secrete antibody in others. T-cells are, however, also affected; each lymphocyte has a low surface 5-nucleotidase, the T-cells lack the small agranular characteristic nonspecific esterase spot (figure 2.6b),

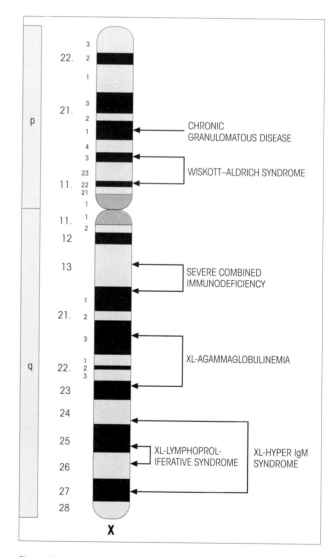

**Figure 15.4. Loci of the X-linked (XL) immunodeficiency syndromes.**

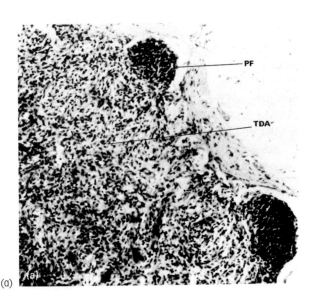
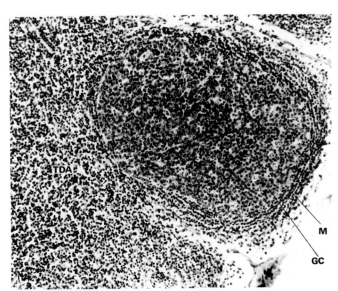

Figure 15.5. Lymph node cortex. (a) From patient with DiGeorge syndrome showing depleted thymus-dependent area (TDA) and small primary follicles (PF); (b) from normal subject: the populated T-cell area and the well-developed secondary follicle with its mantle of small lymphocytes (M) and pale-staining germinal center (GC) provide a marked contrast. (DiGeorge material kindly supplied by Dr D. Webster; photograph by Mr C.J. Sym.) In the murine model, the athymic nude mouse, there is an abnormality in the winged helix protein.

around 30% have poor responses to the polyclonal T-cell activator phytohemagglutinin (PHA) and a small proportion have T-cells of phenotype CD8+, major histocompatibility complex (MHC) class II-positive with marked suppressor activity for B-cells. An excess of such cells, revealed by their ability to suppress pokeweed-driven immunoglobulin synthesis by human leukocyte antigen (HLA)-identical normal lymphocytes, is a feature of the chronic graft-vs-host disease which follows allogeneic bone marrow transplantation in man. The genetic basis of this disease is as yet unknown but a large proportion possess the same HLA haplotypes as patients with IgA deficiency, suggesting a common underlying disorder.

It is exciting to see the molecular basis of diseases being unravelled and an excellent example of nature yielding its secrets has been provided by studies on the **XL hyper-IgM syndrome**, a rare disorder characterized by recurrent bacterial infections, very low levels or absence of IgG, A and E and normal to raised concentrations of serum IgM and IgD. It transpires that point mutations and deletions in the T-cell CD40L map to the part of the molecule thought to be concerned in the interaction with B-cell CD40 (cf. p. 177), thereby rendering the T-cells incapable of transmitting the signals needed for Ig class-switching in B-cells.

**Transient hypo-γ-globulinemia of infancy**, characterized by recurrent respiratory infections, is associated with low IgG levels which often return somewhat abruptly to normal by 4 years of age. There is a deficiency in the number of circulating lymphocytes and in their ability to generate help for Ig production by B-cells activated by pokeweed mitogen, but this becomes normal as the disease resolves spontaneously.

A degree of immunoglobulin deficiency occurs naturally in human infants as the maternal IgG level wanes and may become a serious problem in very premature babies.

## PRIMARY T-CELL DEFICIENCY

The **DiGeorge** and **Nezelof syndromes** are characterized by a failure of the thymus to develop properly from the third and fourth pharyngeal pouches during embryogenesis (DiGeorge children also lack parathyroids and have severe cardiovascular abnormalities). Consequently, stem cells cannot differentiate to become T-lymphocytes and the 'thymus-dependent' areas in lymphoid tissue are sparsely populated; in contrast lymphoid follicles are seen but even these are poorly developed (figure 15.5). Cell-mediated immune responses are undetectable and although the infants can deal with common bacterial infections, they may be overwhelmed by vaccinia (figure 15.6) or measles, or by bacille Calmette–Guérin (BCG) if given by mistake. Humoral antibodies can be elicited but the response is subnormal, presumably reflecting the need for the cooperative involvement of T-cells. (The similarity of this condition to neonatal thymectomy and of B-cell deficiency to neonatal bursectomy in the

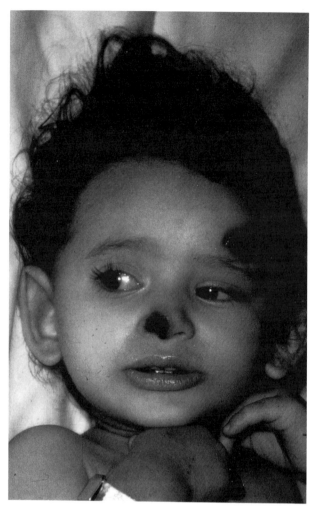

**Figure 15.6. A child with severe combined immunodeficiency** showing skin lesions due to infection with vaccinia gangrenosum resulting from small-pox immunization. Lesions were widespread over the whole body. (Reproduced by kind permission of Professor R.J. Levinsky and the Medical Illustration Department of the Hospital for Sick Children, Great Ormond Street, London.)

chicken should not go unmentioned.) Treatment by grafting neonatal thymus leads to restoration of immunocompetence but some matching between the major histocompatibility antigens on the nonlymphocytic thymus cells and peripheral cells is essential for the proper functioning of the T-lymphocytes (p. 229).

Complete absence of the thymus is pretty rare and more often one is dealing with a 'partial DiGeorge' in which the T-cells may rise from 6% at birth to around 30% of the total circulating lymphocytes by the end of the first year; antibody responses are adequate.

Cell-mediated immunity (CMI) is depressed in immunodeficient patients with **ataxia telangiectasia** or with thrombocytopenia and eczema (**Wiskott–**

**Aldrich syndrome**) and it is of great interest that in both conditions about 10% of the patients so far studied have died of malignancies of the lymphoid system or of epithelial tumors. Wiskott–Aldrich males lack a cell-surface molecule, sialophorin (CD43), which is a ligand for intercellular adhesion molecule-1 (ICAM-1). Normal T-cells proliferate in response to IgG anti-CD43 in the presence of mononuclear phagocytes, independently of the CD3/T-cell receptor (TCR) system. Wiskott–Aldrich is associated with a low IgM and a poor response to many polysaccharides; there are few B-cells bearing surface idiotypes for polysaccharide antigens and they require T-cell help elicited in a nonspecific manner independent of the CD3/TCR receptor. The question arises quite naturally: is CD43 the nonspecific receptor for polysaccharides capable of transducing this message for nonspecific T-cell help? An abnormality in the gene expressing a new cytoplasmic and nuclear transcription factor (WASP) should provide a valuable clue.

Ataxia telangiectasia is a human autosomal recessive disorder of childhood characterized by progressive cerebellar ataxia with degeneration of Purkinje cells, and a hypersensitivity to X-rays, which, together with the unduly high incidence of cancer, has been laid at the door of a defect in DNA repair mechanisms. This presumably accounts for the clustering of breaks on chromosome 11 around genes of the Ig supergene family, especially TCR and IgH, and the associated cellular and Ig deficiency. The abnormal gene has a striking sequence similarity to the phosphatidylinositol-3 kinases (PI-3 kinases) involved in signal transduction. It also possesses a region of homology with the Rad3 protein required for control of a cell cycle checkpoint in yeast where it monitors DNA damage repair.

Isolated cases of T-cell deficiency have been described where the serum contains a lymphocytotoxic antibody which presumably must be selective for T- rather than B-lymphocytes. T-cells from some patients with mucocutaneous candidiasis are unable to produce the cytokine, macrophage migration inhibition factor (MIF), when stimulated *in vitro* and it is conceivable that other selective failures of lymphokine synthesis may be uncovered.

Also for the collector are the rare cases of deficiency arising from mutation in the γ-chains of the CD3 complex and the ZAP-70 kinase which preferentially impair the differentiation of CD8 T-cells. Another small subgroup with CMI deficiency has a defect in the nuclear transcription factor of activated T-cells, NFAT.

# COMBINED IMMUNODEFICIENCY

## Mutation in the common cytokine receptor $\gamma_c$ chain causes SCID

Over half of the cases of severe combined immunodeficiency (SCID), which affects both B- and T-cell development, derive from mutations in the $\gamma_c$ chain of the receptors for interleukins IL-2, 4, 7, 9 and 15. Of these, IL-7R is the most crucial for lymphocyte differentiation. One is on the lookout for the human equivalent of the murine SCID mutation in the Ku80 subunit of the DNA protein kinase responsible for the repair of DNA double-strand breaks and hence the proper *VDJ* joining of lymphocyte receptors (p. 47). Isolated cases of human SCID involving mutations in the *RAG* genes which catalyse the introduction of the double-strand breaks (pp. 47, 48) have been reported.

These children suffer recurrent infections early in life. Prolonged diarrhea resulting from gastrointestinal infections and pneumonia due to *Pneumocystis carinii* are common; *Candida albicans* grows vigorously in the mouth or on the skin. If vaccinated with attenuated organisms (figure 15.6) they usually die of progressive infection. SCID infants must be rescued by a bone marrow transplant if they are to survive.

## SCID can be due to mutations in purine salvage pathway enzymes

Many SCID patients have a genetic deficiency of the purine degradation enzymes, purine nucleoside phosphorylase (PNP) or adenosine deaminase (ADA), which results in the accumulation of metabolites (dGTP and dATP respectively) that are toxic to lymphoid stem cells. The comparable immunodeficiency seen in acute lymphocytic leukemia patients treated with the ADA inhibitor deoxycoformacin attests to the validity of this analysis. Half the ADA-deficient SCID patients do reasonably well on transfusions of normal red cells containing the enzyme, whereas others with a longer-standing more severe deficiency which might have affected the thymus epithelium, also require treatment with the enzyme modified by polyethylene glycol which extends its half-life. These patients are excellent candidates for gene therapy. Children have been treated with periodic infusion of their own T-cells corrected by transfection with the *ADA* gene linked to a retroviral vector. Significant reconstitution of antibody responses and delayed-type skin tests to environmental antigens have been achieved without apparent complications. Hemopoietic stem cells from umbilical cord blood transfected with the *ADA* gene could be detected up to 18 months of age but the level of expression was very low and until the technology is improved, such patients must be maintained on enzyme replacement therapy.

## Other SCID variants

The rapidly fatal variant of severe combined immunodeficiency associated with lack of myeloid cell precursors is termed **reticular dysgenesis**. A recent intriguing piece of detective work on the autosomal recessive MHC class II immunodeficiency known as the **'bare lymphocyte syndrome'**, involving both CMI and humoral immunity, has traced the defect to reaction of a factor with the transacting regulatory protein, RF-X, which binds to the HLA class II promoter. Expression of class II is preserved on thymic medullary, but not cortical, cells, and this leads to the establishment of self-tolerance, a situation so closely parallel with that described in mice carrying an H-2E construct with a 5'-flanking region lacking the X-box (p. 74).

An attempt has been made to summarize the cellular basis of the various deficiency states in figure 15.7.

# RECOGNITION OF IMMUNODEFICIENCIES

Defects in immunoglobulins can be assessed by quantitative estimations; levels of 2 g/l arbitrarily define the practical lower limit of normal. The humoral immune response can be examined by first screening the serum for natural antibodies (A and B isohemagglutinins, heteroantibody to sheep red cells, bactericidins against *E. coli*) and then attempting to induce active immunization with diphtheria, tetanus, pertussis and killed poliomyelitis — but no live vaccines. CD19, 20 and 22 are the main markers used to enumerate B-cells by immunofluorescence.

Patients with T-cell deficiency will be hypo- or unreactive in skin tests to such antigens as tuberculin, *Candida*, tricophytin, streptokinase/streptodornase and mumps. Active skin sensitization with dinitrochlorobenzene may be undertaken. The reactivity of peripheral blood mononuclear cells to phytohemagglutinin is a good indicator of T-lymphocyte reactivity as is also the one-way mixed lymphocyte reaction (see Chapter 17). Enumeration of T-cells is most readily achieved by cytofluorimetry using CD3 monoclonal antibody.

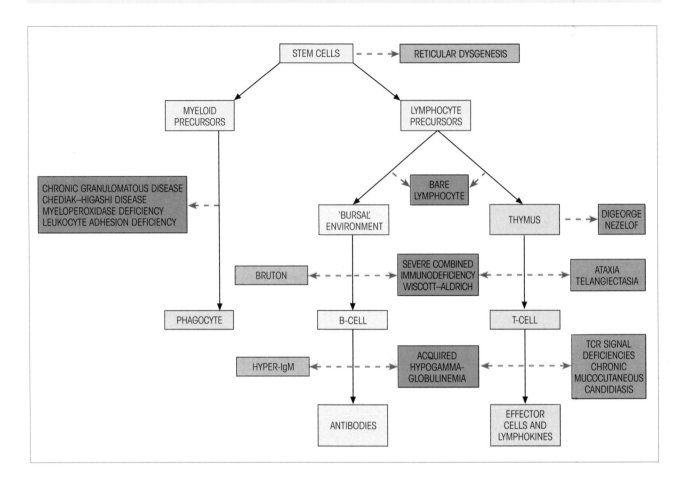

**Figure 15.7. The cellular basis of immunodeficiency states.** The red arrows indicate the cell type or differentiation process which is defective. Complement deficiencies have not been included.

*In vitro* tests for complement and for the bactericidal and other functions of polymorphs are available, while the reduction of nitroblue tetrazolium (NBT) or the stimulation of superoxide production provides a measure of the oxidative enzymes associated with active phagocytosis.

## SECONDARY IMMUNODEFICIENCY

Immune responsiveness can be depressed nonspecifically by many factors. CMI in particular may be impaired in a state of malnutrition, even of the degree which may be encountered in urban areas of the more affluent regions of the world. Iron deficiency is particularly important in this respect.

Viral infections are not infrequently immunosuppressive, and in the case of measles in man, Newcastle disease in chickens and rinderpest in cattle, this has been attributed to a direct cytotoxic effect of virus on the lymphoid cells. The most notorious immuno-suppressive virus, human immunodeficiency virus (HIV), will be elaborated upon in the next major section. In lepromatous leprosy and malarial infection there is evidence for a constraint on immune responsiveness imposed by distortion of the normal lymphoid traffic pathways and, additionally, in the latter instance, macrophage function appears to be aberrant. Skewing of the balance between TH1 and TH2 cells as a result of infection may also depress the subset most appropriate for immune protection.

Many therapeutic agents such as X-rays, cytotoxic drugs and corticosteroids, although often used in a nonimmunological context, can nonetheless have dire effects on the immune system (see p. 364). **B-lymphoproliferative disorders** like chronic lymphatic leukemia, myeloma and Waldenström's macroglobulinemia are associated with varying degrees of hypo-γ-globulinemia and impaired antibody responses. Their common infections with pyogenic bacteria contrast with the situation in Hodgkin's disease where the patients display all the hallmarks of defective CMI — susceptibility to tubercle bacillus, *Brucella, Cryptococcus* and herpes zoster virus.

## ACQUIRED IMMUNODEFICIENCY SYNDROME (AIDS)

AIDS is a particularly unpleasant, fatal disease which has reached endemic proportions and has thereby caused widespread alarm (and knowledge of immunology) amongst the public. In parts of Africa where the incidence is frightful, transmission is largely by heterosexual contact. Prostitutes constitute a pivotal major initial reservoir of the infection unlike their counterparts in developed countries such as Japan, Australia, New Zealand and the West, where the prevalence of AIDS has remained surprisingly low, and the majority of cases have occurred in male homosexuals, with other groups at risk including intravenous drug abusers, hemophiliacs receiving factor VIII derived from pooled plasma and infants of sexually promiscuous or drug-addicted mothers. Nevertheless, the number of infected heterosexuals is increasing. Death is usually due to pulmonary infection, but serious complications involving the nervous system are appearing in about 30% of cases. In essence, there is a sudden onset of immunodeficiency associated with opportunistic infections involving, most commonly, *Pneumocystis carinii*, but also cytomegalovirus (figure 15.8), Epstein–Barr (EB) and herpes simplex viruses, fungi such as *Candida*, *Aspergillus* and *Cryptococcus*, and the protozoon *Toxoplasma*; additionally, there is exceptional susceptibility for Kaposi's sarcoma. There is also an AIDS-related complex (ARC), characterized by fever, weight loss and lymphadenopathy.

## AIDS results from infection by a human immunodeficiency virus (HIV)

Transmission of the disease is usually through infection with blood or semen containing the HIV-1 virus or the related HIV-2, which have been isolated from various body fluids of AIDS patients. HIV-1 shows considerable resemblance to the oncogenic human T-cell leukemia virus (HTLV-1) which is closely linked to the production of a T-cell leukemia of high prevalence in Japan. Whereas HTLV-1 induces lymphoproliferation, HIV-1/2 are members of the lentivirus group, which produce disease with a long latency and are adept at evading the immune system. These include simian immunodeficiency viruses isolated from sooty mangabeys (SIV SM) and rhesus macaques (SIV MAC) which are similar to HIV-2, and a chimpanzee form of the virus with close homology to HIV-1; these are thought to provide the possible gene pools from which the AIDS viruses might have originated. Other examples are the visna virus responsible for central nervous system and lung lesions in sheep, and viruses which cause equine infectious anemia and caprine arthritis. HIV is a budding virus whose genome is relatively complex and tightly compressed (figure 15.9a,d). The many virion proteins are generated by RNA splicing and cleavage by the viral protease.

### The infection of cells by HIV

The envelope glycoprotein gp120 of HIV **binds**

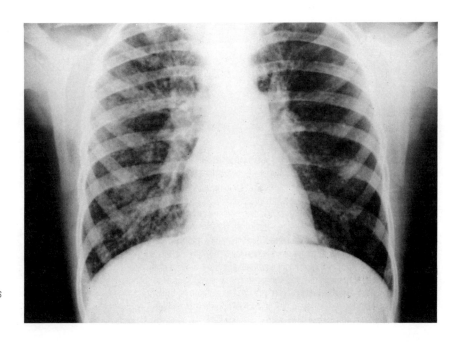

**Figure 15.8. Viral pneumonia due to cytomegalovirus**; radiograph showing extensive diffuse pneumonitis in both lung fields, characteristic of viral infection. (Reproduced from Lambert H.P. & Farrar W.E. (eds) (1982) *Infectious Diseases Illustrated*, p. 2.2. W.B. Saunders and Gower Medical Publishing, with permission.)

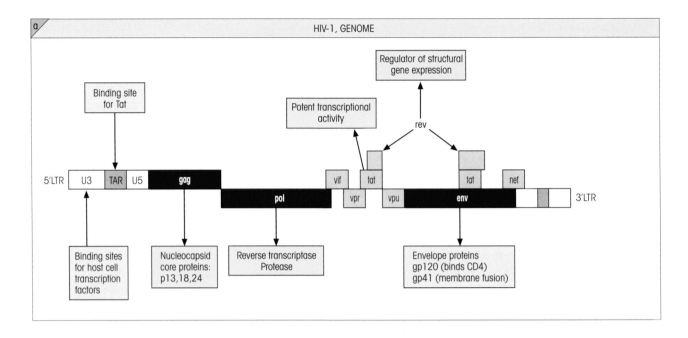

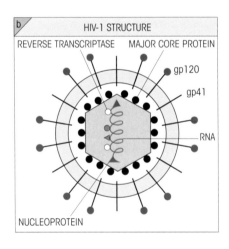

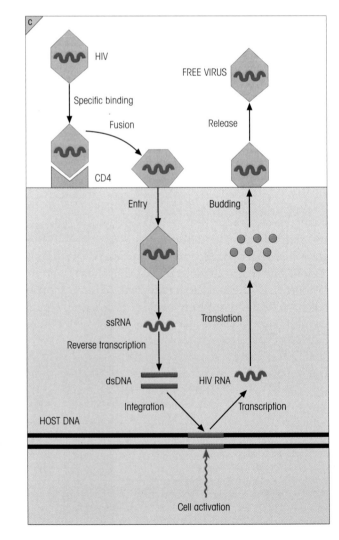

**Figure 15.9. Characteristics of the HIV-1 AIDS virus**. (a) HIV-1 genome and gene products. *tat* = master switch, turns on all viral gene expression; *rev* = gene responsible for expression of structural proteins; *vif* = gene controlling infectivity by free, not cell-bound, virus; *vpr* = weak transcriptional activator; *vpu* = required for efficient virion budding and env processing; *nef* = uncertain function linked to pathogenesis *in vivo*; *LTR* = long terminal repeats concerned in regulation of viral expression, contains regions reacting with products of *tat* and *nef* genes and in addition the *TATAAA* (the TATA box) promoter sequence, NFκB core enhancer elements and Sp-1 binding sites. Mice bearing the *tat* transgene develop Kaposi sarcoma-like skin lesions. (b) HIV-1 structure. (c) Intracellular life cycle of HIV. (d) Electron micrograph of mature and budding HIV-1 particles at the surface of human PHA blasts. (Courtesy of Drs Carol Upton and S. Martin.)

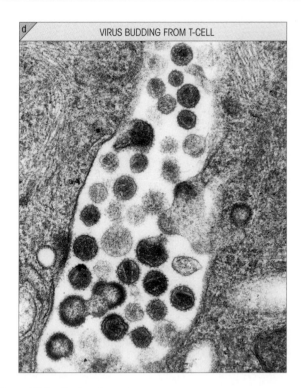

VIRUS BUDDING FROM T-CELL

Figure 15.9. *(Continued)*.

avidly to cell-surface CD4 molecules and initiates fusion with the cell, involving gp41, and infection (figure 15.9c). Helper T-cells with their abundant CD4 are a major target for infection but the presence of even relatively low densities of CD4 on macrophages and microglia makes them susceptible to infection, and in the latter case is suspected to be a major factor in the cerebral complications of the disease. Different virus isolates vary in their relative tropism for T-cells and macrophages, and binding sites for the two cell types have been localized to distinct but overlapping regions on the gp120 molecule. CD4 itself is not sufficient; witness the inability of the virus to infect mouse cells transfected with human CD4. Fusin, an integral membrane glycoprotein and member of a chemokine receptor family, acts as a cofactor with CD4 to bind gp120 and bring about the exposure of the gp41 fusion peptide. Antibodies to the N-terminus of fusin block fusion and infection of CD4 T-cells — but not macrophages whose cofusion factor is still to be revealed. There is also a worry that complexes of virus with antibody may facilitate entry into cells through Fc receptors. Possibly of crucial importance has been the discovery that suspensions of single follicular dendritic cells (FDCs) from human tonsil can be directly infected with HIV by a process which does not involve CD4. The infected cells permit viral repli-

cation and can reinfect T-cells *in vitro*. As we shall see, FDCs are a major reservoir of HIV in AIDS. Note also that the dendritic cells which present antigen to T-cells can also be infected by HIV.

HIV is an RNA retrovirus which utilizes a **reverse transcriptase** to convert its genetic RNA into the corresponding DNA which is integrated into the host genome where it can remain latent for long periods (figure 15.9c). Stimulation of latently infected T-cells or macrophages activates HIV replication through an increase in the intracellular concentration of NFκB dimers, which bind to consensus sequences in the HIV enhancer region (figure 15.10). It is significant that α-tumor necrosis factor (TNFα) which upregulates HIV replication through this NFκB pathway is present in elevated concentrations in the plasma of HIV-infected individuals, particularly, in the advanced stage. Perhaps also, the greater susceptibility of Africans to AIDS may be linked to activation of the immune system through continual microbial insult.

## The AIDS infection depletes helper T-cells

### Natural history of the disease

The sequence of events following HIV-1 infection is

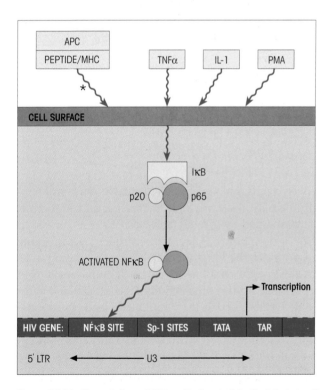

Figure 15.10. Upregulation of HIV replication in latently infected cell through external stimulation. (* = T-cells only; IκB = inhibitor of NFκB.)

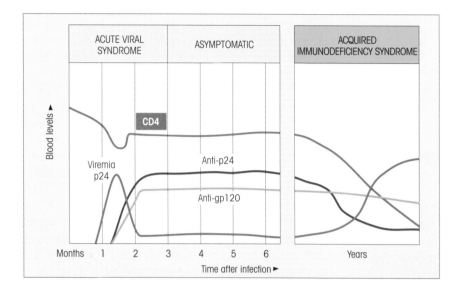

**Figure 15.11. The natural history of HIV-1 infection.** The changes in p24 antigen and antibody shown late in disease are seen in some but not all patients.

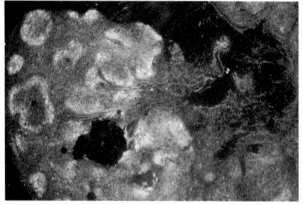

(a)

(b)

**Figure 15.12. Abundance of HIV in lymphoid tissue** demonstrated by *in situ* hybridization of lymph node sections from a representative HIV-infected patient in early-stage disease. (a) Darkfield image of a lymph node section after protease digestion. Location of HIV RNA is indicated by the silver grains which appear as white dots. An intense hybridization signal is predominantly restricted to the area of the germinal centers. (b) Higher magnification of a protease digested section showing the intense distribution of silver grains in the light zone of a germinal center. (Reproduced from photos kindly provided by Dr. A.S. Fauci with permission. cf. Pantaleo G., Graziosi C. & Fauci A.S. (1993) The role of the lymphoid organs in the pathogenesis of HIV infection. *Seminars in Immunology* **5**, 157–163.)

charted in figure 15.11. An acute early retroviral syndrome with fever, myalgia, arthralgia and so forth is accompanied by viremia and positive tests for blood p24, a dominant nucleocapsid antigen. An immune response to the virus identifiable by circulating antibodies to p24 and the envelope proteins gp120 and gp41, and by the production of gp120-specific cytotoxic T-cells, curtails the viremia and leads to **sequestration of HIV in lymphoid tissue**. Trapping of viral particles complexed with antibody and complement stimulates follicular hyperplasia and infection of the FDC. In effect the follicles become the principal site for viral replication and infection of other cells of the immune system (figure 15.12). Eventually, follicular involution leads to a gradual degeneration of the FDC network with an increase in viral burden and replication in peripheral blood mononuclear cells. Crucially, **circulating CD4 T-cell numbers fall progressively** but only when there is profound depletion with levels below, say, 50 mm$^{-3}$, do the consequences for CMI responses, as exemplified by the depressed delayed-type skin reactivity to common antigens (figure 15.13) and the failure to produce cytomegalovirus-specific cytotoxic T-cells (Tc), become quite devastating. The patient is now wide open to life-threatening infections caused by normally nonpathogenic (i.e. opportunistic) agents such as *Pneumocystis carinii* and cytomegalovirus characteristic of AIDS.

## Mechanisms of depletion

After first treatment with antiviral drugs before mutant resistant strains arise, the fall in viral levels showed the rate of removal by the immune system to be of the order of $1 \times 10^8$ to $7 \times 10^9$ viral particles per day. Since there was a steady state, this must also have been the rate of production. At the same time, the rise in levels of CD4 T-cells shows that the total rate of production, and, by extension, destruction, must originally have been approximately $2 \times 10^9$ cells daily. This means that there is one hell of a **battle between the virus and the immune system** before the fulminant HIV production eventually overwhelms the prodigious powers of regeneration of the immune system and produces the dramatic fall in CD4 T-cells with a corresponding change in the CD4:CD8 ratio. There is certainly no shortage of hypotheses to account for CD4 depletion. These include:

**1** A direct cytopathic effect by the virus either on single cells or through the production of syncitia between CD4 T-cells. Correlations between *in vitro* and *in vivo* performance of different isolates are not particularly convincing.

**2** Behavior of HIV as a superantigen like the mammary-tumor retroviruses in mice (cf. p. 100), combining with and deleting certain TCR families. In one study, $V\beta_{12}$ T-cell lines yielded 100-fold more p24 than $V\beta_{6.7}$ lines established from the same patient, which is suggestive.

**3** Susceptibility to programmed cell death (apoptosis). Stimulation of CD4 T-cells in asymptomatic HIV-infected individuals leads to apoptosis. Dendritic cells infected with HIV actively support viral replication and are downregulated with respect to class II MHC and B7; conceivably, multiple copies of gp120 present on the surface during viral budding, could induce apoptosis by ligating and cross-linking CD4 on the T-cell without delivering costimulatory signals.

**4** Suppression of protective TH1 cells, but not of HIV-susceptible TH2 cells, by a conserved retroviral 17mer peptide (CKS-17) present in the HIV gp41 envelope molecule. This peptide inhibits TH1 cells by upregulating IL-10 and downregulating IL-12 (cf. p. 184), it inhibits protein kinase C by a novel Arg. Arg. mechanism, and it boosts intracellular cAMP which impairs proliferation of TH1 but not TH2 cells.

**5** Failure of infected antigen-presenting cells. Dendritic cells and macrophages lose their ability to present soluble antigens to CD45RO T-cells in asymptomatic HIV infection and it may be of significance that studies in the SCID mouse model indicate a close relationship between the CD4-depleting ability of different viral isolates and their tropism for macrophages. Failure to maintain the activated memory pool of CD45RO cells through defective antigen-presenting cells (APC) will lead to shrinkage and subsequently the quiescent CD45RA memory

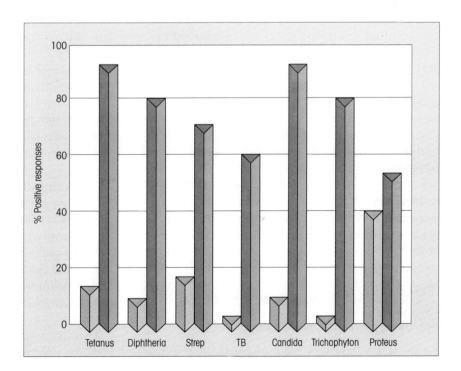

**Figure 15.13. Skin test reactivity to common microbial antigens among AIDS patients (■; n=20) and controls (■; n=10).** Other studies with more advanced patients have reported completely negative skin tests. (Reproduced from Lane H.C. & Fauci A.S. (1985) *Annual Reviews of Immunology* **3**, 477, with permission.)

pool will also shrink due to few re-entrants. These changes may also underly the skewing of the T-helpers towards the TH2 subset seen as the disease progresses.

**6** Induction of an autoimmune response due to cross-reactions between HIV proteins and cryptic epitopes (cf. p. 202) on activated T-cells, or through interference with normal intrathymic tolerance mechanisms.

**7** Opsonic loss due to coating CD4 with gp120 immune complexes.

It is likely that a combination of several of these mechanisms will ultimately act to tip the balance in favor of the virus.

AIDS patients also have hyper-γ-globulinemia and large numbers of B-cells which spontaneously secrete Ig in culture, suggesting that they are polyclonally stimulated. A small proportion of HIV-infected T-cells express membrane TNFα and these can induce polyclonal B-cell activation. Expression of viral proteins on the surface of these T-cells would focus their activity on B-cells expressing antiviral Ig receptors and would account for the predominance of antibodies to HIV in the culture supernatants of unstimulated B-cells from seropositive patients. This could also be a reflection of the domination of FDCs in the germinal centers by virus.

## Diagnosis of AIDS

An individual with opportunistic infections, lymphopenia, low CD4 but relatively normal CD8 in the peripheral blood, raised IgG and IgA levels and poor skin tests to common recall antigens may well have AIDS, particularly if they come from a group at risk. γ-Interferon (IFNγ) and neopterin, a degradation product of guanosine triphosphate (GTP) induced in macrophages by IFNγ, are good indicators of CMI and are significantly increased in AIDS infection preceding subsequent loss of CD4 cells. Confirmation of the diagnosis comes from lymph node biopsy, showing profound abnormalities and drastic changes in germinal centers, and the demonstration of viral antibodies by enzyme-linked immunosorbent assay (ELISA) and by 'immunoblotting' (cf. pp. 113 and 118). Serum p24 antigen is often positive in active disease but isolation of virus or demonstration of HIV genome provides the final confirmation of infection.

## The control of AIDS

*Identifying protective immune responses*

We are still a long way from understanding which immune responses might afford protection and hence could form a basis for rational vaccine design. After inadvertent transfusion of infected plasma, the first antibodies to appear are directed to the gp120 envelope glycoprotein; antibodies to core proteins p24 and 18 may be seen later. Most antibodies are non-neutralizing, in that they fail to prevent infection of susceptible cells in culture, and in the rare instances when they are neutralizing, the titers tend to be disappointingly low and usually type-specific. A resistant variant can be generated by a single mutation and it must be said that the gp120 gene is highly susceptible to mutation, a feature of other lentiviruses with hypervariable envelope regions which prevent immunization with any one variant from protecting against the new variants which emerge rapidly during infection. In the HIV-1 gp120 molecule, it is the V3 region located between residues 307 and 330 within a loop formed by two highly conserved cysteine residues which is subject to extremely high mutation rates. Needless to say, it is this region, important for the fusion process, that provides the dominant epitopes for the development of type-specific neutralizing antibodies. To add further gloom and despondency, it has been shown that FDC can transfer infectious HIV to CD4 T-cells even in the presence of anti-gp120 neutralizing antibodies which are capable of preventing the entry of *free* virus. We have already mentioned the strange susceptibility of FDC to infection by a CD4-independent mechanism, and their function as reservoirs of infection; there have to be some crucial events occurring in these cells which must be uncovered. Interest has also focused on the other surface protein, gp41. The 735–752 peptide from the conserved transmembrane region, when inserted into polio virus, induces antibodies which neutralize HIV and have a wide ability to block fusion and, as an antigen, is said to remove a major fraction of the group-specific neutralizing and fusion-inhibiting antibodies from some sera. This has the makings of a dominant target.

Preventing the virus from gaining entry to the body in the first place is a worthy aim and more attempts are being made to induce mucosal immunity by oral immunization. A multicomponent antigen composed of HIV-1 peptides from the CD4 binding site, the *gag* region and the V3 loops of different strains, linked to cholera toxin was given orally and found to give rise to antigen-specific fecal sIgA capable of neutralizing the virus.

There is a strong school of thought that looks to CMI for effective defense. The temporal association between HIV-specific Tc cells and a reduction in viral load during primary infection suggests a role for these cells in the clearance of the initial viremia. Tc cells have also been observed in seronegative individuals who have been exposed to repeated infection and they could be conferring long-term protection. However, escape mutants readily arise and permit persistence of virus in asymptomatic individuals despite the presence of Tc cells specific for the wild-type strain. The story can take a further turn because in some cases, peptides derived from the mutants can block Tc lysis of cells bearing the wild-type peptide epitope.

The CD8 T-cell population also mounts a non-cytolytic attack on HIV. Remove CD8 from the peripheral blood lymphocytes of asymptomatic HIV-infected subjects and the virus can now readily be isolated; reconstitute with the autologous CD8 cells and HIV replication is suppressed. The active agent has been tracked down to a CD8 T-cell antiviral factor, CAF, which is not identical with IL-16 or other known cytokines and is effective against a broad range of strains. It is not detected in control immune activated CD8 cells but so far only in cells from individuals with a previous HIV infection. By inhibiting viral replication and presumably expression of a Tc target on infected cells, this noncytolytic mechanism can prevent the widespread damage caused by extensive Tc activity. IL-2 sustains CD8 production of CAF, which, in turn, will maintain the function of CD4 cells, further highlighting the importance of TH1 activity.

One gallant human was immunized by intravenous injection of paraformaldehyde-fixed autologous cells infected *in vivo* with recombinant vaccinia expressing the complete gp160 (used by the virus to provide gp120 and gp41), followed by gp160 derived from an HIV-1 clone. High levels of neutralizing antibody and CMI to divergent HIV-1 strains developed, but naturally there was no rush to test for resistance to infection. For this and many other reasons animal models are vital.

## The development of animal models

Rabbits can be infected with HIV but they do not develop disease, although they are useful for testing the responses to recombinant vaccinia-HIV vaccines. Monkeys would seem likely candidates but, like chimpanzees, they show no sign of disease after infection with HIV-1. The less pathogenic HIV-2 does produce lymphadenopathy but nothing more. A good model is the AIDS-like disease produced by simian immunodeficiency virus (SIV). Macaque monkeys could be protected against challenge with a high i.v. dose of the pathogenic SIV by vaccination with a recombinant vaccinia virus expressing the nef protein. Prolonged protection was also obtained using an attenuated strain of SIV with a deletion in the *nef* gene. However, long-term studies revealed some form of disease in these animals suggesting the need for considerable caution with this approach.

## Other therapeutic strategies

The reverse transcriptase enzyme and the HIV protease responsible for cleaving gp160 into the gp120 and p41 components are good targets for antiviral drug therapy but resistant strains emerge with depressing rapidity through mutation. Currently, a triple therapy combining two reverse scriptase antagonists and a protease inhibitor is achieving worthwhile success.

Soluble CD4 molecules bind robustly to HIV and block its infectivity but only have a short half-life. A classy recombinant molecule consisting of the binding CD4 domains linked to two Fcγ domains has been synthesized; it has a much longer half-life and could be a useful therapeutic agent. A new 'super-immunoadhesin' which is a thousand times more potent than soluble CD4 in syncitium inhibition assays has been created by stitching 10 CD4 domains into a single IgM chimeric molecule. I am especially attracted to the strategy of 'intracellular immunization', in which bone marrow cells are transfected with an anti-HIV molecule which will protect the future differentiated CD4 T-cell from infection. In one approach, bone marrow cells are transfected with a sequence of the CD4 gene coding for an HIV-blocking peptide; on regrafting, some of the stem cells will become CD4+ T-cells, secreting a surrounding barrier of the blocking peptide which protects the lymphocyte from infection by the virus. Another group have transfected the stem cells with an scFv (cf. p. 124) gene encoding a single HIV-specific antibody combining site which disrupts the viral replication cycle. Using a similar system, one could also envisage the transfection of antisense genes to block the expression of HIV regulatory genes. Despite this frantic activity a change in social behavior patterns must make a difference to the spread of AIDS.

# SUMMARY

## Primary immunodeficiency states

- These occur in the human, albeit somewhat rarely, as a result of a defect in almost any stage of differentiation in the whole immune system.
- Rare X-linked mutations produce disease in males.
- Defects in phagocytic cells, the complement pathways or the B-cell system lead in particular to infection with bacteria which are disposed of by opsonization and phagocytosis.
- Patients with T-cell deficiencies are susceptible to viruses and moulds which are normally eradicated by CMI.

## Deficiency of innate immunity

- Chronic granulomatous disease results from mutations in the NADPH oxidase of phagocytic cells.
- Leukocyte adhesion deficiency involves mutations in the CD18 subunit of $\beta_2$-integrins.
- Defects in the complement control proteins DAF, homologous restriction factor and CD59 underlie paroxysmal nocturnal hemoglobinuria.
- Lack of C1 inhibitor leads to hereditary angioedema.
- Deficiencies in C1, 4 or 2 are associated with SLE-like syndromes.

## Primary B-cell deficiency

- Congenital X-linked a-$\gamma$-globulinemia (Bruton), involving differentiation arrest at the pre-B stage, is caused by mutations in a novel tyrosine kinase gene.
- Patients with IgA deficiency and common variable immunodeficiency share similar HLA haplotypes.
- Deletions in the T-cell CD40L gene provide the basis for hyper-IgM syndrome.

## Primary T-cell deficiency

- DiGeorge syndrome results from failure of thymic development.
- Defective DNA repair mechanisms are found in patients with ataxia telangiectasia who have mutations in a gene strikingly similar to PI-3 kinase.
- Wiskott–Aldrich males lack sialophorin (CD43), a ligand for ICAM-1. An abnormal gene encoding a transcription factor (WASP) has been identified.

## Severe combined immunodeficiency

- Half the patients with SCID have mutations in the gene for the $\gamma_c$ chain common to receptors for IL-2, 4, 7, 9 and 15.
- Many SCID patients have a genetic deficiency of the purine degradation enzymes PNP and ADA, which leads to accumulation of toxic products. Patients with ADA deficiency are being corrected by transfection of autologous T-cells with the normal gene.

## Secondary immunodeficiency

- Immunodeficiency may arise as a secondary consequence of malnutrition, lymphoproliferative disorders, agents such as X-rays and cytotoxic drugs, and viral infections.

## Acquired immunodeficiency syndrome (AIDS)

- AIDS results from infection by the RNA retroviruses HIV-1 and HIV-2.
- HIV infects T-helper cells through binding of its envelope gp120 to CD4 with the help of a cofactor molecule, fusin. It also infects macrophages, microglia, T-cell stimulating dendritic cells and FDCs, the latter through a CD4 independent pathway.
- Within the cell, the RNA is converted by the reverse transcriptase to DNA which can be incorporated into the host's genome where it lies dormant until the cell is activated by stimulators such as TNFα which increase NFκB levels.
- There is usually a long asymptomatic phase after the early acute viral infection has been curtailed by an immune response and the virus is sequestered to the FDC in the lymphoid follicles where it progressively destroys the dendritic cell meshwork.
- A disastrous fall in CD4 T-helpers destroys cell-mediated defenses and leaves the patient open to life-threatening infections through opportunist organisms such as *Pneumocystis carinii* and cytomegalovirus.
- There is a tremendous battle between the immune system and the virus, with extremely high rates of viral destruction and CD4 T-cell replacement.
- CD4 T-cell depletion may eventually occur as a result of direct pathogenicity, syncitium formation, defective antigen-presenting cells making T-cells susceptible to apoptosis and failing to maintain the CD45RO memory population, suppression of protective TH1 cells, induction of autoimmunity by cross-reaction with HIV proteins, or coating of surface CD4 by gp120 immune complexes.
- AIDS is diagnosed in an individual with opportunistic infections by low CD4 but normal CD8 T-cells in blood,

(Continued)

poor delayed-type skin tests, positive tests for viral antibodies and p24 antigen, lymph node biopsy and isolation of live virus or demonstration of HIV genome by the polymerase chain reaction (PCR).

• To summarize a slightly confusing situation: it is thought that as the disease supervenes, protective and resistant CD4 TH1 cells lose way to susceptible and nonprotective TH2, that CD8 cells offer protection through cytolytic and noncytolytic pathways, that neutralizing antibodies are difficult to raise and may not be very effective, and last, that prophylactic mucosal immunity against viral invasion should be possible.

• A good model for studying candidate vaccines is infection of monkeys with simian immunodeficiency virus.

• Other approaches include synthetic molecules which block gp120–CD4 interaction and transfection of bone marrow cells with potential HIV inhibitors.

# FURTHER READING

Austen K.F., Burakoff S.J., Rosen F.S. & Strom T.B. (eds) (1996) *Therapeutic Immunology*. Blackwell Science, Oxford.

Bolognesi D.P. & Cooper M.D. (eds) (1995) Immunodeficiency. *Current Opinion in Immunology* **7**, 433–470.

Brostoff J., Scadding G.K., Male D. & Roitt I.M. (eds) (1991) *Clinical Immunology*, Chs 23–25. Gower Medical Publishing, London.

Chapel H. & Haeney M. (1993) *Essentials of Clinical Immunology*, 3rd edn. Blackwell Scientific Publications, Oxford.

Fauci A.S. (1996) Host factors and the pathogenesis of HIV-induced disease. *Nature* **384**, 529–534.

Fischer A. (ed.) (1996) Genetic effects on immunity. *Current Opinion in Immunology* **8**, 510.

Haynes B.F., Pantaleo G. & Fauci A.S. (1996) Toward an understanding of the correlates of protective immunity to HIV-infection. *Science* **271**, 324–328.

Ho D.D., Neumann A.U., Perelson A.S., Chen W., Leonard J.M. & Markowitz M. (1995) *Nature* **373**, 123 and Wei X., Ghosh S.K., Taylor M.E. *et al.* (1995) *Nature* **373**, 117. (Both study the effect of initial treatment with antiviral drugs and show the very high rate of viral replication and CD4 repletion.)

Huss R. (1996) Inhibition of cyclophilin function in HIV-1 infection by cyclosporin A. *Immunology Today* **17**, 259–260.

Lokki M.-L. & Colten H.R. (1995) Genetic deficiencies of complement. *Annals of Medicine* **27**, 451.

Pantaleo G., Graziosi C. & Fauci A.S. (1993) The immunology of HIV infection. *Seminars in Immunology* **5**, 147–223.

Poignard P., Klasse P.J. & Sattentau Q.J. (1996) Antibody neutralization of HIV-1. *Immunology Today* **17**, 239–246.

Stiehm E.R. (ed.) (1989) *Immunological Disorders in Infants and Children*, 3rd edn. W.B. Saunders, Philadelphia.

# C H A P T E R  16

# HYPERSENSITIVITY

## C O N T E N T S

## INAPPROPRIATE IMMUNE RESPONSES CAN LEAD TO TISSUE DAMAGE

When an individual has been immunologically primed, further contact with antigen leads to secondary boosting of the immune response. However, the reaction may be excessive and lead to gross tissue changes (hypersensitivity) if the antigen is present in relatively large amounts or if the humoral and cellular immune state is at a heightened level. It should be emphasized that the mechanisms underlying these inappropriate reactions are those normally employed by the body in combating infection as discussed in Chapter 13. We speak of **hypersensitivity reactions** and a state of **hypersensitivity**. Coombs and Gell defined four types of hypersensitivity, to which can be added a fifth, viz. 'stimulatory', which they mention. Types I, II, III and V depend on the interaction of antigen with humoral antibody and tend to be called 'immediate' type reactions although some are more immediate than others! Type IV involves T-cell recognition and because of the longer time-course this has in the past been referred to as 'delayed-type sensitivity'. Hypersensitivity can also arise from direct interaction of the inciting agent with elements of the innate immune system without intervention by acquired responses.

# TYPE I—ANAPHYLACTIC HYPERSENSITIVITY

## The phenomenon of anaphylaxis

The earliest accounts of inappropriate responses to foreign antigens relate to **anaphylaxis** (Milestone 16.1). The phenomenon can be readily reproduced in guinea-pigs which, like man, are a highly susceptible species. A single injection of 1 mg of an antigen such as egg albumin into a guinea-pig has no obvious effect. However, if the injection is repeated 2–3 weeks later, the sensitized animal reacts very dramatically with the symptoms of generalized anaphylaxis;

almost immediately the guinea-pig begins to wheeze and within a few minutes dies from asphyxia. Examination shows intense constriction of the bronchioles and bronchi and generally there is: (i) contraction of smooth muscle and (ii) dilatation of capillaries. Similar reactions can occur in human subjects and have been observed following wasp and bee stings or injections of penicillin in appropriately sensitive individuals. In many instances only a timely injection of epinephrine to counter the smooth muscle contraction and capillary dilatation can prevent death.

Sir Henry Dale recognized that histamine mimics the systemic changes of anaphylaxis and furthermore that the uterus from a sensitized guinea-pig releases histamine and contracts on exposure to antigen (Schultz–Dale technique). Serum from such an animal can passively sensitize the uterus from a normal guinea-pig so that it, too, will contract on addition of the specific antigen. Contraction is associated with an explosive degranulation of the mast cells (figure 1.14) which is responsible for the release of histamine and a number of other mediators (figure 1.15). Passive transfer of anaphylactic sensitivity can be observed locally in the skin using Ovary's **passive cutaneous**

## Milestone 6.1—The Discovery of Anaphylaxis

People are not equal. Idiosyncratic responses to given stimuli have been recognized from time immemorial and hypersensitive reactions in some individuals to normally innocuous environmental agents were frequently observed. As Lucretius remarked two thousand years ago, 'Differences are so great that one man's meat is another man's poison'. Sir Thomas More records that the future King Richard III was aware that strawberries gave him urticaria and arranged to be served a bowl of the fruit at a banquet attended by an arch-enemy. When he broke out in a spectacular rash, he accused his guest of attempted poisoning and had him summarily executed.

Scientific interest in hypersensitivity was aroused by the observations of Richet and Portier. During a South Sea cruise on Prince Albert of Monaco's yacht, the Prince, presumably smarting from an encounter with *Physalia* (the jelly-fish known as the Portugese-Man-of-War with very nasty tentacles), suggested that toxin production by the fish might be of interest. Let Richet and Portier take up the story in their own words (1902):

'On board the Prince's yacht, experiments were carried out proving that an aqueous glycerin extract of the filaments of *Physalia* is extremely toxic to ducks and rabbits.

On returning to France, I could not obtain *Physalia* and decided to study comparatively the tentacles of *Actinaria* (sea anemone). While endeavouring to determine the toxic dose (of extracts), we soon discovered that some days must elapse before fixing it; for several dogs did not die until the fourth or fifth day after administration or even later. We kept those that had been given insufficient to kill, in order to carry out a second investigation upon these when they had recovered. At this point an unforeseen event occurred. The dogs which had recovered were intensely sensitive and died a few minutes after the administration of small doses. The most typical experiment, that in which the result was indisputable, was carried out on a particularly healthy dog. It was given at first 0.1 ml of the glycerin extract without becoming ill: 22 days later, as it was in perfect health, I gave it a second injection of the same amount. In a few seconds it was extremely ill; breathing became distressful and panting; it could scarcely drag itself along, lay on its side, was seized with diarrhea, vomited blood and died in 25 minutes.'

The development of sensitivity to relatively harmless substances was termed by these authors **anaphylaxis**, in contrast to **prophylaxis**.

**anaphylaxis** (PCA) technique; high dilutions of guinea-pig serum containing anaphylactic antibodies may be injected into the skin of a normal animal and, following the intravenous injection of antigen with a dye such as Evans' Blue, the anaphylactic reaction in the skin will lead to release of vasoactive amines and hence a local 'blueing'.

## Human anaphylactic antibodies are mainly IgE

Anaphylaxis is mediated by the reaction of allergen with IgE antibodies bound strongly to the surface of the mast cell.

Switching of B-cells to the IgE isotype is controlled by interleukin-4 (IL-4) acting in concert with a costimulatory signal on the T-cell, probably membrane-bound α-tumor necrosis factor (TNFα). IL-4 stimulation of IgE synthesis is potentiated by IL-5 and IL-6, and by CD23, the soluble form of the low affinity FcεRII which ligates B-cell CD21 (CR2/Epstein–Barr virus (EBV) receptor), but is modulated by α-interferon (IFNα), IFNγ, transforming growth factor-β (TGFβ) and IL-10.

## Anaphylaxis is triggered by clustering of IgE receptors on mast cells through cross-linking

**Two main types of mast cell** have been recognized, exemplified in the rat by those in the intestinal mucosa and those in the peritoneum and other connective tissue sites. They differ in a number of respects, for example in the type of protease and proteoglycan in their granules, and in the proliferative response of the mucosal mast cell to the T-cell lymphokine IL-3 (table 16.1). This last point is made rather tellingly by the striking proliferation of mast cells in the intestinal mucosa during infection with certain parasites in intact, but not in T-depleted rodents, the effect being mediated by a combination of IL-3 and IL-4. The two types have common precursors and are interconvertible depending upon the environmental conditions, with mucosal $MC_t$ (*tryptase*) phenotype favored by IL-3 and that of connective tissue $MC_{tc}$ (*tryptase chymotryptase*) being promoted by a fibroblast factor. However, both types display a high affinity receptor for the Cε2:Cε3 junction region of IgE Fc (FcεRI: cf. figures 3.14 and 3.18), a property shared with their circulating counterpart, the basophil. The strength of binding to the mast cell is evident from the retention of IgE antibodies at a site of intradermal injection for several weeks; IgG4 in the human also binds to the mast cell receptor but more weakly and disperses from the injection site within a

Table 16.1. Comparison of two types of mast cell.

| CHARACTERISTICS | MUCOSAL MAST CELL | CONNECTIVE TISSUE MAST CELL |
|---|---|---|
| **GENERAL** | | |
| Abbreviation* | $MC_t$ | $MC_{tc}$ |
| Distribution | Gut & lung | Most tissues** |
| Differentiation favored by | IL-3 | Fibroblast factor |
| T-cell dependence | + | − |
| High affinity Fcε receptor | $2 \times 10^5$/cell | $3 \times 10^4$/cell |
| **GRANULES** | | |
| Alcian blue and Safranin staining | Blue & brown | Blue |
| Ultrastructure | Scrolls | Gratings/lattices |
| Protease | Tryptase | Tryptase & chymase |
| Proteoglycan | Chondroitin sulfate | Heparin |
| **DEGRANULATION** | | |
| Histamine release | + | + + |
| $LTC_4$: $PGD_2$ release | 25 : 1 | 1 : 40 |
| Blocked by disodium cromoglycate/theophylline | − | + |

*=based on protease in granules; **=predominate in normal skin and intestinal submucosa.

day or so. It has long been established that the anaphylactic antibodies in the human are mainly of the IgE class.

Cross-linking of IgE antibodies bound to a mast cell by a multivalent hapten will trigger mediator release; trimers are more effective than dimers and tetramers even more so. The critical event is aggregation of the receptors by cross-linking as clearly shown by the ability of antibodies reacting directly with the receptor to trigger the mast cell (figure 16.1).

The FcεRI γ subunit resembles the ζ-chain of the T-cell receptor (TCR) and part of the low affinity FcγRIII on macrophages. The cytoplasmic domain on the β and γ subunits shares a common motif with CD3γ, δ, ε, TCR ζ, η and IgM-associated IgM-α and Ig-β, and truncation of this domain abolishes receptor-mediated activation in a reconstituted system. Receptor aggregation activates the associated Lyn protein tyrosine kinase and if the aggregates persist, this leads to transphosphorylation of β- and γ-chains of other receptors within the cluster and subsequent recruitment of other kinases such as Syk.

Activation is rapidly followed by the breakdown of phosphatidylinositol to inositol triphosphate (IP3), the generation of diacylglycerol (DAG) and an increase in intracytoplasmic free calcium. The biochemical cascade produces membrane-active 'fusogens' such as lysophosphatidic acid which may facilitate granular membrane fusion and degranulation, and the series of arachidonic acid metabolites formed by the cyclo-oxygenase and lipoxygenase pathways (cf. figure 1.15). To recapitulate, the pre-

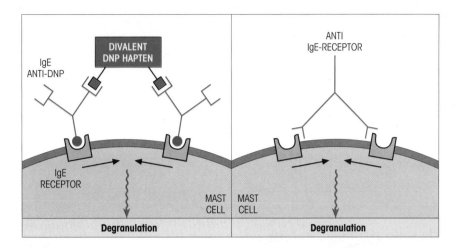

**Figure 16.1. Clustering of IgE receptors** either by multivalent hapten or antibody to the receptors themselves leads to mast cell degranulation. Studies using preformed aggregates of IgE of known size which stimulate mast cells showed that the reaction could be terminated by addition of selective kinase inhibitors. Small stable clusters of receptors continue to initiate signals for at least 1 hour. Lyn, which is the first tyrosine kinase to be activated, is normally present in caveolae membrane domains and only cosediment with the FcεRI when the latter are aggregated.

formed mediators released from the granules include histamine, heparin, neutral protease, eosinophil and neutrophil chemotactic factors, and platelet activating factor, while leukotrienes LTB4, LTC4 and LTD4, the prostaglandin PGD2 and thromboxanes are all newly synthesized. We now know that IL-3, IL-4, IL-5 and IL-6 and granulocyte–macrophage colony-stimulating factor (GM-CSF), a pattern of cytokines typical of TH2 cells, are also released.

Under normal circumstances, these mediators help to orchestrate the development of a defensive acute inflammatory reaction (and in this context let us not forget that complements C3a and C5a can also trigger mast cells, although not through IgE receptors). When there is a massive release of these mediators under abnormal conditions as in atopic disease, their bronchoconstrictive and vasodilatory effects predominate and become distinctly threatening.

## Atopic allergy

### Clinical responses to inhaled allergens

Nearly 10% of the population suffer to a greater or lesser degree with allergies involving localized IgE-mediated anaphylactic reactions to extrinsic allergens such as grass pollens, animal danders, the feces from mites in house dust (figure 16.2) and so on. An increasing number of allergens have now been cloned and expressed including **Der p1** from mites and **Lol**

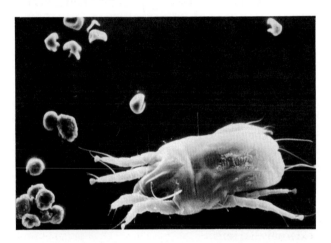

**Figure 16.2. House dust mite**—a major cause of allergic disease. The electron micrograph shows the rather nasty looking mite graced by the name *Dermatophagoides pteryonyssinus* and fecal pellets on the bottom left which are the major source of allergen. The biconcave pollen grains (top left) shown for comparison indicate the size of particle which can become airborne and reach the lungs. The mite itself is much too large for that. (Reproduced by courtesy of Dr E. Tovey.)

**pI-V** from rye grass pollen. Short cuts to allergen purification can be achieved by screening cDNA libraries for IgE binding proteins using immunoblotting techniques. This was a godsend for the purification of the allergen from the venom of the Australian jumper ant, *Myrmecia pilosula*; just think of trying to accumulate ants by the kilogram to isolate the allergen using conventional protein fractionation.

Contact of the allergen with cell-bound IgE in the bronchial tree, the nasal mucosa and the conjunctival tissues releases mediators of anaphylaxis and produces the symptoms of **asthma** or **allergic rhinitis and conjunctivitis** (hay fever) as the case may be (figure 16.3).

The evocation of a local anaphylactic reaction by injection of antigen into a passively sensitized site is short-lived and resolves within an hour or so. But

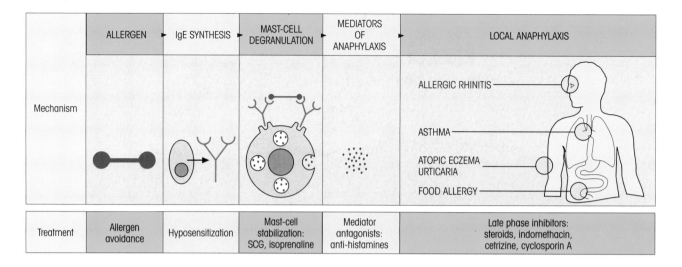

| Mechanism | ALLERGEN | IgE SYNTHESIS | MAST-CELL DEGRANULATION | MEDIATORS OF ANAPHYLAXIS | LOCAL ANAPHYLAXIS |
|---|---|---|---|---|---|
| | | | | | ALLERGIC RHINITIS<br>ASTHMA<br>ATOPIC ECZEMA URTICARIA<br>FOOD ALLERGY |
| Treatment | Allergen avoidance | Hyposensitization | Mast-cell stabilization: SCG, isoprenaline | Mediator antagonists: anti-histamines | Late phase inhibitors: steroids, indomethacin, cetrizine, cyclosporin A |

**Figure 16.3. Atopic allergies**: sites of local responses and possible therapies. SCG = sodium cromoglycate.

many atopic patients develop long-lasting symptoms after exposure to allergen and we should now explore the reason for this by examining the events associated with **asthma**. Patients fall into three main categories:

**1** The majority who are **extrinsic asthmatics** associated with **atopy**, i.e. the genetic predisposition to synthesize inappropriate levels of IgE specific for external allergens.

**2** Nonatopic intrinsic asthmatics.

**3 Occupational asthmatics** exposed to specific proteins or small molecular weight chemicals.

Bronchial biopsy and lavage of asthmatic patients reveal an unequivocal involvement of **mast cells and eosinophils** as the major mediator secreting effector cells, while T-cells provide the microenvironment required to sustain the inflammatory response which is an essential feature of the histopathology in each category (figure 16.4). The resulting variable airflow obstruction and bronchial hyper-responsiveness are the cardinal clinical and physiological features of the disease.

The preferential accumulation of eosinophils derives from the actions of IL-3, IL-5 and GM-CSF; particularly IL-5 which primes eosinophils for enhanced locomotor attraction towards mast cell platelet activating factor (PAF) and leukotriene B$_4$ (LTB$_4$), and bronchial epithelial cell-derived RANTES (regulated upon activation normal T-cell expressed and secreted) and eotaxin (cf. p. 257). IL-5 also inhibits the natural apoptosis of eosinophils which regulates their normal lifespan, it increases adhesion to vascular endothelium via β$_2$ integrins, and lowers thresholds to stimuli causing granule release.

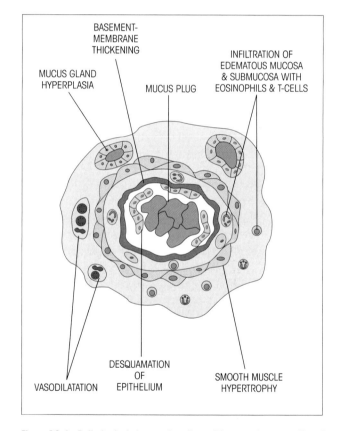

**Figure 16.4. Pathological changes in asthma**. Diagram of cross-section of an airway in severe asthma.

The source of the IL-5 which is such a major player in the eosinophil infiltration could come partly from local mast cells but this would not happily account for chronicity of the response. It now seems certain that T-helper TH2 type cells producing IL-4 and IL-5 are also a major factor in the disease. IL-5 mRNA transcripts are detectable in the T-cells in ongoing steady-state asthma and atopic patients tend to make TH2 type responses to allergens, whereas the same antigen given to normal subjects elicits T<sub>H</sub>1 (figure 16.5a). Reinforcement of this T<sub>H</sub>2 bias is provided by NO· produced by cytokine-stimulated airway epithelial cells. NO· suppresses T<sub>H</sub>1 cells with concomitant reduction in IFNγ, proliferation of T<sub>H</sub>2 and increase in IL-10 which further constrains the T<sub>H</sub>1 cells. Another consequence is that the high level of IL-4 will drive the switch to IgE production by B-cells.

We are happy when the eosinophil is batting for our side and turns its destructive firepower onto an invading parasite, but we are less impressed (to put it at its best) when these micro-'Schwarzeneggers' turn against the loving frame which gave them life. The eosinophil major basic protein causes bronchial hyperresponsiveness and is toxic for respiratory epithelial cells, a property shared with the granule peroxidase operating in the presence of peroxide and halide. There is a strong correlation between bronchial irritability, the number of desquamated epithelial cells in bronchoalveolar lavage fluid and the concentration of major basic protein. It is relevant that cetrizine, a drug which interferes with eosinophil function, has a beneficial effect in asthma. Further pathogenic factors are provided by the mediators PAF and LTC$_4$ which are bronchoconstrictors, the latter also being a potent mucus secretagogue.

The atopic trait can also manifest itself as an **atopic dermatitis** with house dust mite, domestic cats and German cockroaches often proving to be the environmental offenders. Recalling the inflammation in asthma, skin patch tests with *Der p1* in these eczema patients produce an infiltrate of eosinophils, T-cells, mast cells and basophils.

### Food allergy

Awareness of the importance of IgE sensitization to food allergens in the gut has increased dramatically. Sensitization to egg white and cows' milk may even occur in early infancy through breast-feeding, with antigen passing into the mother's milk. Food additives such as sulfiting agents can also cause adverse reactions. Contact of the food with specific IgE on mast cells in the gastrointestinal tract may produce local reactions such as diarrhea and vomiting or may allow the allergen to enter the body by causing a change in gut permeability through mediator release; the allergen may complex with antibodies and cause distal lesions by depositing in the joints, for example, or it may diffuse freely to other sensitized sites such as skin (figure 16.8b) or lungs where it will cause a further local anaphylactic reaction. Thus eating strawberries may produce urticarial reactions and egg may precipitate an asthmatic attack in appropriately sensitized individuals. The role of the sensitized gut acting as a 'gate' to allow entry of allergens is strongly suggested by experiments in which oral sodium cromoglycate, a mast cell stabilizer, prevents subsequent asthma after ingestion of the provoking food (figure 16.6).

### Etiological factors in the development of atopic allergy

There is a strong familial predisposition to the development of atopic allergy (figure 16.7a) but although this is linked to inheritance of a given human leuko-

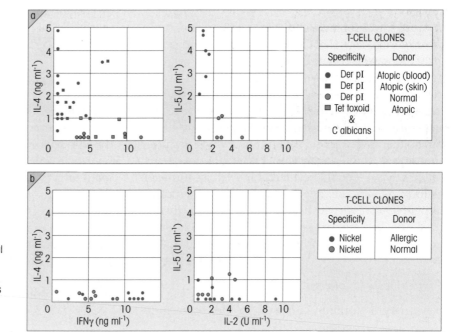

**Figure 16.5. Cytokine profiles of antigen-specific CD4+ T-cell clones** from: (a) patients with type I atopic allergy and (b) subjects with type IV contact sensitivity, compared with normal controls. Each point represents the value for an individual clone. Archetypal T<sub>H</sub>1 clones have high IFNγ, IL-2 and low IL-4 and IL-5; T<sub>H</sub>2 clones show the converse. (Data from Kapsenberg M.L., Wierenga E.A., Bos J.D. & Jansen H.M. (1991) *Immunology Today* **12**(11), 392.)

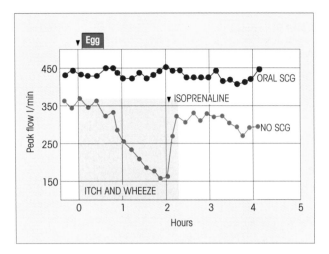

**Figure 16.6. The role of gut sensitivity in the development of asthma to food allergens.** A patient challenged by feeding with egg developed asthma within hours as shown here by the depressed lung function test of measuring peak air flow; the symptoms at the end-organ stage were counteracted by isoprenaline. However, oral sodium cromoglycate (SCG), which prevents antigen-specific mast cell triggering, also prevented the onset of asthma after oral challenge with egg. Note that SCG taken orally has no effect on the response of an asthmatic to inhaled allergen. (From Brostoff J. (1986) In Brostoff J. and Challacombe S.J. (eds) *Food Allergy*, p. 441. Baillière Tindall, London, reproduced with permission.)

cyte antigen (HLA) haplotype within any one family, no association with specific HLA types has so far come to light. There does seem to be a genetic link to the IL-4 gene cluster on chromosome 5 which includes IL-4, 13, 3, 5, 6, GM-CSF and IL-9. One factor is undoubtedly the overall ability to synthesize the IgE isotype—the higher the level of IgE in the blood the greater the likelihood of becoming atopic (figure 16.7b).

Atopic disease tends to start in childhood and there is some evidence that T-cells may be sensitized *in utero*, perhaps through exposure to allergen or allergen fragments crossing the placenta. It should also be borne in mind that allergic patients have a higher expression of histamine H1 receptor mRNA and consequently a lower threshold for triggering by histamine, the minimum concentration which induces sneezing being relatively low. The reason for this is unknown but it could be a factor in exercise-induced asthma, where the hyperventilation may produce hyper-osmolar airway lining fluid which activates mast cells and afferent nerves through stimulation of volume-sensitive chloride channels.

### Clinical tests for allergy

Sensitivity is normally assessed by the response to intradermal challenge with antigen. The release of histamine and other mediators rapidly produces a **wheal and erythema** (figure 16.8a), maximal within 30 minutes and then subsiding. The responsible IgE antibodies can be demonstrated by passive cutaneous anaphylaxis by testing the ability of patient's serum passively to sensitize the skin of normal humans (Prausnitz–Kustner or 'P–K' test) or preferably of monkeys. This passive sensitization of human skin can be blocked most effectively by prior injection of a myeloma of IgE rather than of any other class. The interpretation is that the specialized sites on the skin mast cells become fully saturated by binding to the Fc regions of the IgE myeloma globulin which blocks the subsequent attachment of specific IgE antibodies.

There is an increasing recognition that immediate wheal and flare reactions may be followed by a late phase reaction (cf. figure 16.8a) which sometimes lasts for 24 hours; it is characterized by dense infiltration with eosinophils and T-cells and is more edematous than the early reaction. The similarity to the histopathology of the inflammatory infiltrate in chronic asthma is obvious and these late phase reactions can also be seen following challenge of the bronchi and nasal mucosa of allergic subjects.

The correlation between skin prick test responses and the **radioallergosorbent test (RAST, see p. 113)** for allergen-specific serum IgE is fairly good. In some instances, intranasal challenge with allergen may provoke a response even when both these tests are negative, probably as a result of local synthesis of IgE antibodies.

The presence of proteins secreted from mast cells or eosinophils in the serum or urine could provide important surrogate markers of disease and might predict exacerbations.

### Therapy

*Allergen avoidance.* If one considers the sequence of reactions from initial exposure to allergen right through to the production of atopic disease, it can be seen that several points in the chain provide legitimate targets for therapy (figure 16.3). Avoidance of contact with *potential* allergens is often impractical, although, to give one example, feeding infants cows' milk at too early an age is discouraged. After sensitization, avoidance where possible is obviously worthwhile but the reluctance of some parents to dispose of the family cat to stop little Algernon's wheezing is sometimes quite surprising.

*Modulation of the immunological response.* Attempts to desensitize patients immunologically by repeated treatment with allergen have at least the merit of a long history and, in a significant but as yet unpredictable proportion of patients, can lead to worthwhile improvement. It has generally been supposed that the purpose of these inoculations was to boost the synthesis of 'blocking' antibodies whose function was to divert the allergen from contact with tissue-bound IgE. These were assumed to be of the IgG or IgA isotype but even autoantibodies to IgE have been proposed. This would be of unquestioned value were the increase in protective antibody (?particularly IgA) to occur locally at the sites vulnerable to allergen exposure. However, if T-lymphocyte cooperation is important for IgE synthesis and eosinophil-mediated pathogenesis, the beneficial effects of antigen injection may also be mediated through induction of tolerant, anergic or suppressor T-cells. A switch from TH2 to TH1 or the administration of antagonist peptide epitopes are other possibilities. Fortunately, most patients respond to a remarkably limited number of T-cell epitopes on any given allergen so it may not be necessary to tailor the therapeutic peptide to each individual. Trials with high doses of Fel d 1 derived peptides from cat allergen have resulted in decreased sensitivity and are now entering phase 3. A case can be made for future prophylactic hyposensitization of

children with two asthmatic parents who have a 70–80% probability of developing the disease.

Features of human atopic disease can be fairly readily produced in Brown Norway rats. If they are injected i.m. with the gene for the minor house dust mite allergen DERpV spliced into a plasmid expression vector, there is a transient IgG response and no IgE. On subsequent priming and challenge with the DERpV *protein*, the Ig and airway responses, and the release of histamine from broncheolar lavage cells were grossly reduced. The transfer of this phenomenon by CD8 cells may open an entirely new window on the mechanism of desensitization. Other strategies attempt to inhibit the binding of IgE to its mast cell receptor using either a humanized anti-IgE which does not cross-link, or a small blocking peptide.

*Mast cell stabilization.* At the drug level, much relief has been obtained with agents such as inhalant isoprenaline and **sodium cromoglycate**, a member of the chromone family, which render mast cells resistant to triggering. Sodium cromoglycate blocks chloride channel activity and maintains cells in a normal resting physiological state which probably accounts for its inhibitory effects on a wide range of cellular functions such as mast cell degranulation, eosinophil and neutrophil chemotaxis and mediator release, and reflex bronchoconstriction. Some or all of these effects

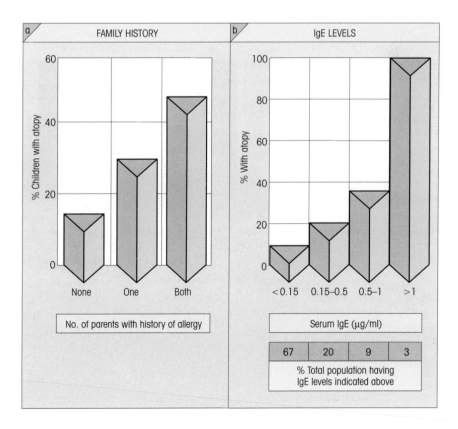

**Figure 16.7. Risk factors in allergy**: (a) family history; (b) IgE levels—the higher the serum IgE concentration, the greater the chance of developing atopy.

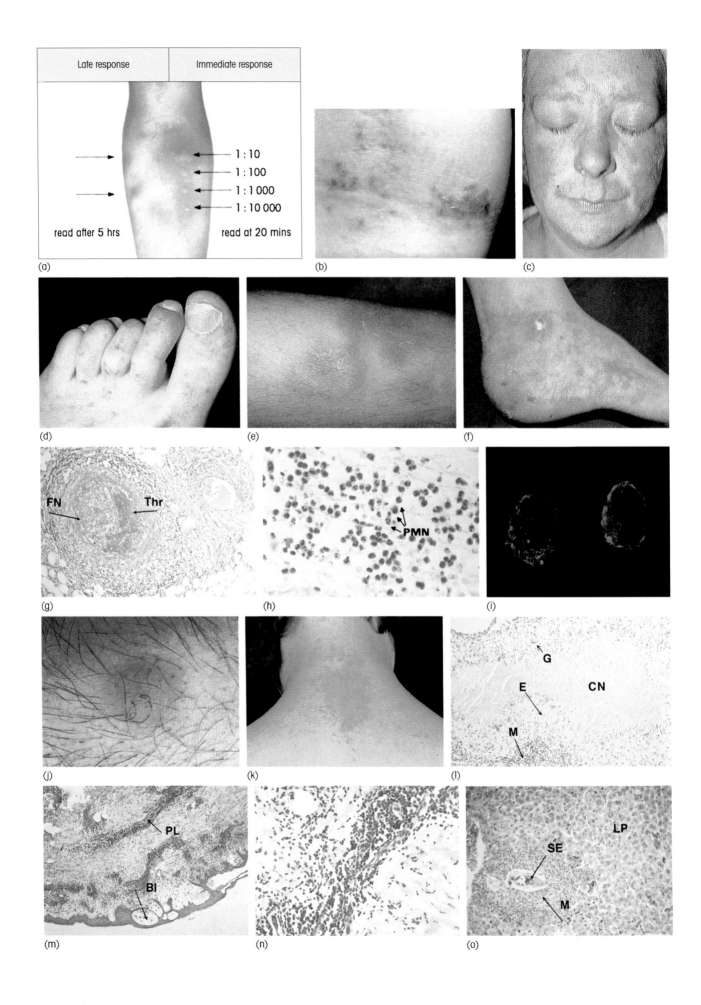

are responsible for its anti-asthmatic actions. Strangely, it also inhibits release of IgE from tonsils of nonatopic subjects stimulated with IL-4.

*Mediator antagonism.* An important recent advance has been the introduction of long-acting inhaled β₂-agonists such as salmeterol and formoterol which are bronchodilators and protect against bronchoconstriction for over 12 hours. Potent **leukotriene antagonists** such as zafirlukast also block constrictor challenges and clinical trials are encouraging. At the experimental level, an antibody to IL-5 had an effect on an allergy model in primates lasting several months.

**Theophylline** has been introduced for the treatment of asthma over more than 50 years and remains the single most prescribed drug for asthma worldwide. As a **phosphodiesterase (PDE) inhibitor** it increases intracellular cAMP, thereby causing bronchodilatation, inhibition of IL-5-induced prolongation of eosinophil survival and probably suppression of eosinophil migration into the bronchial mucosa. Good news for the patient. There are many isoenzyme forms of PDE and bronchodilators such as benafentrine are currently being developed.

*Attacking chronic inflammation.* Mild asthma involving mainly mast cell activation and eosinophil recruitment is treated with short-acting β₂-agonists and chromones but with increasing severity, activated T-cells dominate and **topical steroids** in increasing doses supplemented by long-acting β₂-agonists and theophylline are administered. More serious trials of inhaled cyclosporin A and other T-cell specific drugs are overdue.

## TYPE II — ANTIBODY-DEPENDENT CYTOTOXIC HYPERSENSITIVITY

Where an antigen is present on the surface of a cell, combination with antibody will encourage the demise of that cell by promoting contact with phagocytes, either by reduction in surface charge, by **opsonic adherence** directly through the Fc, or by **immune adherence** through bound C3. Cell death may also occur through activation of the full **complement** system up to C8 and C9 producing **direct membrane damage** (figure 16.9). Although in the case of hemolytic antibodies the generation of a single active complement site is enough to cause erythrocyte lysis, other cells appear to have repair mechanisms and it is likely that several complement sites need to be recruited in order to overwhelm the cell's defenses.

The operation of a quite distinct cytotoxic mechanism derives from the finding that target cells coated with low concentrations of IgG antibody can be killed 'nonspecifically' through an extracellular nonphagocytic mechanism involving nonsensitized leukocytes which bind to the target by their specific receptors for the Cγ2 and Cγ3 domains of IgG Fc (figures 16.9 and 16.10). It should be noted that this so-called **antibody-dependent cell-mediated cytotoxicity (ADCC)** may be exhibited by both phagocytic and nonphagocytic myeloid cells (polymorphs and monocytes) and by large granular lymphocytes with Fc receptors dubbed 'K-cells', which are almost certainly identical with the natural killer (NK) cells (see p. 19). Contact between the effector and target cells is essential and activity is inhibited by cytochalasin B which interferes with cell

---

**Figure 16.8. Hypersensitivity reactions.**

**Type I** (a) Skin prick tests with grass pollen allergen in a patient with typical summer hay fever. Skin tests were performed 5 hours (left) and 20 minutes (right) before the photograph was taken. The tests on the right show a typical end-point titration of a type I immediate wheal and flare reaction. The late phase skin reaction (left) can be clearly seen at 5 hours, especially where a large immediate response has preceded it. Figures for allergen dilution are given. (b) An atopic eczema reaction on the back of a knee of a child allergic to rice and eggs.

**Type III** (c) Facial appearance in systemic lupus erythematosus (SLE). Lesions of recent onset are symmetrical, red and edematous. They are often most pronounced on the areas of the face which receive most light exposure, i.e. the upper cheeks and bridge of the nose, and the prominences of the forehead. (d) Vasculitic lesions in SLE. Small purpuric macules are seen. (e) Erythema nodosum leprosum, forearm. The patient has lepromatous leprosy with superimposed erythema nodosum leprosum. These acutely inflamed nodules were extremely tender and the patient was pyrexial. (f) Polyarteritis nodosa, ankle and foot. Livedo reticularis with chronic painful ulceration is sometimes seen in this disease. (g) Histology of acute inflammatory reaction in polyarteritis nodosa associated with immune complex formation with hepatitis B surface (HBs) antigen. A vessel showing thrombus (Thr) formation and fibrinoid necrosis (FN) is surrounded by a mixed inflammatory infiltrate, largely polymorphs. (h) High-power view of acute inflammatory response in loose connective tissue of patient with polyarteritis nodosa —

polymorphs (PMN) are prominent. (i) Immunofluorescence studies of immune complexes in the renal artery of a patient with chronic hepatitis B infection stained with fluoresceinated antihepatitis B antigen (left) and rhodaminated anti-IgM (right). The presence of both antigen and antibody in the intima and media of the arterial wall indicate the deposition of the complexes at this site. IgG and C3 deposits are also detectable with the same distribution.

**Type IV** (j) Mantoux test showing cell-mediated hypersensitivity reaction to tuberculin, characterized by induration and erythema. (k) Type IV contact hypersensitivity reaction to nickel caused by the clasp of a necklace. (l) Chronic type IV inflammatory lesion in tuberculous lung showing caseous necrosis (CN), epithelioid cells (E), giant cells (G) and mononuclear inflammatory cells (M). (m) Perivascular lymphocytic infiltrates (PL) and blister (Bl) formation characterize a contact sensitivity reaction of the skin. (n) High-power view to show the lymphocytic nature of the infiltrate in a contact hypersensitivity reaction. (o) Essentially Tн2-type hypersensitivity lesion of inflammatory cells (M) around schistosome egg (SE) within the liver parenchyma (LP). ((a), (b) and (j) kindly provided by Dr J. Brostoff; (c), (d), (e) and (f) by Dr G. Levene; (g), (h), (m) and (n) by Professor N. Woolf; (i) by Professor A. Nowoslowski; (l) by Dr R. Barnetson and (o) by Dr M. Doenhoff; (k) reproduced from British Society of Immunology teaching slides with permission of the Society and Dermatology Department, London Hospital.)

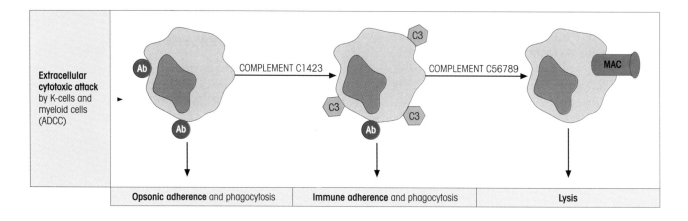

| Extracellular cytotoxic attack by K-cells and myeloid cells (ADCC) | | | |
|---|---|---|---|
| **Opsonic adherence** and phagocytosis | **Immune adherence** and phagocytosis | **Lysis** | |

**Figure 16.9. Type II—antibody-dependent cytotoxic hypersensitivity.** Antibodies directed against cell surface antigens cause cell death not only by C-dependent lysis but also by adherence reactions leading to phagocytosis or through nonphagocytic extracellular killing by certain lymphoid and myeloid cells (antibody-dependent cell-mediated cytotoxicity).

movement, and aggregated IgG which binds firmly to the Fc receptors and blocks their ability to interact with antibody on the surface of the target.

So far, ADCC has been studied exclusively as a phenomenon *in vitro*; to give examples, human K-cells have been shown to be strikingly unpleasant to chicken red cells coated with rabbit antibody and schistosomules coated with either IgG or IgE can be killed by eosinophils (cf. figure 13.21). Whether ADCC is merely a curiosity of the laboratory test-tube or plays a positive role *in vivo* remains an open question. Functionally, this extracellular cytotoxic mechanism would be expected to be of significance where the target is too large for ingestion by phagocytosis, e.g. large parasites and solid tumors. It could also act as a back-up system for T-cell killing.

## Type II reactions between members of the same species (alloimmune)

### Transfusion reactions

Of the many different polymorphic constituents of the human red cell membrane, **ABO blood groups** form the dominant system. The antigenic groups A and B are derived from H substance (figure 16.11) by the action of glycosyl transferases encoded by A or B genes respectively. Individuals with both genes (group AB) have the two antigens on their red cells, while those lacking these genes (group O) synthesize H substance only. Antibodies to A or B occur when the antigen is absent from the red cell surface; thus a person of blood group A will possess anti-B and so on. These **isohemagglutinins** are usually IgM and probably belong to the class of 'natural antibodies'; they would be boosted through contact with antigens of the gut flora which are structurally similar to the blood group carbohydrates, so that the antibodies

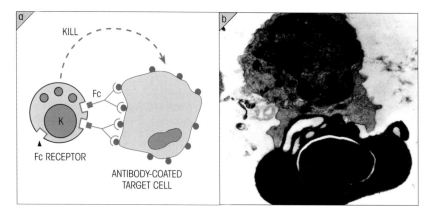

**Figure 16.10. Killing of Ab-coated target by antibody-dependent cell-mediated cytotoxicity (ADCC).** Fcγ receptors bind the effector to the target which is killed by an extracellular mechanism. Human monocytes and IFNγ-activated neutrophils kill Ab-coated tumor cells using their FcγRI and FcγRII receptors; lymphocytes (NK cells) kill hybridoma targets through FcγRIII receptors. (a) Diagram of effector and target cells. (b) Electron micrograph of attack on Ab-coated chick red cell by a mouse large granular lymphocyte showing close apposition of effector and target and vacuolation in the cytoplasm of the latter. ((b) Courtesy of P. Penfold.)

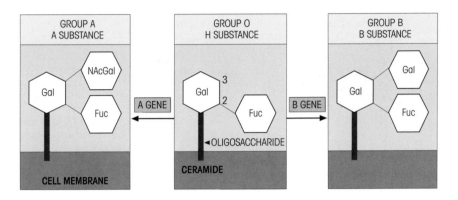

**Figure 16.11. The ABO system.** The allelic genes A and B code for transferases which add either *N*-acetylgalactosamine (NAcGal) or galactose (Gal) respectively to H substance (Fuc, fucose). The oligosaccharide is anchored to the cell membrane by coupling to a sphingomyelin called ceramide. Eighty-five per cent of the population secrete blood group substances in the saliva, where the oligosaccharides are present as soluble polypeptide conjugates formed under the action of a secretor (*se*) gene.

formed cross-react with the appropriate red cell type. If an individual is blood group A, they would be tolerant to antigens closely similar to A and would only form cross-reacting antibodies capable of agglutinating B red cells; similarly an O individual would make anti-A and anti-B (table 16.2). On transfusion, mismatched red cells will be coated by the isohemagglutinins and cause severe reactions.

Clinical refractoriness to platelet transfusions is frequently due to HLA alloimmunization but one can usually circumvent this problem by depleting the platelets of leukocytes.

### Rhesus incompatibility

The **rhesus (Rh) blood groups** form the other major antigenic system, the RhD antigen being of the most consequence for isoimmune reactions. A mother with an RhD–ve blood group (i.e. *dd* genotype) can readily be sensitized by red cells from a baby carrying RhD antigens (*DD* or *Dd* genotype). This occurs most often at the birth of the first child when a placental bleed can release a large number of the baby's erythrocytes

into the mother. The antibodies formed are predominantly of the IgG class and are able to cross the placenta in any subsequent pregnancy. Reaction with the D-antigen on the fetal red cells leads to their destruction through opsonic adherence, giving hemolytic disease of the newborn (figure 16.12).

These anti-D antibodies fail to agglutinate RhD+ve red cells *in vitro* ('incomplete antibodies') because the low density of antigenic sites does not allow sufficient antibody bridges to be formed between the negatively charged erythrocytes to overcome the electrostatic repulsive forces. Erythrocytes coated with anti-D can be made to agglutinate by addition of albumin or of an anti-immunoglobulin serum (Coombs' reagent; figure 16.13).

If a mother has natural isohemagglutinins which can react with any fetal erythrocytes reaching her circulation, sensitization to the D antigens is less likely due to 'deviation' of the red cells away from the antigen-sensitive cells. For example, a group O RhD–ve mother with a group A RhD+ve baby would destroy any fetal erythrocytes with her anti-A before they could immunize to produce anti-D. In an extension of this principle, **RhD–ve mothers are now treated prophylactically** with small amounts of avid IgG anti-D at the time of birth of the first child, and this greatly reduces the risk of sensitization. Another success for immunology.

Another example of disease resulting from transplacental passage of maternal antibodies is **neonatal alloimmune thrombocytopenia**. The fall in platelet numbers is greatly ameliorated by high-dose i.v. injections of pooled human IgG, the mechanism being thought to involve anti-idiotype networks (cf. p. 208).

### Organ transplants

A longstanding allograft which has withstood the first onslaught of the cell-mediated reaction can evoke

**Table 16.2. ABO blood groups and serum antibodies.**

| BLOOD GROUP (PHENOTYPE) | GENOTYPE | ANTIGEN | SERUM ANTIBODY |
|---|---|---|---|
| A | *AA,AO* | A | ANTI-B |
| B | *BB,BO* | B | ANTI-A |
| AB | *AB* | A and B | NONE |
| O | *OO* | H | ANTI-A ANTI-B |

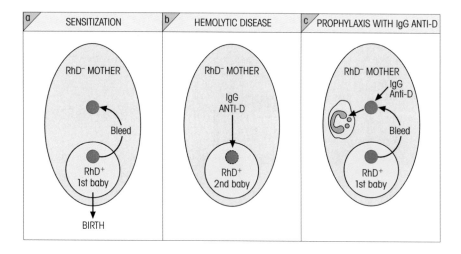

**Figure 16.12. Hemolytic disease of the newborn due to rhesus incompatibility.** (a) RhD+ve red cells from the first baby sensitize the RhD–ve mother. (b) The mother's IgG anti-D crosses the placenta and coats the erythrocytes of the second RhD+ve baby causing type II hypersensitivity hemolytic disease. (c) IgG anti-D given prophylactically at the first birth removes the baby's red cells through phagocytosis and prevents sensitization of the mother.

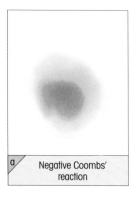

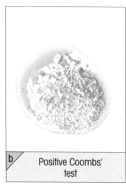

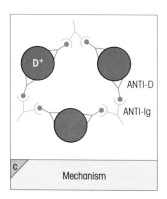

**Figure 16.13. The Coombs' test for antibody-coated red cells** used for detecting rhesus antibodies and in the diagnosis of autoimmune hemolytic anemia (cf. table 19.2, Note 5, p. 403). (Photographs courtesy of Dr A. Cooke.)

humoral antibodies in the host directed against surface transplantation antigens on the graft. These may be directly cytotoxic or cause adherence of phagocytic cells or 'nonspecific' attack by K-cells. They may also lead to platelet adherence when they combine with antigens on the surface of the vascular endothelium (figure 17.6, p. 359). Hyperacute rejection is mediated by preformed antibodies in the graft recipient.

## Autoimmune type II hypersensitivity reactions

Autoantibodies to the patient's own red cells are produced in **autoimmune hemolytic anemia**. They react at 37°C with epitopes on antigens of the Rhesus complex distinct from those which incite transfusion reactions. Red cells coated with these antibodies have a shortened half-life, largely through their adherence to phagocytic cells in the spleen. Similar mechanisms account for the anemia in patients with cold hemagglutinin disease who have monoclonal anti-I after infection with *Mycoplasma pneumoniae*, and in some cases of paroxysmal cold hemoglobinuria associated with the actively lytic Donath–Landsteiner antibodies specific for blood group P. These antibodies are primarily of IgM isotype and only react at temperatures well below 37°C.

The serums of patients with Hashimoto's thyroiditis contain antibodies which, in the presence of complement, are directly cytotoxic for isolated human thyroid cells in culture. In Goodpasture's syndrome (included here for convenience), antibodies to kidney glomerular basement membrane are present. Biopsies show these antibodies together with complement components bound to the basement membranes where the action of the full complement system leads to serious damage (figure 16.14a). I suppose one could also include the stripping of acetylcholine receptors from the muscle end-plate by autoantibodies in myasthenia gravis as a further example of type II hypersensitivity.

## Type II drug reactions

This is complicated. Drugs may become coupled to body components and thereby undergo conversion from a hapten to a full antigen which will sensitize certain individuals (we don't know which). If IgE antibodies are produced, anaphylactic reactions can result. In some circumstances, particularly with topi-

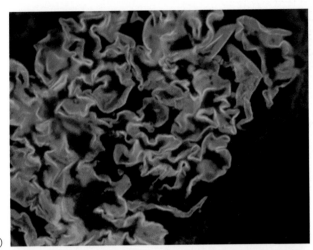

(a)

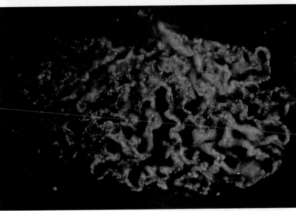

(b)

**Figure 16.14. Glomerulonephritis:** (a) due to linear deposition of antibody to glomerular basement membrane here visualized by staining the human kidney biopsy with a fluorescent anti-IgG, and (b) due to deposition of antigen–antibody complexes, which can be seen as discrete masses lining the glomerular basement membrane following immunofluorescent staining with anti-IgG. Similar patterns to these are obtained with a fluorescent anti-C3. (Courtesy of Dr S. Thiru.)

cally applied ointments, cell-mediated hypersensitivity may be induced. In other cases where coupling to serum proteins occurs, the possibility of type III complex-mediated reactions may arise. In the present context we are concerned with those instances where the drug appears to form an antigenic complex with the surface of a formed element of the blood and evokes the production of antibodies which are cytotoxic for the cell–drug complex. When the drug is withdrawn, the sensitivity is no longer evident. Examples of this mechanism have been seen in the **hemolytic anemia** sometimes associated with continued administration of chlorpromazine or phenacetin, in the **agranulocytosis** associated with the taking of amidopyrine or of quinidine, and the now classic situation of **thrombocytopenic purpura** which may be produced by Sedormid, a sedative of yesteryear. In the latter case, freshly drawn serum from the patient

will lyse platelets in the presence, but not in the absence, of Sedormid; inactivation of complement by preheating the serum at 56°C for 30 minutes abrogates this effect.

## TYPE III — IMMUNE COMPLEX-MEDIATED HYPERSENSITIVITY

The body may be exposed to an excess of antigen over a protracted period in a number of circumstances, persistent infection with a microbial organism, autoimmunity to self-components and repeated contact with environmental agents. The union of such antigens and antibodies to form an insoluble complex at fixed sites within the body may well give rise to acute inflammatory reactions (figure 16.15). If complement is fixed, anaphylatoxins will be released as split products of C3 and C5 and these will cause release of mast cell mediators with vascular permeability changes. The chemotactic factors also produced will lead to an influx of polymorphonuclear leukocytes which begin the phagocytosis of the immune complexes; this in turn results in the extracellular release of the polymorph granule contents, particularly when the complex is deposited on a basement membrane and cannot be phagocytosed (so-called 'frustrated phagocytosis'). The proteolytic enzymes (including neutral proteinases and collagenase), kinin-forming enzymes, polycationic proteins and reactive oxygen and nitrogen intermediates which are released will of course damage local tissues and intensify the inflammatory responses. Further damage may be mediated by reactive lysis in which activated C5,6,7 becomes adventitiously attached to the surface of nearby cells and binds C8,9. Under appropriate conditions, platelets may be aggregated with two consequences: they provide yet a further source of vasoactive amines and may also form microthrombi which can lead to local ischemia. (The discerning reader will appreciate the need for the system of inhibitors present in the body.) Insoluble complexes taken up by macrophages cannot readily be digested and provide a persistent activating stimulus leading to release of the cytokines IL-1 and TNF, reactive oxygen intermediates and nitric oxide (figure 16.15).

The outcome of the formation of immune complexes *in vivo* depends not only on the absolute amounts of antigen and antibody, which determine the intensity of the reaction, but also on their *relative* proportions which govern the nature of the complexes (cf. figure 6.2) and hence their distribution within the body. Between **antibody excess** and **mild**

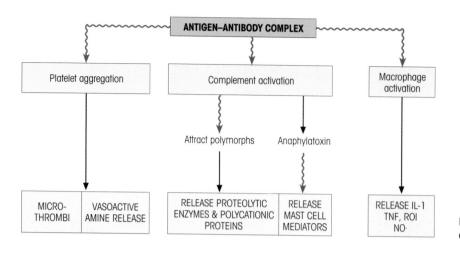

Figure 16.15. Type III immune complex-mediated hypersensitivity.

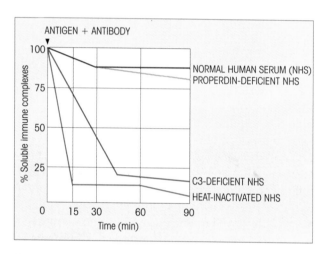

**Figure 16.16. Complement inhibits the formation of insoluble complexes as antigen and antibody combine.** Serum deficient in C3 or in which complement had been inactivated by heating, failed to block the formation of precipitating complexes. Deficiency of the alternative pathway component properdin had no effect. (Data reproduced with permission from Schifferli J.A., Ng Y.C. & Peters D.K. (1986) *New England Journal of Medicine* **315**, 488.)

**antigen excess**, the complexes are rapidly precipitated and tend to be localized to the site of introduction of antigen, whereas in **moderate** to **gross antigen excess**, soluble complexes are formed.

The fate of these complexes is bound up closely with the operation of the classical complement pathway. Fixation of complement inhibits the precipitation of immune complexes by covalent attachment of C3b which prevents the Fc–Fc interactions required to form large insoluble aggregates (figure 16.16). These small complexes containing C3b bind by immune adherence to CR1 complement receptors on the human erythrocyte and are transported to fixed macrophages in the liver where they are safely inactivated. If there are defects in this system, for example

deficiencies in classical pathway components (cf. p. 313; figure 16.16) or perhaps if the system is overloaded, then the immune complexes are free in the plasma and widespread disease involving deposition in the kidneys, joints and skin may result.

## Inflammatory lesions due to locally formed complexes

### The Arthus reaction

Maurice Arthus found that injection of soluble antigen intradermally into hyperimmunized rabbits with high levels of precipitating antibody, produced an erythematous and edematous reaction reaching a peak at 3–8 hours and then usually resolving. The lesion was characterized by an intense infiltration with polymorphonuclear leukocytes (cf. figure 16.8h). The injected antigen precipitates with antibody often within the venule, too fast for the classical complement system to prevent it; subsequently the complex binds complement and, using fluorescent reagents, antigen, immunoglobulin and complement components can all be demonstrated in this lesion (figure 16.8i). Anaphylatoxin is soon generated and causes mast cell degranulation. Local intravascular complexes will also cause platelet aggregation and vasoactive amine release and, as a result, erythema and edema increase. The formation of chemotactic factors leads to the influx of polymorphs. The Arthus reaction can be blocked by depletion of complement or of the neutrophil polymorphs (by nitrogen mustard or specific antipolymorph serum).

### Reactions to inhaled antigens

**Intrapulmonary Arthus-type reactions** to exogenous

inhaled antigen appear to be responsible for a number of hypersensitivity disorders in man. The severe respiratory difficulties associated with **farmer's lung** occur within 6–8 hours of exposure to the dust from mouldy hay. The patients are found to be sensitized to thermophilic actinomycetes which grow in the mouldy hay, and extracts of these organisms give precipitin reactions with the subject's serum and Arthus reactions on intradermal injection. Inhalation of bacterial spores present in dust from the hay introduces antigen into the lungs and a complex-mediated hypersensitivity reaction occurs. Similar situations arise in pigeon-fancier's disease where the antigen is probably serum protein present in the dust from dried feces, in rat handlers sensitized to rat serum proteins excreted in the urine (figure 16.17) and in many other quaintly named cases of **extrinsic allergic alveolitis** resulting from continual inhalation of organic particles, e.g. cheese washer's disease (*Penicillium casei* spores), furrier's lung (fox fur proteins) and maple bark stripper's disease (spores of *Cryptostroma*). Evidence that an immediate anaphylactic type I response may sometimes be of importance for the initiation of

an Arthus reaction comes from the study of patients with allergic bronchopulmonary aspergillosis who have high levels of IgE and precipitating IgG antibodies to *Aspergillus* species.

### Reactions to internal antigens

Type III reactions are often provoked by the local release of antigen from infectious organisms within the body; for example, living filarial worms such as *Wuchereria bancrofti* are relatively harmless, but the dead parasite found in lymphatic vessels initiates an inflammatory reaction thought to be responsible for obstruction of lymph flow and the ensuing, rather monstrous, elephantiasis. Chemotherapy may cause an abrupt release of microbial antigens in individuals with high antibody levels, producing quite dramatic immune complex-mediated reactions such as **erythema nodosum leprosum** in the skin of dapsone-treated lepromatous leprosy patients (figure 16.8e) and the Jarisch–Herxheimer reaction in syphilitics on penicillin.

An interesting variant of the Arthus reaction is seen

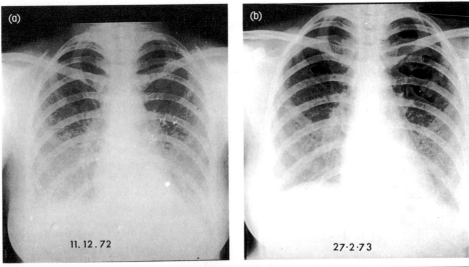

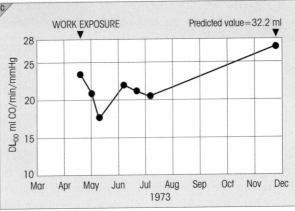

Figure 16.17. **Extrinsic allergic alveolitis due to rat serum proteins** in a research assistant handling rats (type III hypersensitivity). Typical systemic and pulmonary reactions on inhalation and positive prick tests were elicited by rat serum proteins; precipitins against serum proteins in rat urine were present in the patient's serum. (a) Bilateral micronodular shadowing during acute episodes. (b) Marked clearing within 11 days after cessation of exposure to rats. (c) Temporary fall in pulmonary gas exchange measured by $DL_{CO}$ (gas transfer, single breath) following a 3-day exposure to rats at work (arrowed). (From Carroll K.B., Pepys J., Longbottom J.L., Hughes D.T.D. & Benson H.G. (1975) *Clinical Allergy* **5**, 443; figures by courtesy of Professor J. Pepys.)

in rheumatoid arthritis where complexes are formed locally in the joint due to the production of self-associating IgG anti-IgG by synovial plasma cells (cf. p. 432).

It has also been recognized that complexes could be generated at a local site by a quite different mechanism involving nonspecific adherence of an antigen to tissue structures followed by the binding of soluble antibody—in other words, the antigen becomes fixed in the tissue *before* not *after* combining with antibody. Although it is not clear to what extent this mechanism operates in patients with immune complex disease, let me describe the experimental observation on which it is based. After injection with bacterial endotoxin, mice release DNA into their circulation which binds specifically to the collagen in the basement membrane of the glomerular capillaries: the endotoxin also polyclonally activates B-cells making anti-DNA which gives rise to antigen–antibody complexes in the kidney.

## Disease resulting from circulating complexes

### Serum sickness

Injection of relatively large doses of foreign serum (e.g. horse antidiphtheria) used to be employed for various therapeutic purposes. It was not uncommon for a condition known as 'serum sickness' to arise some 8 days after the injection. A rise in temperature, swollen lymph nodes, a generalized urticarial rash and painful swollen joints associated with a low serum complement and transient albuminuria (cf. figure 16.18) could be encountered. These result from the deposition of soluble antigen–antibody complexes formed in antigen excess.

Some individuals begin to synthesize antibodies against the foreign protein—usually horse globulin. Since the antigen is still present in gross excess at that time, circulating soluble complexes of composition $Ag_2Ab$, $Ag_3Ab_2$, $Ag_4Ab_3$, etc. will be formed (cf. figure 6.2). To be pathogenic, the complexes have to be of the right size — too big and they are snapped up smartly by the macrophages of the mononuclear phagocyte system, too small (<19S) and they fail to induce an inflammatory reaction. Even when they are the right size, it seems that they will only localize in vessel walls if there is a change in vascular permeability. This may come about through release of 5-hydroxytryptamine (5HT) from platelets reacting with larger complexes or through an IgE or complement-mediated degranulation of basophils and mast cells to produce histamine,

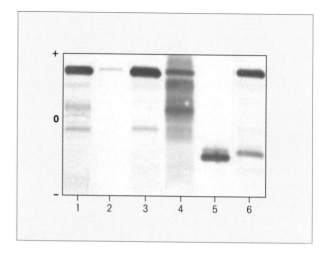

**Figure 16.18. Proteinuria demonstrated by electrophoresis.** Lane 1: Normal serum as reference. The major band nearest to the cathode is albumin. Lane 2: Normal urine showing a trace of albumin. Lane 3: Glomerular proteinuria showing a major albumin component. Lane 4: Proteinuria resulting from tubular damage with a totally different electrophoretic pattern. Lane 5: Bence-Jones proteinuria representing excreted paraprotein light chains (cf. p. 390). Lane 6: Bence-Jones proteinuria with a trace of the intact paraprotein. Some of the samples have been concentrated. (Electropherograms kindly supplied by T. Heys.)

leukotrienes and PAF. The effect on the capillaries is to cause separation of the endothelial cells and exposure of the basement membrane to which the appropriately sized complexes attach, the skin, joints, kidneys and heart being particularly affected. As antibody synthesis increases, antigen is cleared and the patient normally recovers.

### Immune complex glomerulonephritis

The deposition of complexes is a dynamic affair and long-lasting disease is only seen when the antigen is persistent, as in chronic infections and autoimmune diseases. Experimentally, Dixon produced chronic glomerular lesions by repeated administration of foreign proteins to rabbits. Not all animals showed the lesion and perhaps only those genetically capable of producing low affinity antibody (Soothill & Steward) or antibodies to a restricted number of determinants (Christian) formed soluble complexes in the right size range. **The smallest complexes reach the epithelial side** but progressively **larger complexes are retained in or on the endothelial side of the glomerular basement membrane** (figure 16.19). They build up as 'lumpy' granules staining for antigen, immunoglobulin and complement (C3) by immunofluorescence (figure 16.14b) and appear as large amorphous masses in the electron microscope (cf. figure 20.7). The inflammatory process damages

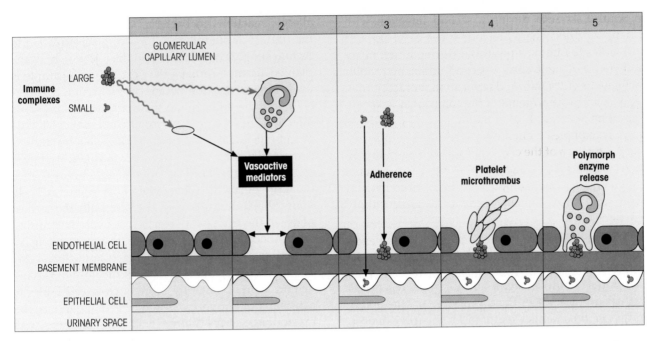

**Figure 16.19. Deposition of immune complexes in the kidney glomerulus**. (1) Complexes induce release of vasoactive mediators from basophils and platelets which cause (2) separation of endothelial cells, (3) attachment of larger complexes to exposed basement membrane, smaller complexes passing through to epithelial side, (4) complexes induce platelet aggregation, (5) chemotactically attracted neutrophils release granule contents in 'frustrated phagocytosis' to damage basement membrane and cause leakage of serum proteins. Complex deposition is favored in the glomerular capillary because it is a major filtration site and has a high hydrodynamic pressure. Deposition is greatly reduced in animals depleted of platelets or treated with vasoactive amine antagonists.

the basement membrane, causing leakage of serum proteins and consequent proteinuria (figure 16.18, lane 3). Serum albumin being small, appears in the urine even with minor degrees of glomerular damage.

Many cases of glomerulonephritis are associated with circulating complexes and biopsies give a fluorescent staining pattern similar to that of figure 16.14b which depicts DNA/anti-DNA/complement deposits in the kidney of a patient with SLE (cf. p. 429). Well known is the disease which can follow infection with certain strains of so-called 'nephritogenic' streptococci and the nephrotic syndrome of Nigerian children associated with quartan malaria where complexes with antigens of the infecting organism have been implicated. Immune complex nephritis can arise in the course of chronic viral infections; for example, mice infected with lymphocytic choriomeningitis virus develop a glomerulonephritis associated with circulating complexes of virus and antibody. This may well represent a model for many cases of glomerulonephritis in man.

*Deposition of immune complexes at other sites*

The choroid plexus being a major filtration site is also

favored for immune complex deposition and this could account for the frequency of central nervous disorders in SLE. Neurologically affected patients tend to have depressed C4 in the cerebrospinal fluid (CSF) and at post-mortem, SLE patients with neurologic disturbances and high titer anti-DNA were shown to have scattered deposits of immunoglobulin and DNA in the choroid plexus. Subacute sclerosing panencephalitis is associated with a high CSF to serum ratio of measles antibody, and deposits containing Ig and measles Ag may be found in neural tissue.

The vasculitic skin rashes which are a major feature of serum sickness are also characteristic of systemic and discoid lupus erythematosus (figure 16.8c and d) and biopsies of the lesions reveal amorphous deposits of Ig and C3 at the basement membrane of the dermal epidermal junction.

The necrotizing arteritis produced in rabbits by experimental serum sickness closely resembles the histology of polyarteritis nodosa (figure 16.8g and h) and it has recently been reported that in some of these patients (figure 16.8f), immune complexes containing the HBs antigen of hepatitis B virus are present in the lesions (figure 16.8i). Another example is the hemorrhagic shock syndrome found with some frequency in South-East Asia during a second infection with a dengue virus. There are four types of virus, and antibodies to one type produced during a first infection may not neutralize a second strain but rather facilitate its entry into, and replication within, human monocytes by attachment of the complex to Fc receptors. The enhanced production of virus leads to immune complex formation and a massive intravascular activation of the classical complement pathway. In some instances drugs such as penicillin become antigenic after conjugation with body proteins and form complexes which mediate hypersensitivity reactions.

It should be said that persistence of circulating complexes does not invariably lead to type III hypersensitivity (e.g. in many cancer patients and in individuals with idiotype–anti-idiotype reactions). Perhaps in these cases the complexes lack the ability to initiate the changes required for complex deposition, but some hold the view that complexes detected in the serum may sometimes be artifacts released from their *in vivo* attachment to the erythrocyte CR1 receptors by the action of factor I during processing of the blood.

## Treatment

The avoidance of exogenous inhaled antigens inducing type III reactions is obvious. Elimination of microorganisms associated with immune complex disease by chemotherapy may provoke a further reaction due to copious release of antigen. Suppression of the accessory factors thought to be necessary for deposition of complexes would seem logical; for example, the development of serum sickness is prevented by histamine and 5HT antagonists. Disodium cromoglycate, heparin and salicylates are often used, the latter being an effective platelet stabilizer as well as a potent anti-inflammatory agent. Corticosteroids are particularly powerful inhibitors of inflammation and are immunosuppressive. In many cases, particularly those involving autoimmunity, conventional immunosuppressive agents may be justified. Where type III hypersensitivity is thought to arise from an inadequate immune response, the more aggressive approach of immunopotentiation to boost avidity is being advocated, but that is a path that will be trodden gently.

## TYPE IV — CELL-MEDIATED (DELAYED-TYPE) HYPERSENSITIVITY

This form of hypersensitivity is encountered in many

allergic reactions to bacteria, viruses and fungi, in the contact dermatitis resulting from sensitization to certain simple chemicals and in the rejection of transplanted tissues. Perhaps the best known example is the **Mantoux reaction** obtained by injection of tuberculin into the skin of an individual in whom previous infection with the mycobacterium had induced a state of cell-mediated immunity (CMI). The reaction is characterized by erythema and induration (figure 16.8j) which appears only after several hours (hence the term 'delayed') and reaches a maximum at 24–48 hours, thereafter subsiding. Histologically the earliest phase of the reaction is seen as a perivascular cuffing with mononuclear cells followed by a more extensive exudation of mono- and polymorphonuclear cells. The latter soon migrate out of the lesion leaving behind a predominantly mononuclear cell infiltrate consisting of lymphocytes and cells of the monocyte-macrophage series (figure 16.8l). This contrasts with the essentially 'polymorph' character of the Arthus reaction (figure 16.8h).

Comparable reactions to soluble proteins are obtained when sensitization is induced by incorporation of the antigen into complete Freund's adjuvant (see p. 193). In some, but not all cases, if animals are primed with antigen alone or in incomplete Freund's adjuvant (which lacks the *Mycobacteria*), the delayed hypersensitivity state is of shorter duration and the dermal response more transient. This is known as 'Jones–Mote' sensitivity but has recently been termed **cutaneous basophil hypersensitivity** on account of the high proportion of basophils infiltrating the skin lesion.

## The cellular basis of type IV hypersensitivity

Unlike the other forms of hypersensitivity which we have discussed, delayed-type reactivity cannot be transferred from a sensitized to a nonsensitized individual with serum antibody; lymphoid cells, in particular the T-lymphocytes, are required. Transfer has been achieved in the human using viable white blood cells and, interestingly, by a low molecular weight material extracted from them (Lawrence's transfer factor). The nature of this substance is, however, a mystery. The extracts contain a variety of factors which appear capable of stimulating precommitted T-cells mediating delayed hypersensitivity, but whether there is also an informational molecule conferring antigen-specific reactivity is still a highly contentious issue.

It cannot be stressed too often that the hypersensitivity lesion results from an exaggerated interaction between antigen and the *normal* cell-mediated immune mechanisms (cf. p. 186). Following earlier priming, memory T-cells recognize the antigen together with class II major histocompatibility complex (MHC) molecules on an antigen-presenting cell and are stimulated into blast cell transformation and proliferation. The stimulated T-cells release a number of cytokines which function as mediators of the ensuing hypersensitivity response, particularly by attracting and activating macrophages if they belong to the TH1 subset, or eosinophils if they are TH2; they also help Tc precursors to become killer cells which can cause tissue damage (figure 16.20).

## Tissue damage produced by type IV reactions

### Infections

The development of a state of cell-mediated hypersensitivity to bacterial products is probably responsible for the lesions associated with bacterial allergy such as the cavitation, caseation and general toxemia seen in human tuberculosis and the granulomatous skin lesions found in patients with the borderline

form of leprosy. When the battle between the replicating bacteria and the body defenses fails to be resolved in favor of the host, persisting antigen provokes a chronic local delayed hypersensitivity reaction. Continual release of cytokines from sensitized T-lymphocytes leads to the accumulation of large numbers of macrophages, many of which give rise to arrays of epithelioid cells, while others fuse to form giant cells. Macrophages bearing bacterial antigen on their surface may become targets for killer T-cells and be destroyed. Further tissue damage will occur as a result of indiscriminate cytotoxicity by lymphokine-activated macrophages (and natural killer (NK) cells?). Morphologically, this combination of cell types with proliferating lymphocytes and fibroblasts associated with areas of fibrosis and necrosis is termed a **chronic granuloma** and represents an attempt by the body to wall off a site of persistent infection (figures 16.8l and 16.20). It should be noted that granulomas can also arise from the persistence of indigestible antigen–antibody complexes or inorganic materials such as talc within macrophages, although nonimmunological granulomas may be distinguished by the absence of lymphocytes.

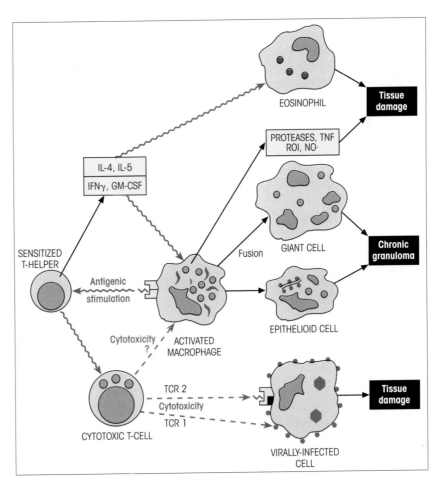

Figure 16.20. The cellular basis of type IV hypersensitivity.

The skin rashes in smallpox and measles and the lesions of herpes simplex may be largely attributed to delayed-type allergic reactions with extensive damage to virally infected cells by Tc cells. Cell-mediated hypersensitivity has also been demonstrated in the fungal diseases, candidiasis, dermatomycosis, coccidioidomycosis and histoplasmosis, and in the parasitic disease, *Leishmania*.

Sarcoidosis is a disease of unknown etiology affecting lymphoid tissue and involving the formation of chronic granulomas. Evidence for atypical mycobacteria has been obtained but delayed-type hypersensitivity is depressed and the patients are anergic on skin testing with tuberculin; curiously they give positive responses if cortisone is injected together with the antigen and it has been suggested that cortisone-sensitive T suppressors might be responsible for the anergy. The patients develop a granulomatous reaction a few weeks after intradermal injection of spleen extract from another sarcoid patient — the **Kweim reaction**.

### Contact dermatitis

The epidermal route of inoculation tends to favor the development of a T-cell response through processing by class II-rich dendritic Langerhans' cells (cf. figure 2.6i) which migrate to the lymph nodes and present antigen to T-lymphocytes. Thus, delayed-type reactions in the skin are often produced by foreign materials capable of binding to body constituents, possibly surface molecules of the Langerhans' cell, to form new antigens. The reaction is characterized by a mononuclear cell infiltrate peaking at 12–15 hours, accompanied by edema of the epidermis with microvesicle formation (figure 16.8m and n). Contact hypersensitivity can occur in people who become sensitized while working with chemicals such as picryl chloride and chromates, or who repeatedly come into contact with the substance urushiol from the poison ivy plant. *p*-Phenylene diamine in certain hair dyes, neomycin in topically applied ointments, and nickel salts formed from articles such as nickel jewellery clasps (figure 16.8k), can provoke similar reactions. T-cell clones specific for nickel salts isolated from the latter group produce a T$_{H1}$-type profile of cytokines (IFN$\gamma$, IL-2) on antigen stimulation (figure 16.5b).

### T$_{H2}$-mediated hypersensitivity

The examples of type IV hypersensitivity we have discussed so far are centered essentially on the T$_{H1}$-macrophage pathway, but it is now clear that excessive responses by T$_{H2}$-cells can damage tissues through activation of eosinophils (figure 16.20). As recounted earlier, T-cells synthesizing IL-5 are largely responsible for the influx of eosinophils in asthma and atopic dermatitis, and in the late phase reaction to allergen challenge in allergic rhinitis and atopic asthma (cf. p. 332). They also essentially account for the liver pathology in schistosomiasis which has been attributed to a reaction against soluble enzymes derived from the eggs which lodge in the capillaries (figure 16.8o).

### Other examples

Delayed hypersensitivity contributes significantly to the prolonged reactions which result from insect bites. The possible implication of allograft rejection by Tc cells as a mechanism for the control of cancer cells is discussed in Chapter 18. In certain organ-specific autoimmune diseases, such as type I diabetes, cell-mediated hypersensitivity reactions undoubtedly provide the major engine for tissue destruction.

**Psoriasis** involves marked proliferation of epidermal keratinocytes and accelerated incomplete epidermal differentiation. There is inflammation in the skin with pockets of micro-abscesses containing neutrophils and, in all instances, CD4 cells in the psoriatic dermis and CD8 in the lesional epidermis. A reversal of epidermal dysfunction, and a marked reduction in intra-epidermal CD8 T-cells was achieved by systemic administration of a fusion protein of IL-2 and fragments of diphtheria toxin which selectively blocks the growth of activated lymphocytes but not keratinocytes. This shows that the disorder is primarily immunological rather than a dysfunction of keratinocytes which secondarily activate T-cells through, say, TGF$\beta$. The party line now would be that CD8 T-cells attack the skin, activating injury repair programmes associated with wound healing while cytokines act directly as mitogens for epidermal keratinocytes.

## TYPE V — STIMULATORY HYPERSENSITIVITY

Many cells are signaled by agents such as hormones through surface receptors to which they specifically bind the external agent presumably through complementarity of structure. For example, when thyroid-stimulating hormone (TSH) of pituitary origin binds to the thyroid cell receptors, adenyl cyclase is activated and the cAMP 'second messenger' which is generated acts to stimulate the thyroid cell. The **thyroid stimulating antibody** present in the sera of thyrotoxic patients (cf. p. 425) is an autoantibody directed against a site on the TSH receptor which produces the changes required for adenyl cyclase activation. The situation is analogous to lymphocyte stimulation; B-lymphocytes with immunoglobulin surface receptors can be stimulated by changes induced through the receptor molecules either by binding of specific multimeric antigen or by an antibody to the immunoglobulin (even anti-Fc) as shown in figure 16.21. Intriguingly, there are indications that cimetidine-resistant duodenal ulcer patients might have stimulatory antibodies directed to H2-histamine receptors.

Other experimental examples of stimulation by antibodies to cell surface antigens may be cited: the transformation of human T-lymphocytes by monoclonal antibodies to the CD3 antigen; the production of cell division in thyroid cells by 'growth' autoantibodies; the induction of pinocytosis by anti-macrophage serum; and the mitogenic effect of antibodies to sea-urchin eggs. It is worthy of note that although antibodies to enzymes directed against determinants near to the active site can exert a blocking effect, combination with more distant determinants can sometimes bring about allosteric conformational changes which are associated with a considerable increase in enzymic activity as has been described for certain variants of penicillinase and β-galactosidase.

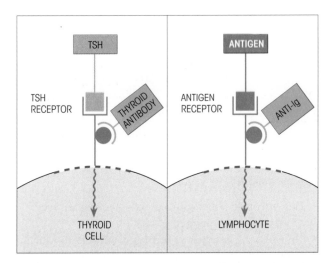

**Figure 16.21. Stimulation of thyroid cell and of lymphocyte by physiological agent or by antibody**, both of which cause comparable membrane changes leading to cell activation by reacting with surface receptors.

## 'INNATE' HYPERSENSITIVITY REACTIONS

Many infections provoke a **'toxic shock syndrome'** characterized by hypotension, hypoxia, oliguria and microvascular abnormalities and mediated by elements of the innate immune system independently of the operation of acquired immune responses.

Septicemia associated with **Gram-negative bacteria** results in excessive release of TNF, IL-1 and IL-6 through stimulation of macrophages and endothelial cells by the lipopolysaccharide (LPS) endotoxin (cf. figure 13.6). Normally this would enhance host defenses, aiding the recruitment of phagocytes by promoting adherence to endothelium, priming neutrophils for subsequent release of reactive oxygen intermediates, inducing febrile responses (immune responses improve steadily from 33 to 44°C) and so on. Unfortunately, the excess of circulating LPS and the cytokines released by it lead to unwanted pathophysiology at distant sites such as the **adult respiratory distress syndrome** brought about by an overwhelming invasion of the lung by neutrophils. There is a prolonged pathologically high concentration of nitric oxide but, additionally, LPS can activate the alternative complement pathway and this may be linked to its ability to induce release of thromboxane $A_2$ and prostaglandin from platelets leading to **disseminated intravascular coagulation**.

Whereas the major culprit in Gram-negative sepsis is LPS, **Gram-positive organisms** possess a variety of components which act on host defense elements to initiate septic shock. Thus adherence of *Staphylococcus aureus* to macrophages induces TNFα synthesis and peptidoglycan-mediated aggregation of platelets by the same organism leads to disseminated intravascular coagulation. The staphylococcal and streptococcal enterotoxins induce toxic shock syndrome by quite different means. By functioning as **superantigens** (cf. p. 100), they react directly with particular T-cell receptor families and give rise to massive cytokine release, including of course TNF. Various treatments are under investigation. Pentoxifylline blocks TNF production by macrophages. Humanized monoclonal antibodies to TNF, IFNγ and IL-6 will be tried and an intriguing naturally occurring IL-1 receptor antagonist has been cloned.

The reader's attention has already been drawn to the unusual susceptibility of erythrocytes to lysis in **paroxysmal nocturnal hemoglobinuria** resulting from deficiency in complement control proteins on the red cell surface (see p. 313). Undue C3 consumption is associated with mesangiocapillary glomerulonephritis and partial lipodystrophy in patients with the so-called **C3 nephritic factor**, which appears to be an IgG autoantibody capable of activating the alternative pathway by combining with and stabilizing the C3bBb convertase.

We should include **idiopathic pulmonary fibrosis** in this section. It is a chronic fatal disorder characterized by diffuse fibrosis of the alveolar walls in which local macrophages play a central role. On activation they produce an early G1 competence growth signal such as platelet-derived growth factor and fibronectin, and then a late G1 progression growth signal such as insulin-like growth factor 1. As a result, the fibroblasts multiply and become embedded in a collagen matrix to the respiratory detriment of the host.

The neuropathological hallmarks of Alzheimer's disease are extracellular plaques and intracellular neurofibrillary tangles. One of the constituents of senile plaques is β-amyloid composed of a hydrophobic fragment of amyloid precursor protein (APP). Normally APP is cleaved by an α-secretase into soluble products which cannot form β-amyloid but members of a family diagnosed with Alzheimer's disease and having a pathogenic mutation at residues 670–671 of APP, had very low levels of this soluble cleaved form compared with noncarriers. This could also represent a new and promising diagnostic marker.

---

## SUMMARY

- Excessive stimulation of the normal effector mechanisms of the immune system can lead to tissue damage and we speak of hypersensitivity reactions of which several types can be distinguished.

### Type I—anaphylactic hypersensitivity

- Anaphylaxis involves contraction of smooth muscle and dilatation of capillaries.
- This depends upon the reaction of antigen with specific IgE antibody bound through its Fc to the mast cell.
- Cross-linking and clustering of the IgE receptors activates the Lyn protein tyrosine kinase, recruits other kinases and leads to release from the granules of mediators including histamine, leukotrienes and platelet activating factor, plus eosinophil and neutrophil chemotactic factors and the cytokines IL-3, 4, 5 and GM-CSF.
- IL-4 is involved in isotype switch to IgE.

### Atopic allergy

- Atopy stems from an excessive IgE response to extrinsic antigens (allergens) which leads to local anaphylactic reactions at sites of contact with allergen.
- Hay fever and extrinsic asthma represent the most common atopic allergic disorders resulting from exposure to inhaled allergens.
- Serious prolongation of the response to allergen is caused by T-cells of TH2-type which recruit tissue-damaging eosinophils through release of IL-5. This TH2 bias is reinforced by NO· produced by cytokine-stimulated airway epithelial cells.
- Many food allergies involve type I hypersensitivity.

- Strong genetic factors include the propensity to make the IgE isotype.
- The offending antigen is identified by intradermal prick tests giving immediate wheal and erythema reactions, by provocation testing and by RAST.
- Where possible, allergen avoidance is the best treatment.
- Symptomatic treatment involves the use of long-acting β₂-agonists and newly developed leukotriene antagonists. Chromones such as sodium cromoglycate block chloride channel activity thereby stabilizing mast cells and inhibiting bronchoconstriction. Theophylline, the single most prescribed drug for asthma, is a phosphodiesterase inhibitor which raises intracellular calcium; this causes bronchodilatation and inhibition of IL-5 effects on eosinophils. Chronic asthma is dominated by activated TH2 cells and is treated with topical steroids, supplemented where necessary by long-acting β₂-agonists and theophylline.
- Courses of antigen injection may desensitize by formation of blocking IgG or IgA antibodies or through T-cell regulation. T-cell epitope peptides may be manipulated to modulate the atopic state.

### Type II—antibody-dependent cytotoxic hypersensitivity

- This involves the death of cells bearing antibody attached to a surface antigen.
- The cells may be taken up by phagocytic cells to which they adhere through their coating of IgG or C3b or lysed by the operation of the full complement system.
- Cells bearing IgG may also be killed by polymorphs

*(Continued)*

and macrophages or by K-cells through an extracellular mechanism (antibody-dependent cell-mediated cytotoxicity).

• Examples are: transfusion reactions, hemolytic disease of the newborn through rhesus incompatibility, antibody-mediated graft destruction, autoimmune reactions directed against the formed elements of the blood and kidney glomerular basement membranes, and hypersensitivity resulting from the coating of erythrocytes or platelets by a drug.

## Type III—complex-mediated hypersensitivity

• This results from the effects of antigen–antibody complexes through (i) activation of complement and attraction of polymorphonuclear leukocytes which release tissue-damaging mediators on contact with the complex, and (ii) aggregation of platelets to cause microthrombi and vasoactive amine release.

• Where circulating antibody levels are high, the antigen is precipitated near the site of entry into the body. The reaction in the skin is characterized by polymorph infiltration, edema and erythema maximal at 3–8 hours (Arthus reaction).

• Examples are farmer's lung, pigeon-fancier's disease and pulmonary aspergillosis where inhaled antigens provoke high antibody levels, reactions to an abrupt increase in antigen caused by microbial cell death during chemotherapy for leprosy or syphilis, and an element of the synovial lesion in rheumatoid arthritis.

• In relative *antigen excess*, soluble complexes are formed which are removed by binding to the CR1 C3b receptors on red cells. If this system is overloaded or if the classical complement components are deficient, the complexes circulate in the free state and are deposited under circumstances of increased vascular permeability at certain preferred sites, the kidney glomerulus, the joints, the skin and the choroid plexus.

• Examples are: serum sickness following injection of large quantities of foreign protein, glomerulonephritis associated with systemic lupus erythematosus (SLE) or infections with streptococci, malaria and other parasites, neurological disturbances in SLE and subacute sclerosing panencephalitis, polyarteritis nodosa linked to hepatitis B virus, and hemorrhagic shock in dengue viral infection.

## Type IV—cell-mediated or delayed-type hypersensitivity

• This is based upon the interaction of antigen with primed T-cells and represents tissue damage resulting from inappropriate cell-mediated immunity reactions.

• A number of soluble cytokines including IFNγ are released which activate macrophages and account for the events which occur in a typical delayed hypersensitivity response such as the Mantoux reaction to tuberculin, that is, the delayed appearance of an indurated and erythematous reaction which reaches a maximum at 24–48 hours and is characterized histologically by infiltration with mononuclear phagocytes and lymphocytes.

**Table 16.3. Comparison of types of hypersensitivity involving acquired responses.**

| | I<br>Anaphylactic | II<br>Cytotoxic | III<br>Complex-mediated | IV<br>Cell-mediated | V<br>Stimulatory |
|---|---|---|---|---|---|
| Antibody mediating reaction | Homocytotropic Ab<br>Mast-cell binding | Humoral Ab<br>± CF* | Humoral Ab<br>± CF* | Receptor on<br>T-lymphocyte | Humoral Ab<br>Non-CF* |
| Antigen | Usually exogenous<br>(e.g. grass pollen) | Cell surface | Extracellular | Associated with MHC<br>on macrophage<br>or target cell | Cell surface |
| Response to intradermal antigen: Max. reaction Appearance | 30 min (+ late reaction)<br>Wheal and flare | – | 3–8 h<br>Erythema and<br>edema | 24–48 h<br>Erythema and indura-<br>tion | – |
| Histology | Degranulated mast<br>cells; edema;<br>(late reaction<br>cellular including<br>eosinophils) | – | Acute inflammatory<br>reaction; pre-<br>dominant<br>polymorphs | Perivascular inflamma-<br>tion: polymorphs<br>migrate out leaving<br>predominantly mono-<br>nuclear cells | – |
| Transfer sensitivity to normal subject | ←————————— Serum antibody —————————→ | | | Lymphoid cells<br>Transfer factor | Serum antibody |
| Examples: | Atopic allergy,<br>e.g. hay fever | Hemolytic disease<br>of newborn (Rh) | Complex glomerulo-<br>nephritis<br>Farmer's lung | Mantoux reaction to TB<br>Granulomatous reaction<br>to TB<br>Contact sensitivity | Thyrotoxicosis |

* CF = complement fixation.

*(Continued on p. 352)*

- Continuing provocation of delayed hypersensitivity by persisting antigen leads to formation of chronic granulomas.
- TH2-type cells producing IL-4 and IL-5 can also produce tissue damage through their ability to recruit eosinophils.
- CD8 T-cells are activated by class I major histocompatibility antigens to become directly cytotoxic to target cells bearing the appropriate antigen.
- Examples are: tissue damage occurring in bacterial (tuberculosis, leprosy), viral (smallpox, measles, herpes), fungal (candidiasis, histoplasmosis) and parasitic (leishmaniasis, schistosomiasis) infections, contact dermatitis from exposure to chromates and poison ivy, insect bites and psoriasis.

## Type V—stimulatory hypersensitivity

- The antibody reacts with a key surface component such as a hormone receptor and 'switches on' the cell.

- An example is the thyroid hyperreactivity in Graves' disease due to a thyroid-stimulating autoantibody.

Features of these five types of hypersensitivity are compared in table 16.3.

## 'Innate' hypersensitivity reactions

- Many infections provoke a 'toxic shock syndrome' involving excessive release of TNF, IL-1 and IL-6 and intravascular activation of complement.
- Septic shock associated with Gram-negative bacteria is primarily due to the lipopolysaccharide (LPS) endotoxin.
- Gram-positive organisms cause release of TNF through direct action on macrophages and stimulation of selected T-cell families by the enterotoxin superantigens. Aggregation of platelets by *S. aureus* induces disseminated intravascular coagulation.
- Aberration of innate mechanisms may underly idiopathic pulmonary fibrosis and contribute to the β-amyloid plaques in Alzheimer's disease.

# FURTHER READING

Chapel H. & Haeney M. (1993) *Essentials of Clinical Immunology*, 3rd edn. Blackwell Scientific Publications, Oxford. (Very broad account of the diseases involving the immune system. Good illustration by case histories and the laboratory tests available. Also MCQ. One reviewer questions the adequacy of the treatment of allergy.)

Chauhan A.J., Krishna M.T. & Holgate S.T. (1996) Aetiology of asthma: how public health and molecular medicine work together. *Molecular Medicine Today* **2**, 192–197.

Dale M.M. & Foreman J.C. (eds) (1989) *Textbook of Immunopharmacology*, 2nd edn. Blackwell Scientific Publications, Oxford.

Haeney M. (1985) *Introduction to Clinical Immunology*. Butterworths-Update, London. (In vivid technicolor; suitable for the busy clinician.)

Holgate S.T. & Church M.K. (1993) *Allergy*. Gower Medical Publishing, London.

Lachmann P., Peters D.K., Rosen F.S. & Walport M.J. (eds) (1993) *Clinical Aspects of Immunology*, 5th edn. Blackwell Scientific Publications, Oxford.

Metzger H. (1995) Initiation of signal transduction by multi-chain immune response receptors. *The Immunologist* **3**, 129.

Rich R.R., Fleisher T.A., Schwartz B.D., Shearer W.T. & Strober W. (eds) (1996) *Clinical Immunology, Principles and Practice*. Mosby, St Louis.

Stiehm E.R. (ed.) (1989) *Immunologic Disorders in Infants and Children*, 3rd edn. W.B. Saunders, Philadelphia.

Thompson R.A. (ed.) (1985) Laboratory investigation of immunological disorders. *Clinics in Immunology and Allergy* **5**. W.B. Saunders, London.

Thompson R.A. (series ed.) *Recent Advances in Clinical Immunology*. Churchill Livingstone, Edinburgh.

# CHAPTER 17

# TRANSPLANTATION

## GRAFT REJECTION IS IMMUNOLOGICAL

The replacement of diseased organs by a transplant of healthy tissue has long been an objective in medicine but has been frustrated to no mean degree by the uncooperative attempts by the body to reject grafts from other individuals. Before discussing the nature and implications of this rejection phenomenon, it would be helpful to define the terms used for transplants between individuals and species.

*Autograft* — tissue grafted back on to the original donor.

*Isograft* — graft between syngeneic individuals (i.e. of identical genetic constitution) such as identical twins or mice of the same pure line strain.

*Allograft* (old term, homograft)—graft between allogeneic individuals (i.e. members of the same species but different genetic constitution), e.g. man to man and one mouse strain to another.

*Xenograft* (heterograft) — graft between xenogeneic individuals (i.e. of different species), e.g. pig to man.

It is with the allograft reaction that we have been most concerned, although there is now a serious interest in the use of grafts from other species. The most common allografting procedure is probably blood transfusion where the unfortunate consequences of mismatching are well known. Considerable attention has been paid to the rejection of solid grafts such as skin and the sequence of events is worth describing. In mice, for example, the skin allograft settles down and becomes vascularized within a few days. Between 3 and 9 days the circulation gradually diminishes and there is increasing infiltration of the graft bed with lymphocytes and monocytes but very few plasma cells. Necrosis begins to be visible macroscopically and within a day or so the graft is sloughed completely (figure M17.1.1). As we shall see, the process has all the hallmarks of an immunological response.

### First and second set reactions

It would be expected, if the reaction has an immuno-

logical basis, that the second contact with antigen would represent a more explosive event than the first and indeed the rejection of a second graft from the same donor is much accelerated (Milestone 17.1). The initial vascularization is poor and may not occur at all. There is a very rapid invasion by polymorphonuclear leukocytes and lymphoid cells including plasma cells. Thrombosis and acute cell destruction can be seen by 3–4 days.

### Specificity

Second set rejection is not the fate of all subsequent allografts but only of those derived from the original donor or a related strain (figure M17.1.2). Grafts from unrelated donors are rejected as first set reactions.

### Role of the lymphocyte

Neonatally thymectomized animals have difficulty in

## Milestone 17.1—The Immunological Basis of Graft Rejection

The field of transplantation owes a tremendous debt to Sir Peter Medawar, the outstanding scientist who kickstarted and inspired its development. Even at the turn of the century it was an accepted paradigm that grafts between unrelated members of a species would be unceremoniously rejected after a brief initial period of acceptance (figure M17.1.1). That there was an underlying genetic basis for rejection became apparent from Padgett's observations in Kansas City in 1932 that skin allografts between family members tended to survive for longer than those between unrelated individuals and J.B. Brown's critical demonstration in St Louis in 1937 that monozygotic (i.e. genetically identical) twins accepted skin grafts from each other. However, it was not until Medawar's research in the early part of the Second World War, motivated by the need to treat aircrew with appalling burns, that rejection was laid at immunology's door. He showed that a second graft from a given donor was rejected more rapidly and more vigorously than the first and further, that an unrelated graft was rejected with the kinetics of a first set reaction (figure M17.1.2). This **second set rejection** is characterized by **memory** and **specificity** and thereby bears the hallmarks of an immunological response. This of course was later confirmed by transferring the ability to express a second set reaction with lymphocytes.

The message was clear: to achieve successful transplan-

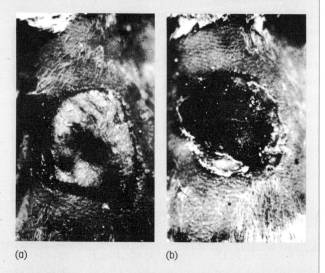

(a)        (b)

**Figure M17.1.1.** Rejection of CBA skin graft by strain A mouse. (a) Ten days after transplantation; discolored areas caused by destruction of epithelium and drying of the exposed dermis. (b) Thirteen days after transplantation; the scabby surface indicates total destruction of the graft. (Photographs courtesy of Professor L. Brent.)

tation of tissues and organs in the human, it would be necessary to overcome this immunogenetic barrier. Limited success was obtained by Murray at the Peter Bent Brigham Hospital and Hamburger in Paris, who grafted kidneys between dizygotic twins using sublethal X-

(Continued)

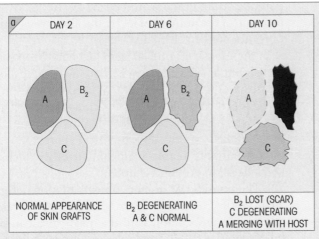

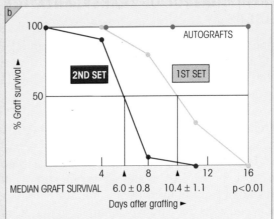

**Figure M17.1.2.** Memory and specificity in skin allograft rejection in rabbits. (a) Autografts and allografts from two unrelated donors B and C are applied to the thoracic wall skin of rabbit A which has already rejected a first graft from B (B$_1$). While the autograft A remains intact, graft C seen for the *first* time undergoes 1st set rejection, whereas a second graft from B (B$_2$) is sloughed off very rapidly. (b) Median survival times of 1st and 2nd set skin allografts showing faster 2nd set rejection. (From Medawar P.B. (1944) The behavior and fate of skin autografts and skin homografts (allografts) in rabbits. *Journal of Anatomy* **78**, 176.)

irradiation. The key breakthrough came when Schwartz and Damashek's report on the immunosuppressive effects of the antimitotic drug 6-mercaptopurine was applied independently by Calne and Zukowski in 1960 to the prolongation of renal allografts in dogs. This was fol-

lowed very rapidly by Murray's successful grafting in 1962 of an unrelated cadaveric kidney under the immunosuppressive umbrella of azathioprine, the more effective derivative of 6-mercaptopurine devised by Hutchings and Elion.

This story is studded with Nobel Prize winners and readers of a historical bent will gain further insight into the development of this field and the minds of the scientists who gave medicine this wonderful prize in *History of Transplantation; thirty-five recollections*, Terasaki P.I. (ed.) (1991) UCLA Tissue Typing Laboratory, Los Angeles, CA.

rejecting skin grafts but their capacity is restored by injection of lymphocytes from a syngeneic normal donor, suggesting that T-cells are implicated. The recipient of T-cells from a donor which has already rejected a graft will give accelerated rejection of a further graft of the same type (figure 17.1), showing that the lymphoid cells are primed and retain memory of the first contact with graft antigens.

### Production of antibodies

After rejection, humoral antibodies with specificity for the graft donor may be recognized. In the mouse, where the erythrocytes carry transplantation antigens, hemagglutination tests become positive; in the human, lymphocytotoxins are found. A Jerne plaque test using donor strain thymocytes in place of sheep erythrocytes will often demonstrate the presence of antibody-forming cells in the lymphoid tissues of grafted animals.

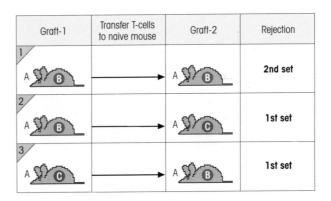

**Figure 17.1. Graft rejection induces memory which is specific and can be transferred by T-cells.** In experiment 1, an A strain recipient of T-cells from another A strain mouse which had rejected a graft from strain B, will give accelerated (i.e. 2nd set) rejection of a B graft. Experiments 2 and 3 show the specificity of the phenomenon with respect to the genetically unrelated third party strain C.

## GENETIC CONTROL OF TRANSPLANTATION ANTIGENS

The specificity of the antigens involved in graft rejection is under genetic control. Genetically identical individuals such as mice of a pure strain or uniovular twins have identical transplantation antigens and grafts can be freely exchanged between them. The Mendelian segregation of the genes controlling these antigens has been revealed by interbreeding experiments between mice of different pure strains. Since these mice breed true within a given strain and always accept grafts from each other, they must be homozygous for the 'transplantation' genes. Consider two such strains A and B with allelic genes differing at one locus. In each case paternal and maternal genes will be identical and they will have a genetic constitution of, say, $A/A$ and $B/B$ respectively. Crossing strains A and B gives a first familial generation (F1) of constitution $A/B$. Now all F1 mice accept grafts from either parent showing that they are tolerant to both A and B due to the fact that the transplantation antigens from each parent are codominantly expressed (figure 4.15). By intercrossing the F1 generation one would expect an average distribution of genotypes for the F2s as shown in figure 17.2; only 1 in 4 would have no $A$ genes and would therefore reject an A graft because of lack of tolerance, and 1 in 4 would reject B grafts for the same reason. Thus for each locus, 3 out of 4 of the F2 generation will accept parental strain grafts. Extending the analysis, if instead of one locus with a pair of allelic genes there were $n$ loci, the fraction of the F2 generation accepting

parental strain grafts would be $(3/4)^n$. In this way an estimate of the number of loci controlling transplantation antigens can be made.

In the mouse around 40 such loci have been established, but as we have seen earlier, the complex locus termed H-2 (HLA in the human) predominates in the sense that it controls the 'strong' transplantation antigens which provoke intense allograft reactions. We have looked at the structure (cf. figure 4.9) and biology of this **major histocompatibility locus** in some detail in previous chapters (see Milestone 4.2, p. 72). The non-H-2 or 'minor' transplantation antigens such as the male H-Y are recognized as processed peptides in association with the major histocompatibility complex (MHC) molecules on the cell surface by T-cells but not at all by B-cells. One should not be misled by the term 'minor' into thinking that these antigens do not give rise to serious rejection problems, albeit more slowly than the MHC.

## SOME OTHER CONSEQUENCES OF MHC INCOMPATIBILITY

### Class II MHC differences produce a mixed lymphocyte reaction (MLR)

When lymphocytes from individuals of different class II haplotype are cultured together, blast cell transformation and mitosis occurs (MLR), the T-cells of each population of lymphocytes reacting against MHC class II determinants on the surface of the other population. For the 'one-way MLR', the stimulator cells are made unresponsive by treatment with mitomycin C or X-rays and then added to the responder lymphocytes from the other donor. The responding cells belong predominantly to a population of CD4+ T-lymphocytes and are stimulated by the class II determinants present mostly on B-cells, macrophages and especially dendritic antigen-presenting cells. Thus, the MLR is inhibited by antisera to class II determinants on the stimulator cells.

### The graft-vs-host (g.v.h.) reaction

When competent T-cells are transferred from a donor to a recipient which is incapable of rejecting them, the grafted cells survive and have time to recognize the host antigens and react immunologically against them. Instead of the normal transplantation reaction of host against graft, we have the reverse, the so-called graft-vs-host (g.v.h.) reaction. In the young rodent there can be inhibition of growth (runting), spleen enlargement and hemolytic anemia (due to

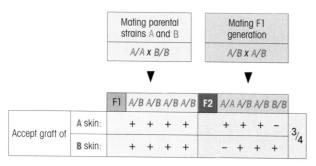

**Figure 17.2. Inheritance of genes controlling transplantation antigens.** $A$ represents a gene expressing the A antigen and $B$ the corresponding allelic gene at the same genetic locus. The pure strains are homozygous for $A/A$ and $B/B$ respectively. Since the genes are codominant, an animal with $A/B$ genome will express both antigens, become tolerant to them and therefore accept grafts from either A or B donors. The illustration shows that for each gene controlling a transplantation antigen specificity, three-quarters of the F2 generation will accept a graft of parental skin. For $n$ genes the fraction is $(3/4)^n$. If F1 $A/B$ animals are back-crossed with an $A/A$ parent, half the progeny will be $A/A$ and half $A/B$; only the latter will accept B grafts.

production of red cell antibodies). In the human, fever, anemia, weight loss, rash, diarrhea and splenomegaly are observed, with cytokines, especially tumor necrosis factor (TNF), being thought to be the major mediators of pathology. The 'stronger' the transplantation antigen difference, the more severe that reaction. Where donor and recipient differ at HLA or H-2 loci, the consequences can be fatal, although it should be noted that reactions to dominant minor transplantation antigens, or combinations of them, may be equally difficult to control.

Two possible situations leading to g.v.h. reactions are illustrated in figure 17.3. In the human this may arise in immunologically anergic subjects receiving bone marrow grafts, e.g. for combined immunodeficiency (see p. 317), for red cell aplasia after radiation accidents, or as a possible form of cancer therapy. Competent T-cells in blood or present in grafted organs given to immunosuppressed patients may give g.v.h. reactions; so could maternal cells which adventitiously cross the placenta, although in this case there is as yet no evidence of diseases caused by such a mechanism in the human.

## MECHANISMS OF GRAFT REJECTION

### Lymphocytes can mediate rejection

A great deal of the work on allograft rejection has involved transplants of skin or solid tumors because

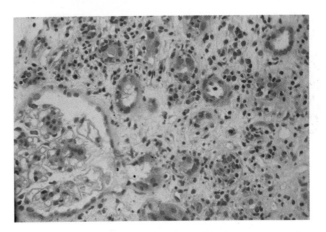

**Figure 17.4. Acute rejection of human renal allograft** showing dense cellular infiltration of interstitium by mononuclear cells. (Photograph courtesy of Drs M. Thompson & A. Dorling.)

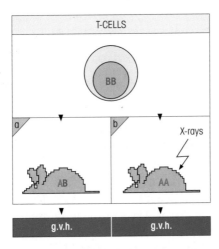

**Figure 17.3. Graft-vs-host reaction**. When competent T-cells are inoculated into a host incapable of reacting against them, the grafted cells are free to react against the antigens on the host's cells which they recognize as foreign. The ensuing reaction may be fatal. Two of many possible situations are illustrated: (a) the hybrid AB receives cells from one parent (BB) which are tolerated but react against the A antigen on host cells; (b) an X-irradiated AA recipient restored immunologically with BB cells cannot react against the graft and a g.v.h. reaction will result.

their fate is relatively easy to follow. In these cases there is little support for the view that humoral antibodies are instrumental in destruction of the graft, although, as we shall see later, this is not necessarily so with transplants of other organs such as the kidney. Whereas passive transfer of *serum* from an animal which has rejected a skin allograft cannot usually accelerate the rejection of a similar graft on the recipient animal, injection of *lymphoid* cells (particularly recirculating small lymphocytes) is effective in shortening graft survival (cf. figure 17.1).

A primary role of lymphoid cells in first set rejection would be consistent with the histology of the early reaction showing infiltration by mononuclear cells with very few polymorphs or plasma cells (figure 17.4). The dramatic effect of neonatal thymectomy on prolonging skin transplants, as mentioned earlier, and the long survival of grafts on children with thymic deficiencies implicate the T-lymphocytes in these reactions. In the chicken, homograft rejection and g.v.h. reactivity are influenced by neonatal thymectomy but not bursectomy. More direct evidence has come from *in vitro* studies showing that T-cells taken from mice rejecting an allograft could kill target cells bearing the graft antigens *in vitro*. Recent work on the importance of murine and human CD4+ cells as effectors has cast some doubt, probably wrongly, on the role of CD8 cytotoxic cells in graft rejection *in vivo*; although sometimes CD4 cells have cytotoxic potential for class II targets, as a rule they are associated with helper activity, in this case particularly for Tc precursors, and with the production of lymphokines mediating delayed hypersensitivity reactions. Perhaps they act to encourage access of Tc cells to their targets? We do know that γ-interferon (IFNγ) upregulates antigen expression on the target graft cell, so increasing its vulnerability to CD8 cyto-toxic cells.

## The allograft response is powerful

Remember, we defined the MHC by its ability to provoke the most powerful rejection of grafts between members of the same species. The frequency of allograft-specific T-helpers can be established by limiting dilution analysis by culturing a fixed number of irradiated allogeneic stimulator cells with serial dilutions of responder lymphocytes (cf. MLR above); the generation of IL-2 in positively reacting cultures is monitored by addition of an IL-2-dependent cell line. It transpires that **normal individuals have a very high frequency of alloreactive cells** (i.e. cells which react with allografts), which presumably accounts for the intensity of MHC mismatched rejection. Whereas merely a fraction of a per cent of the normal T-cell population is specific for a given single peptide, upwards of 10% of the T-cells react with alloantigens. What is the basis for this remarkable phenomenon? Three main hypotheses are current.

1 *Alloreactive T-cells recognize allo-MHC plus self-peptides* (figure 17.5a). If the allogeneic MHC differs from the recipient in the groove residues which contact processed peptide but not in those in the helices which are recognized by the TCR, the allo-MHC will be able to bind a number of peptides derived from proteins common to donor and host which might be unable to fit the groove in self-MHC and therefore fail to induce self-tolerance. Thus the T-cells which recognize allo-MHC plus common peptides will not have been eliminated and will be available to react with a large number of different peptides binding to the allo-groove. This seems to be the main explanation for the abundance of alloreactive T-cells.

2 *T-cells directly recognize the allo-MHC molecule* (figure 17.5b). The polymorphic residues may lie within the regions of the MHC helices which contact TCR directly and, by chance, a proportion of the T-cell repertoire cross-reacts and binds to the donor MHC with high affinity. In this situation, attachment of the T-cell to the antigen-presenting cell (APC) will be particularly strong since the TCRs will bind to all the donor MHC molecules on the APC, whereas, in the case of normal MHC-peptide recognition, only a small proportion of the MHC grooves will be filled by the specific peptide in question. Some T-cells react in this manner with empty allo-MHC molecules but they probably only represent a relatively small proportion of the total. These two mechanisms involve

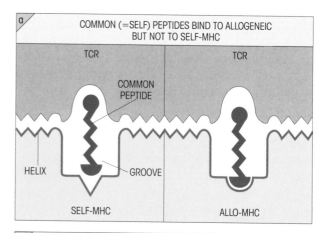

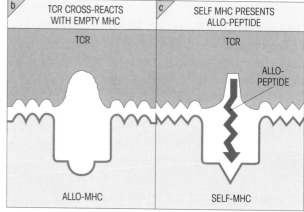

**Figure 17.5. Hypotheses to account for the high frequency of alloreactive T-cells.** (a) Polymorphic differences affect peptide binding but not T-cell receptor (TCR) contact by the donor MHC. Under these circumstances, the donor MHC molecule will be seen as 'self' by the T-cells. Unlike the self-MHC, however, the donor MHC groove will bind different sets of processed serum and cellular peptides common to graft and recipient to which the responder T-cells have not been rendered tolerant and which can therefore provoke a reaction. (b) Some T-cells may cross-react adventitiously with polymorphic residues in the allo-MHC helices which contact the TCR. Binding to large numbers of MHC molecules on the antigen-presenting cell (APC) will give a powerful signal to the T-cells. (c) Polymorphic peptides derived from the graft may be presented on self-MHC to an initially small population of T-cells which will expand with time. The regions differing in polymorphic residues are indicated in red.

**direct immunization** by the allograft MHC usually initiated by the most powerful APC, the dendritic cell. Since early sensitization in general can be blocked by antibodies to the *allo*-MHC class II, these direct mechanisms would seem to predominate. However, with time, as the donor APCs in the graft are replaced by recipient cells, a third mechanism based on **indirect sensitization** becomes possible.

3 *Allogeneic peptides are presented on self-MHC* (figure 17.5c). T-cells recognizing peptides derived from polymorphic graft proteins would be expected to be present in low frequency comparable to that observed with any foreign antigen. Nonetheless, a graft which has been in place for an extended period

will have the time to expand this small population significantly so that later rejection will depend progressively on this indirect pathway. In these circumstances, anti-recipient MHC class II can now be shown to prolong renal allografts in rats.

## The role of humoral antibody

It has long been recognized that isolated allogeneic cells such as lymphocytes can be destroyed by cytotoxic (type II) reactions involving humoral antibody. However, although earlier experience with skin and solid tumor grafts suggested that they were not readily susceptible to the action of cytotoxic antibodies, it is now clear that this does not hold for all types of organ transplants. Consideration of the different ways in which kidney allografts can be rejected illustrates the point.

*Hyperacute rejection* within minutes of transplantation, characterized by sludging of red cells and microthrombi in the glomeruli, occurs in individuals with pre-existing humoral antibodies—either due to blood group incompatibility or presensitization to class I MHC through blood transfusion.

*Acute early rejection* occurring up to 10 days or so after transplantation is characterized by dense cellular infiltration (figure 17.4) and rupture of peritubular capillaries, and appears to be a cell-mediated hypersensitivity reaction mainly involving CD8 cytotoxic attack on graft cells whose MHC antigen expression has been upregulated by γ-interferon.

*Acute late rejection*, which occurs from 11 days onwards in patients suppressed with prednisone and azathioprine, is probably caused by the binding of immunoglobulin (presumably antibody) and complement to the arterioles and glomerular capillaries, where they can be visualized by immunofluorescent techniques. These immunoglobulin deposits on the vessel walls induce platelet aggregation in the glomerular capillaries leading to acute renal shutdown (figure 17.6). The possibility of damage to antibody-coated cells through antibody-dependent cell-mediated cytotoxicity must also be considered.

*Insidious and late rejection* is associated with subendothelial deposits of immunoglobulin and C3 on the glomerular basement membranes which may sometimes be an expression of an underlying immune complex disorder (originally necessitating the transplant) or possibly of complex formation with soluble antigens derived from the grafted kidney.

The complexity of the action and interaction of cellular and humoral factors in graft rejection is therefore

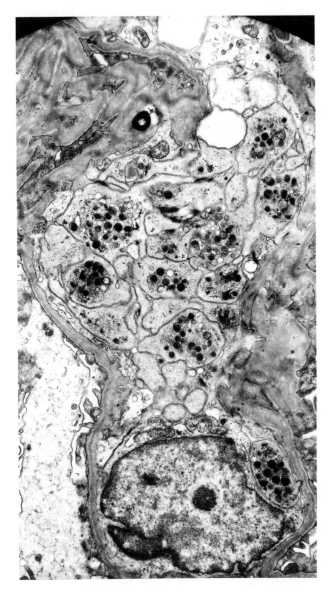

Figure 17.6. **Acute late rejection of human renal allograft showing platelet aggregation in a glomerular capillary** induced by deposition of antibody on the vessel wall (electron micrograph). (Photograph courtesy of Professor K. Porter.)

considerable and an attempt to summarize the postulated mechanisms involved is presented in figure 17.7.

There are also circumstances when antibodies may actually *protect* a graft from destruction, a phenomenon termed *enhancement*.

## THE PREVENTION OF GRAFT REJECTION

### Matching tissue types on graft donor and recipient

Since MHC differences provoke the most vicious

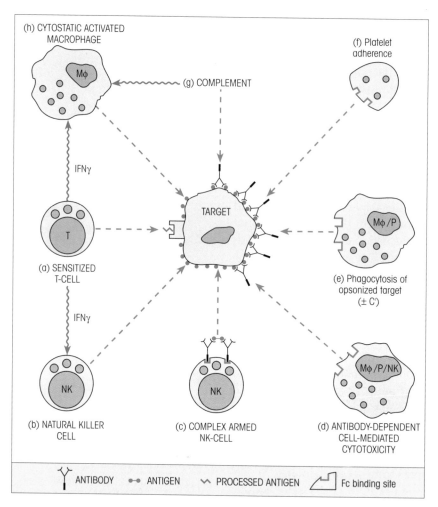

**Figure 17.7. Mechanisms of target cell destruction.** Mφ = macrophage; P = polymorph; NK = natural killer cell. (a) Direct killing by Tc cells and indirect tissue damage through release of cytokines from delayed-type hypersensitivity T-cells. (b) Killing by NK cells (see p. 19) enhanced by interferon. (c) Specific killing by immune-complex-armed NK cell which recognizes target through free antibody valencies in the complex. (d) Attack by antibody-dependent cell-mediated cytotoxicity (in a–d the killing is extracellular). (e) Phagocytosis of target coated with antibody (heightened by bound C3b). (f) Sticking of platelets to antibody bound to surface of graft vascular endothelium leading to formation of microthrombi. (g) Complement-mediated cytotoxicity. (h) Macrophages activated nonspecifically by agents such as BCG, endotoxin, poly-I:C, IFNγ and possibly C3b are cytostatic and sometimes cytotoxic for dividing tumor cells, perhaps through extracellular action of TNF and O₂-derived radicals generated at the cell surface (see p. 9).

rejection of grafts, a prodigious amount of effort has gone into defining these antigen specificities, in an attempt to minimize rejection by matching graft and recipient in much the same way that individuals are cross-matched for blood transfusions (incidentally, the ABO group provides strong transplantation antigens).

*Methods for tissue typing*

Alleles (tissue types) at the three most allelic class I loci, the so-called 'classical' MHC-loci, **HLA-A, -B and -C** (cf. figure 4.11, p. 74) are identified by complement-dependent cytotoxic reactions (figure 4.15) using operationally monospecific sera which are selected from patients transfused with whole blood and multigravidas who often become immunized with fetal antigens having specificities defined by paternally derived genes absent from the mother's genome. An individual is typed by setting up their lymphocytes against a panel of such sera in the presence of complement, cell death normally being judged by the inability to exclude Trypan Blue or eosin (figure 17.8a). Each different antigen is arbitrarily assigned a numerical specificity (figure 17.9); an individual heterozygous at each locus must express four major class I HLA specificities and two minor ones (HLA-C) derived from both the maternal and paternal chromosomes.

The original class II locus, **HLA-D**, was defined by MLR using homozygous stimulating cells for typing (figure 17.8b); if an individual fails to respond to a

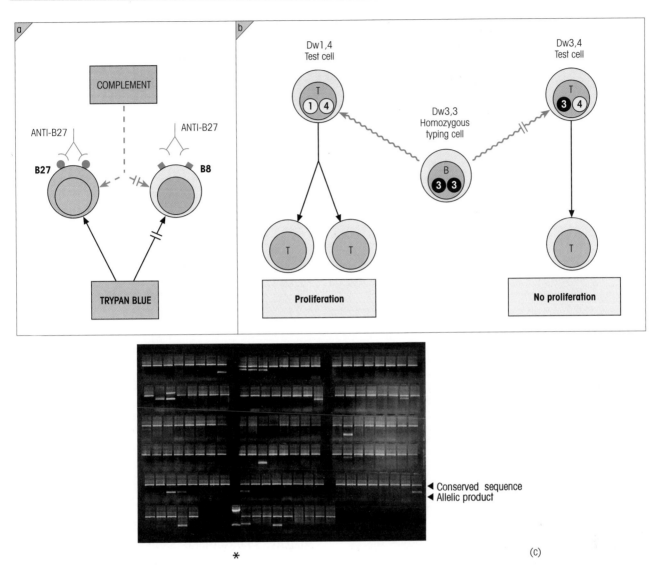

**Figure 17.8. Tissue typing.** (a) Serologic testing. Complement-mediated killing by monospecific antibody allows entry of Trypan Blue. (b) Mixed lymphocyte reaction. Cells bearing the HLA-D specificity of the homozygous typing cell are tolerant to that antigen and do not respond. Cells lacking this specificity give a proliferative response measured by incorporation of [³H]thymidine. (c) HLA typing by polymerase chain reaction (PCR) amplification using sequence-specific primers. The photograph shows reactions of 96 primer pairs specific for each allele as listed in the protocol given by Bunce M. *et al.* (1995) *Tissue Antigens* **46**, 355. A DNA sample to be typed was added to each PCR mix consisting of a pair of control primers (796 base pair product from a conserved DRB1 intron sequence) and primers to produce allele specific products. After DNA amplification, the product was electrophoresed on ethidium bromide prestained gel and visualized by ultra violet light. All lanes contain a band corresponding to the control product while positive reactions are those lanes containing an additional allele specific band of predetermined size. This sample has the HLA type: A*2501,2601-04; B*1401/02,1801/02; Cw*0802,1203; DRB1*1501-05,0701; DRB4*0101-03; DRB5*0101/02/0201/02; DQB1*0201/02,0602. *This lane contains a DNA base pair ladder. The advantages of the method are correct assignment of homozygosity, higher resolution and improved accuracy. (Photograph kindly supplied by Dr D. Briggs.)

given typing cell then his lymphocytes must be tolerant to those specificities on the typing cells because they are already present on his own body cells. These specificities defined by T-cell recognition are designated by a Dw number (table 17.1). As serological reagents were developed it transpired that the locus could be split into DR and DQ, each encoding heterodimer class II molecules with homology for murine H-2E and H-2A respectively. Subsequently a new locus, HLA-DP, was discovered (figure 17.9).

HLA alleles are now defined by their gene sequences and individuals can be typed by the polymerase chain reaction (PCR) using discriminating pairs of primers (figure 17.8c). However, it is vitally important to bear in mind the important distinction between typing based on T-cell discrimination and all

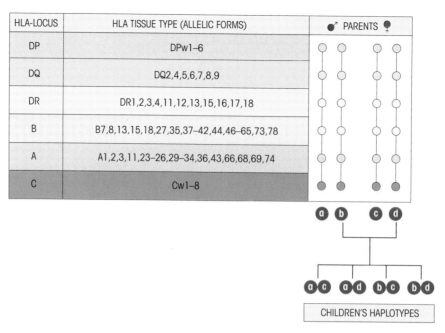

| HLA-LOCUS | HLA TISSUE TYPE (ALLELIC FORMS) | ♂ PARENTS ♀ |
|-----------|--------------------------------|-------------|
| DP | DPw1–6 | |
| DQ | DQ2,4,5,6,7,8,9 | |
| DR | DR1,2,3,4,11,12,13,15,16,17,18 | |
| B | B7,8,13,15,18,27,35,37–42,44,46–65,73,78 | |
| A | A1,2,3,11,23–26,29–34,36,43,66,68,69,74 | |
| C | Cw1–8 | |

ⓐ ⓑ   ⓒ ⓓ

ⓐⓒ  ⓐⓓ  ⓑⓒ  ⓑⓓ

CHILDREN'S HAPLOTYPES

**Figure 17.9. Serologically defined HLA specificities and their inheritance.** The complex lies on chromosome 6, the DP locus being closest to the centromere. The numbers at the A and B loci do not overlap. For brevity, each number preceded by a stop has the w designation, e.g. w46.47, 49 = w46, w47, 49. The small 'w' before a number stands for 'workshop' and indicates that the specificity concerned has not yet been characterized sufficiently for upgrading to full HLA-status. Each individual phenotypic tissue type defined by the relevant antibody may be present on HLA molecules with minor allelic variations at the DNA sequence level (see Table 17.1) which do not affect the epitope concerned. Since there are several possible alleles at each locus, the probability of a random pair of subjects from the general population having identical HLA specificities is very low. However, there is a 1:4 chance that two siblings will be identical in this respect because each group of specificities on a single chromosome forms a haplotype which will be inherited en bloc, giving four possible combinations of paternal and maternal chromosomes. Parent and offspring can only be identical (1 : 2 chance) if the mother and father have one haplotype in common.

other types of analysis because **the important initial event for transplantation is the recognition of the graft antigens by T-cells**, and antibodies do not necessarily define the same epitopes. Thus, individuals bearing the serologically defined DR4 specificities can be subdivided by T-lymphocyte typing into several different subgroups (table 17.1). Ultimately these T-cell specificities are related to specific allelic gene sequences which encode the linear T-cell epitopes.

### The polymorphism of the human HLA system

With so many alleles at each locus and so many loci in each individual (figure 17.9), it will readily be appreciated that this gives rise to an exceptional degree of polymorphism which is compounded further by the existence of multiple allotypic forms of the class III MHC complement components C2, C4a, C4b and factor B.

This remarkable polymorphism is of great potential value to the species since the need for T-cells to recognize their own individual specificities provides a defense against microbial molecular mimicry in which a whole species might be put at risk by its inability to recognize as foreign an organism which displays determinants similar in structure to these crucial MHC conformations. It is also possible that in some way the existence of a high degree of polymorphism helps to maintain the diversity of antigenic recognition within the lymphoid system of a given species and also ensures heterozygosity (hybrid vigor).

### The value of matching tissue types

Improvements in operative techniques and the use of drugs such as cyclosporin A have greatly diminished the effects of mismatching HLA specificities on solid graft survival but, nevertheless, most transplanters favor a reasonable degree of matching especially at the DR locus (see figure 17.9). The consensus is that matching at the DR loci is of greater benefit than the B loci, which in turn are of more relevance to graft survival than the A loci. In addition, the need for crossmatching to detect presensitized recipients is now taken very seriously. Bone marrow grafts, however, require a high degree of compatibility and the greater accuracy of DNA typing methods can be most helpful in this respect.

Because of the many thousands of different HLA phenotypes possible (figure 17.9), it is usual to work with a large pool of potential recipients on a continen-

**Table 17.1.** **Genetic and T-cell defined** subdivision of the main serologically identified DR specificities using new nomenclature.

| HLA alleles | HLA-DR specificities (antibody-defined) | | HLA-D associated (T-cell defined) |
|---|---|---|---|
| | Old | New | |
| DRB1*0101 | DR1 | DR1 | Dw1 |
| DRB1*0102 | DR1 | DR1 | Dw20 |
| DRB1*0103 | DR1 | DR103 | Dw'BON' |
| DRB1*0104 | — | DR1 | — |
| DRB1*1501 | DR2 | DR15 | Dw2 |
| DRB1*1502 | DR2 | DR15 | Dw12 |
| DRB1*1601 | DR2 | DR16 | Dw21 |
| DRB1*1602 | DR2 | DR16 | Dw22 |
| DRB1*0301 | DR3 | DR17 | Dw3 |
| DRB1*0302 | DR3 | DR18 | Dw'RSH' |
| DRB1*0401 | DR4 | DR4 | Dw4 |
| DRB1*0402 | DR4 | DR4 | Dw10 |
| DRB1*0403 | DR4 | DR4 | Dw13 |
| DRB1*0404 | DR4 | DR4 | Dw14 |
| DRB1*0405 | DR4 | DR4 | Dw15 |
| DRB1*0406 | DR4 | DR4 | Dw'KT2' |
| DRB1*0407 | DR4 | DR4 | Dw13 |
| DRB1*0408 | DR4 | DR4 | Dw14 |
| DRB1*1101 | DR5 | DR11 | Dw5 |
| DRB1*1102 | DR5 | DR11 | Dw'JVM' |
| DRB1*1103 | DR5 | DR11 | — |
| DRB1*1104 | DR5 | DR11 | Dw'FS' |
| DRB1*1201 | DR5 | DR12 | Dw'DB6' |
| DRB1*1301 | DRw6 | DR13 | Dw18 |
| DRB1*1302 | DRw6 | DR13 | Dw19 |
| DRB1*1303 | DRw6 | DR13 | Dw'HAG' |
| DRB1*1401 | DRw6 | DR14 | Dw9 |
| DRB1*1402 | DRw6 | DR14 | Dw16 |
| DRB1*0701 | DR7 | DR7 | Dw17 |
| DRB1*0702 | DR7 | DR7 | Dw'DBl' |
| DRB1*0801 | DRw8 | DR8 | Dw8.1 |
| DRB1*0802 | DRw8 | DR8 | Dw8.2 |
| DRB1*0803 | DRw8 | DR8 | Dw8.3 |
| DRB1*0901 | DR9 | DR9 | Dw23 |
| DRB1*1001 | DRw10 | DR10 | — |

The nomenclature works as follows. To give an example: DRB1*0302 = HLA-DR β-chain locus no. 1, main gene sequence no. *3, minor sequence variant no. 2. In addition to the B1 locus, certain haplotypes contain an extra locus which expresses a DR product; DR15 or 16 individuals have an additional B5 locus and are DR51 positive, DR3, 11, 12, 13 or 14 subjects have an additional B3 locus and are DR52 positive, while those which are DR4, 7 or 9 positive possess an extra B4 locus with a DR53 product. Clearly a group of alleles can encode molecules bearing a common B-cell epitope as defined serologically by an appropriate typing serum or antibody while at the same time giving rise to different peptide products which are the basis for the individual T-cell specificities. At the time of writing there are 106 known DRB1 alleles. The DRA locus is invariant.

The DQA chain is allelic and gives rise to a variety of T-cell specificities but serologically defined types are associated only with the DQβ chain. DP specificities are all T-cell defined and based entirely on the DPβ chain. (Based on Bodmer J.G. *et al.* (1994) *Tissue Antigens* **44**, 1.)

tal basis (Eurotransplant), so that when graft material becomes available the best possible match can be made. The position will be improved when the pool of available organs can be increased through the development of long-term tissue storage banks, but techniques are not good enough for this at present, except in the case of bone marrow cells which can be kept viable even after freezing and thawing. With a paired organ such as the kidney, living donors may be used; siblings provide the best chance of a good match (cf. figure 17.9). However, the use of living donors poses difficult ethical problems and there has been encouraging progress in the use of cadaver material. Some groups are looking at the possibility of animal organs (see below) or mechanical substitutes, while some are even trying to prevent the disease in the first place!

## Agents producing general immunosuppression

Graft rejection can be held at bay by the use of agents which nonspecifically interfere with the induction or expression of the immune response (figure 17.10). Because these agents are nonspecific, patients on immunosuppressive therapy tend to be susceptible to infections; they are also more prone to develop lymphoreticular cancers, particularly those of viral etiology.

### Targeting lymphoid populations

Anti-CD3 monoclonals are in widespread use as anti-T-cell reagents to reverse successfully acute graft rejection. They produce a complex 'flu-like clinical syndrome which includes fever, chills, headache and gastrointestinal discomfort associated with an increase in serum γ-interferon (IFNγ), α-tumour necrosis factor (TNFα) and often interleukin-2 (IL-2), presumably resulting from T-cell activation. Like other monoclonal antibodies reacting with cell-surface antigens, the anti-CD3 immunoglobulins have a propensity to evoke neutralizing anti-idiotypes, but this problem can be circumvented by using a succession of different anti-CD3s. Xenosensitization to the mouse monoclonal can be avoided either by 'humanizing' the antibody (see p. 124) or by injecting under an umbrella of anti-CD4 which allows the host to become tolerant to the murine Ig epitopes. An IgM monoclonal to conserved regions on the TCR now available seems to provoke fewer untoward reactions than the anti-CD3.

The IL-2 receptor β-chain represents another potential target and attachment of a chelate containing β-

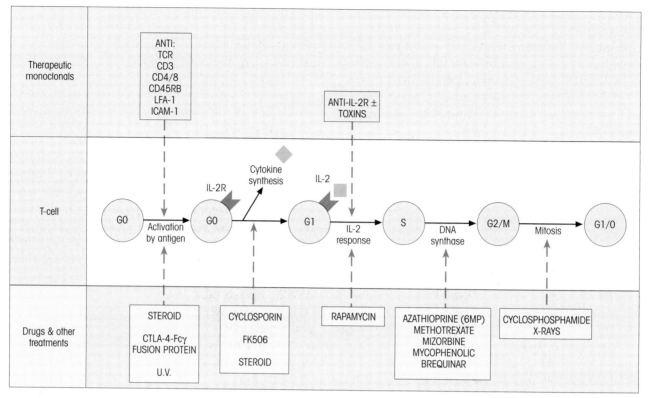

**Figure 17.10. Immunosuppressive agents used to control graft rejection.** The new name for FK506 is tacrolimus and for rapamycin, sirolimus. Mycophenolic acid, a purine analog produced by metabolism of mycophenolate mofetil, is a powerful new immunosuppressant undergoing early trials, as is deoxyspergualin which interferes with lymphocyte function in an, as yet, ill-understood manner. Leflunomide effectively blocks T-dependent and -independent antibody synthesis *in vivo* by inhibiting dihydroorotate dehydrogenase, an enzyme required for *de novo* synthesis of uridine 5'-PO₄. Simultaneous treatment with agents acting at sequential stages in development of the rejection response would be expected to synergize strongly and this is clearly seen with cyclosporin A and rapamycin.

emitting isotopes to monoclonal anti-IL-2R gave marked prolongation of heart xenografts in monkeys. Results with conjugates of the monoclonal with ricin A-chain toxin are not too encouraging because, although the molecule is internalized slowly in coated pits and thence into endosomic vesicles, it does not pass easily into the cytosol where it has its toxic action on elongation of factor-2. A somewhat similar strategy is to construct a fusion protein of IL-2 itself with PE-40, the truncated *Pseudomonas* exotoxin which should be taken up selectively by cells bearing IL-2 receptors. Following the relative ease of engraftment of allogeneic bone marrow in patients with a deficiency of the 'adhesin' molecule LFA-1 (see p. 170), attention is now turning to the use of anti-LFA-1 as an immunosuppressant for such grafts.

An antibody to the CD45RB phosphatase isoform blocked renal allograft rejection in mice and reversed acute rejection even when therapy was delayed until day 4. Note that the treatment increased tyrosine phosphorylation of phospholipase Cγ1 which is a property of anergic T-cells. The simultaneous block-ade of the CD28 and CD40 costimulatory pathways by a CTLA-4-Fcγ fusion protein and anti-CD40L (cf. p. 177) effectively aborts T-cell clonal expansion, promotes long-term survival of fully allogeneic skin grafts and inhibits the chronic vascular rejection of primarily vascularized cardiac allografts.

### Total lymphoid irradiation (TLI)

Fractionated irradiation focused on the lymphoid tissues, with shielding of marrow, lungs and other vital nonlymphoid tissue, has been used in humans to treat Hodgkin's disease for over 20 years. When mice given similar treatment are injected with allogeneic bone marrow, they fully accept the graft and show no signs of g.v.h. disease which would normally occur. Furthermore, the chimerism (coexistence of both donor and host cells) is permanent and such mice will accept grafts of other tissue from the bone marrow donor strain. The irradiation induces the formation of large granular lymphocytes lacking T, B and macrophage markers which nonspecifically suppress the antigen-specific cytolytic arm of allogeneic immune reactions, while at the same time facilitating the development of antigen-specific suppressors which maintain tolerance. That TLI can induce true transplantation tolerance to renal allografts in the human is suggested by the fact that three patients receiving this form of therapy prior to engraftment had still not rejected their kidneys after 6 years without any further immunosuppression.

Another form of radiation, UV-B light, is absorbed by skin urocanic acid and undergoes isomerization to a *cis* form which induces suppression through an effect on dendritic antigen-presenting cells.

### Immunosuppressive drugs

The development of an immunological response requires the active proliferation of a relatively small number of antigen-sensitive lymphocytes to give a population of sensitized cells large enough to be effective. Many of the immunosuppressive drugs now employed were first used in cancer chemotherapy because of their toxicity to dividing cells. Aside from the complications of blanket immunosuppression mentioned above, these antimitotic drugs are especially toxic for cells of the bone marrow and small intestine and must therefore be used with great care.

A most commonly used drug in this field is **azathioprine** which has a preferential effect on T-cell-mediated reactions. It is broken down in the body first to 6-mercaptopurine and then converted to the active agent, the ribotide. Because of the similarity in shape, this competes with inosinic acid for enzymes concerned in the synthesis of guanylic and adenylic acids; it also inhibits the synthesis of 5-phosphoribosyl-amine, a precursor of inosinic acid, by a feedback mechanism. The net result is inhibition of nucleic acid synthesis. Another drug, **methotrexate**, through its action as a folic acid antagonist also inhibits synthesis of nucleic acid. The N-mustard derivative **cyclophosphamide** probably attacks DNA by alkylation and cross-linking, so preventing correct duplication during cell division. These agents appear to exert their damaging effects on cells during mitosis and for this reason are most powerful when administered after presentation of antigen at a time when the antigen-sensitive cells are dividing.

An exciting and entirely new group of fungal metabolites (figure 17.11) are having a dramatic effect in human transplantation and in the therapy of immunological disorders, through their ability to target T-cells. **Cyclosporin A** (CsA), a neutral hydrophobic cyclical peptide containing 11 amino acids which is extremely insoluble, selectively blocks the transcription of IL-2 in activated T-cells. Resting cells which carry the vital memory for immunity to microbial infections are spared and there is little toxic-

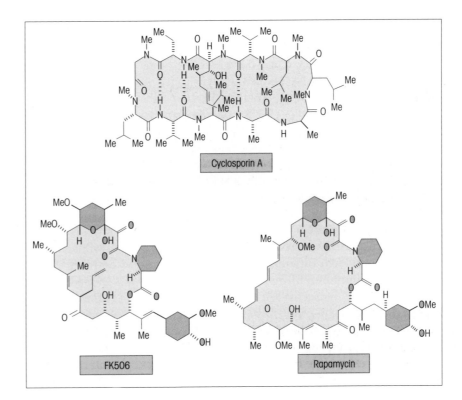

**Figure 17.11. Structures of cyclosporin, FK506 and rapamycin.** Note the complex, slightly sinister, hydrophobic ring structures, circular peptide in the case of cyclosporin, macrolide in the other two. The highlighting draws attention to similarities between FK506 and rapamycin.

Cyclosporin A

FK506

Rapamycin

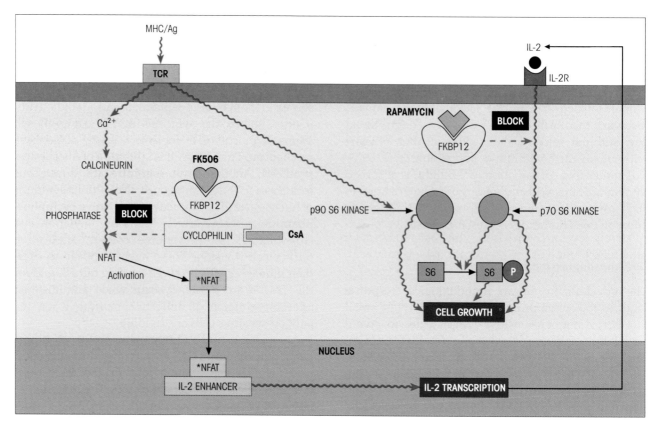

**Figure 17.12. The mode of action of cyclosporin, FK506 and rapamycin.** The complexes of CsA with cyclophilin and of FK506 with FKBP12 (one of a family of FK506-binding proteins), bind to and inactivate the phosphatase calcineurin responsible for activating nuclear factor of activated T-cells (NFAT) (and possibly OAP and Oct-1) which is a transcription factor for IL-2 synthesis. Transfection with calcineurin decreases the inhibitory powers of CsA and FK506. On binding to cyclophilin, CsA undergoes an awesome conformational change enabling it to exteriorize hydrophobic side-chains to form a patch which can bind calcineurin, rather like double-sided tape. Aminodextran derivatized with approximately 10 molecules of CsA agglutinated T-cells and although it cannot penetrate the lymphocytes, it inhibited phorbol ester-induced IL-2 synthesis, suggesting a reaction with cyclophilin on the cell membrane rather than in the cytoplasm. The rapamycin–FKBP12 complex blocks the activation of p70 S6 kinase by transduced IL-2 signals, thereby inhibiting cell growth.

*antigen presenting cell.*

ity for dividing cells in gut and bone marrow. Some studies also point to an 'exquisite' sensitivity of dendritic APC to the drug. Another T-cell-specific immunosuppressive drug, **FK506**, recently isolated from a species of *Streptomyces*, also blocks lymphokine production. The latest addition to the stable is **rapamycin**, a product of the fungus *Streptomyces hygroscopicus*, which is a macrolide like FK506, but in contrast acts to block signals induced by combination of IL-2 with its receptor.

We now have greater insight into the mode of action of these drugs (figure 17.12). Both CsA and FK506 complex with different specific binding proteins termed **immunophilins** (cyclophilin and FK-binding protein respectively), which for obscure reasons have peptidyl-prolyl isomerase activity; these complexes then interact with and inhibit the calcium and calmodulin-dependent phosphatase, calcineurin A, which is responsible for producing the transcription factors for IL-2, apoptosis and exocytosis in activated T-cells. Transcription of IL-10 is spared

suggesting that switching from TH1 to TH2 responses may be a consequence. Although rapamycin also binds to the FK-binding protein, the complex has a quite different biological activity in that it blocks the IL-2-induced activation of the p70 S6 kinase which phosphorylates ribosomal S6 prior to cell proliferation.

Cyclosporin now has a proven place as first-line therapy in the prophylaxis and treatment of transplant rejection. Figure 17.13 gives an example of its use in kidney transplantation but it has also been evaluated in a wide range of disorders where T-cell-mediated hypersensitivity reactions are suspected. Indeed, the benefits of cyclosporin in diseases such as idiopathic nephrotic syndrome, type 1 insulin-dependent diabetes, Behçet's syndrome, active Crohn's disease, aplastic anemia, severe corticosteroid-dependent asthma and psoriasis have been interpreted to suggest or confirm a pathogenic role for the immune system. However, effects not only on Langerhans' dendritic cells but also on proliferation of normal and transformed keratinocytes *in vitro* may contribute to the favorable outcome in psoriasis. A rapid onset of benefit, and relapse when treatment is stopped, are common features of cyclosporin therapy.

There are, of course, side-effects. It has to be used at doses below those causing nephrotoxicity so that blood levels have to be monitored regularly by radioimmunoassay. There is also some cause for concern that cyclosporin may make patients susceptible to EB virus-induced lymphomas since the drug inhibits T-cells which control EB virus transformation of B-cells *in vitro*; however, the latest results suggest that the incidence of lymphoma is relatively low in comparison with that reported for allografted patients on conventional immunosuppressive therapy.

FK506 is greatly superior to CsA on a molar basis *in vitro* but is not substantially more effective when used in kidney grafting; however its tropism for liver could be exploited. Because they act at different stages in the activation of the T-cell, CsA and rapamycin show a most impressive degree of synergy.

Steroids such as prednisone intervene at many points in the immune response, affecting lymphocyte recirculation and the generation of cytotoxic effector cells, for example; in addition, their outstanding anti-inflammatory potency rests on features such as inhibition of neutrophil adherence to vascular endothelium in an inflammatory area and suppression of monocyte/macrophage functions such as microbicidal activity and response to lymphokines.

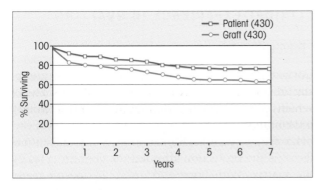

**Figure 17.13. Actuarial survival of primary cadaveric kidney grafts** in 430 patients treated at the Oxford Transplant Centre with triple therapy. **Cyclosporin**: 10 mg/kg/day orally given as a single dose (first dose given before surgery) and reduced according to whole-blood trough levels (200–400 ng/ml in first 3 months and then maintained at 100–200 ng/ml). **Azathioprine**: 100 mg/day orally; reduced if leukocyte count <5000. **Prednisolone**: 20 mg/day given in divided doses orally and reduced to a maintenance dose of 10 mg/day by 6 months. The initial dose is reduced to 15 mg/day in patients less than 60 kg body weight. In patients with stable renal function at 1 year, prednisolone is discontinued over a period of some months. (Data reproduced from Morris P.J. (ed.) *Kidney Transplantation: Principles and Practice* (4th edn). W.B. Saunders Company, Philadelphia, USA, with permission of the author and publishers.)

Corticosteroids form complexes with intracellular receptors which then bind to regulatory genes and block transcription of TNF, IFNγ, IL-1, 2, 3, 6 and MHC class II, i.e. they block expression of lymphokines and monokines whereas cyclosporin has its main action on lymphokines.

In parentheses, the immunophilins may be involved in other cellular functions such as regulation of the *N*-methyl-ᴅ-aspartate subtype of neural glutamate receptors and the augmentation of neuronal process extension by growth-associated protein-43 leading to the propositions that FK506 could be clinically employed in stroke patients and in treatment of nerve degeneration. A close association of FKBP12 with the surface receptor for transforming growth factor-β (TGFβ) has also been revealed. With good fortune these drugs will take us down some very unexpected and intriguing pathways.

## Strategies for antigen-specific depression of allograft reactivity

If the disadvantages of blanket immunosuppression are to be avoided, we must aim at knocking out only the reactivity of the host to the antigens of the graft, leaving the remainder of the immunological apparatus intact – in other words, the induction of **antigen-specific tolerance**. Total lymph node irradiation plus bone marrow (see above) is known to induce T-suppression in mice, and grafts of skin and heart from the same donor enjoy prolonged survival.

It turns out that bone marrow represents a privileged source of tolerogenic alloantigens and the production of stable lymphohematopoietic mixed chimerism by bone marrow engraftment is proving to be a potent means of inducing robust specific transplantation tolerance to solid organs across major MHC mismatches. Despite the role of the *mature* dendritic cell as the champion stimulator of resting T-cells, the dendritic cell *precursors* which display little or no MHC class II or B7 costimulators appear to bear the primary responsibility for tolerance induction. A major subpopulation of dendritic cells, particularly in the thymus, expresses the CD8α homodimer and the apoptosis-inducing Fas ligand, FasL. These could act as 'veto' cells capable of killing activated CD4+ T-cells and inducing tolerance by clonal deletion. With a lower inoculum of allogeneic bone marrow, there is evidence for the establishment of tolerance through the induction of active suppression by regulatory T-cells.

Such microchimerism, which can be brought about by nondepleting anti-CD4 and -8, gave specific and indefinite acceptance of mouse skin grafts across class

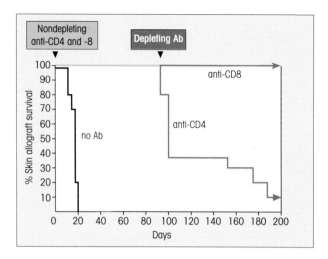

**Figure 17.14. Induction of allograft tolerance by non-depleting anti-CD4 plus anti-CD8.** Tolerance to skin grafts from donors with multiple minor transplantation antigen mismatches was achieved by concurrent injection of IgG2a monoclonal antibodies to CD4 and CD8 which do not induce cell depletion. The maintenance of tolerance depends upon the continued presence of antigen which enables the unresponsive cells to interact with newly arising immunocompetent cells on the surface of the same antigen-presenting cells and render them unresponsive through an infectious tolerance mechanism (cf. figure 11.8, 12.8 and 20.22). Whether the mechanism involves 'infectious anergy', direct suppression, 'immune deviation' of potentially aggressive TH1 cells by suppressor TH2, downregulation of the antigen-presenting cell or all four in various combinations, is unresolved. Loss of tolerance on depletion of CD4 but not CD8 cells shows that active tolerance is maintained by the CD4 subset. (Figure synthesized from data kindly provided by Dr S.P. Cobbold and Prof. H. Waldmann.)

I or multiple minor transplantation antigen barriers (figure 17.14). Grafting of organs such as heart, which are less fastidious than skin require less aggressive immunotherapy.

Full-frontal attack by antigen alone is also possible provided it is presented in a non-costimulatory tolerogenic form. Thus, syngeneic mouse tumor cells transfected with the H-2K^b antigen were able to prolong the survival of H-2^b heart allografts in H-2^k mice. In a novel approach, peptides corresponding to residues 75–84 on the α-helix of the α1-domain of MHC class I can bind heat shock protein 70 and cause a rise in intracellular calcium accompanied by the development of T-cell anergy. Given together with a subtherapeutic dose of cyclosporin A during the pre- or post-transplant period, the peptide fostered indefinite survival of cardiac allografts in rats.

## IS XENOGRAFTING A PRACTICAL PROPOSITION?

Because the supply of donor human organs for transplantation lags seriously behind the demand, a widespread interest in the feasibility of using animal

organs is emerging. Pigs are more favored than primates as donors both on grounds of ethical acceptability and the hazards of zoonoses. The first hurdle to be overcome is **hyperacute rejection** due to xenoreactive natural antibodies in the host. Humans lack α-1,3-galactosyl transferase and generally develop antibodies to galactose which react with the galactosyl α-1,3-galactose expressed abundantly on the xenogeneic vascular endothelium. This activates complement in the absence of regulators of the human complement system such as decay accelerating factor, CD59 and MCP (cf. figure 15.2) and precipitates the hyperacute rejection phenomenon. Novel genetic engineering strategies for the solution of this problem are outlined in figure 17.15.

The next crisis is acute vascular rejection as antibodies are formed to the xenoantigens on donor epithelium. Brequinar sodium (figure 17.10), an inhibitor of pyrimidine biosynthesis and suppressor of both B- and T-cell mediated responses, has been evaluated for efficacy but induction of tolerance would clearly be more desirable. Stable multilineage xenogeneic chimerism and donor specific transplantation tolerance have been achieved using injection of mixed rat and mouse bone marrow into lethally or sublethally conditioned mouse recipients; an ill-understood two-way interaction is responsible.

Even when the immunological problems are overcome, it remains to be seen whether the xenograft will be compatible with human life over a prolonged period.

## CLINICAL EXPERIENCE IN GRAFTING

### Privileged sites

Corneal grafts survive without the need for immunosuppression. Because they are avascular they do not sensitize the recipient, although they become cloudy if the individual has been presensitized. Grafts of cartilage are successful in the same way but an additional factor is the protection afforded the chondrocytes by the matrix. With bone and artery it doesn't really matter if the grafts die because they can still provide a framework for host cells to colonize.

### Kidney grafts

Thousands of kidneys have been transplanted and with improvement in patient management there is a high survival rate. Matching at the HLA-D locus has a strong effect on graft survival (figure 17.16) but in the long term (5 years or more) the desirability of reason-

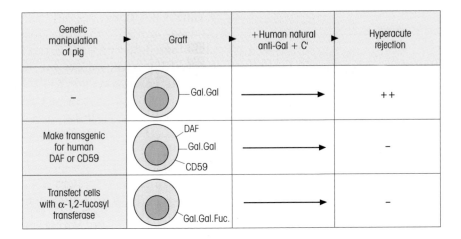

**Figure 17.15. Strategies for avoiding complement-mediated hyperacute rejection of a xenograft** caused by reaction of natural anti-galactose antibodies with Galα-1,3-Gal on the surface of the pig graft cells. Heart xenografts from transgenic pigs expressing the human complement regulatory proteins decay accelerating factor (DAF) or CD59 functioned for prolonged periods in baboons. Transfection of pig cells with α-1,2-fucosyl transferase converted the terminal sugars into the blood group H and rendered the cells resistant to lysis by the anti-galactose.

able HLA-B, and to a lesser extent HLA-A, matching also becomes apparent.

Patients are partially immunosuppressed at the time of transplantation because uremia causes a degree of immunological anergy. The combination of azathioprine and prednisone was commonly employed in the long-term management of kidney grafts but is now supplemented by cyclosporin A in the so-called **triple therapy** (figure 17.13). One hopes that the synergy between cyclosporin and rapamycin will emerge as a powerful new therapeutic regimen. If kidney function is poor during a rejection crisis, renal dialysis can be used. As mentioned above, there is active interest in the possibility of xenografting. When transplantation is performed because of immune

complex-induced glomerulonephritis, the immunosuppressive treatment used may help to prevent a similar lesion developing in the grafted kidney. Patients with glomerular basement membrane antibodies (e.g. Goodpasture's syndrome) are likely to destroy their renal transplants unless first treated with plasmapheresis and immunosuppressive drugs.

## Heart transplants

The overall 1-year survival figure for heart transplants has moved up to over the 70% mark (figure 17.17), helped considerably by the introduction of cyclosporin A therapy. Its nephrotoxicity is a drawback, although the analog cyclosporin G is better in this respect. Full HLA matching is of course not practical but single DR mismatches gave 90% survival at 3 years compared with a figure of 65% for two DR mismatches. Aside from the rejection problem it is likely that the number of patients who would benefit from cardiac replacement is much greater than the number dying with adequately healthy hearts. More attention will have to be given to the possibility of xenogeneic grafts and mechanical substitutes.

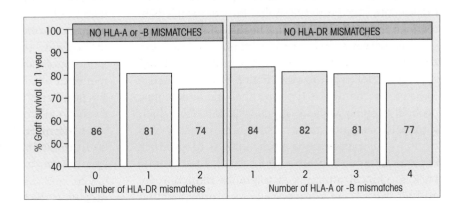

**Figure 17.16. First cadaveric kidney graft survival in Europe on the basis of mismatches for HLA-A, B and DR.** There is a significant influence of matching. (Data kindly supplied by Drs G. Opelz and Jacqueline Smits of the Eurotransplant International Foundation.)

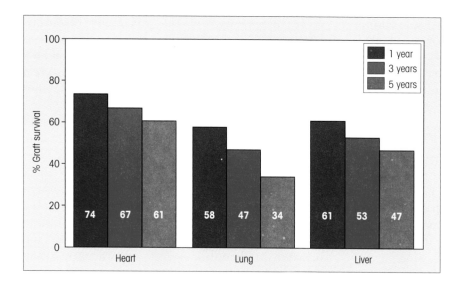

**Figure 17.17. Graft survival rates for first heart, liver and lung transplantations in Eurotransplant.** (Data kindly supplied by Dr Jacqueline Smits, Eurotransplant International Foundation.)

## Liver transplants

Survival rates for orthotopic liver grafts are not quite as high as those achieved with heart transplants (figure 17.17). The hepatotrophic capacity of FK506 is an added bonus which makes it the preferred drug for liver transplantation. Rejection crises are dealt with by high dose steroids and, if this proves ineffective, antilymphocyte globulin. The use of a totally synthetic colloidal hydroxyethyl starch solution containing lactobionate as a substitute for chloride, allows livers to be preserved for 24 hours or more and has revolutionized the logistics of liver transplantation. To improve the prognosis of patients with primary hepatic or bile duct malignancies which were considered to be inoperable, transplantation of organ clusters with liver as the central organ has been designed, e.g. liver and pancreas, or liver, pancreas, stomach and small bowel or even colon. Nonetheless, the outcome is not very favorable in that up to three-quarters of the patients transplanted for hepatic cancer have had recurrence of their tumor within 1 year.

Experience with liver grafting between pigs revealed an unexpected finding. Many of the animals retained the grafted organs in a healthy state for many months without any form of immunosuppression and enjoyed a state of unresponsiveness to grafts of skin or kidney from the same donor. True tolerance is induced by the donor type intrahepatic leukocytes, probably a subset of dendritic cells (see above), which form microhematopoietic clusters, and possibly also by the liver parenchyma itself, known to produce copious amounts of soluble MHC class I. This takes us back to clinical attempts at tolerance induction by adding extra bone marrow cells to supplement the small number of passenger leukocytes in a kidney graft or perhaps a preconditioning manipulation with bone marrow plus a small course of cyclosporin (and maybe soluble class I thought to induce apoptosis in specific cytotoxic CD8 T-cells?).

Work is in progress on the transfer of isolated hepatocytes attached to collagen-coated microcarriers injected i.p. for the correction of isolated deficiencies such as albumin synthesis. This attractive approach could have much wider applications, although in the distant future it will presumably run into competition from gene therapy.

## Bone marrow grafting

Patients with certain immunodeficiency disorders and aplastic anemia are obvious candidates for treatment with bone marrow stem cells, as are acute leukemia patients treated radically with intensive chemotherapy and possibly whole-body irradiation in attempts to eradicate the neoplastic cells (table 17.2). Good results are being obtained with stem cell transplantation *in utero* for inherited blood disorders using CD34-enriched populations from paternal bone marrow. From the practical standpoint, it has been recognized that cord blood contains sufficient hematopoietic stem cells for bone marrow replacement but what is even more convenient is to enhance the number of CD34-positive progenitor cells in relatively small volumes of peripheral blood by recombinant stem cell factor, IL-1β, IL-3, IL-6 and erythropoietin *ex vivo* prior to transplantation. It is encouraging also that both colony-stimulating factors G-CSF and GM-CSF greatly accelerate the return of myeloid cells after lethal doses of myelotoxic agents preceding autologous bone marrow transplantation; there are fewer infections, less use of i.v. antibodies and earlier discharge from hospital. They also accelerate the engraftment of allogeneic bone marrow without exacerbating g.v.h. disease.

### Graft-vs-host disease is a major problem in bone marrow grafting

G.v.h. disease resulting from recognition of recipient antigens by allogeneic T-cells in the bone marrow inoculum represents a serious, sometimes fatal complication. If possible, it is of benefit to make a quantitative assessment of IL-2 precursors in the donor marrow by limiting dilution analysis, since a frequency >1:100 000 predicts grade 2–4 acute g.v.h. The incidence of g.v.h. disease is reduced if T-cells in the grafted marrow are first purged with a cytotoxic cocktail of anti-T-cell monoclonals. Unexpectedly, there is an alarmingly high incidence of graft failure, apparently due to natural killer cell (NK) recognition of the recessive hematopoietic histocompatibility (Hh) antigen system, which in mice is responsible for paradoxical rejection of parental bone marrow by F1 generation recipients.

Successful results with bone marrow transfers require highly compatible donors if fatal g.v.h. reactions are to be avoided, and here siblings offer the best chance of finding a matched donor (figure 17.9). Undoubtedly nonHLA minor transplantation antigens are important and are more difficult to match. Acute g.v.h. disease occurring within the first 100 days following infusion of allogeneic marrow primarily affects the skin, liver and gastrointestinal tract. Antibodies to TNF or IL-1R block mortality. Current therapy uses cyclosporin with prednisone but inclusion of methotrexate in this regimen is said to improve efficacy. There are also indications that selective depletion of CD8 cells from the graft inhibits

g.v.h. disease without the potentially disastrous effects of whole T-cell purging on engraftment mentioned above. Chronic g.v.h. disease (i.e. later than 100 days) has a relatively good prognosis if limited to skin and liver, but if multiple organs are involved, clinically resembling progressive systemic sclerosis, the outcome is poor. Patients are treated with cyclosporin and prednisone but recently thalidomide has been found to be very helpful. The pathogenesis is not straightforward and chronic disease could arise by a curious mechanism involving the sneaking through of autoreactive T-cells which fail to be deleted in the thymus possibly because of thymic damage due to pre- or post-transplant therapy, e.g. associated viral infection, irradiation or even cyclosporin itself. It may be significant that cyclosporin inhibits the programmed cell death of immature thymocytes which occurs on activation by anti-CD3 and it is known that an autologous 'g.v.h.' supervenes on termination of prolonged cyclosporin administration to young irradiated rats which had received syngeneic bone marrow.

## Other organs

It is to be expected that improvement in techniques of control of the rejection process will encourage transplantation in several other areas — not cases of endocrine disorders where exogeneous replacement therapy is convenient, but, for example, in diabetes where the number of transplants recorded is rising rapidly and the current success rate is around 40%, although a major problem still is inadequate ouput of insulin by the grafted islets. The 5-year survival rate of 34% for lung transplants is still less than satisfactory. In particular, one also looks forward one day to the successful transplantation of skin for lethal burns.

Reports are coming in of experimental foray into

Table 17.2. Bone marrow transplants: summary of survival and relapse data from many centers.

| DISEASE | | PROBABILITY | |
|---|---|---|---|
| TYPE | STAGE | LONG-TERM SURVIVAL | DISEASE RECURRENCE |
| Acute leukemia | Relapse | 0.1–0.3 | 0.60 |
| Acute nonlymphocytic leukemia | 1st remission | 0.6 | 0.25 |
| Acute lymphocytic leukemia | 2nd remission | 0.3 | 0.25 |
| Chronic granulocytic leukemia | Blastic phase | 0.2 | 0.70 |
| Chronic granulocytic leukemia | Accelerated phase | 0.2 | 0.50 |
| Chronic granulocytic leukemia | Chronic phase | 0.6 | 0.30 |
| Severe combined immunodeficiency | — | 0.5 | — |
| Severe aplastic anemia | — | 0.8 | — |
| Thalassemia major | — | 0.7 | 0.3 |

the grafting of **neural tissues**. Mutant mice with degenerate cerebellar Purkinje cells which mimic the human condition, cerebellar ataxia, can be restored by engraftment of donor cerebellar cells at the appropriate sites; these express insulin growth factor-1 (IGF-1), migrate to form a layer in lieu of the missing cells, induce sprouting in host neurons and become synaptically integrated. Clinical trials with transplantation of human embryonic dopamine neurons to reverse the neurological deficit in Parkinson's disease have been severely hampered by the excessive death of the grafted cells. The hypothesis that this was due to oxidative stress led to a study showing that grafted neurons from transgenic mice overexpressing Cu/Zn superoxide dismutase (cf. p. 9) had a greatly increased survival rate.

Work proceeds apace to produce a successful prosthetic vascular graft which would remain patent as a blood conduit, prevent thrombosis of the blood in low flow or adverse states and control anastomotic cellular hyperplasia with overgrowth of smooth muscle cells and matrix production. This has proved difficult to achieve but there are encouraging attempts to engineer a composite vascular graft in which microvessel endothelial cells present in a small sample of subcutaneous abdominal wall fat obtained by the relatively simple cosmetic liposuction technique, grow as an antithrombotic endothelial layer to line the surface of an expanded polytetrafluoroethylene tube. Expect development in this field, particularly for the replacement of arteries.

## ASSOCIATION OF HLA TYPE WITH DISEASE

### Linkage disequilibrium and disease susceptibility

An impressive body of data is accumulating which links specific HLA antigens with particular disease states in the human (table 17.3) and even more striking relationships may be uncovered as the complexity of the HLA-D region is unravelled (please note that in this section, the old DR nomenclature, table 17.1, has been used). The relationships are influenced by **linkage disequilibrium**, a state where closely linked genes on a chromosome tend to remain associated rather than undergo genetic randomization in a given population, so that the frequency of a pair of alleles occurring together is greater than the product of the individual gene frequencies (figure 17.18a). This could result from natural selection favoring a particular haplotype or from insufficient time elapsing since the first appearance of closely located alleles to allow

them to become randomly distributed throughout the population. Be that as it may, a significant association between a disease and a given HLA specificity does not imply that we have identified the disease susceptibility gene, because we might find an even better correlation with another HLA gene in linkage disequilibrium with the first. To take an example: in multiple sclerosis, an association with the B7 allele was first established but when patients were typed for the D locus, a much stronger correlation with DR2 emerged (figure 17.18b). The initial correlation with B7 resulted from linkage disequilibrium between B7 and DR2. We still cannot be sure that DR2 itself is the disease susceptibility gene since, carrying the argument a stage further, one cannot exclude the possibility of finding an even greater association with another closely linked gene and indeed recent studies reveal an even tighter relationship to DQB1*0602. However,

Table 17.3. Association of HLA with disease.

| DISEASE | HLA ALLELE | RELATIVE RISK |
|---|---|---|
| **a  Class II associated** | | |
| Hashimoto's disease | *DR5 | 3.2 |
| Primary myxedema | DR3 | 5.7 |
| Thyrotoxicosis (Graves') | DR3 | 3.7 |
| Insulin-dependent diabetes | DQ8 | 14 |
| | DQ2/8 | 20 |
| | DQ6 | 0.2 |
| Addison's disease (adrenal) | DR3 | 6.3 |
| Goodpasture's syndrome | DR2 | 13.1 |
| Rheumatoid arthritis | DR4 | 5.8 |
| Juvenile rheumatoid arthritis | DR8 | 8.1 |
| Sjögren's syndrome | DR3 | 9.7 |
| Chronic active hepatitis (autoimmune) | DR3 | 13.9 |
| Multiple sclerosis | DR2,DR6 | 12 |
| Narcolepsy | DQ6 | 38 |
| Dermatitis herpetiformis | DR3 | 56.4 |
| Celiac disease | DQ2 | 250 |
| Tuberculoid leprosy | DR2 | 8.1 |
| **b  Class I, HLA-B27 associated** | | |
| Ankylosing spondylitis | B27 | 87.4 |
| Reiter's disease | B27 | 37.0 |
| Post-salmonella arthritis | B27 | 29.7 |
| Post-shigella arthritis | B27 | 20.7 |
| Post-yersinia arthritis | B27 | 17.6 |
| Post-gonococcal arthritis | B27 | 14.0 |
| Uveitis | B27 | 14.6 |
| Amyloidosis in rheumatoid arthritis | B27 | 8.2 |
| **c  Other class I associations** | | |
| Subacute thyroiditis | B35 | 13.7 |
| Psoriasis vulgaris | Cw6 | 13.3 |
| Idiopathic hemochromatosis | A3 | 8.2 |
| Myasthenia gravis | B8 | 4.4 |

(Data mainly from Ryder *et al.*: see legend to figure 17.18, and Thorsby E. (1995) *The Immunologist* **3**, 51.)
*DR specificities relate to 'old nomenclature' table 17.1.

in those instances where two susceptibility genes encoding α and β chains synergize *and* are in the *trans* configuration (i.e. on different chromosomes) linkage disequilibrium is less likely to be the explanation.

Ethnic studies may help by making available recombination events which alter haplotypes and permit the identification of susceptibility determinants outside their normal context. Thus, the DQα (DQA1*0201) linked to DR7 on the Caucasian haplotype has a neutral effect on diabetes susceptibility but, in the black population, DR7 is associated with a high risk DQα (DQA1*0301) and now becomes a susceptibility haplotype.

## Association with immunological diseases

With the odd exceptions such as idiopathic hemochromatosis and congenital adrenal hyperplasia resulting from a 21-hydroxylase deficiency which

| HLA GENES | SINGLE GENE | GENE FREQUENCY % | |
|---|---|---|---|
| | | PAIRED GENES | |
| | | EXPECTED | OBSERVED |
| A1 | 16 | 1.6 | 8.8 |
| B8 | 10 | | |
| A3 | 13 | 1.3 | 2.8 |
| B7 | 10 | | |

(a)

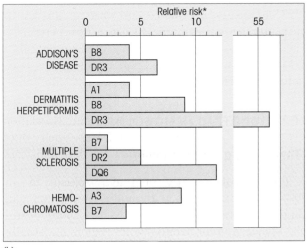

(b)

**Figure 17.18. Linkage disequilibrium and the association between HLA and disease.** (a) Two examples of linkage disequilibrium. The expected frequency for a pair of genes is the product of each individual gene frequency. B8 and DR3 are in linkage disequilibrium as are B7 and DR2; thus the haplotypes A1, B8, DR3 and A3, B7, DR2 are relatively common. (b) Influence of linkage disequilibrium on disease association. *Relative risk=the increased chance of contracting the disease for individuals bearing the antigen relative to those lacking it. (Data from Ryder L.P., Andersen E. & Svejgaard A. (1979) HLA and disease Registry 1979. *Tissue Antigens*, supplement.)

only gain membership of this august club through linkage disequilibrium, HLA-linked diseases are intimately bound up with immunological processes. By and large, the HLA-D-related disorders are autoimmune with a tendency for DR3 or linked genes to be associated with organ-specific diseases. It has been suggested that HLA antigens might affect the susceptibility of a cell to viral attachment or infection, thereby influencing the development of autoimmunity to associated surface components. Inevitably though, because class II genes tend to dominate these relationships, the temptation is to think in terms of immune response genes controlling the nature of the reaction to the relevant autoantigen or to whatever might be a causative agent, perhaps through an ability to bind certain antigenic peptides. A given HLA-D allele may permit the binding of foreign peptides and cross-reacting self-epitopes; alternatively the complex with particular self-peptides could positively or negatively select either reactive or suppressive T-cells.

**Insulin-dependent diabetes mellitus** is associated with DQ8 (DQA1*0301,DQB1*0302) and DQ2 (DQA1*0501,DQB1*0201) but the strongest susceptibility is seen in the **DQ2/8 heterozygote** arguing in favor of a role for the *trans* encoded DQ molecule(s) in these individuals, most probably DQ(α1*0301, β1*0201). The fact that two genes are necessary to determine the strongest susceptibility and the universality of this finding in all populations studied, implies that the DQ molecules themselves, not other molecules in linkage disequilibrium, are primarily involved in disease susceptibility. Possession of some subtypes of DQ6 gives a dominantly protective effect (Table 17.3). Thus the degree of HLA-associated predisposition to type 1 diabetes will be a composite of the effects of the particular combination of *cis*- or *trans*- encoded DQ molecules. To get down to the molecular level, different polymorphic amino acids at residues DQα52 and DQβ57 have a powerful influence on disease susceptibility.

DR4 and, to a lesser extent, DR1 are risk factors for **rheumatoid arthritis** in white Caucasians. Analysis of DR4 subgroups, and of other ethnic populations where the influence of DR4 is minimal, has identified a particular linear T-cell sequence from residues 67–74 as the disease susceptibility element and the variations observed are based on sharing of this sequence with other HLA-DR specificities, which presumably arose from the recombination and gene conversion events responsible for MHC polymorphism (table 17.4). This stretch of amino acids is highly polymorphic and forms pockets 4 and 7 of the peptide-binding

**Table 17.4. Shared sequences on the DRβ1 α-helix in different haplotypes confer susceptibility to rheumatoid arthritis.** (Data from Bell J.I. & McMichael A.J. (1993) In Lachmann P.J., Peters D.K., Rosen F.S. & Walport M.J. (eds) *Clinical Aspects of Immunology*, p.748. Blackwell Scientific Publications, Oxford.)

| | HLA-DR SPECIFICITY | DRβ1 GENE | HLA-DRβ RESIDUES IN THE THIRD ALLELIC HYPERVARIABLE REGION | | | | | | | | | |
|---|---|---|---|---|---|---|---|---|---|---|---|---|
| | | | 66 | | | | 70 | | | 74 | | |
| **Susceptible to RA** | DR1 | *0101 | Asp | Leu | Leu | Glu | Gln | Arg | Arg | Ala | Ala | Val |
| | DR4 | *0404 | – | – | – | – | – | – | – | – | – | – |
| | DR4 | *0405 | – | – | – | – | – | – | – | – | – | – |
| | DR4 | *0401 | – | – | – | – | – | Lys | – | – | – | – |
| | DR10 | *1001 | – | – | – | – | Arg | – | – | – | – | – |
| **Not susceptible to RA** | DR4 | *0402 | – | Ile | – | – | Asp | Glu | – | – | – | – |
| | DR4 | *0407 | – | – | – | – | – | – | – | – | Glu | – |
| | DR7 | *0701 | – | Ile | – | – | Asp | – | – | Gly | Gln | – |
| **Nucleotide sequences** | DR1 | *0101 | GAC | CTC | CTG | GAG | CAG | AGG | CGG | GCC | GCG | GTG |
| | DR4 | *0401 | --- | --- | --- | --- | --- | -A- | --- | --- | --- | --- |

cleft. There are striking differences between the sets of peptides bound by DR subtypes associated with rheumatoid arthritis and those that are not; notably, differences involved the amino acid charge at residues 4 or 5 of the peptide sequence bound to the cleft. Analysis of the peptides bound spontaneously to the DR molecules from patients could yield an important clue to pathogenesis. As in diabetes, the DR2 allele is underrepresented and DR2-positive patients have less severe disease, implying that a DR2-linked gene might be protective in some way (through interaction with a heat-shock protein maybe?).

The association with HLA in **ankylosing spondylitis** is quite remarkable; up to 95% of patients are of B27 phenotype as compared with around 5% in controls. The incidence of B27 is also markedly raised in other conditions when accompanied by sacroiliitis, e.g. Reiter's disease, acute anterior uveitis, psoriasis and other forms of infective sacroiliitis such as *Yersinia*, gonococcal and *Salmonella* arthritis. The extraordinarily close association with B27 and the development of a somewhat similar disease in rodents made transgenic for the B27 gene speaks for the B27 molecule itself as a central pathogenic factor. There are nine subtypes of B27 encoded by the B*2701–2708 alleles, all of which are associated with ankylosing spondylitis and have a 'B' pocket in their cleft which is very exclusive with respect to binding the arginine side chain. The hunt should be on for a nonapeptide with an arginine at residue 2. The involvement of infective agents may provide a clue. The cross-reaction of B27 with *Klebsiella pneumoniae* nitrogenase reported by Ebringer and colleagues is certainly provocative in this respect. One suggestion is that a bacterial peptide may cross-react with a B27-derived sequence and provoke an autoreactive T-cell response.

Deficiencies in C4 and C2, which are MHC class III molecules, clearly predispose to the development of **immune complex disease** (see p. 313) and so it would be expected that the inheritance of null genes or alleles coding for the less active complement allotypes would increase the risk of rheumatological disorders and add yet further complexity to the correlations between HLA types and disease.

Last, it is worthy of note that the relationship of MHC to disease resistance and vaccine efficacy in farm animals is beginning to preoccupy veterinary scientists; it is known for instance, that susceptibility to Marek's disease in White Leghorn chickens is associated with distinct MHC haplotypes.

## REPRODUCTIVE IMMUNOLOGY

### The fetus is a potential allograft

A further consequence of polymorphism in an outbred population is that mother and fetus will almost certainly have different MHCs. Some examples of selection for heterozygotes (where maternally and paternally derived haplotypes are different) over homozygotes (both fetal haplotypes identical with the mother's) in viviparous animals suggest that this is beneficial. Likewise, the placentae of F1 offspring are larger than normal when mothers are preimmunized to the paternal H-2 haplotype and smaller when mothers are tolerant to these antigens.

The threat posed to the fetus as a potential graft due to the possession of paternal transplantation antigens so intrigued Lewis Thomas that he was moved to suggest that rejection of the fetus might initiate parturition, although it would be difficult to account for the normal birth of female offspring to pure-strain mating pairs where fetus and mother would have identical histocompatibility antigens without further postulating a placenta-specific surface antigen.

Nonetheless, in the human hemochorial placenta, maternal blood with immunocompetent lymphocytes does circulate in contact with the fetal trophoblast and we have to explain how the fetus avoids allograft rejection, despite the development of an immunological response in a proportion of mothers as evidenced by the appearance of anti-HLA antibodies and cytotoxic lymphocytes. In fact, prior sensitization with a skin graft fails to affect a pregnancy, showing that trophoblast cells are immunologically protected and indeed they are resistant to most cytotoxic mechanisms although susceptible to IL-2-activated NK cells. Some of the many speculations which have been aired on this subject are summarized in figure 17.19.

Undoubtedly, the most important factor is the well-documented lack of both conventional class I and class II MHC antigens on the placental villous trophoblast which protects the fetus from allogeneic attack. These fundamental changes in the regulation of MHC genes also lead to the unique expression of the nonclassical HLA-G protein on the extravillous cytotrophoblast. This may protect the trophoblast from killing by uterine endometrial large granular lymphocytes which are an NK cell subset, since HLA-null lymphoblastoid cells transfected with HLA-G are resistant to NK lysis. This would be consistent with the 'missing self hypothesis' which postulates that MHC class I inhibits a positive signal from a potential target to the NK cell. On the other hand, the placenta is vulnerable to IL-2 activated uterine NK cells, which may therefore fine tune overaggressive invasion by the trophoblast early in pregnancy and may control the normal development of the blastocyst in the decidualized uterus, in contrast with the excessive trophoblast proliferation and tissue destruction produced by transfer of blastocysts to mouse kidney.

Maternal IgG antipaternal MHC is found in 20% of first pregnancies and this figure rises to 75–80% in multiparous women. Some of these antibodies cross-react with HLA-G but the vulnerability of the trophoblast cells to complement is blocked by the presence on their surface of the control proteins, decay accelerating factor (DAF) and membrane cofactor protein (MCP), which inactivate C3 convertase (cf. p. 313).

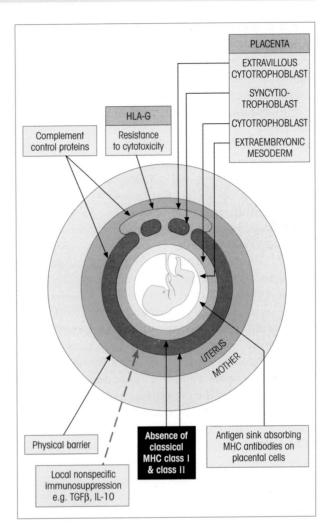

**Figure 17.19.** Mechanisms postulated to account for the survival of the fetus as an allograft in the mother.

Cytokines seem to have a complex role in postimplantation pregnancy given the production of growth factors such as CSF-1 and GM-CSF, which have a trophic influence on the placenta, and of transforming growth factor-β (TGFβ) which could help to damp down any activation of NK cells by potentially abortive events such as intrauterine exposure to lipopolysaccharide (LPS) or to interferons. The placenta itself produces IL-10, the importance of which was revealed by IL-10 'knock-out' experiments (cf. p. 144) which caused runting of the fetus compared with its littermate controls — incidentally this is a slick demonstration that IL-10 is synthesized by the embryo rather than the trophoblast.

## Fertility can be controlled immunologically

Notwithstanding the complacent attitudes of some members of the chattering classes, informed opinion recognizes the enormity of the problems posed by the world population explosion. That being so, a rich variety of strategic approaches are being followed, one of which involves the targeting of key hormones (figure 17.20a) by the production of neutralizing autoantibodies.

Immunization, actually autoimmunization, with diphtheria toxoid-linked **luteinizing hormone releasing hormone** (LHRH), which regulates gonadotropin synthesis, impairs fertility in male animals and causes a marked atrophy of the prostate accompanied by a devastating fall in testosterone levels — immunological castration no less. The therapy may have a role in androgen-dependent prostatic carcinoma, while in postpartum women it should prevent ovulation and prolong lactational amenorrhea without adverse effects. Internal image anti-idiotype Ab$_{2b}$ (cf. p. 208) has been raised against monoclonal antiprogesterone and shown to provoke **progesterone neutralizing antibodies** in experimental animals.

Most attention has focused on a human vaccine based on **human chorionic gonadotropin** (hCG) which is made by the preimplantation blastocyst and is essential for the establishment of early pregnancy (figure 17.20a); it is also the antigen assayed in the urine tests for pregnancy which cause so much plea-sure or consternation as the case may be. The α-chain of hCG is common to follicle-stimulating hormone (FSH), thyroid-stimulating hormone (TSH) and LH while the β-subunit shows around 80% homology with LH (figure 17.20b). Clearly immunization with whole hCG would elicit some exceedingly unwelcome reactions and two vaccines try to avoid them wholly or in part. Both couple the antigen to tetanus or diphtheria toxoid carriers. The WHO vaccine uses the 37-amino acid C-terminal peptide (CTP) which is wholly specific for hCG but not exciting as an immunogen. The Indian vaccine combines β-hCG with ovine α-chain. This evokes much better antibody responses and in Phase 2 clinical trials only one pregnancy was observed in 128 cycles when neutralizing antibodies were above a certain level. Despite strong cross-reactions with LH there was said to be no disturbance of ovulation or loss of libido. As contraceptive cover while antibodies were rising, cell-mediated hypersensitivity was induced by local intrauterine implantation of purified extracts from Neem, an ancient Indian tree. As antibody levels fall, fertility is regained. Long-term maintenance of adequate antibody titers should be possible with biodegradable microspheres or a recombinant *Salmonella* construct incorporating the β-hCG gene.

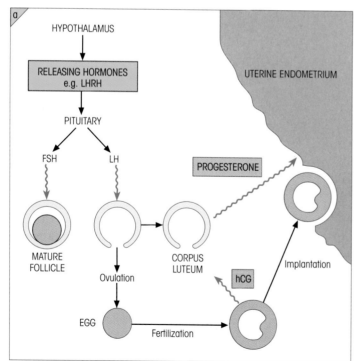
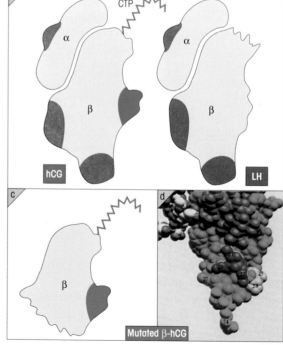

**Figure 17.20. Immunological contraception**. (a) Target hormones. (b) Purely diagrammatic representation of human chorionic gonadotropin (hCG) showing epitopes specific for hCG (green) and structures similar if not identical to luteinizing hormone (LH) (dark red). (c) β-hCG mutant in which the hCG-specific epitopes have been preserved but epitopes shared with LH lost. As a candidate vaccine this should avoid the problem of inducing antibodies cross-reacting with LH. (d) Structure of β-hCG showing some of the residues altered (magenta, yellow and cyan) to produce epitope-loss mutants, fulfilling the criteria in (c). (Reproduced from Jackson A.M. *et al.* (1996) *Journal of Reproductive Immunology* **31**, 21, with permission from Elsevier Science, Ireland Ltd.)

# SUMMARY

## Graft rejection is an immunological reaction

• It shows specificity, the second set response is brisk, it is mediated by lymphocytes, and antibodies specific for the graft are formed.

## Genetic control of transplantation antigens

• In each vertebrate species there is a major histocompatibility complex (MHC) which is responsible for provoking the most intense graft reactions.
• Parental MHC antigens are codominantly expressed on cell surfaces.

## Other consequences of MHC incompatibility

• Class II MHC molecules provoke a mixed lymphocyte reaction of proliferation and blast transformation when genetically dissimilar lymphocytes interact.
• Class II differences are largely responsible for the reaction of tolerated grafted lymphocytes against host antigen (graft vs host (g.v.h.) reaction).
• Siblings have a 1:4 chance of identity with respect to MHC.

## Mechanisms of graft rejection

• CD8 lymphocytes play a major role in the acute early rejection of first set responses.
• The strength of allograft rejection is due to the surprisingly large number of allospecific precursor cells. These derive mainly from the variety of T-cells which recognize allo-MHC plus self-peptides plus a small number which directly recognize the allo-MHC molecule itself; later rejection increasingly involves allogeneic peptides presented by self-MHC.
• Preformed antibodies cause hyperacute rejection within minutes.
• Acute late rejection of organ grafts from 11 days onwards is caused by Ig and C binding to graft vessels.
• Insidious and late rejection may be due to immune complex deposition.

## Prevention of graft rejection

• This can be minimized by cross-matching donor and graft for ABO and MHC tissue types. Individual MHC antigens are typed on lymphocytes using cytotoxic antisera. HLA-DR specificities can now be identified by the PCR.

• Rejection can be blocked by agents producing general immunosuppression such as antimitotic drugs (e.g. azathioprine), anti-inflammatory steroids and antilymphocyte monoclonals. Cyclosporin A, FK506 and rapamycin represent exciting new groups of T-cell specific drugs; complexes of cyclosporin and FK506 with their cellular ligands, block calcineurin, a phosphatase which activates the IL-2 transcription factor NFAT, while rapamycin complexes with the FK binding protein to block kinases involved in cell proliferation.
• Antigen-specific depression through tolerance induction can be achieved by injection of bone marrow or dendritic cell precursors into conditioned recipients.

## Xenografting

• Strategies are being developed to prevent hyperacute rejection of pig grafts in humans due to reaction of natural antibodies in the host with galactose epitopes on pig cells.

## Clinical experience in grafting

• Cornea and cartilage grafts are avascular and comparatively well tolerated.
• Kidney grafting gives excellent results and has been the most widespread, although immunosuppression must normally be continuous.
• High success rates are also being achieved with heart and liver transplants particularly helped by the use of cyclosporin.
• Bone marrow grafts for immunodeficiency and aplastic anemia are accepted from matched siblings but it is difficult to avoid g.v.h. disease with allogeneic marrow, although this can be reduced by purging CD8 T-cells in the graft and by cyclosporin treatment. Recombinant G-CSF and GM-CSF accelerate the return of myeloid cells after grafting.
• Experimental studies on transplantation of neural tissue and the production of prosthetic vascular grafts have been described.

## Association of HLA type with disease

• HLA specificities are often associated with particular diseases, e.g. HLA-B27 with ankylosing spondylitis, B8 with myasthenia gravis, DR3 with Sjögren's syndrome, DR4 with rheumatoid arthritis, DQ2 and 8 with insulin-dependent diabetes mellitus and DR2,DQ6 with multiple sclerosis.

(Continued on p. 378)

- The association may be related to an ability to bind particular antigenic peptides or to cross-react with certain infectious agents.

### The fetus as an allograft

- Differences between MHC of mother and fetus may be beneficial to the fetus but as a potential graft it must be protected against transplantation attack by the mother.
- A major defense mechanism is the lack of classical class I and II MHC antigens on syncytiotrophoblast and cytotrophoblast which form the outer layers of the placenta.
- The extravillous cytotrophoblast expresses a nonclassical nonpolymorphic MHC class I protein, HLA-G, which may act to inhibit cytotoxicity by maternal NK cells.

- Syncitio- and cytotrophoblasts bear surface DAF and MCP which break down C3 convertase and so block any complement-mediated damage.
- Local production of IL-10 and TGFβ may suppress unwanted reactions.

### Immunological contraception

- Autoimmunization against hormones such as LHRH, progesterone and hCG which play a key role in reproduction, can block fertility.
- The C-terminal peptide of β-hCG and a complex of human β-hCG with sheep α-chain has been used in human trials. If antibody titers are sufficiently high, prevention of pregnancy is close to 100%. As antibody levels fall, fertility is regained.

## FURTHER READING

Austen K.F., Burakoff S.J., Rosen F.S. & Strom T.B. (eds) (1996) *Therapeutic Immunology*. Blackwell Science, Oxford.

Bach F.H., Winkler H., Ferran C., Hancock W.W. & Robson S.C. (1996) Delayed xenograft rejection. *Immunology Today* **17**, 379.

Bodmer J.G., Marsh S.G., Albert E.D. *et al.* (1994) Nomenclature for factors of the HLA system. *Tissue Antigens* **44**, 1–8.

Borel J.F. *et al.* (1996) *In vivo* pharmacological effects of cyclosporin and some analogues. *Advances in Pharmacology* **35**, 115. (An in-depth review of the field by the discoverer of cyclosporin and his colleagues.)

Carosella E.D., Dausset J. & Kirszenbaum M. (1996) HLA-G revisited. *Immunology Today* **17**, 407.

Claman H.N. (1993) *The Immunology of Human Pregnancy*. Humana Press, Totowa, New Jersey. (Said in a review to give clinicians an easily readable, albeit superficial overview that will serve as a useful introduction.)

Lachmann P.J., Peters D.K., Rosen F.S. & Walport M.J. (eds) (1993) *Clinical Aspects of Immunology*, 5th edn, chapters on Transplantation, pp. 1687–1758. Blackwell Scientific Publications, Oxford.

Morris P.J. (ed.) (1994) *Kidney Transplantation: Principles and Practice*, 4th edn. W.B. Saunders Company, Philadelphia, USA.

Pazmanty L., Mandelboim O., Vales-Gomes M. *et al.* (1996) Protection from natural killer cell-mediated lysis by HLA-G expression on target cells. *Science* **274**, 792–793.

Rowe P. (1996) Xenotransplantation: from animal facility to the clinic. *Molecular Medicine* **2**, 10.

Sachs D.H. (ed.) (1996) Transplantation. *Current Opinion in Immunology* **8**, 671–728.

Sandberg P.R., Borlongan C.V., Saporta S. & Cameron D.F. (1996) Testis-derived Sertoli cells survive and provide localized immunoprotection for xenografts in rat brain. *Nature Biotechnology* **14**, 1692–1695.

Sriwatanawongsa V., Davies H.S. & Calne R.Y. (1995) The essential roles of parenchymal tissues and passenger leukocytes in the tolerance induced by liver grafting in rats. *Nature Medicine* **1**, 428–432.

Steptoe R.J. & Thomson A.W. (1996) Dendritic cells and tolerance. *Clinical Experimental Immunology* **105**, 397–402.

Talwar G.P. *et al.* (1992) Vaccines for control of fertility. In Gergely *et al.* (eds) *Progress in Immunology* **VIII**, pp. 849–856. Springer-Verlag, Budapest.

Thorsby E. (1995) HLA-associated disease susceptibility. *The Immunologist* **3**, 51.

Vince G.S. & Johnson P.M. (1996) Reproductive immunology: conception, contraception, and the consequences. *The Immunologist* **4(5)**, 172.

Wilson S.E. & Aston R. (1994) Overview: recent developments in macrolide immunosuppressants. *Expert Opinion on Therapeutic Patents* **4**, 1445. (Academics should be aware of the enormous amount of data in the patent literature.)

Yu Y.Y.L., Kumar V. & Bennet M. (1992) Murine NK cells and marrow graft rejection. *Annual Review of Immunology* **10**, 189–213. (Problems associated with engraftment.)

# CHAPTER 8

# TUMOR IMMUNOLOGY

## CONTENTS

For as long as I can recollect, immunologists have wanted to believe that they would be the chosen ones to knock the stuffing out of the cancer problem. The fortunes of tumor immunology have fluctuated widely, flavor of the month at one time, a subject fit only for no-hopers at another. It looks as though its time has come at last.

The ability to reject transplants of tissue may be traced back a long way down the evolutionary tree—back even as far as the annelid worms. Long before the studies on the involvement of self-major histocompatibility complex (MHC) in immunological responses, Lewis Thomas suggested that the allograft rejection mechanism represented a means by which the body's cells could be kept under **immunological surveillance** so that altered cells with a neoplastic potential could be identified and summarily eliminated. For this to operate, cancer cells must display some new discriminating surface structure which can be recognized by the immune system.

## CHANGES ON THE SURFACE OF TUMOR CELLS (Figure 18.1)

### Virally controlled antigens

A substantial minority of tumours arises through infection with **oncogenic viruses**, Epstein–Barr viruses (EBV) in lymphomas, human T-cell leukemia virus-1 (HTLV-1) in leukemia and papilloma virus in cervical cancers. After infection, the viruses express genes homologous with cellular oncogenes which encode factors affecting growth and cell division. Failure to control these genes therefore leads to potentially malignant transformation. Virally derived peptides associated with surface MHC on the surface of the tumor cell behave as powerful transplantation antigens which generate haplotype-specific cytotoxic T-cells (Tc). All tumors induced by a given virus should carry the same surface antigen, irrespective of their cellular origin, so that immunization with any one of these tumors would confer resistance to subsequent challenge with the others provided there were no artful mutations by the virus. Unfortunately viruses are not innately friendly.

### Expression of normally silent genes

The dysregulated uncontrolled cell division of the cancer cell creates a milieu in which the products of normally silent genes may be expressed. Sometimes these encode differentiation antigens normally associated with an earlier fetal stage. Thus tumors derived from the same cell type are often found to express such **oncofetal antigens** which are also present on embryonic cells. Examples would be α-fetoprotein in

hepatic carcinoma and carcino-embryonic antigen (CEA) in cancer of the intestine. Certain monoclonal antibodies also react with tumors of neural crest origin and fetal melanocytes. Another monoclonal antibody defines the SSEA-1 antigen found on a variety of human tumors and early mouse embryos but absent from adult cells with the exception of human granulocytes and monocytes.

But the exciting quantum leap forward stems from the original observation that cytosolic viral nucleoprotein could provide a target for Tc cells by appearing on the cell surface as a processed peptide associated with MHC class I (cf. p. 95). This established the general principle that the intracellular proteins which are not destined to be positioned in the surface plasma membrane can still signal their presence to T-cells in the outer world by the processed peptide/MHC mechanism. Cytotoxic T-cells specific for tumor cells obtained from mixed cultures of peripheral blood cells with tumor, can be used to establish the identity of the antigen using the strategy described in figure 18.2. By something of a *tour de force* a gene encoding a melanoma antigen, MAGE-1, was identified. It belongs to a family of 12 genes, six of which are expressed in a significant proportion of melanomas as well as head and neck tumors, non-small cell lung cancers and bladder carcinomas. MAGE-1 is *not* expressed in normal tissues except for germ-line cells in testis and gives rise to antigenic T-cell epitopes which in light of the absence of class I MHC on the testis cells, must be considered tumor-specific. This exciting research reveals the tumor-specific antigen as an expression of a normally silent gene.

### Mutant antigens

The seminal work on tum- mutants (see Milestone 18.1) has persuaded us that single point mutations in oncogenes can account for the large diversity of antigens found on carcinogen-induced tumors. The gene encoding the p53 cell cycle inhibitor is a hot spot for mutation in cancer, while the oncogenic human *ras* genes differ from their normal counterpart by point mutations usually leading to single amino acid substitutions in positions 12, 13 or 61. Such mutations have been recorded in 40% of human colorectal cancers and their preneoplastic lesions, in more than 90% of pancreatic carcinomas, in acute myelogenous leukemia and in preleukemic syndromes. The mutated *ras* peptide can induce proliferative T-cell lines *in vitro*. Tumors produced by UV light produce individual Tc cells not reacting with other tumors or normal cells

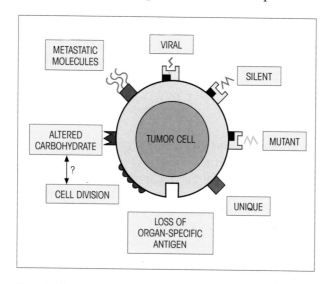

**Figure 18.1. Tumor-associated surface changes.**

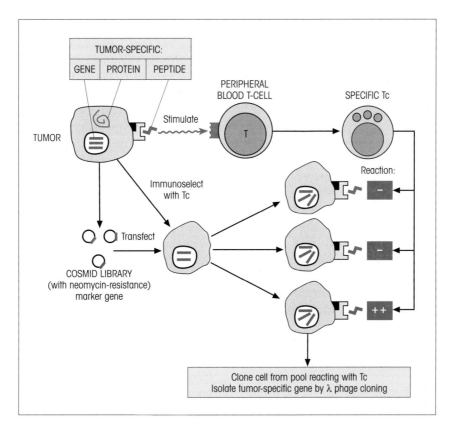

**Figure 18.2. Identification of tumor-specific gene using tumor-specific cytotoxic T-cell (Tc) clones derived from mixed tumor–lymphocyte culture.** A cosmid library incorporating the tumor DNA is transfected into an antigen-negative cell line derived from the wild-type tumor by immunoselection with the Tc. Small pools of transfected cells are tested against the Tc. A positive pool is cloned by limiting dilution and the tumor-specific gene (*MAGE-1*) cloned from the antigen-positive well(s). (Based on van der Bruggen P., Tra-versari C., Chomez P., Lurquin C., de Plaen E., van den Eynde B., Knuth A. & Boon T. (1991) A gene encoding an antigen recognized by cytolytic T lymphocytes on a human melanoma. *Science* **254**, 1643. Copyright 1991 by the AAAS.) The original MAGE-1 belongs to a family of 12 genes. A further two melanoma-specific gene families, BAGE and GAGE, have been discovered and like the MAGE cluster are silent in normal tissues except testis, but are expressed in several tumor types.

and it would be surprising if this were not a further example of tumor-specific mutant peptide antigenicity.

## Changes in carbohydrate structure

The chaotic internal control of metabolism within neoplastic cells often leads to the presentation of abnormal surface carbohydrate structures. Sometimes one sees blocked synthesis, e.g. deletion of blood group A. In other cases there may be enhanced synthesis of structures absent in progenitor cells: thus some gastrointestinal cancers express the Lewis Le^a antigen in individuals who are Le(a−,b−) and others produce extended chains bearing dimeric Le^a or Le(a,b).

Abnormal mucin synthesis can have immunological consequences. Consider the mucins of pancreatic and breast tissue. These consist of a polypeptide core of 20 amino acid tandem repeats with truly abundant O-linked carbohydrate chains. A monoclonal anti-body SM-3 directed to the core polypeptide reacts poorly with normal tissue where the epitope is masked by glycosylation but well with breast and pancreatic carcinomas possessing shorter and fewer O-linked chains. Tc cells specific for tumor mucins are not MHC restricted and the slightly heretical suggestion has been made that the T-cell receptors (TCRs) are binding multivalently to closely spaced SM-3 epitopes on unprocessed mucins; alternatively, and closer to the party line, recognition is by γδ cells.

## Changes on the surface of cycling cells

In some instances it is possible that the changes which occur in the carbohydrate moiety of tumor surface membrane glycoproteins are a natural consequence of cell division. For example, Thomas found that the density of surface sugar determinants cross-reacting with blood group H fell as murine mastocytoma cells moved into the G1 phase of the division cycle, while, reciprocally, group B determinants increased. Surface components binding the lectin, wheat-germ agglutinin are poorly represented on resting T- and B-cells, but within 24 hours of stimulation by lymphocyte polyclonal activators and before DNA synthesis begins, high concentrations of lectin binding sites appear on the surface.

Unusual events may be observed in active cells associated with tumor growth and spread. For example, the 95 kDa surface glycoprotein, F19, is expressed in sarcomas and the **reactive stromal fibroblasts** in more than 90% of carcinomas of the colon, breast, lung and pancreas, making them a novel target for immunological attack since normal adult tissues and benign epithelial tumors express zero or very low levels. In like vein, the highly sialylated cell surface glycoprotein endosialin (FB5) is present in the vasculature of a significant proportion of malignant tumors but not in blood vessels of normal tissues.

## Molecules related to metastatic potential

Changes in surface carbohydrates can have a dramatic effect on malignancy. For example, colonic cancers expressing sialyl Lewis$^x$ have a poor prognosis and higher propensity to metastasize. Lung cancer patients whose tumors showed deletion of blood group A had a much worse prognosis than those with continuous A expression (figure 18.3); the finding that

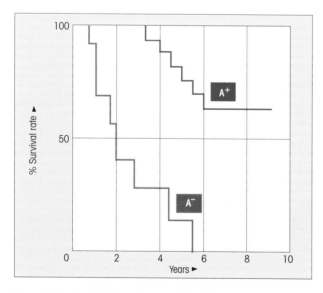

**Figure 18.3.  Survival of lung tumor patients with and without expression of the blood group A antigen**. (From Lee J.S., Ro J.Y., Sahin A.A., Hong H.W., Brown B.W., Mountain C.F. & Hittelman W.N. (1991) Expression of blood group antigen A—a favorable prognostic factor in non-small-cell lung cancer. *New England Journal of Medicine* **324**, 1084–1090.)

patients expressing H/Le$^y$/Le$^b$ also had a poorer prognosis than antigen-negative subjects is consistent with this observation.

The role of **CD44** (HERMES/Pgp-1; cf. p. 152) in cell trafficking based on its interaction with vascular endothelium has afforded it some prominence in the facilitation of metastatic spread. CD44 occurs in several isoforms with a varying number of exons between the transmembrane and common N-terminus. Normal epithelium expresses the CD44H isoform with hyaluran binding domains, but lacking the intervening v1–v10 exons; expression of certain of these exons on tumors is indicative of a growth advantage, since it is present with higher frequency on more advanced cancers. Stable transfection of a nonmetastatic tumor with a CD44 cDNA clone encompassing exons v6 and v7 induced the ability to form metastatic tumors — a most striking effect. Further, injection of a monoclonal anti-CD44 v6 prevented the formation of lymph node metastases. Exons v6 and v10 have now been shown to bind blood group H and chondroitin 4-sulfate respectively and the latest hypothesis is that these carbohydrates can bind to CD44H on endothelium and thence homotypically to each other so generating a metastatic nidus.

Changes have quite frequently been observed in the expression of class I MHC molecules. For example, oncogenic transformation of cells infected with adenovirus 12 is associated with highly reduced class I as a consequence of very low levels of Tap-1 and -2 mRNA. Mutation frequently leads to diminished or absent class I expression linked in most cases to increased metastatic potential, presumably reflecting their decreased vulnerability to T-cells but not NK cells. In breast cancer, for example, around 60% of metastatic tumors lack class I.

## Unique (idiotypic) determinants

The occurrence of single point mutations in oncogenic proteins such as ras and p53 endows each tumor with a potential T-cell epitope specificity which will tend to be as characteristic of the individual tumor as the mutation itself.

An unequivocal example of a truly unique tumor-specific antigen is provided by the immunoglobulin (Ig) idiotype on the surface of chronic lymphocytic leukemic cells which represent an expansion of individual B-cell clones whose differentiation has been arrested by neoplastic transformation. There will be no dispute about the idiotypic B-cell epitopes on the native Ig receptor but what is less obvious is the potential for processed Ig peptides to act as unique T-cell epitopes.

The seemingly unique T-cell antigens displayed by chemically induced tumors (Milestone 18.1) are peptides derived from a glycoprotein gp110 presented on heat-shock protein gp96. Heat-shock proteins (hsp)

never fail to surprise and hsp gp96 isolated from tumor cells and injected into mice generates systemic tumor-specific immunity. Whether the individuality of each different tumor antigen results from mutations in the gp110, or a natural polymorphism, remains to be seen.

## Milestone 18.1—Tumors Can Induce Immune Responses

The first convincing evidence for tumor-associated antigens comes from the work of Prehn and Main who demonstrated quite clearly that **chemically induced cancers** can induce immune responses to themselves but not to other tumors produced by the same carcinogen (figure M18.1.1a). Tumors induced by **oncogenic viruses** are different in that processed viral peptides are present on the surface of all neoplastic cells bearing the viral genome so that Tc cells raised to one tumor will cross-react with all others produced by the same virus (figure M18.1.1b).

Dramatic advances were made by Boon and colleagues. First they showed that random mutagenesis of transplantable tumors, i.e. tumors which can be passaged

within a pure mouse strain without provoking rejection, can give rise to mutant progeny with strong transplantation antigens. As a result they could not be grown in syngeneic animals with a normal immune system; accordingly they were referred to as **tum-** variants. Boon's team developed a powerful technology (cf. figure 18.2) which enabled them to use Tc clones specific for the tum- variant, to screen cosmid clones for the mutant gene. These two breakthroughs, the recognition that mutation in tumors can generate strong transplantation reactions, and development of the technique for identifying the relevant antigens with Tc cells, herald really profound developments in tumor immunology and put it firmly on the map as a key area for cancer research.

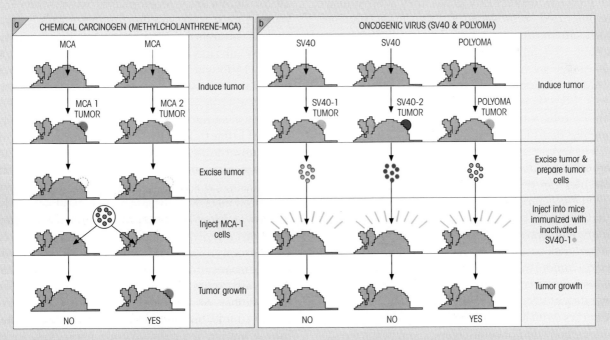

**Figure M18.1.1.** The specificity of immunity induced by tumors. (a) A chemically induced tumor MCA-1 can induce resistance to an implant of itself but not to a tumor produced in a syngeneic mouse by the same carcinogen. Thus each tumor has an individual antigen. (b) Tumors produced by a given oncogenic virus immunize against tumors produced in syngeneic mice by the same but not other viruses. Thus tumors produced by an oncogenic virus share a common antigen.

## IMMUNE RESPONSE TO TUMORS

### Immune surveillance against strongly immunogenic tumors

When present, many of these antigens can provoke immune responses in experimental animals which lead to resistance against tumor growth but they vary tremendously in their efficiency. Powerful antigens associated with tumors induced by oncogenic viruses or ultraviolet light generate strong resistance, while the transplantation antigens on chemically induced tumors (Milestone 18.1) are weaker and somewhat variable; disappointingly, tumors which arise spontaneously in animals produce little or no response. The **immune surveillance theory** would predict that there should be more tumors in individuals whose immune systems are suppressed. This undoubtedly seems to be the case for **strongly immunogenic tumors**. There is a considerable increase in skin cancer in immunosuppressed patients living in high sunshine regions north of Brisbane and, in general, transplant patients on immunosuppressive drugs are unduly susceptible to skin cancers, largely associated with papilloma virus, and EBV-positive lymphomas. Likewise, the lymphomas which arise in children with T-cell deficiency linked to Wiskott–Aldrich syndrome or ataxia telangiectasia, express EBV genes; they show unusually restricted expression of EBV latent proteins which are the major potential target epitopes for immune recognition, while cellular adhesion molecules such as intercellular adhesion molecule-1 (ICAM-1) and lymphocyte function associated molecule-3 (LFA-3), which mediate conjugate formation with Tc cells, cannot be detected on their surface. Knowing that most normal individuals have highly efficient EBV-specific Tc cells, this must be telling us that only by downregulating appropriate surface molecules can the lymphoma cells escape even the limited T-cell surveillance operating in these patients. Mutations in the oncogenic virus itself can increase its tumorigenic potential. Thus the frequent association of a high risk variant of human papilloma virus with cervical tumors in HLA-B7 individuals is attributed to the loss of a T-cell epitope which would otherwise generate a protective B7-mediated cytolytic response.

Cancers which express neoantigens of low immunogenicity do not come creeping out of the woodwork when patients are radically immunosuppressed and, although T-cell responses can often be rescued from tumor-infiltrating lymphocytes or peripheral blood, they may be functionally deficient due to suppression by local IL-10. This line of reasoning leads one to reinterpret a 30-year-old 'discriminant function' test which held that a low ratio of urinary androgen to glucocorticoids was a marker for women who subsequently developed breast cancer. In the current intellectual climate, since the adrenal androgen dehydroepiandrosterone (DHA) and its sulfate (cf. figure 11.22) encourage activity of TH1 cells, decreased production of the androgen would be associated with a bias towards TH2 responses which may be inappropriate for the control of a neoplasm.

Mutation of p53 and its overexpression are very common events in human cancer and is often associated with production of antibodies; but while these could prove to have a diagnostic utility, it is most unlikely that they are of benefit to the patient. Reluctantly, one has to accept the view that with tumors of weak immunogenicity, we are dealing with low-key reactions which clearly play little role in curbing the neoplastic process. That is not to say that these 'weak' antigens cannot be exploited for therapeutic purposes as we shall soon see.

### A role for innate immunity?

Perhaps in speaking of immunity to tumors, one too readily thinks only in terms of acquired responses, whereas it is now accepted that innate mechanisms are of significance. Macrophages which often infiltrate a tumor mass, can destroy tumor cells in tissue culture through the copious production of reactive oxygen intermediates (ROI) and tumour necrosis factor (TNF) when activated by a diversity of factors, bacterial lipopolysaccharide, double-stranded RNA, T-cell γ-interferon (IFNγ) and so forth.

There is an uncommon flurry of serious interest in **natural killer (NK)** cells. It is generally accepted that they subserve a function as the earliest cellular effector mechanism against dissemination of blood-borne metastases. Let's look at the evidence. Patients with advanced metastatic disease often have abnormal NK activity and low levels appear to predict subsequent metastases. In experimental animals, removal of NK cells from mice with surgically resected B16 melanoma resulted in uncontrolled metastatic disease and death. Acute ethanol intoxication in rats boosted the number of metastases from an NK-sensitive tumor 10-fold but had no effect on an NK-resistant cancer, hinting at a possible underlying cause for the association between alcoholism, infectious disease and malignancies. (Those who enjoy the odd Bacchanalian splurge should not be too upset—be comforted by the beneficial effect in heart disease, but no excesses please!) Powerful evidence implicating these cells in protection against cancer is provided by beige mice which congenitally lack NK cells. They die with spontaneous tumors earlier than their nondeficient +/bg littermates and the incidence of radiation-induced leukemia is reduced by prior injection of cloned isogeneic NK cells which could be suppressing preleukemic cells. Note however that tumors induced chemically or with murine leukemia virus were handled normally.

Resting NK cells are spontaneously cytolytic for certain, but by no means all, tumor targets; IL-2-activated cells display a wider lethality. Recognition involves two types of receptor: NKR-P1 receptors sense the surface structures, probably carbohydrate(?), characteristic of the tumor, while a second set of p58 molecules belonging to the human Ig superfamily, bind to supertypic public specificities on MHC class I. I mentioned earlier, and must emphasize again, recognition of class I imparts a **negative inactivating** signal to the NK cell implying conversely that downregulation of MHC class I, which tumors employ as a strategy to escape Tc cells, would make them **more susceptible to NK attack**.

Divisions are surfacing in the NK ranks. The NK cells, which remarkably constitute up to 50% of the liver-associated lymphocytes in man, have a higher level of expression of IL-2 receptor and adhesion molecules such as integrins compared with NK cells in peripheral blood. They are precursors of a subset of activated adherent NK cells (A-NK) which adhere rapidly to solid surfaces under the influence of IL-2 and are distinguished from their nonadherent counterparts by their superiority in entering solid tumors and in prolonging survival following adoptive transfer with IL-2 into animal models of tumor growth or metastasis. The nonadherent NK variety are better at killing antibody-coated cancer cells through antibody-dependent cell-mediated cytotoxicity (ADCC), mediated by their CD16 FcγRIII receptor.

Be kind to your NK cells. Really late nights which involve major curtailment of slow-wave sleep, lead to drastic falls in NK cells and levels of IL-2, quite apart from bleary eyes.

## UNREGULATED DEVELOPMENT GIVES RISE TO LYMPHOPROLIFERATIVE DISORDERS

We should now turn our attention to the manner in which cells involved in immune responses themselves may undergo malignant transformation, giving rise to leukemia, lymphoma or myeloma characterized by uncontrolled proliferation. An obvious example is the subset of adult human T-cell leukemia associated with **HTLV1** (human T-cell lymphotropic virus type 1). After infection of the T-cell, the viral tax protein which is constitutively expressed, stimulates transcription of IL-2, IL-2R etc., leading to vigorous proliferation; however, only if there is a subsequent chromosome abnormality (see below) does malignant transformation take place.

### Deregulation of protooncogenes is a characteristic feature of many lymphocytic tumors

The realization that viral oncogenes are almost certainly derived from normal host genes concerned in the regulation of cellular proliferation, has led to the identification of many of these so-called protooncogenes. One of them, c-*myc*, appears to be of crucial importance for entry of the lymphocyte, and probably many other cells, from the resting G0 stage to the cell cycle (cf. figure 10.1), while shutdown of c-*myc* expression is linked to exit from the cycle and return to G0. Thus deregulation of c-*myc* expression will prevent cells from leaving the cycle and consign them to a fate of continuous replication. This is just what is seen in many of the neoplastic B-lymphoproliferative disorders, where the malignant cells express high levels of c-*myc* protein usually associated with a reciprocal chromosomal translocation involving the c-*myc* locus. For example, Burkitt's lymphoma is a B-cell neoplasia with a relatively high incidence among African children in whom there is an association with the EBV; in most cases studied, the c-*myc* gene located on chromosome 8 band q24 is joined by a reciprocal translocation event to the μ-heavy chain gene on chromosome 14 band q32 (figure 18.4). It is suggested that the normal mechanisms which downregulate c-*myc* can no longer work on the translocated gene and so the cell is held in the cycling mode. Less frequently, c-*myc* translocates to the site of the κ (chromosome 2) or λ (chromosome 22) loci.

### Chromosome translocations are common in lymphoproliferative disorders

Most lymphomas and leukemias have visible chromosome abnormalities bound up with translocations to B-cell immunoglobulin or T-cell receptor gene loci but not necessarily involving c-*myc*. A reciprocal translocation between the μ-chain gene on chromosome 14 and the *bcl*-2 oncogene on chromosome 18 has been identified in almost all follicular B-cell lymphoma, and another between the T-cell gene on chromosome 14 (q11) and another presumed oncogene on

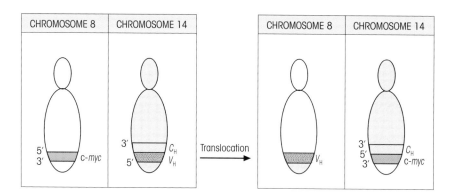

**Figure 18.4.** Translocation of the c-*myc* gene to the μ-chain locus in Burkitt's lymphoma.

chromosome 11 in a T-cell acute lymphoblastic leukemia (T ALL).

Lymphomagenesis is a multistep process. The lack of proliferative control engendered by deregulation of c-*myc* and other similar events induced by chromosomal translocations is permissive for the vulnerability to induction of neoplasia but is not in itself sufficient to bring about malignant transformation. Thus, transgenic mice harboring a c-*myc* gene driven by the μ-heavy chain enhancer ($E_\mu$-*myc* mice) have hyperplastic expansions of the pre-B-cell population in the bone marrow and spleen during the preneoplastic period and yet do not develop tumors until 6–8 weeks of age and then they are monoclonal not polyclonal, suggesting that a random second event is required before autonomy is achieved. Indeed, if the $E_\mu$-*myc* transgenic mice are now infected with viruses carrying the v-*raf* oncogene, they rapidly develop lymphomas. It is generally thought that whereas factors like c-myc can make a cell competent for mitosis, it is only the additional upregulation of **cell cycle progression genes** like *fos*, *jun* and *myb* or the loss of **cell cycle suppressor gene products** like p53 which allow cell division to occur. Deregulation of two such events may synergize in the process of malignant transformation and the associated unfettered cell proliferation.

Transgenic mice with a susceptibility to the development of cancer may be exploited to supplement the Ames' test for potential carcinogens. Conversely, mice with disrupted *p53* which develop tumors very smartly are ideal for studying treatments which might impede tumorigenesis. The protective effect of caloric restriction on neoplastic change was admirably confirmed in this system.

## Different lymphoid malignancies show maturation arrest at characteristic stages in differentiation

Lymphoid cells at almost any stage in their differenti-

ation or maturation may become malignant and proliferate to form a clone of cells which are virtually 'frozen' at a particular developmental stage because of defects in maturation. The malignant cells bear the markers one would expect of normal lymphocytes reaching the stage at which maturation had been arrested. Thus, chronic lymphocytic leukemia cells resemble mature B-cells in expressing surface class II and Ig, albeit of a single idiotype in a given patient. Using monoclonal antibodies directed against the terminal deoxynucleotidyl transferase (see figure 18.6a), class II MHC, Ig and specific antigens on cortical thymocytes, mature T-cells and non-T, non-B acute lymphoblastic leukemia cells, it has been possible to classify the lymphoid malignancies in terms of the phenotype of the equivalent normal cell (figure 18.5).

Susceptibility to malignant transformation is high in lymphocytes at an early stage in ontogeny. If we look at Burkitt's lymphoma, the EBV-induced translocation of the c-*myc* to bring it under control of the *IgH* gene complex is most likely to occur at the pro-B-cell stage since the chromatin structure of the Ig locus opens up for transcription as signaled by the appearance of sterile $C_\mu$ transcripts. Furthermore, the cell is likely to escape immunological recognition because in its undifferentiated resting form it has downregulated its EBV-encoded antigens and MHC class I polymorphic specificities, and the adhesion molecules LFA-1, LFA-3 and ICAM-1, as mentioned above.

At one time it was thought that maturation arrest occurred at the stage when the cell first became malignant, but we now know that the tumor cells can be forced into differentiation by agents such as phorbol myristate acetate and the current view is that cells may undergo a few differentiation steps after malignant transformation before coming to a halt. The demonstration of a myeloma protein idiotype on the cytoplasmic μ-chains of pre-B-cells in the same patient certainly favors the idea that the malignant event had occurred in a pre-B-cell whose progeny formed the plasma cell tumor. However, an alternative explanation could be transfection of normal pre-B-cells by an oncogene complex from the myeloma cells, possibly through a viral vector. With the exciting discovery of retroviruses associated with certain human T-cell leukemias, this is an interesting possibility.

## Immunohistological diagnosis of lymphoid neoplasias

With the availability of a range of monoclonal antibodies and improvements in immuno-enzymic technology, great strides have been made in exploiting, for diagnostic purposes, the fact that malignant lymphoid cells display the markers of the normal lymphocytes which are their counterpart.

### Leukemias

This point can be made rather well if one looks at the markers used to distinguish between the various types of leukemia (table 18.1). Whereas T ALL and B ALL cases have a poor prognosis, the patients positive for the common acute lymphoblastic leukemia

Table 18.1. Classification of lymphocytic leukemia by immuno-enzymatic staining.

| Lymphocyte marker | Common ALL | Pre-B ALL | B-cell ALL | T-cell ALL | Chronic lymphocytic leukemia |
|---|---|---|---|---|---|
| *CALLA (CDIO) | + | + | – | – | – |
| Cytoplasmic μ | – | + | – | – | – |
| Surface μ | – | – | + | – | + |
| Surface κ + λ | – | – | – | – | – |
| Pan-B | – | + | + | – | + |
| TdT | + | + | – | + | – |
| CD5 | – | – | – | + | + |
| CD2 | – | – | – | + | – |
| HLA-DR | + | + | + | – | + |

* Antigen-specific for lymphoid precursor cells and pre-B-cells.

antigen (CALLA; figure 18.6b), who include most childhood leukemias, belong to a prognostically favorable group, many of whom are curable with standard therapeutic combinations of vincristine, prednisone and L-asparaginase. Bone marrow transplantation may help in the management of patients with recurrent ALL provided a remission can first be achieved.

Earlier results suggesting that expression of the lymphoid lineage markers CD2 and CD19 on leukemic blasts predicted a poor outcome in childhood acute myeloid leukemia have been called into question but they are indicators of a good prognosis in adults with the disease.

Chronic lymphocytic leukemia is uncommon in people under 50 and is usually relatively benign, although the 10–20% of patients with a circulating monoclonal Ig have a bad prognosis. Excessive numbers of CLL small lymphocytes are found in the blood (figure 18.6c–e) and, being derived from a single clone, they can be stained only with anti-κ or anti-λ. Their weak expression of CD5 strongly suggests that they may be derived from the equivalent of the Ly1 (CD5) B-cell population in the mouse, especially since they can be encouraged to make the IgM polyspecific autoantibodies typical of this subset, if pushed by phorbol ester stimulation.

### Lymphomas

The extensive use of markers has greatly helped in the diagnosis of non-Hodgkin lymphomas. In the first place, the sometimes difficult distinction between a lymphoproliferative condition and carcinoma can be

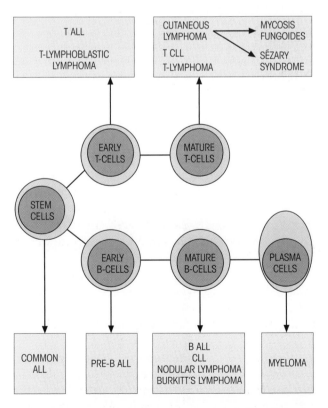

**Figure 18.5. Cellular phenotype of human lymphoid malignancies.** ALL=acute lymphoblastic leukemia; CLL=chronic lymphocytic leukemia. (After Greaves M.F. & Janossy G, personal communication.)

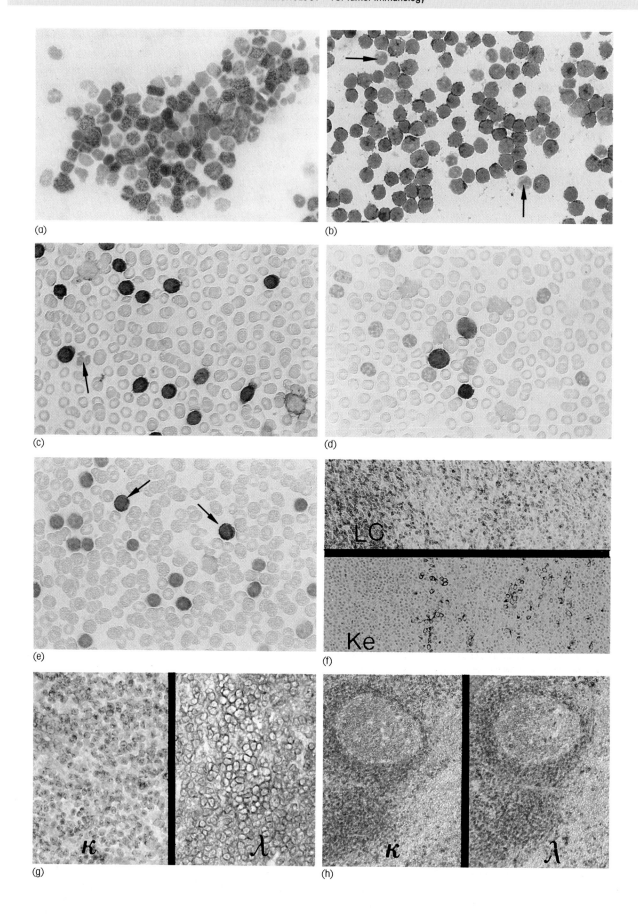

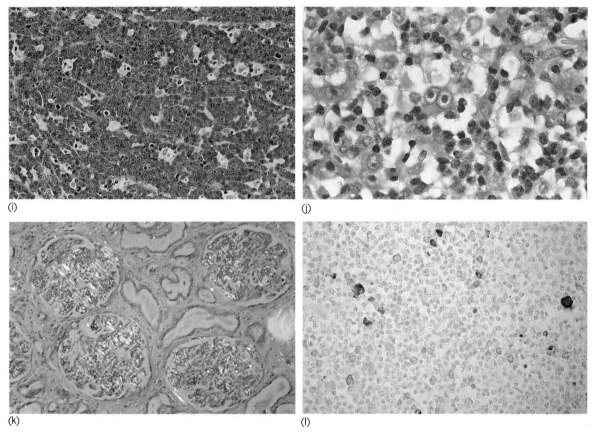

(i)
(j)
(k)
(l)

**Figure 18.6. Immunodiagnosis of lymphoproliferative disorders**. (a) Cytocentrifuged blast cells from a case of acute lymphoblastic leukemia stained by anti-terminal deoxynucleotidyl transferase (TdT) using an immuno-alkaline phosphatase method (cells treated first with mouse monoclonal anti-TdT, then anti-mouse Ig and finally with an immune complex of mouse anti-alkaline phosphatase + alkaline phosphatase before developing the enzymic reddish-purple color reaction). Many strongly stained blast cells are seen together with unlabeled normal marrow cells. (b) Immuno-alkaline phosphatase staining of bone marrow cells from a case of acute lymphoblastic leukemia, using monoclonal antibody specific for the common-acute lymphoblastic leukemia antigen (anti-CALLA; antibody J5). The majority of cells are strongly labeled. Two nonreactive cells are indicated by arrows. (c, d, e) Immuno-alkaline phosphatase labeling of blood smears from a case of chronic lymphocytic leukemia with three monoclonal antibodies (anti-HLA-DR, anti-CD3 antigen, and anti-CD1 antigen); (c) HLA-DR antigen is present on all the leukemic cells seen, but absent from a polymorph (arrowed); (d) three normal T-cells are labeled for the CD3 antigen, but the leukemic cells are negative; (e) CD1 antigen is strongly expressed on two normal lymphocytes (arrowed), but also weakly expressed on the chronic lymphocytic leukemia (CLL) cells. This pattern is typical of CLL. (f) A case of gastric carcinoma (stained at the bottom using anticytokeratin, Ke) with a heavy lymphocytic infiltrate (top, stained with antileukocyte common antigen, LC). (g) Diffuse follicle center type B-cell lymphoma showing λ light chain restriction; compare with (h) a reactive lymph node staining for both κ and λ light chains. (i) Burkitt's lymphoma showing 'starry sky' appearance. (j) Hodgkin's disease showing mixed cellularity and characteristic binucleate Reed–Sternberg cell with massive prominent nucleoli in the center of the figure. (k) Amyloid deposits in kidney glomeruli visualized by Congo Red staining under polarized light. (l) A case of malignant lymphoma associated with macroglobulinemia, showing lymphoplasmacytoid cells stained by the brown immunoperoxidase reaction for cytoplasmic IgM.

((a)–(e) Very kindly provided by Dr D. Mason, and (f)–(l) by Professor P. Isaacson.)

made with ease by using monoclonal antibodies to the leukocyte common antigen which will react with all lymphoid cells, whether in paraffin or cryostat sections, and antibodies to cytokeratin which recognize most carcinomas (figure 18.6f). Second, the cell of origin of the lymphoma can be ascertained by panels of monoclonals which differentiate the cellular elements which form normal lymphoid tissue (table 18.2).

The majority of non-Hodgkin lymphomas are of B-cell origin and the feature which gives the game away to the diagnostic immunohistologist is the synthesis of monotypic Ig, i.e. of one light chain only (figure 18.6g); in contrast, the population of cells at a site of reactive B-cell hyperplasia will stain for both κ and λ chains (figure 18.6h).

Follicle center cell lymphomas (figure 18.6g) imitating the reactive germinal center account for over 50% of the B-lymphomas. They exhibit monotypic surface Ig and the larger centrocytes and centroblasts which make up two-thirds of the cases contain cytoplasmic Ig. They stain for MHC class II and weakly for CALLA (cf. table 18.2). Morphologically similar cells make up tumors variously labeled 'mantle zone

| Marker | Follicle center cells | Mantle zone cells | Plasma cells | T-cells | Macrophages | Interdigit-ating cells (T-cell area) | Follicular dendritic cells |
|---|---|---|---|---|---|---|---|
| Cytoplasmic Ig | ± | – | + | – | – | – | – |
| J chain | ± | – | ± | – | – | – | – |
| Leukocyte common antigen (LCA) | + | + | + | + | + | + | ? |
| HLA-DR | + | + | – | – | ± | + | ? |
| CALLA | + | – | – | – | – | – | – |
| Lysozyme | – | – | – | – | + | – | – |
| α1-Antitrypsin | – | – | – | – | + | – | – |
| S-100 | – | – | – | – | – | + | – |
| Surface Ig | + | + | – | – | – | – | – |
| T-cell | – | – | – | + | – | ± | – |
| Pan B-cell | + | + | ± | – | – | – | – |
| C3b receptor | – | ± | – | – | – | – | + |

Table 18.2. Immunohistochemical markers of normal lymphoid tissue. (From Isaacson P.G. & Wright D.H. (1986) In Polak J.M. & van Noorden S. (eds) *Immunochemistry: Modern Methods and Applications*, 2nd edn. Wright, Bristol, with permission.)

lymphoma' or 'small cleaved cell lymphoma' but differ from follicle center cells in positive surface staining for IgM *and* IgD, and CD5 and negativity for CALLA. Burkitt lymphoma lymphoblastoid cells (figure 18.6i) exhibit the common ALL antigen and surface IgM.

The overall prognosis for patients with non-Hodgkin lymphoma is poor, even though improved by combined chemotherapy. Transplanted patients are 35 times more likely to develop lymphoma than normals, and there are indications that this cannot necessarily be attributed to the long-term immuno-suppression.

Hodgkin's disease attacks the gross architecture of lymphoid tissue and is characterized by the binucle-ate giant cells known as Reed–Sternberg cells (figure 18.6j) which appear to have a germinal center B-cell lineage. Therapy depends upon the stage of the disease; patients with disease localized to lymphoid tissue above the diaphragm respond well to radio-therapy, while those with more widespread disease are treated more aggressively.

## Plasma cell dyscrasias

### Multiple myeloma

This is defined as a malignant proliferation of a clone of plasma cells in the bone marrow secreting a mono-clonal Ig. The myeloma or 'M' component in serum is recognized as a tight band on paper electrophoresis (figure 18.7) as all molecules in the clone are of course identical and have the same mobility. Since Ig-secreting cells produce an excess of light chains, free

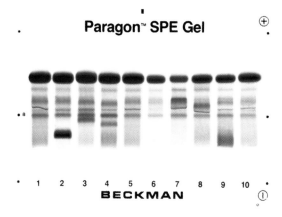

Figure 18.7. Myeloma paraprotein demonstrated by gel electrophoresis of serum. Lane 1, normal; lane 2, γ-paraprotein; lane 3, near β-paraprotein; lane 4, fibrinogen band in the γ-region of a *plasma* sample; lane 5, normal serum; lane 6, immunoglobulin deficiency (low γ); lane 7, nephrotic syndrome (raised $\alpha_2$-macroglobulin, low albumin and Igs); lane 8, hemolysed sample (raised hemoglobin/haptoglobin in $\alpha_2$ region); lane 9, polyclonal increase in Igs (e.g. infection, autoimmune disease); lane 10, normal serum. (Gel kindly provided by Mr. A. Heys.)

light chains are present in the plasma of multiple myeloma patients, and can be recognized in the urine as Bence-Jones protein (cf. figure 16.18) and give rise to amyloid deposits (see below). The characteristic 'punched out' osteolytic lesions in bones are thought to be due to release of osteoclastic factors such as IL-6 by the abnormal plasma cells in the marrow. If untreated, the disease is rapidly progressive. With chemotherapy, the mean survival time from diagnosis is now about 5 years.

'M' bands have been found in the sera of a number of individuals who have no clinical signs of myeloma; the comparative rarity with which invasive multiple myeloma develops in these people and the constant level of the monoclonal protein over a period of years suggests the presence of benign tumors of the lymphocyte-plasma cell series.

*Amyloid.* Between 10% and 20% of patients with myeloma develop widespread amyloid deposits which contain the variable region of the myeloma light chain. Being identical, the variable region fragments polymerize and form the characteristic amyloid fibrils which are recognizable by their birefringence on staining with Congo Red (figure 18.6k). Other components in amyloid have not yet been characterized. The fibrils are relatively resistant to digestion and accumulate in the ground substance of connective tissue where they can lead to pathological changes in the kidneys, heart and brain. Amyloid can also be formed secondarily to chronic inflammatory conditions such as rheumatoid arthritis and familial Mediterranean fever, but in this case involves the polymerization of a unique substance, Amyloid A (AA) protein derived from the N-terminal part of a serum precursor (SAA) of molecular weight 90 kDa. SAA behaves as an acute phase protein in that its concentration increases rapidly in response to tissue injury or inflammation. Levels rise with age and the minority of individuals with high values are those most likely to develop amyloid.

### Waldenström's macroglobulinemia

This disorder is produced by the unregulated proliferation of cells of an intermediate appearance called lymphoplasmacytoid cells which secrete a monoclonal IgM, the Waldenström macroglobulin (figure 18.6l). Remarkably, many of the monoclonal proteins have autoantibody activity, anti-DNA, anti-IgG (rheumatoid factor) and so on. It has been suggested that they are of the same lineage as CLL cells. Since the IgM is secreted in large amounts and is confined to the intravascular compartment, there is a marked rise in serum viscosity, the consequences of which can be temporarily mitigated by vigorous plasmapheresis. The disease runs a fairly benign course and the prognosis is quite good, although the appearance of lymphoplasmacytoid tumor cells in the blood is an ominous sign.

### Heavy chain disease

Heavy chain disease is a rare condition in which quantities of abnormal heavy chains are excreted in the urine — γ-chains in association with malignant lymphoma and α-chains in cases of abdominal lymphoma with diffuse lymphoplasmacytic infiltration of the small intestine. The amino acid sequences of the N-terminal regions of these heavy chains are normal but they have a deletion extending from part of the variable domain through most of the $C_H1$ region so that they lack the structure required to form cross-links to the light chains. One idea is that the defect arises through faulty coupling of *V* and *C* region genes (cf. p. 46).

## Immunodeficiency secondary to lymphoproliferative disorders

Immunodeficiency is a common feature in patients with lymphoid malignancies. The reasons for this are still obscure but it seems as though the malignant cells interfere with the development of the corresponding normal cells, almost as though they were producing some cell-specific chalone or transfecting suppressor factor. Thus in multiple myeloma the levels of normal B-cells and of nonmyeloma Ig may be grossly depressed and the patients susceptible to infection with pyogenic bacteria.

## APPROACHES TO CANCER IMMUNOTHERAPY

Although immune surveillance seems to operate only against strongly immunogenic tumors, the exciting new information on the antigenicity of mutant and previously silent proteins and the changes in carbohydrate structures should be of tremendous encouragement to any red-blooded investigator with an eye to develop new immunotherapies for cancer which exploit these antigens.

On one point all are agreed, if immunotherapy is to succeed, it is essential that the tumor load should first be reduced by surgery, irradiation or chemotherapy, since not only is it unreasonable to expect the immune system to cope with a large tumor mass, but considerable amounts of antigen released by shedding would tend to prevent the generation of any significant response in some cases due to the stimulation of T-suppressors. This leaves the small secondary deposits as the proper target for immunotherapy.

### Exploitation of acquired immune responses

#### The antigen is known

Based on the not unreasonable belief that certain forms of cancer (e.g. lymphoma) are caused by oncogenic viruses, attempts are being made to isolate the virus and prepare a suitable vaccine from it. In fact, large-scale protection of chickens against the development of Marek's disease lymphoma has been successfully achieved by vaccination with another herpes virus native to turkeys. In human Burkitt's lymphoma, work is in progress to develop a vaccine to exploit the ability of Tc cells to target **EBV-related antigens** on the cells of all Burkitt tumors. It may be an advantage to treat the patient at the same time with cytokines to upregulate the expression of ICAM-1, LFA-3 and possibly of the virus itself.

The unique **idiotype** on monoclonal B-cell tumors with surface Ig also offers a potentially feasible target for immunotherapy and a particularly intriguing approach has been to immunize with a novel construct in which GM-CSF molecules are fused at the C-terminus of each heavy chain of the idiotypic Ig molecule. The presence of two GM-CSF molecules to each Ig could increase the affinity to cellular receptors and prove to be more potent biologically than recombinant GM-CSF itself. The immunogen effectively protected mice from challenge with tumor cells bearing the idiotype without the need for adjuvants (figure 18.8). An alternative *modus operandi* which also bypasses the need for adjuvant is to pulse autologous

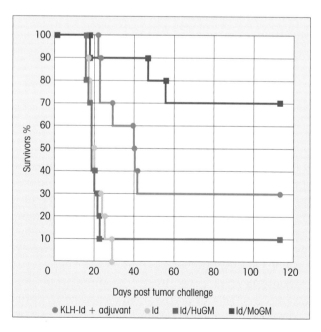

**Figure 18.8. Immunotherapy of B-cell leukemia using an idiotype/GM-CSF construct.** Two weeks after a second immunization with 10 mg of antigen, mice were challenged with 200 idiotype-bearing tumor cells. Good survival was observed. KLH = keyhole limpet hemocyanin (T-cell carrier); Id = idiotype; HuGM = human GM-CSF (granulocyte–macrophage colony-stimulating factor); MoGM = mouse GM-CSF. (Reproduced with permission from Tao M.-H. & Levy R. (1993) *Nature* **362**, 755–758. Copyright © 1993, Macmillan Magazines Ltd.)

immature dendritic cells, expanded from peripheral blood by culture in GM-CSF, interleukin-4 (IL-4) and α-tumor necrosis factor (TNFα), with the idiotypic protein. No anti-idiotypic antibodies are formed but very good cell-mediated proliferative responses and clinical benefit (figure 18.9) were observed. This tactic of harnessing the powerful immunogenicity of antigen-pulsed dendritic cells is obviously of universal applicability to other protein antigens. Watch out also for methods targeting antigen to the cellular arm of the immune response by uptake into phagocytes after conjugating to iron beads or coupling to *Listeria monocytogenes*, which escapes into the cytosol; i.m. injection of naked DNA also has enormous potential and is rather straightforward.

The other tumor-specific antigens and mutant peptide sequences are all possible candidates for immunotherapy. Thus, peptides derived from a mutated connexin 37 gap junction protein from a malignant murine lung carcinoma, induced Tc cells, protected mice from spontaneous metastases and reduced pre-established metastases. Trials are in progress using the human melanoma-specific MAGE antigenic peptides. Normal differentiation antigens expressed only on the tumor and a tissue of origin which is not crucial for survival, represent legitimate immunotherapeutic targets. This would be true of the tyrosinase, Melan-A, gp100 and gp75 melanoma antigens; given the choice I would readily opt for vitiligo if the alternative was growth of the melanoma. The same considerations would hold for prostatic cancer. Looking to exploitation of recent findings, perhaps we will see some progress with the use of heat shock protein complexes as tumor immunogens.

However, if we are dealing with a set of tumors bearing a multiplicity of individual mutant antigens, it would not be a practical proposition economically to identify each one and make a customized vaccine for every patient. We may be able to get away with using conserved cryptic epitope sequences but otherwise, we may have to augment the immunogenicity of the individual tumor cell, which does have the advantage that we do not necessarily have to know the identity of the antigen concerned.

### The antigen is unknown

The 'weaker' tumors may sometimes establish a mild immune response and one line of attack is to expand the lymphocytes infiltrating a tumor or present in a draining lymph node by treatment *in vitro* with a mixture of anti-CD3 and anti-CD28; reinjection should take these smartly to the site of the residual

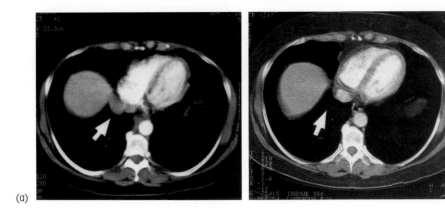

(a)                    (b)

**Figure 18.9. Clinical response to autologous vaccine utilizing dendritic cells pulsed with idiotype from a B-cell lymphoma.** Computed tomography scan through patient's chest (a) prevaccine and (b) 10 months after completion of three vaccine treatments. The arrow in (a) points to a paracardiac mass. All sites of disease had resolved and the patient remained in remission 24 months after beginning treatment. (Photography kindly supplied by Professor R. Levy from the article by Hsu F.J. et al. (1996) *Nature Medicine* **2**, 52; reproduced by kind permission of Nature America Inc.)

tumor, the supposition being that these populations contain some antigen-specific cytolytic T-cells.

Another approach is to make the tumor cells more immunogenic. This has a fairly respectable history covering manipulations such as viral infection of the tumor or coupling purified protein derivative (PPD) to the surface. The problem is the **barrier to activation of** *resting T-cells*. Remember the MHC–peptide complex on its own is not enough; costimulation with molecules such as B7-1 and -2 and possibly certain cytokines is required to push the G0 T-cell into active proliferation and differentiation. Once we get to this

stage, however, **the activated T-cell no longer requires the accessory costimulation** to react with its target, for which it has a greatly increased avidity due to upregulation of accessory binding molecules such as CD2 and LFA-1 (cf. p. 170; figure 18.10). The system works! Vaccination with B7-transfected murine melanoma generated CD8+ cytolytic effectors which protected against subsequent tumor challenge. Success was also obtained with a sarcoma cell line, although here it was necessary to transfect with genes for truncated MHC class II in addition to B7, implying participation of CD4 T-cells in the antitumor response. A further telling observation was that an irradiated nonimmunogenic melanoma line which had been transfected with a retroviral vector carrying the GM-CSF gene stimulated potent and specific antitumor immunity, almost certainly by enhancing the differentiation and activation of host antigen-presenting cells. It would be exciting to suppose that in the future we might expose a tumor surgically and then

**Figure 18.10. Immunotherapy by transfection with costimulatory molecules.** The tumor can only stimulate the resting T-cell with the costimulatory help of B7-1 and -2 and/or cytokines such as GM-CSF, γ-interferon (IFNγ) and interleukins IL-2,4 and 7. Once activated, the T-cell with upregulated accessory molecules can now attack the original tumor lacking costimulators.

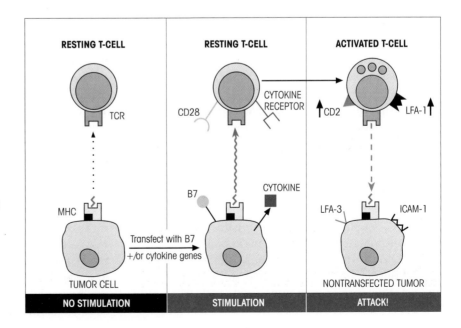

transfect it *in situ* by firing gold particles (cf. p. 144) bearing appropriate gene constructs such as B7, IFNγ (to upregulate MHC class I and II), GM-CSF, IL-2 and so on (figure 18.10). There is a theoretical risk of inducing autoimmune responses to cryptic epitopes (cf. p. 410) shared with other normal tissues which the prudent investigator will not overlook.

## Monoclonal antibodies as magic bullets

Immunologists have for long been bemused by the idea of eliminating tumor cells by specific antibody linked to a killer molecule. Not surprisingly, the 'magic bullet' devotees were greatly encouraged by experiments in which guinea-pig B lymphoma cells were killed *in vitro* by anti-idiotype conjugated with ricin, a toxin of such devastating potency that one molecule entering the cell is lethal (those readers who still maintain contact with the outside world will recollect that minute amounts of **ricin** on the end of a pointed walking stick provide a favorite weapon for the liquidation of unwanted intelligence agents!). There is optimism that by using monoclonal antibodies, it may be feasible to apply this approach to the human but the pathway to success is not without its difficulties. The immunotoxins must have a reasonable half-life in the circulation, penetrate into tumors and not bind significantly ·to nontumor cells; they must also be internalized efficiently and delivered to the correct intracellular department, e.g. ricin must go to the transgolgi network or a postgolgi compartment. Another problem is the heterogeneity of tumors with respect to the putative antigen. Encouraging results have been obtained in patients bearing solid tumors treated with a monoclonal specific for the Ley carbohydrate epitope and in breast cancer patients injected with an scFv fragment directed to the overexpressed c-erbB2 antigen; both agents were coupled to *Pseudomonas* exotoxin either as a conjugate or a fusion protein.

Nothing daunted, there is a plethora of ingenious initiatives. For example, a mixture of **two bispecific heteroconjugates** of antitumor/anti-CD3 and antitumor/anti-CD28 should act synergistically to induce contact between a T-cell and the tumor to activate direct cytotoxicity even though the T-cell itself will not have conventional specificity for the tumor target (figure 18.11). **Radioimmunoconjugates** which carry a radiation source such as Tc-99 and In-111 to the tumor site for therapy or diagnosis are being intensively developed and have two advantages over toxins: they are nonimmunogenic and they can destroy adjacent tumor cells which have lost antigen

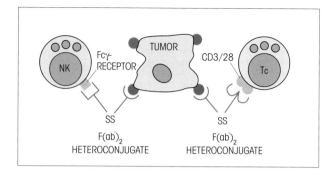

**Figure 18.11. Focusing effector cells by heteroconjugates**. Coupling F(ab') fragments of monoclonal antibodies specific for the tumor and an appropriate molecule on the surface of NK or Tc cells, provides the specificity to bring the effectors into intimate contact with the target cell. Many variants are possible: the second Fab' can be directed to a bacterial superantigen or a hapten which chelates a radionuclide. This allows clearance of nontargeted primary antibody before treatment with the effector molecule and produces good tumor localization with reduced liver and bone marrow uptake.

through heterogeneity. Higher tumor binding can be achieved by increasing blood flow or vascular permeability. Host toxicity can be reduced by pretargeting the tumor and clearing unbound antibody. In one study, following a preliminary injection of the monoclonal antibody conjugated to streptavidin, the nontargeted antibody was cleared by a biotin conjugate after which administration of a radiotherapeutic yttrium-labeled molecule coupled to biotin led to focusing of the isotope onto the tumor-bound streptavidin. The nontargeted primary antibody could also be cleared by an anti-idiotype. A bright idea is to inject specific antibody coupled to alkaline phosphatase followed later by phosphorylated derivatives of three anticancer drugs.

Unmodified monoclonal antibodies which seek out a tumor-specific surface target may be as effective in recruiting NK cells for ADCC as the bifunctional heteroconjugates described above because, being bivalent, they bind to the tumor with greater avidity. They would not be very effective in promoting complement-mediated lysis of the tumor because of the regulatory proteins, DAF, MCP, CD59 and HRF (cf. p. 313), which normally protect host cells from complement-dependent damage. These considerations do not come into play when monoclonal antibodies are used to **purge bone marrow grafts** of unwanted cells *in vitro* in the presence of complement from a foreign species. Thus, differentiation antigens present on leukemic cells but absent from bone marrow stem cells, even though not tumor-specific, can be used to prepare tumor-free autologous stem cells to restore function in patients treated with chemotherapy or X-irradiation which destroys both their tumor cells and their hematopoietic tissue (figure 18.12). Recombinant GM-CSF, G-CSF and IL-3, which enhance hematopoiesis, are of great value in shortening the period of neutropenia following chemotherapy. The difficulty is to cope with the few remaining tumor cells and autologous grafts do not provide the little understood beneficial 'graft-versus-leukemia' effect obtained with allogeneic marrow, albeit the potential is there for more generalized g.v.h. disease. Anti-CD33 would seem to be uniquely specific for myeloid leukemias in relation to other hematopoietic stem cells and has been used successfully for bone marrow purging and also for therapy. It localizes rapidly to all areas of leukemia involvement followed by internalization by the target cell; using a radionuclide conjugate, more than 99% of leukemic cells can be killed.

For solid tumors, the focus is upon two main targets. The first would be **minimal residual micrometastases in the bone marrow** which occur in one-third to one-half of patients with epithelial cancer after curative radical treatment of the primary lesion. The second would be the **reactive tissue evoked by the malignant process**, stromal fibroblasts expressing the F19 glycoprotein and blood vessels positive for the FB5 endosialin.

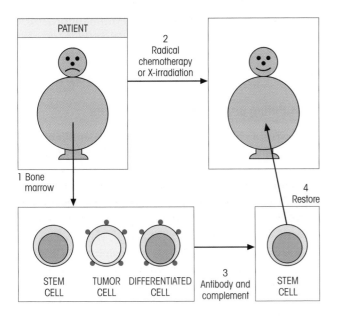

**Figure 18.12. Treatment of leukemias by autologous bone marrow rescue.** By using cytotoxic antibodies to a differentiation antigen ( ● ) present on leukemic cells and even on other normal differentiated cells, but absent from stem cells, it is possible to obtain a tumor-free population of the latter which can be used to restore hematopoietic function in patients subsequently treated radically to destroy the leukemic cells. Another angle is positive selection of stem cells utilizing the CD34 marker.

## Harnessing innate immunity

It is over 100 years since the physician Coley gave his name to the mixture of microbial products termed **Coley's toxin**. This concoction certainly livens up the innate immune system and does produce remission in a minority of patients. The suggestion has been made that these beneficial effects are due to release of TNF since the vascular endothelium of tumors is unduly susceptible to damage by this cytokine and hemorrhagic necrosis is readily induced. It is questionable whether the critical levels of TNF are reached in the human since these would be very toxic, although one study involving perfusion of an isolated limb with TNF, IFNγ and melphalan provoked lesions in the tumor endothelium without affecting the normal vasculature. Opinion is coming round to the view that the Coley phenomenon may be linked more to boosting a pre-existing weak antitumor immunity.

### Lymphokine activated killer cells

We earlier drew attention to the cytolytic activity of NK cells for a number of cultured tumor lines. On activation by IL-2, NK cells are capable of killing a variety of fresh tumor cells *in vitro*. These so-called 'lymphokine-activated killer' (LAK) cells probably include the A-NK set described above. Administration of autologous LAK cells together with high doses of IL-2 has led, in one study, to a considerable reduction in evaluable tumor in renal cancer patients (figure 18.13). Other cancers are less sensitive to this treatment which is cumbersome, gruesome for the patient, and has significant side-effects.

### Interferon therapy

In trials using IFNα and IFNβ, a 10–15% objective response rate was seen in patients with renal carcinoma, melanoma and myeloma, an approximate 20% response rate among patients with Kaposi's sarcoma, about 40% positive responders in patients with various lymphomas and a remarkable response rate of 80–90% among patients with hairy cell leukemia and mycosis fungoides.

With regard to the mechanisms of the antitumor effects, in certain tumors IFNs may serve primarily as antiproliferative agents, in others, activation of NK cells and macrophages may be important, while augmenting the expression of class I MHC molecules may make the tumors more susceptible to control by immune effector mechanisms. In some circumstances the antiviral effect could be contributory.

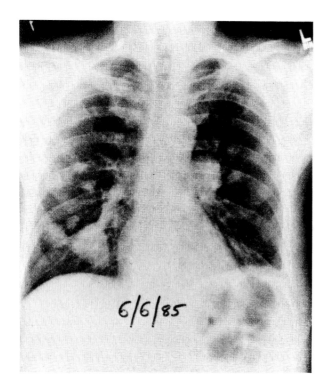
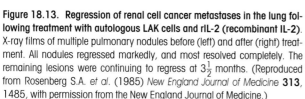
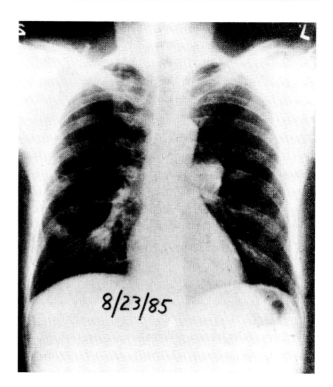

**Figure 18.13. Regression of renal cell cancer metastases in the lung following treatment with autologous LAK cells and rIL-2 (recombinant IL-2).** X-ray films of multiple pulmonary nodules before (left) and after (right) treatment. All nodules regressed markedly, and most resolved completely. The remaining lesions were continuing to regress at 3½ months. (Reproduced from Rosenberg S.A. *et al.* (1985) *New England Journal of Medicine* **313**, 1485, with permission from the New England Journal of Medicine.)

For diseases like renal cell cancer and hairy cell leukemia, IFNs have induced responses in a significantly higher proportion of patients than conventional therapies. However, in the wider setting, most investigators consider that their role will be in combination therapy, e.g. with active immunotherapy or with various chemotherapeutic agents where synergistic action has been observed in murine tumor systems. IFNα and β synergize with IFNγ and the latter synergizes with TNF. IFNα acts as a radiation sensitizer and its ability to increase the expression of estrogen receptors on cultured breast cancer cells suggests the possibility of combining IFN with anti-estrogens in this disease.

*Colony-stimulating factors*

Normal cell development proceeds from an immature stem cell with the capacity for unlimited self-renewal, through committed progenitors to the final lineage-specific differentiated cells with little or no potential for self-renewal. Therapy aimed at inducing tumor cell differentiation is founded on the idea that the induction of cell maturation decreases and possibly abrogates the capacity of the malignant clone to divide. Along these lines, GM-CSF has been shown to enhance the differentiation, decrease the self-renewal capacity and suppress the leukemogenicity of murine myeloid leukemias. Recombinant human products are now undergoing trials.

## IMMUNODIAGNOSIS OF SOLID TUMORS

### Circulating and cellular tumor markers

Analysis of blood for the oncofetal antigens, α-fetoprotein in hepatoma and carcinoembryonic antigen in tumors of the colon has provided valuable diagnostic information, but enthusiasm has been slightly curtailed by the knowledge that there is a high incidence of so-called 'false positives'. Reappearance of these proteins after surgical removal of the primary is strongly indicative of fresh tumor growth. The GM1 monosialoganglioside has been demonstrated in the blood of 96% of patients with pancreatic carcinoma and 64% of colorectal carcinomas as against 2% in normal subjects.

Identification of the cell type by monoclonal antibodies is of value for the diagnosis and treatment of an increasing number of tumors, including the lymphoproliferative disorders as discussed earlier (see p. 387).

## Tumor imaging *in vivo*

The same principles which govern the localization of monoclonal antibodies for tumor therapy apply equally to imaging. Maximizing the binding to tumor relative to normal tissue and surrounding fluids is the name of the game. For example, the use of a bifunctional antibody which targets the tumor and an isotope chelator can be followed 24–120 hours later with the chelate containing radionuclide which allows clearance of uncombined antibody (cf. legend figure 18.11).

The Thomson–Friedenreich (T) antigen (Galβ1–3-GalNAcα-O-Ser) expressed in the mucins of various types of epithelial cancer has proved to be a highly successful target for antibody imaging. So has the F19 glycoprotein associated with proliferating fibroblasts in the stroma of many carcinomas.

## Detection of micrometastases in bone marrow

Because of the difficulty in detecting individual tumor cells in distant organs, the diagnosis of early disseminated cancer has not been possible so that attempts to identify earlier stages and to monitor the immunotherapy of early disease have been hindered. A major advance was made when micrometastases

**Table 18.3. Detection of bone marrow micrometastases by staining for epithelial cytokeratin in colorectal cancer patients.** (From data of Schlimok G. *et al.* (1990), see Further Reading.)

| Dukes' Stage | | Positive reaction with mAb CK2 for cytokeratin in bone marrow aspirate | |
|---|---|---|---|
| | | No. patients | % Positive |
| A | Limited to mucosa | 3 | 0 |
| B | Extending into muscularis propria | 58 | 14 |
| C | Involving local nodes | 62 | 34 |
| D | With distant metastatic spread | 33 | 39 |

were demonstrated by immunocytochemistry in the bone marrow of patients with colorectal cancer and were related to more widespread disease (table 18.3) and a high relapse rate. The method involves scanning pelvic crest bone marrow aspirates taken at surgery for epithelial cells by staining for cytokeratin (cf. figure 18.6f) and proliferation markers such as the Ki67 nuclear antigen and receptors for transferrin and epidermal growth factor. Detection of micrometastases in the marrow of patients with small-cell lung carcinoma also predicted early relapse.

## SUMMARY

### Changes on the surface of tumor cells

• Processed peptides derived from oncogenic viruses are powerful MHC-associated transplantation antigens.
• Some tumors express genes which are silent in normal tissues: sometimes they have been expressed previously in embryonic life (oncofetal antigens).
• Many tumors express weak antigens associated with point mutations in oncogenes such as *ras* and *p53*.
• Dysregulation of tumor cells frequently causes structural abnormalities in surface carbohydrate structures.
• Some surface changes are a consequence of cell division *per se*.
• The v6 and v10 exons of CD44 are intimately involved with metastatic potential. Loss of blood group A determinants leads to a poor prognosis.
• The idiotype of the Ig receptor on chronic lymphocytic leukemia (CLL) cells is a unique tumor-specific antigen. Peptides presented by heat-shock protein gp96 represent the unique chemically induced tumor antigens.

### Immune response to tumors

• T-cells generally mount effective surveillance against tumors associated with oncogenic viruses or UV induction which are strongly immunogenic.
• More weakly immunogenic tumors are not controlled by T-cell surveillance, although sometimes low-grade responses are evoked.
• NK cells probably play a role in containing tumor growth and metastases. They can attack MHC class I negative tumor cells because the class I molecule imparts a negative inactivation signal to NK cells. The A-NK subset which express high levels of adhesion molecules are more cytolytic for fresh tumor cells.

### Unregulated development gives rise to lymphoproliferative disorders

• Deregulation of the c-*myc* protooncogene is a characteristic feature of many B-cell tumors.
• Chromosome translocations are common.

(Continued on p. 398)

• Lymphoid malignancies show maturation arrest at characteristic stages in differentiation.
• The surface markers of leukemias and lymphomas identified by monoclonal antibodies are important aids in diagnosis. Most non-Hodgkin lymphomas are of B-cell origin, are associated with EBV and express a monoclonal surface Ig.
• Multiple myeloma represents a malignant proliferation of a single clone of plasma cells producing a single 'M' band on electrophoresis. 10–20% have widespread amyloid deposits containing the variable region of the myeloma light chain.
• Waldenström's macroglobulinemia is produced by unregulated proliferation of a clone producing monoclonal IgM causing a marked rise in serum viscosity.
• Malignant lymphoid cells produce secondary immunodeficiency by suppressing differentiation of the corresponding normal lineage.

### Approaches to cancer immunotherapy

• Cancer vaccines based on oncogenic viral proteins can be expected.
• Immunization with a CLL idiotype provides protection against the tumor. Effective melanoma-specific antigens have been identified. Immunogenic potency of a tumor antigen is greatly enhanced by pulsing dendritic cells.
• Weakly immunogenic tumors provoke effective anticancer responses if transfected with costimulatory molecules such as B7 and cytokines IFNγ, IL-2,4 and 7.

• Monoclonal antibodies conjugated to toxins or radionuclides can target tumor cells or antigens on the reactive stromal fibroblasts associated with malignancy. Encouraging therapeutic results have been obtained with antibodies to the Le$^y$ epitope expressed on many solid tumors, and c-erbB2 overexpressed on breast cancers. Bifunctional antibodies can bring effectors such as NK and T$_c$ close to the tumor target.
• Innate immune mechanisms can be harnessed. IL-2-stimulated NK cells (LAK) are active against renal carcinoma. IFNγ and β are very effective in the T-cell disorders, hairy cell leukemia and mycosis fungoides, less so but still significant in Kaposi's sarcoma and various lymphomas; they may be used in synergy with other therapies. GM-CSF enhances proliferation and decreases leukemogenicity of murine myeloid leukemias.

### Immunodiagnosis of solid tumors

• Many circulating tumor markers are diagnostic, e.g. α-fetoprotein in hepatic carcinoma and carcino-embryonic antigen in colorectal carcinoma.
• Monoclonal antibody to tumor surfaces can provide a basis for imaging. Certain tumor mucins and the F19 glycoprotein on reactive stromal fibroblasts around the tumor are good targets.
• Detection of micrometastases in bone marrow by immunocytochemistry provides valuable information on prognosis and the efficacy of new therapies.

## FURTHER READING

Baskar S., Ostrand-Rosenberg S., Nabaro N., Nadler L.M., Freeman G.J. & Glimcher L.H. (1993) Constitutive expression of B7 restores immunogenicity of tumor cells expressing truncated major histocompatibility complex class II molecules. *Proceedings of the National Academy of Sciences (USA)* **90**, 5687–5690.

Begent R.H.J., Verhaar M.J., Chester K.A. *et al.* (1996) Clinical evidence of efficient tumor targeting based on single-chain Fv antibody selected from a combinatorial library. *Nature Medicine* **2(9)**, 979.

Forbes I.J. & Leong A.S.-Y. (1987) *Essential Oncology of the Lymphocyte.* Springer-Verlag, Berlin.

Lanier L.L. & Phillips J.H. (1996) Inhibitory MHC class I receptors of NK cells and T-cells. *Immunology Today* **17**, 86–91.

Leonard R.C.F., Duncan L.W. & Hay F.G. (1990) Immunocytological detection of residual marrow disease at clinical remission predicts metastatic relapse in small cell lung cancer. *Cancer Research* **50**, 6545–6548.

Maio M. & Parmiani G. (1996) Melanoma immunotherapy: new dreams of solid hopes? *Immunology Today* **17**, 405–407.

Mannel D., Murray C., Risau W. & Clauss M. (1996) Tumor necrosis: factors and principles. *Immunology Today* **17**, 254–256.

Moretta L. (ed.) (1995) NK cells: origin, receptors and specificity. *Seminars in Immunology* **7**, 57.

Pardoll D.M. (ed.) (1996) Cancer. *Current Opinion in Immunology* **8**, 619–669.

Pardoll D.M. (ed.) (1996) Cancer and the immune system. *Seminars in Immunology* **8**, 269.

Soussi T. (1996) The humoral response to the tumor-suppressor gene-product p53 in human cancer: implications for diagnosis and therapy. *Immunology Today* **17**, 354–356.

Stein H. & Mason D.Y. (1985) Immunological analysis of tissue sections in diagnosis of lymphoma. In A.V. Hoffbrand (ed.) *Recent Advances in Haematology*, Vol 4, p. 127. Churchill Livingstone, Edinburgh.

Townsend S.E. & Allison J.P. (1993) Tumor rejection after direct co-stimulation of CD8(+) T cells by B7-transfected melanoma cells. *Science* **259**, 368–370.

Witte O.N. & Boon T. (eds) (1995) Cancer. *Current Opinion in Immunology* **7**, 657. (Critical overviews of the whole field, which serious students are highly advised to read.)

# AUTOIMMUNE DISEASES
## 1—Scope and Etiology

C O N T E N T S

## THE SCOPE OF AUTOIMMUNE DISEASES

The monumental repertoire of the adaptive immune system has evolved to allow it to recognize and ensnare virtually any shaped microbial molecules, either at present in existence or yet to come, and in so doing, has been unable to avoid the generation of lymphocytes which react with the body's own constituents. We have already discussed the mechanisms which exist to prevent these self-components from provoking an adaptive immune response but, as with all machinery, there is always a chance that these systems might break down, and the older the individual, the greater the chance of this happening.

Notwithstanding the IgM low affinity **autoantibodies** (i.e. antibodies capable of reacting with 'self' components) produced by CD5+ B-cells as part of the 'natural' antibody spectrum which we will discuss later, we are here concerned more with autoimmune phenomena which appear in relation to certain defined human diseases. Ideally we wish to apply the term **'autoimmune disease'** to those cases where it can be shown that the **autoimmune process contributes to the pathogenesis of the disease** rather than situations where apparently harmless autoantibodies are formed following tissue damage, e.g. heart antibodies appearing after a myocardial infarction. Yet the role of autoimmunity in many disorders is still

# Milestone 19.1—The Discovery of Thyroid Autoimmunity

Although Dacie's studies on red cell autoantibodies in certain forms of hemolytic anemia were amongst the earliest to implicate autoimmunity in the pathogenesis of disease, a direct link to disorders affecting whole organs was not established until 1956 when three major papers on thyroid autoimmunity appeared.

In an attempt to confirm Paul Ehrlich's concept of 'horror autotoxicus'—the body's dread of making antibodies to self—Rose and Witebsky immunized rabbits with rabbit thyroid extract in complete Freund's adjuvant. To what I would hazard was Witebsky's dismay and Rose's delight, this procedure resulted in the production of thyroid autoantibodies and chronic inflammatory destruction of the thyroid gland architecture (figure M19.1.1a and b).

Having noted the fall in serum γ-globulin which followed removal of the goiter in Hashimoto's thyroiditis and the similarity of the histology (figure M19.1.1c) to that of Rose and Witebsky's rabbits, Roitt, Doniach and Campbell tested the hypothesis that the plasma cells in the gland might be making an autoantibody to a thyroid component, so causing the tissue damage and chronic inflammatory response. Sure enough, the sera of the first patients tested had precipitating antibodies to an autoantigen in normal thyroid extracts which was soon identified as thyroglobulin (figure M19.1.2).

In far off New Zealand (depending on your geographical location!), Adams and Purves, in seeking a circulating factor which might be responsible for the hyperthyroidism of Graves' thyrotoxicosis, injected patient's

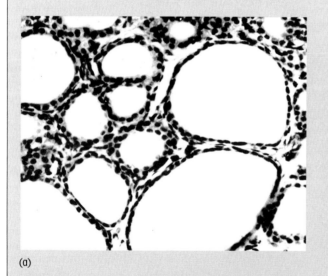

(a)

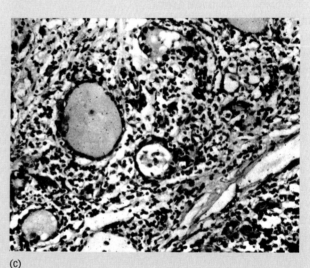

(c)

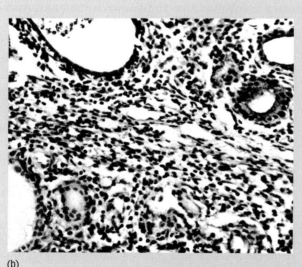

(b)

**Figure M19.1.1. Experimental autoallergic thyroiditis.** (a) Control rat thyroid showing normal follicular architecture. (b) Thyroiditis produced by immunization with rat thyroid extract in complete Freund's adjuvant; the invading chronic inflammatory cells have destroyed the follicular structure. (Based on the experiments of Rose N.R. & Witebsky E. (1956) Studies on organ specificity. V. Changes in the thyroid gland of rabbits following active immunization with rabbit thyroid extracts. *Journal of Immunology* **76**, 417.) (c) Similarity of lesions in spontaneous human autoimmune disease to those induced in the experimental model. Other features of Hashimoto's disease such as the eosinophilic metaplasia of acinar cells (Askenazy cells) and local lymphoid follicles are not seen in this experimental model, although the latter occur in the spontaneous thyroiditis of Obese strain chickens.

*(Continued)*

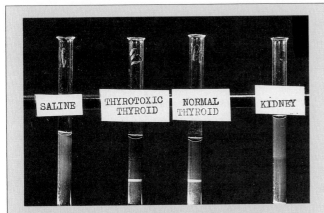

**Figure M19.1.2. Thyroid autoantibodies in the serum of a patient with Hashimoto's disease demonstrated by precipitation in agar.** Test serum is incorporated in agar in the bottom of the tube; the middle layer contains agar only while the autoantigen is present in the top layer. As serum antibody and thyroid autoantigen diffuse towards each other, they form a zone of opaque precipitate in the middle layer. Saline and kidney extract controls are negative. (Based on Roitt I.M., Doniach D., Campbell P.N. & Hudson R.V. (1956) Autoantibodies in Hashimoto's disease. *Lancet* **ii**, 820.)

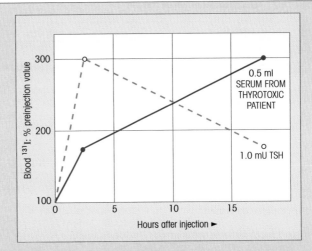

**Figure M19.1.3. The long-acting thyroid stimulator in Graves' disease.** Injection of TSH causes a rapid release of $^{131}$I from the prelabeled animal thyroid in contrast to the prolonged release which follows injection of serum from a thyrotoxic patient. (Based on Adams D.D. & Purves H.D. (1956) Abnormal responses in the assay of thyrotrophin. *Proceedings of the University of Otago Medical School* **34**, 11.)

serum into guinea-pigs whose thyroids had been prelabeled with $^{131}$I, and followed the release of radiolabeled material from the gland with time. Whereas the natural pituitary thyroid-stimulating hormone (TSH) produced a peak in serum radioactivity some 4 hours or so after injection of the test animal, serum from thyrotoxic patients had a prolonged stimulatory effect (figure M19.1.3). The so-called *long-acting thyroid stimulator* (LATS) was ultimately shown to be an IgG mimicking TSH through its reaction with the TSH receptor but differing in its time-course of action, largely due to its longer half-life in the circulation.

not clearly defined, and it is as a matter of convenience that we will refer to all maladies firmly associated with autoantibody formation as 'autoimmune diseases', except where it can be shown that the immunological phenomena are purely secondary findings.

## The spectrum of autoimmune diseases

These disorders may be looked upon as forming a spectrum. At one end we have '**organ-specific diseases**' with organ-specific autoantibodies. **Hashimoto's disease** of the thyroid is an example: there is a specific lesion in the thyroid involving infiltration by mononuclear cells (lymphocytes, histiocytes and plasma cells), destruction of follicular cells and germinal center formation, accompanied by the production of circulating antibodies with absolute specificity for certain thyroid constituents (Milestone 19.1).

Moving towards the center of the spectrum are those disorders where the lesion tends to be localized to a single organ but the antibodies are nonorgan-specific. A typical example would be **primary biliary**

**Table 19.1. Spectrum of autoimmune diseases.**

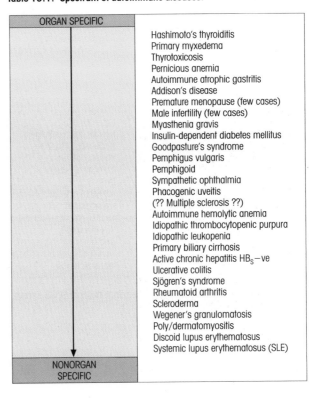

ORGAN SPECIFIC

Hashimoto's thyroiditis
Primary myxedema
Thyrotoxicosis
Pernicious anemia
Autoimmune atrophic gastritis
Addison's disease
Premature menopause (few cases)
Male infertility (few cases)
Myasthenia gravis
Insulin-dependent diabetes mellitus
Goodpasture's syndrome
Pemphigus vulgaris
Pemphigoid
Sympathetic ophthalmia
Phacogenic uveitis
(?? Multiple sclerosis ??)
Autoimmune hemolytic anemia
Idiopathic thrombocytopenic purpura
Idiopathic leukopenia
Primary biliary cirrhosis
Active chronic hepatitis HB$_S$−ve
Ulcerative colitis
Sjögren's syndrome
Rheumatoid arthritis
Scleroderma
Wegener's granulomatosis
Poly/dermatomyositis
Discoid lupus erythematosus
Systemic lupus erythematosus (SLE)

NONORGAN SPECIFIC

**Table 19.2.** Autoantibodies in human disease.

| DISEASE | ANTIGEN | DETECTION OF ANTIBODY |
|---|---|---|
| Hashimoto's thyroiditis | Thyroglobulin | Precipitins; passive hemagglutination; ELISA |
| Primary myxedema | Thyroid peroxidase: Cytoplasmic | IFT on unfixed thyroid; passive hemagglutination; ELISA |
|  |      Cell surface | IFT on viable thyroid cells; C'-mediated cytotoxicity |
| Thyrotoxicosis | Cell surface TSH receptors | Bioassay–stimulation of mouse thyroid *in vivo*; blocking combination TSH with receptors; stimulation adenyl cyclase |
|  | 'Growth' receptors | Induction of cell division in thyroid fragments |
| Pernicious anemia[1] | Intrinsic factor | Neutralization; blocking combination with vit-$B_{12}$; binding to intrinsic factor-$B_{12}$ by coprecipitation |
|  | Parietal cell $H^+$–$K^+$ ATPase | IFT on unfixed gastric mucosa |
| Addison's disease | Cytoplasm adrenal cells ($17\alpha$-/$21$-hydroxylase) | IFT on unfixed adrenal cortex |
| Premature onset of menopause[2] | Cytoplasm steroid-producing cells | IFT on adrenal and interstitial cells of ovary and testis |
| Male infertility (some)[3] | Spermatozoa | Sperm agglutination in ejaculate |
| Insulin-dependent diabetes[4] | Cytoplasm of islet cells | IFT on unfixed human pancreas |
|  | Insulin, GAD and ICA512 | ELISA |
| Type B insulin resistance with acanthosis nigricans | Insulin receptor | Block hormone binding to receptor |
| Atopic allergy (some) | $\beta$-Adrenergic receptor | Blocking radioassay with hydroxybenzylpindolol |
| Myasthenia gravis | Skeletal and heart muscle | IFT on skeletal muscle |
|  | Acetylcholine receptor | Blocking or binding radioassay with $\alpha$-bungarotoxin |
| Lambert–Eaton syndrome | $Ca^{2+}$ channels in nerve endings | IgG produces neuromuscular defects in mice |
| (Multiple sclerosis) | Brain | Cytotoxic effects on cerebellar cultures by serum and lymphocytes (? secondary to disease) |
| Goodpasture's syndrome | Glomerular and lung basement membrane | Linear staining by IFT of kidney biopsy with fluorescent anti-IgG |
|  |  | Radioimmunoassay with purified Ag; ELISA |
| Pemphigus vulgaris | Desmosomes between prickle cells in epidermis (cadherin) | IFT on skin |
| Pemphigoid | Basement membrane | IFT on skin |
| Phacogenic uveitis | Lens | Passive hemagglutination |
| Sympathetic ophthalmia | Uvea | (Delayed skin reaction to uveal extract) |
| Autoimmune hemolytic anemia[5] | Erythrocytes | Coombs' antiglobulin test |
| Idiopathic thrombocytopenic purpura | Platelets | Shortened platelet survival *in vivo* |
| Primary biliary cirrhosis | Mitochondria (pyruvate dehyrogenase) | IFT on mitochondria-rich cells (e.g. distal tubules of kidney) |
| Active chronic hepatitis (HBV & HCV −ve) | Smooth muscle/nuclear lamins/nuclei | IFT (e.g. on gastric mucosa) |
|  | Kidney/liver microsomes (cyt P450) | IFT (kidney) |
| Ulcerative colitis | Colon 'lipopolysaccharide' | IFT; passive hemagglutination (cytotoxic action of lymphocytes on colon cells) |
|  | Colon epithelial cell surface protein | ADCC on colon cancer cell line |
|  |  | Ab data in this disease not universally accepted |
| Sjögren's syndrome[6] | SS-A(Ro) SS-B(La) | IFT; gel precipitation; ELISA |
|  | Ducts/mitochondria/nuclei/thyroid | IFT |
|  | IgG | Antiglobulin (rheumatoid factor) tests |
| Rheumatoid arthritis[7] | IgG | Antiglobulin test; latex agglutination; sheep red cell agglutination test (SCAT; commercial product, RAHA test) and ELISA; agalacto-glycoform |
|  | Collagen | Passive hemagglutination |
| Discoid lupus erythematosus | Nuclear/IgG | IFT/antiglobulin test |
| Scleroderma[8] | Nuclear/IgG/centromere | IFT |
|  | Nuclear/IgG/Scl-70 | IFT; countercurrent electrophoresis; ELISA |
|  | Nuclear/IgG/Jo-1 | IFT; countercurrent electrophoresis; ELISA |
| Dermatomyositis[9] | Extractable nuclear | IFT; countercurrent electrophoresis; ELISA |
| Mixed connective tissue disease[10] | DNA | Radioassay[11]; ELISA |
| Systemic lupus erythematosus | snRNP (Sm & ribonucleoprotein) | IFT; gel precipitation techniques; ELISA |
|  | Nucleoprotein | IFT |
|  | Array of other Ag including formed elements of blood/IgG |  |
|  | Cardiolipin/$\beta$2-glycoprotein1 | Radioassay |
| Wegener's granulomatosis | Neutrophil cytoplasm (ANCA; myeloperoxidase/ serine proteinase)[12] | IFT on alcohol fixed polymorphs; ELISA |

IFT = immunofluorescent test; hemaggln = hemagglutination; ELISA = enzyme-linked immunosorbent assay, cf. p. 113.

**cirrhosis** where the small bile ductule is the main target of inflammatory cell infiltration but the serum antibodies present — mainly mitochondrial — are not liver-specific.

At the other end of the spectrum are the '**nonorgan-specific or systemic autoimmune diseases**' broadly belonging to the class of rheumatological disorders, exemplified by **systemic lupus erythematosus (SLE)**, where both lesions and autoantibodies are not confined to any one organ. Pathological changes are widespread and are primarily lesions of connective tissue with fibrinoid necrosis. They are seen in the skin (the 'lupus' butterfly rash on the face is characteristic), kidney glomeruli, joints, serous membranes and blood vessels. In addition, the formed elements of the blood are often affected. A bizarre collection of autoantibodies are found, some of which react with the DNA and other nuclear constituents of all cells in the body.

An attempt to fit the major diseases considered to be associated with autoimmunity into this spectrum is shown in table 19.1.

## Autoantibodies in human disease

At this stage in the discussion it may be of value to have a more precise account of the major autoantibodies detected in the different diseases to provide a framework for reference. Table 19.2 documents a list of these antibodies and the methods employed in their detection. The notes accompanying the table amplify specific points while some of the tests are illustrated in figures 19.1, 6.7 and 6.8. As antigens are characterized and become available in purified form, the convenient ELISA is becoming a dominant technique.

## Overlap of autoimmune disorders

There is a tendency for more than one autoimmune disorder to occur in the same individual and when this happens the association is often between diseases within the same region of the autoimmune spectrum (cf. table 19.1). Thus patients with autoimmune thyroiditis (Hashimoto's disease or primary myxedema) have a much higher incidence of pernicious anemia than would be expected in a random population matched for age and sex (10% as against 0.2%). Conversely, both thyroiditis and thyrotoxicosis are diagnosed in pernicious anemia patients with an unexpectedly high frequency. Other associations are seen between Addison's disease and autoimmune

---

*Notes to table 19.2*

**1** Two major types of antibody to intrinsic factor are detected, viz. blocking and binding. Binding antibody combines with preformed intrinsic factor–radioactive $B_{12}$ (*$B_{12}$) complex which can then be precipitated at 50% ammonium sulfate and the radioactivity in the precipitate counted. Blocking antibody prevents binding of *$B_{12}$ to intrinsic factor. and the uncombined *$B_{12}$ can then be adsorbed to charcoal and counted.

**2** Antibodies occur in the minority of patients with associated Addison's disease of the adrenal and are directed to the $17\alpha$/21-hydroxylase, the cholesterol side-chain cleavage enzyme and a 51 kDa gonadal antigen.

**3** Only a small percentage show agglutinins. Spermatozoa may be agglutinated head to head, tail to tail or joined through their midpiece. Seen also in a small percentage of infertile women.

**4** Most if not all insulin-dependent diabetics have islet cell antibodies at some stage during the first year of onset but these tend to decline progressively. In contrast islet cell antibodies in diabetic patients with an associated autoimmune polyendocrinopathy persist for many years. GAD (glutamic acid decarboxylase) Ab also occur in Stiff man syndrome. ICA512 is a protein tyrosine kinase.

**5** The Coombs' test involves the demonstration of bound antibody on the washed red cell by agglutination with an antiglobulin (cf. figure 16.13). Erythrocyte autoantibodies, which bind well over the temperature range 0–37°C ('warm' Ab), are mostly IgG; approximately 60% of cases are primary, the remainder being associated with other autoimmune disorders, e.g. SLE and ulcerative colitis. 'Cold' Ab, which react best over the range 0–20°C, are mostly IgM and red cells coated with this Ab can often be agglutinated by anticomplement serum; approximately half are primary, the others being associated with *Mycoplasma pneumoniae* infection or generalized neoplastic disease of the lymphoreticular tissues.

**6** Antibodies specifically reacting with the epithelium of salivary gland excretory ducts are demonstrable by immunofluorescence in over half the cases of secondary Sjögren's associated with RA or SLE. SS-A and SS-B antibodies give a speckled nuclear fluorescence pattern.

**7** The main antiglobulin factors react with the Fc portion of IgG which is usually adsorbed on to latex particles (human IgG) or present in an antigen–antibody complex (sheep red cells coated with a subagglutinating dose of rabbit antibody). In the ELISA test, rabbit IgG is bound to a plastic tube, patient's serum added and the antiglobulin bound assessed by subsequent binding of labeled anti-human IgG or IgM (cf. p. 113). Rheumatoid factors specific for human IgG can be detected by this test using human Fc$\gamma$ to coat the tubes and labeled antihuman Fd$\gamma$ or IgM for the final stage.

**8** In scleroderma (progressive systemic sclerosis) antinucleolar antibodies are frequently found. Scl-70 is topoisomerase 1.

**9** Jo-1 is histidine tRNA synthetase.

**10** This syndrome combines features of scleroderma, RA, SLE and dermatomyositis. The antigens are extractable from the nucleus and give a speckled fluorescence pattern.

**11** Antibodies to single- or double-stranded DNA are assayed by the salt coprecipitation test (cf. figure 6.3) using labeled Ag, or by a DNA-coated tube test similar to the radioassay for antiglobulins (note 7 above).

**12** Component of primary granule, probably serine proteinase III, gives cytoplasmic staining. In periarteritis nodosa, antibodies to myeloperoxidase give perinuclear staining in alcohol-fixed polymorphonuclear neutrophils (PMNs). Some sera react with azurocidin, a potent antibiotic. ANCA (anti-neutrophil cytoplasmic antibody) directed against bactericidal/permeability increasing protein is a marker for inflammatory bowel disease and primary sclerosing cholangitis.

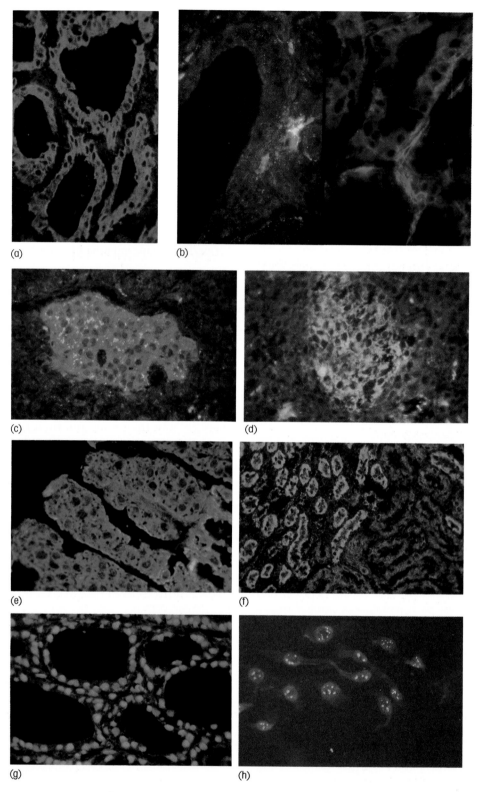

**Figure 19.1. Fluorescent antibody studies in autoimmune diseases.** (a) Thyroid microsomal (thyroid peroxidase) antibodies staining cytoplasm of acinar cells. (b) Human thyroid sections stained for MHC class II: *left*—normal thyroid with unstained follicular cells and an isolated strongly MHC class II positive dendritic cell; *right*—thyrotoxic (Graves' disease) thyroid with abundant cytoplasmic MHC class II indicative of active synthesis. (c) Fluorescence of cells in the pancreatic islets of Langerhans' stained with serum from insulin-dependent diabetic. (d) The same, showing cells stained simultaneously for somatostatin (the yellow cells are stained with rhodamine anti-somatostatin and fluorescein anti-human IgG which localizes the patient's bound autoantibody). (e) Serum of patient with Addison's disease staining cytoplasm of monkey adrenal granulosa cells. (f) Fluorescence of distal tubular cells of the kidney after reaction with mitochondrial autoantibodies. (g) Diffuse nuclear staining on a thyroid section obtained with nucleoprotein antibodies from an SLE patient. (h) Serum of a scleroderma patient staining the nucleoli of SV40-transformed human keratinocytes (K14) in monolayer culture. ((a), (c), (d), (e), (f) and (g) kindly provided by Prof. F. Bottazzo; (b) by Dr R. Pujol-Borrell, and (h) by Dr F.T. Wojnarowska.)

thyroid disease and in the rare cases of juveniles with pernicious anemia and polyendocrinopathy which includes Addison's disease, hypoparathyroidism, diabetes and thyroiditis.

There is an even greater overlap in serological findings. Thirty per cent of patients with autoimmune thyroid disease have concomitant parietal cell antibodies in their serum. Conversely, thyroid antibodies have been demonstrated in up to 50% of pernicious anemia patients. It should be stressed that these are not cross-reacting antibodies. The thyroid-specific antibodies will not react with stomach and vice versa. When a serum reacts with both organs it means that two populations of antibodies are present, one with specificity for thyroid and the other for stomach.

At the nonorgan-specific end of the spectrum, systemic autoimmune disease such as SLE is clinically associated with rheumatoid arthritis and several other disorders which are themselves uncommon: hemolytic anemia, idiopathic leukopenia and thrombocytopenic purpura, dermatomyositis and Sjögren's syndrome. Antinuclear antibodies and antiglobulin (rheumatoid) factors are a general feature.

Sjögren's syndrome occupies an interesting position (table 19.3); aside from the clinical and serological features associated with systemic disease mentioned above, characteristics of an organ-specific disorder are evident. Antibodies reacting with salivary ducts are demonstrable and there is an abnormally high incidence of thyroid autoantibodies; histologically the affected lacrimal and salivary glands reveal changes of a similar nature to those seen in Hashimoto's disease, namely a replacement of the glandular elements by patchy lymphocytic and plasma cell granulomatous tissue. Associations between diseases at the two ends of the spectrum have been reported, but, as might be predicted from the serological data (table 19.3), they are not common.

Patients with organ-specific disorders are slightly more prone to develop cancer in the affected organ,

whereas generalized lymphoreticular neoplasia shows up with uncommon frequency in nonorgan-specific disease.

## Animal models of autoimmune disease

Both spontaneous and induced animal models have given tremendous insights into the nature of human autoimmune disease and, to assist our discussions, I felt it would be helpful to list them (table 19.4).

# NATURE AND NURTURE

## Genetic factors in autoimmune disease

Autoimmune phenomena tend to aggregate in certain families. For example, the first degree relatives (sibs, parents and children) of patients with Hashimoto's disease show a high incidence of thyroid autoantibodies (figure 19.2) and of overt and subclinical thyroiditis. The proportion with autoantibodies is higher in those families where more than one member is clinically affected. Parallel studies have disclosed similar relationships in the families of pernicious anemia patients, in that gastric parietal cell antibodies are prevalent in the relatives who are wont to develop achlorhydria and atrophic gastritis. Familial aggregation of mitochondrial antibodies has been observed, albeit to a lesser extent, in primary biliary cirrhosis. Turning to SLE, disturbances of immunoglobulin synthesis and a susceptibility to develop 'connective tissue diseases' have been reported but there are some conflicting accounts still not resolved.

These familial relationships could be ascribed to environmental factors such as infective microorganisms, but there is powerful evidence that multiple genetic components must be involved. The data on **twins** is unequivocal. When thyrotoxicosis or insulin-dependent diabetes mellitus (IDDM) occurs in twins there is a far greater concordance rate (i.e. both twins

Table 19.3. Organ-specific and nonorgan-specific serological interrelationships in human disease.

| DISEASE | % POSITIVE REACTIONS FOR ANTIBODIES TO: | | | |
|---|---|---|---|---|
| | THYROID* | STOMACH* | NUCLEI* | IgG† |
| Hashimoto's thyroiditis | 99.9 | 32 | 8 | 2 |
| Pernicious anemia | 55 | 89 | 11 | |
| Sjögren's syndrome | 45 | 14 | 56 | 75 |
| Rheumatoid arthritis | 11 | 16 | 50 | 75 |
| SLE | 2 | 2 | 99 | 35 |
| Controls‡ | 0–15 | 0–16 | 0–19 | 2–5 |

*Immunofluorescence test.

†Rheumatoid factor classical tests.

‡Incidence increases with age and females > males.

**Table 19.4.** Spontaneous and induced animal models of autoimmune disease.

| | | MODEL | AUTOIMMUNE DISEASE |
|---|---|---|---|
| **ORGAN-SPECIFIC** | SPONTANEOUS | Nonobese diabetic (NOD) mouse; BB rat<br>Obese strain (OS) chicken; Buffalo rat | Insulin-dependent diabetes<br>Thyroiditis |
| | INDUCED | *Complete Freund's adjuvant incorporating brain<br>*Complete Freund's adjuvant incorporating thyroid,<br>  adrenal, sperm, type II collagen, Ach-R or gbm<br>Cross reaction: heterologous with autologous r.b.c.<br>               Coxsackie B with myosin<br>Thymectomy in 2–4 day old mice<br>Neonatal thymectomy + X-irradiation in rats<br>HgCl$_2$ in rats | Allergic encephalomyelitis<br>Destruction of cell/tissue bearing relevant antigen<br><br>Anemia<br>Myocarditis<br>Widespread organ-specific<br>Thyroiditis<br>'Goodpasture's' |
| **SYSTEMIC** | SPONTANEOUS | New Zealand Black (NZB) mouse strain<br>NZB x W, BXSB<br>MRL/lpr<br>Motheaten mouse strain | Autoimmune hemolytic anemia<br>SLE<br>SLE, arthritis<br>Widespread fatal systemic disease |
| | INDUCED | Parent BM into F1 mice<br>CFA incorporating anti-DNA idiotype<br>CFA incorporating TB hsp | G.v.h., pseudo SLE<br>SLE<br>Adjuvant arthritis |

*Antigen emulsified in water/oil mixture containing killed tubercle bacilli or derivative.

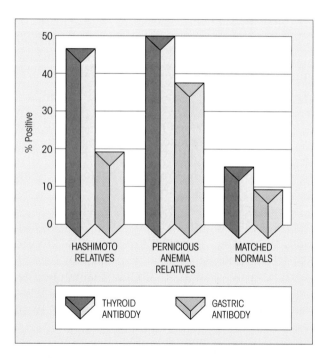

**Figure 19.2. The high incidence of thyroid and gastric autoantibodies in the first degree relatives of patients with Hashimoto's disease or pernicious anemia.** Note the overlap of gastric and thyroid autoimmunity and the higher incidence of gastric autoantibodies in pernicious anemia relatives. In general, titers were much higher in patients than in controls. (Data from Doniach D. & Roitt I.M. (1964) *Seminars in Haematology* **1**, 313.)

affected) in identical than in nonidentical twins. Second, we have already noted that lines of animals have been bred which spontaneously develop autoimmune disease (table 19.4). In other words, **the**

**autoimmunity is genetically programmed**. There is an Obese line of chickens with autoimmune thyroiditis, the nonobese diabetic (NOD) mouse modelling human IDDM and the New Zealand Black (NZB) strain succumbing to autoimmune hemolytic anemia. The hybrid of NZB with another strain, the New Zealand White (B×W hybrid), actually develops antinuclear antibodies including anti-dsDNA and a fatal immune complex-induced glomerulonephritis, key features of human SLE.

These diseases are **genetically complex**. Genome-wide searches for mapping the loci for predisposition to disease by linkage to the many thousand microsatellite markers (polymorphic variable numbers of tandem repeats, VNTR, located by the polymerase chain reaction (PCR) using known flanking sequences), have identified at least 13 susceptibility genes for IDDM and probably more than nine for murine SLE.

Dominant amongst the genetic associations with autoimmune diseases is **linkage to the major histocompatibility complex (MHC)**; of the many examples, we may recall the increased risk of IDDM for DQw8 individuals, and the higher incidence of DR3 in Addison's disease and of DR4 in rheumatoid arthritis (table 17.3, p. 372). Figure 19.3 shows a multiplex family, with IDDM in which the disease is closely linked to a particular HLA-haplotype. Another pointer to the central role of class II structure in determining T-cell responsiveness to self derives from the inability of the NOD mouse to develop pancreatic

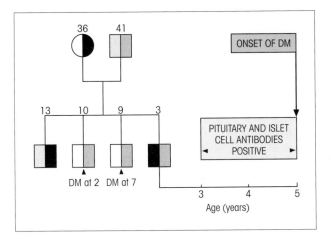

**Figure 19.3. HLA-haplotype linkage and onset of insulin-dependent diabetes (DM).** Haplotypes: ☐ A3, B14, DR6; ■ A3, B7, DR4; ▨ A28, B51, DR4; and ▧ A2, B62, C3, DR4. Disease is linked to possession of the A2, B62, C3, DR4 haplotype. The 3-year-old brother had complement-fixing antibodies to the islet cell surface for 2 years before developing frank diabetes. (From Gorsuch A.N. et al. (1981) Lancet ii, 1363.)

autoimmunity when just a single amino acid residue in the α-helix of the H-2β chain is altered by introduction of a transgene. The close relationship to MHC is not altogether unexpected given that, as we shall see, autoimmune diseases are T-cell-dependent and most T-cell responses are MHC restricted.

Amongst the plethora of non-MHC-linked loci may be genes controlling the pattern of cytokine secretion affecting the milieu in early SLE which permits polyclonal B-cell activation, or influencing the balance of TH1/TH2 subsets which could enhance susceptibility to IDDM or lead to resistance in otherwise predisposed subjects. A mutation in the *IL-2* gene not affecting its functional ability to produce proliferation may be a candidate for *Idd-3* contributing to spontaneous diabetes in the NOD and for *Aod-2* controlling autoimmune ovarian dysgenesis provoked by neonatal thymectomy. Polymorphism at a candidate locus identified in more than one autoimmune disease is interesting. An example is *CTLA-4*, recently linked to IDDM and Graves' disease, both associated with *DR3*. CTLA-4 mediates antigen-specific apoptosis capable of clonally deleting previously activated T-cells, and other 'apoptotic genes' such as *Fas*, *FasL* and *Bcl-2* are all involved in different autoimmune disorders.

Appropriate breeding experiments disclose that the genes predisposing to aggressive autoimmunity, on the one hand, are distinct from those which lead to the selection of autoantigen, on the other. The '**autoimmunity genes**' contribute the common element underlying the overlaps in autoantibodies and disease discussed above, although within this group

the genes which predispose to organ-specific disease must be different from those in nonorgan-specific disorders (as judged by the minimal overlap between them).

Evidence for '**autoantigen selection**' genes derives not only from breeding experiments with NZB×W mice showing separate control of red cell nuclear antibodies, but also from genetic analysis of Obese chickens which has delineated an influence of the MHC, abnormalities in regulatory T-cell control *and* a defect in the thyroid gland expressed as an abnormally high uptake of $^{131}$I (figure 19.4). In the family studies described above (figure 19.2), there must be additional genes which are organ-related in that relatives of patients with pernicious anemia are more prone to gastric autoimmunity than members of Hashimoto kindreds. Further to this point, analysis has mapped the IDDM-2 diabetes susceptibility gene to a VNTR lying 5′ to the insulin gene, which affects the transcriptional activity for insulin production. This could influence the level of thymic expression of insulin during a critical period in the development of self-tolerance, which might subsequently lead to insulin autoreactivity often seen in the early stages of IDDM. (Yes, it looks as though mRNA for a number of 'organ-specific' antigens can be detected in the fetal thymus!)

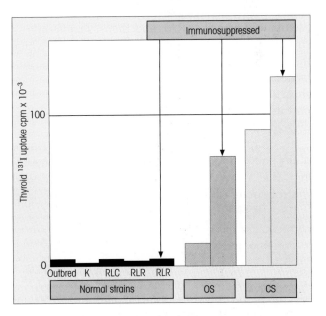

**Figure 19.4. Abnormality in the Obese strain (OS) chicken thyroid.** $^{131}$I uptake in (OS) chickens and the related Cornell strain (CS) from which they were derived, compared with normal strains. Endogenous TSH production was suppressed by administration of thyroxine so that one was measuring TSH-independent $^{131}$I uptake. Immune suppression showed that the abnormally high uptake was not due to immunological stimulation. (From Sundick R.S., Bagchi N., Livezey M.D., Brown T.R. & Mack R.E. (1979) Abnormal thyroid regulation in chickens with autoimmune thyroiditis. Endocrinology (Baltimore) **105**, 493.)

Unravelling complex polygenic conditions is a very tough assignment. If we may take murine SLE as archetypal, genetic analysis of the predisposition to disease is most compatible with a threshold liability model requiring additive contributions of multiple susceptibility genes and dependent on particular allele combinations. These are linked to different stages of disease pathogenesis implying multiple thresholds that must be exceeded, many of which are likely to be influenced by environmental and developmental factors. There is considerable genetic heterogeneity involving a large number of susceptibility genes, different combinations of which predispose to the same phenotype. Many alleles individually make only a small contribution to full expression of disease and in several strains, no particular allele was absolutely required.

## Hormonal influences in autoimmunity

There is a general trend for autoimmune disease to occur far more frequently in women than in men (figure 19.5) probably due, in essence, to differences in hormonal patterns. There is a suggestion that higher estrogen levels are found in patients and administration of male hormones to mice with SLE reduces the severity of disease. Pregnancy is often associated with amelioration of disease severity, particularly in rheumatoid arthritis (RA), and there is sometimes a striking relapse after giving birth, a time at which there are drastic changes in hormones such as prolactin, not forgetting the loss of the placenta. We should also note the frequent development of postpartum hypothyroidism in women with preexisting thyroid autoimmunity.

In Chapter 11, we dwelt on the importance of the neuroendocrine immune feedback encompassing the cytokine–hypothalamic–pituitary–adrenal control circuit. Abnormalities in this feedback loop

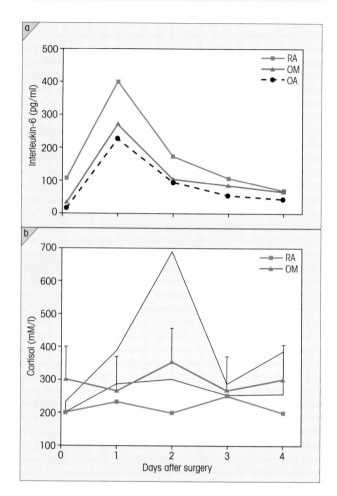

Figure 19.6. Failure of feedback control of cortisol production in rheumatoid arthritis (RA). After surgery (a) RA patients have even higher levels of plasma IL-6 than osteoarthritis and osteomyelitis controls. Nonetheless, (b) they have profoundly deficient production of cortisol which is evidence of faulty feedback control. (Data Kindly provided by Professor G. Panayi from Chikanza I.C. et al. (1992) Defective hypothalamic response to immune and inflammatory stimuli in patients with rheumatoid arthritis. Arthritis & Rheumatism **35**, 1281, with permission from the publishers.)

have now been revealed in several autoimmune disorders. Patients with mild RA have lower corticosteroid levels than normals or patients with osteoarthritis or osteomyelitis despite the presence of inflammation. Moreover, RA patients undergoing surgery manifest grossly inadequate cortisol secretion in the face of high levels of plasma IL-1 and IL-6 (figure 19.6), a phenomenon now attributed to defective hypothalamic control. The OS chicken, several strains of lupus mice and the Lewis rat, which is abnormally susceptible to the induction of autoimmunity, all show blunted IL-1-induced corticosteroid responses. Both T- and B-cells from NOD mice survive for abnormally long periods in culture and their thymocytes are relatively resistant to corticosteroid-induced apoptosis. This would imply that the

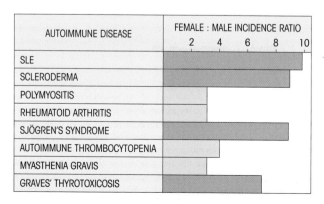

Figure 19.5. Increased incidence of autoimmune disease in females.

feedback cycle is not operating at the lymphocyte level and could cause dysregulated immune function; the ability of IL-1 injections to delay the onset of diabetes would accord with this view.

## Does the environment contribute?

### Twin studies

Although the 50% concordance rate for the development of the autoimmune disease insulin-dependent diabetes mellitus (IDDM) in identical twins is considerably higher than that in dizygotic twins and suggests a strong genetic element, there is still 50% unaccounted for. This is not necessarily all due to environment, since although monozygotic twins have identical germ-line immunoglobulin and T-cell receptor (TCR) genes, the processes of diversification of receptors and of internal anti-idiotype interactions are so complex that the resulting receptor repertoires will be extremely variable and unlikely to be identical. Nonetheless, a later study on concordance rates for IDDM in monozygotic twins gave the extraordinarily high figure of 70% if they were DR3/DR4 heterozygotes, but only 40% if they were not. Thus, in the same disease, the genetic element can be almost completely dominant or be a significant but minor factor in determining the outcome. As we turn to the nonorgan-specific diseases such as SLE we find an even lower genetic contribution with a concordance rate of only 23% in same-sex monozygotic twins, compared with 9% in same-sex dizygotic twins. There are also many examples where clinically unaffected relatives of patients with SLE have a higher incidence of nuclear autoantibodies if they are household contacts than if they live apart from the proband. However, within a given home, the spouse is less likely to develop autoantibodies than blood relatives. Summing up, in some disorders the major factors are genetic, whereas in others, environmental influences seem to dominate.

### Nonmicrobial factors

What environmental agents can we identify? Diet could be one—fish oils containing long-chain, highly polyunsaturated ω-3 fatty acids are reputed to be beneficial for patients with RA; someone must know whether rheumatologists in Greenland are underworked! Sunshine is an undisputed trigger of the skin lesions in SLE. Exposure to organic solvents can initiate the basement membrane autoimmunity which results in Goodpasture's syndrome—witness the high incidence of this disease in HLA-DR2 individuals who work in dry-cleaning shops or syphon petrol from other people's petrol tanks. A more contrived situation is the production of a similar disease in Brown Norway rats by injection of mercuric chloride, but it makes its point, and there are several drug-induced diseases such as SLE, myasthenia gravis, autoimmune hemolytic anemia, and so on.

### Microbes

Of course everyone's favorite environmental agent has to be an infectious microorganism and we do have some clearcut examples of autoimmune disease following infection, usually in genetically predisposed individuals: acute rheumatic fever follows group A streptococcal pharyngitis in 2–3% of patients with a hereditary susceptibility and B3 Coxsackie virus produces autoimmune myositis in certain mouse strains.

In most cases of human chronic autoimmune disease, the problem is the long latency period which makes it difficult to track down the initiating event and, secondly, viable organisms usually cannot be isolated from the affected tissues.

Some groups are focusing down on **very slow-growing forms of mycobacteria** which are exceedingly difficult to culture but appear to be associated with various hypersensitivity states. *M. paratuberculosis* is linked with Jöhne's disease, a chronic granulomatous intestinal infection of cattle similar to Crohn's disease. Genetic probes have identified mycobacterial sequences in sarcoidosis. The granulomatous Takayasu arthritis is often accompanied by very powerful responses to TB. Whipple's disease associated with arthralgias and skin changes evolves so slowly it can often take 10 years for the diagnosis to be made and although organisms can be identified in macrophages at electron microscopy level, none can so far be cultivated. There has been a breakthrough in the HLA-B27 related **reactive arthritis** provoked by infection with *Chlamydia, Yersinia* or *Salmonella*, in that T-cell responses to bacterial fragments present in affected joints can now be demonstrated years after the primary infection.

Given the possibility that we may ultimately identify persistent microorganisms in some disorders, we then have to re-examine the question of whether the hypersensitivity lesions are driven by the microbe or by self-antigen, i.e. are we dealing with a microbially triggered autoimmune disease or autoimmune phenomena secondarily superimposed on an underlying microbial hypersensitivity? Perhaps both circumstances occur. Certainly we know that cross-reactions with microbial components can initiate autoimmunity and recently it has been shown that infection with the helminth *Nippostrongylus brasiliensis* can break tolerance to an unrelated staphylococcal superantigen; perhaps infections of this nature can stimulate such a welter of cytokines as to nonplus and maybe activate anergic, potentially autoreactive T-cells. They can also act as superantigens in bringing about the polyclonal stimulation of certain TCR Vβ families. Further complexity is injected by the knowledge that environmental microbes may sometimes **protect** against spontaneous autoimmune disease; the incidence of diabetes is greatly increased if NOD mice are kept in specific pathogen-free conditions, while Sendai virus inhibits the development of arthritis in the MRL/lpr strain. The extraordinary variation in incidence of diabetes in NOD colonies bred in a wide variety of different animal houses (figure 19.7) testifies to the dramatic influence of environmental flora on the expression of autoimmune disease.

## AUTOREACTIVITY COMES NATURALLY

Tolerance mechanisms do not destroy all self-reactive lymphocytes. Processing of an autoantigen will lead to certain (dominant) peptides being preferentially expressed on antigen-presenting cells (APC) while others (cryptic) only appear in the MHC groove in very low concentrations which may fail to signal for negative selection of the corresponding T-cell in the thymus. Thus autoreactive T-cells specific for **cryptic epitopes** will survive in the repertoire. Also, the reader will recall the B-1 cell population, which starts off early in life by forming a network connected by germ-line idiotypes. The cells are stimulated, presumably by T-independent type 2 idiotypic interactions, to produce so-called '**natural antibodies**', a term applied to those serum antibodies thought to be present before external antigen challenge and therefore arising independently of conventional antigen stimulation. These antibodies are IgM and include a basic set of autoantibodies with low affinity reactivity for multiple specificities and which cross-react with common bacterial antigens usually of a carbohydrate nature. One can see this as a strategy which ensures that preliminary excitation of cells by autoantigens (including idiotypes) will provide bacterial protection, especially since the polymeric nature of the carbohydrate antigens will mean that the IgM antibodies, even though of low affinity, will bind with high avidity to the microbes.

Other functions for these natural antibodies have

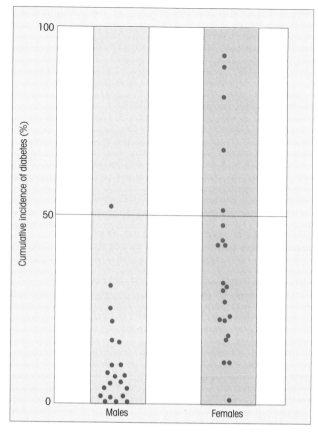

**Figure 19.7. The incidence of spontaneous diabetes in geographically dispersed colonies of NOD mice at 20 weeks of age.** Each point represents a single colony. The extreme spread of values is not attributable to genetic drift to any significant extent. The lower incidence in males is particularly evident. (Data adapted from Pozzilli P, Signore A., Williams A.J.K. & Beales P.E. (1993) NOD mouse colonies around the world. *Immunology Today* **14**, 193–196.)

been proposed which are not mutually exclusive: Grabar viewed them as transporting agents responsible for scavenging effete body components. Others envisage a homeostatic role in which they actually prevent stimulation of autoreactive cells in the conventional B-2 cell population either by masking autoantigen epitopes or by overall idiotype regulation. The latter view receives some encouragement from a report that the IgM fraction of normal serum can block binding of the autologous IgG F(ab')$_2$ fragments to a range of autoantigens; perhaps one should counsel some caution in interpretation of these results because they are based on interaction with solid phase antigens where divalent binding increases avidity and the partial denaturation of protein on the plastic surface exposes internal hydrophobic regions not normally implicated in antibody reactions. This raises an important issue. The IgM autoantibodies produced by the B-1 subset are demonstrable in comparatively low titer in the general population and the incidence of positive results increases steadily with age (figure 19.8) up to around 60–70 years. They are harmless in the sense that they do not cause tissue-damaging hypersensitivity reactions; but under abnormal circumstances, do they give rise to cells which produce the high affinity IgG antibodies characteristic of most autoimmune diseases? This question is difficult to resolve and we will return to it later, but here let us note that in the case of the thyroid and stomach at least, biopsy has indicated that the presence of raised titers of antibody, especially of the IgG class, is almost invariably associated with minor thyroiditis or gastritis lesions (as the case may be), and postmortem examination has identified 10% of middle-aged women with significant degrees of lymphadenoid change in the thyroid, similar in essence to that characteristic of Hashimoto's disease.

As enthusiasts for symmetry and order might have predicted, there appears to be an analogous T-cell population, of phenotype CD3+ CD4⁻8⁻ bearing the B-cell marker B220, containing large internally activated cells which react strongly with self-T-cells and are expanded in early life. It is possible that they connect to the CD5+ B-cell network through idiotype interactions with cells of this lineage present in the thymus. The reader may be surprised to learn that in generating T-cell lines it is not an uncommon experience to isolate cells which proliferate and release IL-2 in response to autologous class II positive feeder cells; even allowing for the fact that the presence of these

feeders in the cultures will tend to select for such autoreactive cells, it would not have been predicted that cells with these specificities would be permitted to roam around freely in the body unless constrained in some way. This brings us back to the ideas of the 'immunological homunculus' in which dominant autoantigens in the body are imprinted on the immune system and the T-cells which recognize them are heavily controlled by regulatory T-cells (cf. p. 209).

Although much evidence suggests that the effector cells of autoimmune disease are present in normal individuals, abnormal conditions must be required for their stimulation. In experimental models of organ-specific disease such as that induced in the thyroid by injection of thyroglobulin in complete Freund's adjuvant, the effector T-cells and the plasma cells making high affinity IgG autoantibodies are generated in normal animals. Complete Freund's will not produce antibodies to double-stranded DNA, Sm or other autoantigens typical of nonorgan-specific disorders and this may be telling us that the appropriate antigen-specific T-cells are not available in the normal repertoire. However, if T-cells are stimulated by radically different approaches, nonorgan-specific antibodies can be coaxed out of normal animals; in one system, allogeneic T-cells inducing a graft-vs-host (g.v.h.) reaction are stimulated by, and thence polyclonally activate, class II-bearing B-cells, while another involves immunization with a public anti-DNA idiotype (16/6) in complete Freund's.

## IS AUTOIMMUNITY DRIVEN BY ANTIGEN?

This is not such a silly question as it might appear since lymphocytes can be stimulated by polyclonal activators and anti-idiotypes as well as by antigen. And if the answer is in the affirmative, is the self molecule an autoimmunogen or just an autoantigen, i.e. does it drive the autoimmune response or is it merely recognized by its products?

### Organ-specific disease

First, some direct evidence straight from the shoulder. The Obese strain (OS) chicken spontaneously develops precipitating IgG autoantibodies to thyroglobulin and a chronic inflammatory antithyroid response which destroys the gland so causing hypothyroidism. If the source of antigen is removed by neonatal thyroidectomy, no autoantibodies are formed. Injection of these animals with normal thyroglobulin then induces antibodies. Thyroidectomy of chickens with

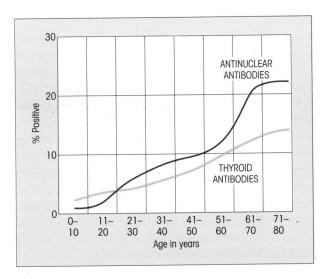

**Figure 19.8. Incidence of autoantibodies in the general population.** A serum was considered positive for thyroid antibodies if it reacted at a dilution of 1/10 in the tanned red cell test or neat in the immunofluorescent test and positive for antinuclear antibodies if it reacted at a dilution of 1/4 by immunofluorescence.

established thyroiditis is followed by a dramatic fall in antibody titer. Conclusions: the spontaneous antithyroglobulin immunity is initiated and maintained by autoantigen from the thyroid gland. Furthermore, since the response is completely T-cell dependent, we can infer both B- and T-cells are driven by thyroglobulin in this model. An entirely parallel study in NOD mice showed that destruction of the β-cells in the pancreas by alloxan, switched off the stimulus to autoantibody production.

As usual, human disease is a tougher nut to crack and one has to rely on more indirect evidence. T-cell lines have been established from thyrotoxic glands and it has been possible to show direct stimulation by whole thyroid cells. The production of high affinity IgG autoantibodies accompanied by somatic mutation is taken as powerful evidence for selection of B-cells by antigen in a T-dependent response. The reason for this, simply, is that high affinity IgG antibodies only arise through mutation and selection by antigen within germinal centers (cf. p. 190). Suffice it to say that ample evidence for somatic mutation and high affinity antibodies has been reported. More indirect is the argument that when antibodies are regularly formed against a cluster of epitopes on a single molecule (e.g. thyroglobulin) or of antigens within a single organ (e.g. thyroglobulin plus thyroid peroxidase), it is difficult to propose a hypothesis which does not depend finally on stimulation by antigen.

## Systemic autoimmunity

The question is even harder to answer here, particularly since antigen removal is impossible. With respect to B-cells, the same arguments marshalled for organ-specific disease obtain, i.e. high affinity mutated IgG autoantibodies directed often to antigen clusters such as the nucleosome.

T-cells are critical for such responses and indeed depletion of CD4 T-cells in NZB or NZB×W mice abrogates autoantibody production. Fine so far, but from there on we are in black box territory since we are woefully ignorant of the antigen specificity of the T-cells. So much so that more radical hypotheses are tendered. One of these postulates that we are really dealing with hypersensitivity responses to microorganisms which are difficult to identify (see above), although one still has to account for the autoantibodies produced and their known pathogenic role in certain diseases (e.g. complexes in SLE). Another view which has been seriously mooted is that the T-cells do not see conventional antigen at all, clearly the

case with DNA responses, but instead are devoted to the recognition of idiotype; SLE for example would be an '**idiotype disease**' resulting from network breakdown. Immunization of mice with monoclonal autoantibodies to DNA, ribonucleoprotein (RNP) and Sm has stimulated production of the corresponding antibody bearing the original idiotype; this must have involved an internal network.

## Is autoantigen available to the lymphocytes?

Our earliest view, with respect to organ-specific antibodies at least, was that the antigens were sequestered within the organ, and through lack of contact with the lymphoreticular system failed to establish immunological tolerance. Any mishap which caused a release of the antigen would then provide an opportunity for autoantibody formation. For a few body constituents this holds true, and in the case of sperm, lens and heart for example, release of certain components directly into the circulation can provoke autoantibodies. But, in general, the experience has been that injection of *unmodified* extracts of those tissues concerned in the organ-specific autoimmune disorders does not readily elicit antibody formation. Indeed detailed investigation of the thyroid autoantigen, thyroglobulin, has disclosed that it is not completely sequestered within the gland but gains access to the extracellular fluid around the follicles and leaves via the thyroid lymphatics (figure 19.9), reaching the serum in normal human subjects at concentrations of approximately 0.01–0.05 mg/ml. In fact, in the majority of cases—e.g. red cells in autoimmune hemolytic anemia, RNP and nucleosome components present as blebs on the surface of apoptotic cells in SLE, and surface receptors in many cases of organ-specific autoimmunity — the autoantigens are readily accessible to circulating lymphocytes.

Presumably, antigens present at adequate concentrations in the extracellular fluid will be processed by professional antigen-presenting cells (APCs), but for autoantigens associated with cells, the derivative peptides will only interact 'meaningfully' with specific T-cells if there are appropriate MHC surface molecules, if the concentration of processed peptide associated with them is significant and, for resting T-cells, if costimulatory signals can be given. As we shall see, these are important constraints.

## CONTROL OF THE T-HELPER CELL IS PIVOTAL

The message then is that we are all sitting on a mine-

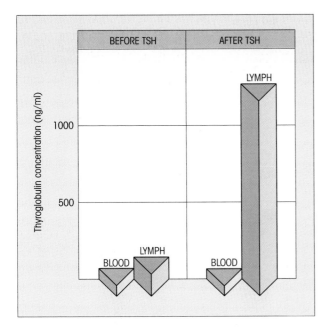

**Figure 19.9. Thyroglobulin in the cervical lymph draining the thyroid in the rat.** The concentration of thyroglobulin is increased after injection of pituitary thyroid-stimulating hormone (TSH), suggesting that the release from thyroid follicles is linked to the physiological activity of the acinar cells. (From Daniel P.N., Pratt D.E., Roitt I.M. & Torrigiani G. (1967) *Quarterly Journal of Experimental Physiology* **52**, 184.)

field of self-reactive cells, with potential access to their respective autoantigens, but since autoimmune disease is more the exception than the rule, the body has homeostatic mechanisms to prevent them being triggered under normal circumstances. Accepting its limitations, figure 19.10 provides a framework for us to examine ways in which these mechanisms may be circumvented to allow autoimmunity to develop. It is assumed that the key to the system is control of the autoreactive T-helper cell since the evidence heavily favors the T-dependence of virtually all autoimmune responses; thus, interaction between the T-cell and MHC-associated peptide becomes the core consideration. We start with the assumption that these cells are

unresponsive because of clonal deletion, clonal anergy, T-suppression or inadequate autoantigen presentation.

## AUTOIMMUNITY CAN ARISE THROUGH BYPASS OF T-HELPERS

### Provision of new carrier determinant

Allison and Weigle argued independently that if autoreactive T-cells are tolerized and thereby unable to collaborate with B-cells to generate autoantibodies (figure 19.11a), provision of new carrier determinants to which no self-tolerance had been established would bypass this mechanism and lead to autoantibody production (figure 19.11b).

### 1 Modification of the autoantigen

A new carrier could arise through some modification to the molecule, for example by defects in synthesis or by an abnormality in lysosomal processing yielding a split product exposing some new groupings (figure 19.11b.1). Experimentally it has been found that large proteolytic fragments of thyroglobulin are autoantigenic when injected alone but no evidence for such a mechanism has yet been uncovered in man. In fact many studies on spontaneous autoimmune disease have failed to reveal an abnormality in the antigen. Remember the experiment in which neonatal thyroidectomized Obese strain chickens make autoantibodies if injected with thyroglobulin prepared from *normal* chickens, suggesting that the immunological response rather than the antigen is abnormal. Nonetheless, there may be defects in the iodine metabolism of the gland itself in this strain and recent work has shown that the severity of thyroiditis is ameliorated when the birds are put on a low iodine diet. There might also be more subtle changes in glycosylation patterns which are not picked up by

**Figure 19.10. Autoimmunity arises through bypass of the control of autoreactivity.** The constraints on the stimulation of self-reactive helper T-cells by autoantigen can be circumvented either through bypassing the helper cell or by disturbance of the regulatory mechanisms.

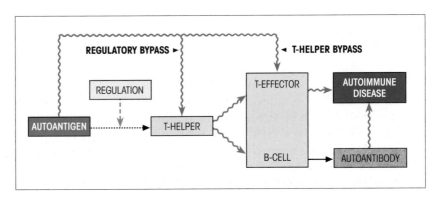

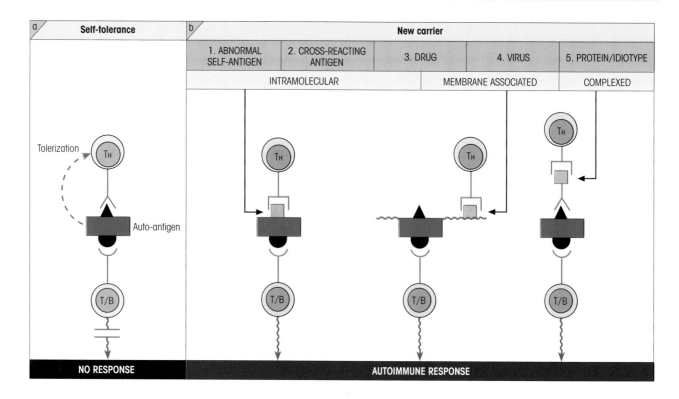

**Figure 19.11. T-helper bypass through new carrier epitope (▢) generates autoimmunity.** For simplicity, processing for MHC association has been omitted from the diagram, but is elaborated in figure 19.12. (a) The pivotal autoreactive T-helper is unresponsive either through tolerance or inability to see a cryptic epitope. (b) Different mechanisms providing a new carrier epitope.

the available serological reagents, the most exciting example being the low galactosylation of the Fcγ sugar chains in rheumatoid arthritis, to be discussed later.

Incorporation into Freund's complete adjuvant frequently endows many autologous proteins with the power to induce autoallergic disease in laboratory animals. It is conceivable that the physical constraints on the proteins at the water–oil interface of the emulsion provide the required alteration in configuration of the 'carrier portions' of the molecules although the intense production of cytokines is likely to be the major influence.

Modification can also be achieved through combination with a drug (figure 19.11b.3). The autoimmune hemolytic anemia associated with administration of α-methyldopa might be attributable to modification of the red-cell surface in such a way as to provide a carrier for stimulating B-cells which recognize the rhesus antigen. This is normally regarded as a 'weak' antigen and would be less likely to induce B-cell tolerance than the 'stronger' antigens present on the ery-

throcyte. Isoniazid may produce arthritis associated with nuclear antibodies and, unlike most other cases of drug-induced autoimmunity, synthesis of these antibodies is said to continue after cessation of drug therapy. A high proportion of patients on continued treatment with procainamide develop nuclear antibodies and 40% present with clinical signs of SLE. Myasthenia gravis and symptoms of pemphigus have been described in some patients on penicillamine. It is not clear in every case whether the drug provides carrier help through direct modification of the autoantigen or of some independent molecule concerned in associative recognition.

## 2 Cross-reactions with B-cell epitopes

Many examples are known in which potential human autoantigenic B-cell epitopes are present on a microbial exogenous cross-reacting antigen which provides the new carrier that provokes autoantibody formation (figure 19.11b.2). The mechanism is spelt out in more detail in figure 19.12a. Two low molecular weight envelope proteins of *Yersinia enterolytica* share epitopes with the extracellular domain of the human thyroid-stimulating hormone (TSH) receptor; in rheumatic fever, antibodies produced to the *Streptococcus* also react with heart, and the sera of 50% of children with the disease who develop Sydenham's chorea give neuronal immunofluorescent staining which can be absorbed out with streptococcal membranes. Colon antibodies present in ulcerative colitis have been found to cross-react with *Escherichia coli* 014. There is also some evidence for the view that antigens common to *Trypanosoma cruzi* and cardiac muscle and peripheral nervous system provoke some of the immunopathological lesions seen in Chagas' disease.

### 3 Molecular mimicry of T-cell epitopes

The drawback with the Allison–Weigle model of

cross-reaction of B-cell epitopes and provision of a new T-cell carrier is that once the cross-reacting agent is eliminated from the body, and with it the T-cell epitope, the only way that the autoimmunity can be sustained is for the activated B-cell to capture circulating autoantigen and after processing, present it to the T-helper (figure 19.12c). This is not possible for **cell-associated antigens** but their special link with T-cell recognition puts them in a totally different ballpark. In this case, if an infecting agent mimics an autoantigen by producing a **cross-reacting T-cell epitope**, the resulting T-cell autoimmunity could theoretically

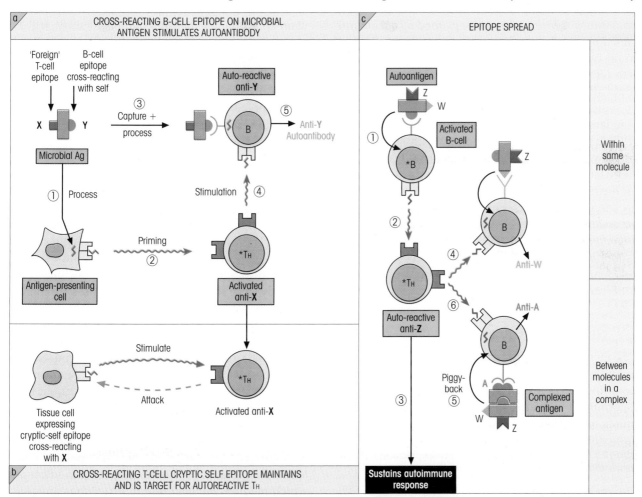

**Figure 19.12. Mechanisms of microbial induction of autoimmunity and epitope spread**. (a) A microbial antigen bearing an epitope Y which cross-reacts with self and a foreign T-cell epitope X is (1) processed by an antigen-presenting cell, (2) activates the T-helper which (3) recognizes the processed X after capture by an anti-Y B-cell and (4) stimulates the B-cell to secrete anti-Y autoantibody. (b) The *activated* anti-X T-helper as distinct from the *resting* cell, may recognize and be stimulated by a cross-reacting cryptic T-cell epitope expressed by a tissue cell. This will maintain the autoimmune response even after elimination of the microbe, because of the persistence of the self-epitope. The tissue expressing the epitope will also be a target for immunological attack. Note also that a T-helper primed nonspecifically by a polyclonal superantigen activator could also fulfil the same function of responding to a cryptic epitope. (c) If the autoantigen is soluble or capable of uptake and processing after capture by the activated autoreactive B-cell (1) (either from (a) or through nonspecific polyclonal activation), a new epitope can be presented on the B-cell class II which now stimulates an autoreactive (anti-Z) T-helper (2) which can now sustain an autoimmune response entirely through autoantigen stimulation (3). It can also produce epitope spread within the same molecule through helping a B-cell which captures the autoantigen through a new epitope W (4). It can also permit epitope spread to another component in an intermolecular complex such as nucleosomal histone/DNA or idiotype positive (Id+) anti-DNA/DNA which is 'piggy-backed' into the B-cell (5) which presents processed antigen to the T-helper (6) in the cases cited, specific for histone or Id respectively. (This is a complex mouthful but digestion is recommended because these ideas are crucial.)

persist even after elimination of the infection. The autoantigen will normally be presented to the resting autoreactive T-cell as a **cryptic epitope** and by definition will be unable to provide an activating signal. The cross-reacting infectious agent will provide abundant antigen on professional APCs which can prime the T-cell and upregulate its adhesion molecules so that it now has the **avidity** to bind to and be persistently activated by the cryptic self epitope presented on the target tissue cell provided that is associated with the appropriate MHC molecule (figure 19.12b). Remember the transgenic cytotoxic T-cells (Tc) which could only destroy the pancreatic β-cells bearing a viral transgene when they were **primed** by a real viral infection (cf. figure 12.9). Also the tumor cells that could only be recognized by primed not resting T-cells (cf. figure 18.10). Theoretically the resting T-cell could also be primed in a nonantigen-specific manner by a microbial **superantigen**.

A large number of microbial peptide sequences with varying degrees of homology with human proteins have been identified (table 19.5) but it should be emphasized at this stage that they only provide clues for further study. The mere existence of a homology is no certainty that infection with that organism will necessarily lead to autoimmunity because everything depends on the manner in which the proteins are processed by the APCs and we cannot predict, as yet, which peptides will be presented and in what concentration.

### 4 'Piggy-back' T-cell epitopes and epitope spread

One membrane component may provide help for the immune response to another (associative recognition). In the context of autoimmunity, a new helper determinant may arise through drug modification as mentioned above, or through the insertion of viral

Table 19.5. Molecular mimicry: homologies between microbes and body components as potential cross-reacting T-cell epitopes.

| Microbial molecule | Body component |
|---|---|
| **Bacteria:** | |
| Arthritogenic *Shigella flexneri* | HLA-B27 |
| *Klebsiella* nitrogenase | HLA-B27 |
| *Proteus mirabilis* urease | HLA-DR4 |
| *Mycobact. tuberculosis* 65 kDa hsp | Joint (adjuvant arthritis) |
| | |
| **Viruses:** | |
| Coxsackie B | Myocardium |
| Coxsackie B | Glutamic acid decarboxylase |
| EBV gp110 ⎱ | RA shared Dw4 T-cell epitope |
| *E.coli* DNAJ hsp ⎰ | |
| HBV octamer | Myelin basic protein |
| HSV glycoprotein | Acetylcholine receptor |
| Measles hemagglutinin | T-cell subset |
| Retroviral gag p32 | U-1 RNA |

antigen into the membrane of an infected cell (cf. figure 19.11b.4). That this can promote a reaction to a preexisting cell component is clear from the studies in which infection of a tumor with influenza virus elicited resistance to uninfected tumor cells. The appearance of cold agglutinins often with blood group I specificity after *Mycoplasma pneumonia* infection could have a similar explanation. In a comparable fashion, T-cell help can be provided for a molecule such as DNA, which cannot itself form a T-cell epitope, by complexing with a T-dependent carrier, in this example a histone, or an anti-DNA idiotype to which T-cells were sensitized. For this mechanism to work, the helper component must still be physically attached to the fragment bearing the B-cell epitope. When this is recognized by the B-cell receptor the helper component will be 'piggy-backed' into the B-cell, processed and presented as an epitope for recognition by T-cells (figure 19.12c). By the same token, the autoimmune response can spread to other epitopes on the same molecule.

### Idiotype bypass mechanisms

We have argued the evidence for internal regulated idiotype networks involving self-reactivity at some length. This raises the possibility of involving autoreactive lymphocytes with responses to exogenous agents through idiotype network connections, particularly since some autoimmune diseases are characterized by major cross-reactive idiotypes.

Thus, knowing that T-helpers with specificity for the idiotype on a lymphocyte receptor can be instrumental in the stimulation of that cell, it is conceivable that an environmental agent such as a parasite or virus which triggered antibody carrying a public idiotype (CRI) which happened to be shared with the receptor of an autoreactive T- or B-cell, could provoke an autoimmune response (figure 19.13b). Similarly, if it is correct that the germ-line idiotypes on autoantibodies generate a whole range of anti-idiotypes which mediate the response to exogenous antigens, then by the same token, it is conceivable that antibodies produced in response to an infection may react with the corresponding idiotype on the autoreactive lymphocyte (figure 19.13b). For example, a hybridoma from a myasthenia gravis patient secreted an anti-Id to an acetylcholine receptor autoantibody; this anti-Id was found to react with the bacterial product 1,3-dextran (figure 19.13a). Finally, it is possible for Id network interactions to allow a viral infection to give rise to autoantibodies reacting with the viral receptor (figure 19.13c). Since viruses all bind to

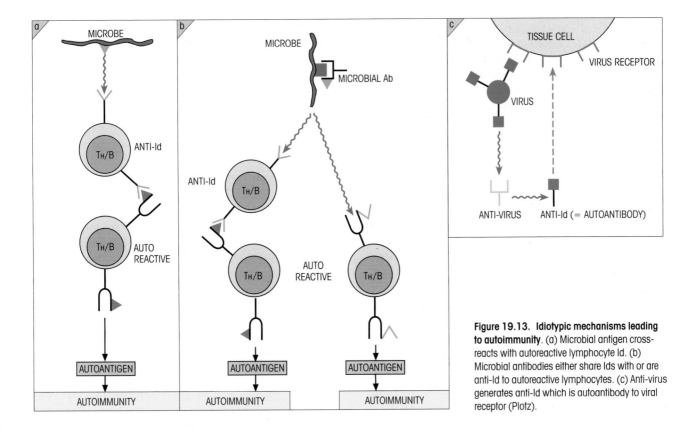

**Figure 19.13. Idiotypic mechanisms leading to autoimmunity.** (a) Microbial antigen cross-reacts with autoreactive lymphocyte Id. (b) Microbial antibodies either share Ids with or are anti-Id to autoreactive lymphocytes. (c) Anti-virus generates anti-Id which is autoantibody to viral receptor (Plotz).

specific complementary receptors on the cells they infect, this sequence of events may have serious consequences; we note for example that β-adrenergic receptors are the surface targets for certain reoviruses and that rabies virus binds to the acetylcholine receptor.

## Polyclonal activation

Microbes often display adjuvant properties through their possession of polyclonal lymphocyte activators such as bacterial endotoxins which act by providing a nonspecific inductive signal for B-cell stimulation, so bypassing the need for specific T-cell help (cf. p. 174). This can occur by direct interaction with the B-lymphocyte or indirectly through stimulating the secretion of nonspecific factors from T-cells or macrophages. The variety of autoantibodies detected in cases with infectious mononucleosis must surely be attributable to the polyclonal activation of B-cells by the Epstein–Barr (EB) virus. They are seen also in lepromatous leprosy where the abundance of mycobacteria reproduces some of the features of Freund's adjuvant. However, unlike the usual situation in human autoimmune disease, these autoantibodies tend to be IgM and, normally, do not persist when the microbial components are cleared from the body. It is

likely that the reactions largely involve B-1 cells. Curiously, lymphocytes from many patients with SLE and from mice with spontaneous lupus produce abnormally large amounts of IgM when cultured *in vitro* as if they were under polyclonal activation. Nevertheless it is difficult to see how a pan-specific polyclonal activation could give rise to the patterns of autoantibodies characteristic of the different autoimmune disorders without the operation of some antigen-directing factor. We have already hinted at scenarios in which polyclonally activated B- or T-cells might contribute to a sustained autoimmune response (see legend figure 19.12b and c).

## AUTOIMMUNITY CAN ARISE THROUGH BYPASS OF REGULATORY MECHANISMS

### Regulatory cells try to damp down autoimmunity

It should be emphasized that these T-helper bypass mechanisms for the induction of autoimmunity do not by themselves ensure the continuation of the response, since normal animals have been shown to be capable of damping down autoantibody production through regulatory T-cell interactions as, for example, in the case of red cell autoantibodies induced in mice by injection of rat erythrocytes (figure 19.14). When T-suppressor activity is impaired by low doses of cyclophosphamide or if strains like the SJL which have prematurely ageing suppressors are used, autoimmunity is prolonged and more severe. Yet another example is the protection against autoimmune diabetes and thyroiditis which develop in irradiated adult thymectomized rats, by injection of CD4, CD45RB[lo], RT6+ T-cells from a normal donor; this is the phenotype of a primed but nonactivated set which includes cells capable of secreting IL-4. Depletion of CD25-positive cells in normal mice provoked the appearance of various types of autoimmunity. From another tack, small numbers of an encephalitogenic T-cell clone **vaccinated** normal recipients against the pathogenic consequences of a subsequent higher dose, hinting strongly at anti-idiotypic control.

Regulatory cells can also be picked out in spontaneously autoimmune strains of mice such as the NOD. Transfer of disease from splenocytes of recently diabetic NOD mice into NOD-SCID congenics could be inhibited by the CD4, CD45RB[lo] (memory) splenic subset of young nondiabetic animals. Along the same lines, it was shown long ago that Coombs' positivity (i.e. the state in which circulating red cells are coated with antibody) can be transferred with the spleen cells of a Coombs' positive NZB to a *young, negative mouse* of the same strain, but the continued production of

red cell antibodies is short-lived unless the recipient's T-cells are first depleted by pretreatment with anti-lymphocyte serum.

## Neonatal thymectomy deletes potential self-regulators

We are surely nodding our grudging assent to the idea that in general, manipulations which reduce regulatory T-cells encourage the development of autoantibodies. Even so, the effect of thymectomy within a narrow window of 2–4 days after birth in the mouse is quite startling in that it gives rise to widespread organ-specific autoimmune disease affecting mainly stomach, thyroid, ovary, prostate and sperm; circulating antibodies are frequently detected and deposits of Ig and complement are often seen around the basement membranes. Spleen cells from intact adult males but not females injected into these 3-day thymectomized mice can prevent the development of prostatitis although both are able to prevent gastritis, from which one concludes that the normal male has additional suppressor T-cells specific for prostate and activated by prostate antigens. We have alluded earlier to the evidence for intrathymic expression of mRNA for a whole set of nominally organ-specific antigens such as insulin, thyroglobulin and myelin basic protein. Presumably the thymus is producing potential organ-specific suppressors between days 2 and 4 and at that time thymectomy upsets the balance between autoreactive and suppressor cells.

If neonatal thymectomy really does greatly deplete the T-suppressor population, the induction or exacerbation of spontaneous autoimmune states in susceptible animals—autoimmune hemolytic anemia in NZB mice and thyroiditis in Obese strain chickens and Buffalo rats—is not entirely unexpected.

## Defects in regulatory cells contribute to spontaneous autoimmunity

The power of normal cells to check the diabetogenic capability of NOD splenocytes and the inability of the NZB to normalize the experimental induction of red cell autoimmunity (figure 19.14) are strong pointers. A progressive loss of regulatory cells with age may account for the increasing resistance to the induction of tolerance to soluble proteins in elderly NZB mice, apparently associated with a sudden fall in the plasma concentration of the thymic peptide thymulin before the onset of disease (note: thymulin is said to inhibit the autoreactive response of spleen cells to syngeneic fibroblasts in culture).

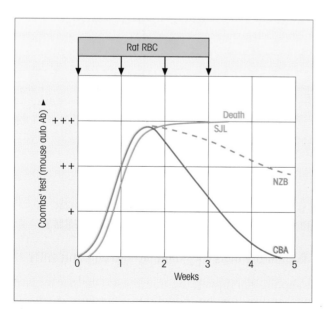

**Figure 19.14. Regulation of self-reactivity.** When CBA strain mice are injected with rat red cells, autoantibodies are produced by this cross-reacting antigen (see p. 414) which coat the host erythrocytes and are detected by the Coombs' antiglobulin test (see p. 340). The SJL strain, in which suppressor activity declines rapidly with age, is unable to regulate the autoimmune response and develops particularly severe disease. The response is also prolonged in the autoimmune NZB strain. (After A. Cooke & P. Hutchings.)

Is there any relationship of defects in apoptotic mechanisms to these regulatory changes? T- and B-cells of NOD mice are resistant to apoptosis, as are lymphocytes of the MRL/lpr lupus mouse strain which has a *fas* gene mutation. This mutation produces the characteristic lymphoproliferation, and possibly failure to eliminate self-reactive B-cells by apoptosis which orchestrates the autoimmune pathology. The *gld* lupus model complements this with mutations in the *fas* ligand.

We have previously drawn attention to the distinctive properties of the B-1 population with respect to its propensity to synthesize IgM autoantibodies and its possible intimate relationship to the setting up of the regulatory idiotype network (cf. p. 209), and one must seriously entertain the hypothesis that unregulated activity by these cells could be responsible for certain autoimmune disorders. The pitifully named motheaten strain is heavily into autoimmunity, and the mice make masses of anti-DNA and anti-polymorphs and die with intense pneumonitis, often before they have tasted the fruits of life. They exhibit reduced catalytic activity of their protein tyrosine phosphatase 1C due to mutation. Their IgM levels rise to a staggering level of 25–50 times normal and—this is quite bizarre—their B-cells are nearly all CD5+, i.e. B-1. This population is also raised in the NZB and largely accounts for the production of the IgM autoantibodies in this strain. Now here is a persuasive experiment. When transgenes encoding an NZB red cell autoantibody were introduced into normal mice, no B-2 cells were present and 50% developed autoimmune disease. Intraperitoneal injection of erythrocytes deleted the B-1 cells and prevented disease. This tells us that the NZB hemolytic anemia is due to red blood cell autoantibodies produced by B-1 cells, that this population is only tolerized properly when the antigen gains access to the peritoneum where they develop, and that some (around 50%), but not all, animals can control the autoreactive clones. Whether B-1 cells escape regulatory control and undergo an unrestrained isotype switch to the pathogenic IgG antibodies responsible for disease in other models such as the NZB×W is still a question on which the jury's verdict is awaited, although depletion of B-1 lymphocytes greatly reduces the immune complex glomerulonephritis. The IdD-23 idiotype characteristic of natural autoantibodies has been identified on a monoclonal IgG anti-DNA—but one idiotype doesn't make a summer, if I can misquote a well-known saying!

In man, a high proportion of B-1 cells make IgM rheumatoid factors (anti-Fcγ) and anti-DNA using germ-line genes. In rheumatoid arthritis patients, although there are increased numbers of circulating B-1 cells, the polyclonal rheumatoid factors synthesized do not, by and large, bear the public idiotypes of this subset. SLE could be different because the 16/6 public idiotype associated with germ-line genes encoding anti-DNA is found on a significant fraction of the IgG anti-DNA in patients' serums. Gene sequencing is required to establish the relationship between B-1 cells and IgG autoantibody synthesis.

Aside from the defective IL-1/6-hypothalamic feedback loop giving rise to low corticosteroid levels in rheumatoid arthritis described earlier (cf. figure 19.6), less is known of regulatory circuits in man, although there is increasing evidence that nonspecific T-suppressor function in SLE may be poorly regulated. B-lymphocytes from patients with active disease secrete larger amounts of Ig when cultured *in vitro* than normal B-cells. Concanavalin-A-induced nonspecific suppressors are reduced or absent and T-cells with Fcγ receptors, which suppress pokeweed mitogen-stimulated lymphocytes are low, the defect being greater the more active the disease. The production of thymulin and of IL-2 is also depressed in these patients. A significant proportion of clinically unaffected close relatives also demonstrate abnormally low levels of nonspecific suppressors, indicating that the deficit in SLE patients is not a consequence of the illness or its treatment and that additional factors must be implicated in the causation of disease.

In any case, it is difficult to account for the antigenic specificity of different autoimmune disorders on the basis of a generalized depression of nonspecific suppressors *alone*, without invoking defects in either antigen- or idiotype-specific suppressor T-cells. There is, however, a further possibility which has aroused much interest.

## Upregulation of T-cell interaction molecules

The majority of organ-specific autoantigens normally appear on the surface of the cells of the target organ in the context of class I but not class II MHC molecules. As such they cannot communicate with T-helpers and are therefore immunologically silent. Pujol-Borrell, Bottazzo and colleagues reasoned that if the class II genes were somehow derepressed and class II molecules were now synthesized, they would endow the surface molecules with potential autoantigenicity (figure 19.15). Indeed, they have been able to show that human thyroid cells in tissue culture can be persuaded to express HLA-DR (class II) molecules on their surface after stimulation with γ-interferon

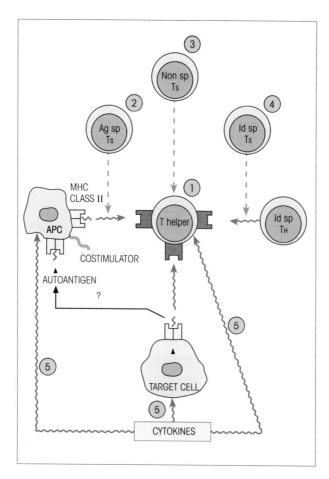

**Figure 19.15. Bypass of regulatory mechanisms leads to triggering of autoreactive T-helper cells through defects** in (1) tolerizability or ability to respond to or induce T-suppressors, or (2) expression of antigen-specific, (3) nonspecific or (4) idiotype-specific T-suppressors, or through (5) imbalance of the cytokine network producing derepression of class II genes with inappropriate cellular expression of class II and presentation of antigen on target cell, stimulation of APC, and possible activation of anergic T-helper. The beneficial effect of pooled whole Ig in certain human autoimmune diseases such as idiopathic thrombocytopenic purpura and of T-cell vaccination in experimental allergic encephalomyelitis (EAE) and adjuvant arthritis in rats lend weight to the idea of idiotype control mechanisms. Evidence for a regulatory CD4 subset comes from studies reporting inflammatory infiltrates in liver, lung, stomach, thyroid and pancreas in athymic rats reconstituted with CD45RBhi/CD4 T-cells but not with unfractionated or CD45RBlo CD4 cells (presumably the regulators).

(IFNγ), and, further, that the cytoplasm of epithelial cells from the glands of patients with Graves' disease (thyrotoxicosis) stains strongly with anti-HLA-DR reagents, indicating active synthesis of class II polypeptide chains (figure 19.1b). Inappropriate class II expression has also been reported on the bile ductules in primary biliary cirrhosis and on endothelial cells and some β-cells in the diabetic pancreas both in the human and in the BB rat model.

Whether adventitious expression of class II on these cells by something like virally induced IFN is responsible for *initiating* the autoimmune process by priming autoreactive T-helpers, or whether reaction with *already activated* T-cells induces class II by release of IFNγ and makes the cell a more attractive target for provoking subsequent tissue damage, is still an unresolved issue. However, transfection of mice with the class II *H-2A* genes linked to the insulin-promoter led to expression of class II on the β-islet cells of the pancreas but did *not* induce autoimmunity. Lack of B7 costimulatory molecules could be responsible for the failure of these class II positive β-cells to activate naive T-cells, a job which may have to be left to the professional APCs.

## Cytokine imbalance may induce autoimmunity

In contrast, transfection with the IFNγ gene on the insulin promoter under the same circumstances produced a local inflammatory reaction in the pancreas with aberrant expression of class II *and* diabetes; this must have been a result of autoimmunity since a normal pancreas grafted into the same animal suffered a similar fate. This implies that unregulated cytokine production producing a local inflammatory reaction can initiate autoimmunity perhaps by increasing the concentration of processed intracellular autoantigens available to professional APCs and increasing their avidity for naive T-cells by upregulating adhesion molecules, or even by making previously anergic cells responsive to antigen (figure 19.15(5)). Once primed, the T-cells can now interact with the islet β-cells which will display increased amounts of class II and adhesion molecules for T-cells on their surface.

We can correct some spontaneous models of autoimmune disease by injection of cytokines: IL-1 cures the diabetes of NOD mice and tumor necrosis factor (TNF) prevents the onset of SLE symptoms in NZB×W hybrids. Transforming growth factor-β1 (TGFβ1) is known to protect against collagen arthritis and relapsing experimental allergic encephalomyelitis (EAE) and, interestingly, 'knockout' mice lacking TGFβ develop multifocal inflammatory disease, although at the time of writing we do not know whether this is due to autoimmunity.

Detailed studies have been made of cytokine synthesis in the battleground of the joint in rheumatoid arthritis. Cultures of synovial cells spontaneously produce high levels of IL-6, TNFα and GM-CSF which strongly activate macrophages, but very little IFNγ or TNFβ even though mRNA was present (perhaps due to TGF?). Does this hot-bed of chronic inflammation nurture the seeds of persistent autoimmune reactivity?

## AUTOIMMUNE DISORDERS ARE MULTIFACTORIAL

I must come back to this. Undoubtedly, the autoimmune diseases have a multifactorial etiology. Perhaps most, if not all, the defects we have discussed may contribute in various combinations to different disorders. Although these defects individually may be not uncommon, their origin remains obscure. Superimposed upon a genetically complex susceptibility, we might be dealing with some ageing process affecting the thymus or the lymphoid stem cells and their internal control of self-reactivity. Sex hormones and defective pituitary adrenal feedback loops may contribute. Now throw into this melange a panoply of environmental factors particularly microbial agents which could have a variety of effects on the target organs, the lymphoid system and the cytokine network.

---

## SUMMARY

The immune system balances precariously between effective responses to environmental antigens and regulatory control of an array of potentially suicidal self molecules.

### The scope of autoimmune diseases

• Autoimmunity is associated with certain diseases which form a spectrum. At one pole, exemplified by Hashimoto's thyroiditis, the autoantibodies and the lesions are **organ-specific** with the organ acting as the target for autoimmune attack; at the other pole are the **nonorgan-specific** or **systemic autoimmune diseases** such as SLE where the autoantibodies have widespread reactivity and the lesions resemble those of serum sickness relating to deposition of circulating immune complexes.
• There is a tendency for organ-specific disorders such as thyroiditis and pernicious anemia to overlap in given individuals, while overlap of rheumatological disorders is greater than expected by chance.
• There are a number of models of organ-specific and systemic autoimmune diseases which occur spontaneously (e.g. nonobese diabetic mice or NZB×W hybrids with SLE) or can be induced experimentally (e.g. thyroiditis by thyroglobulin in complete Freund's adjuvant (CFA) and perhaps SLE by immunization with Id+ anti-DNA monoclonal in CFA).

### Genetic and environmental influences

• Multifactorial genetic factors increase predisposition to autoimmune disease: these include HLA tissue type, the predisposition to aggressive autoimmunity and the selection of potential autoantigens.
• Females have a far higher incidence of autoimmunity than males, perhaps due to hormonal influences.
• Feedback control of lymphocytes through the cytokine–hypothalamus–pituitary and adrenal loop may be defective as shown for rheumatoid arthritis.
• Twin studies indicate a strong environmental influence in many disorders; both microbial and nonmicrobial factors have been suspected.

### Autoreactivity comes naturally

• B-1 cells form a pool of mutually stimulating cells spontaneously producing 'natural antibodies' which interact idiotypically and frequently show multispecific autoreactivity.
• The immune system appears to have a set of T-cells directed to a limited number of dominant autoantigens which are tightly controlled.

### Is autoimmunity driven by antigen?

• In spontaneous models of diabetes and thyroiditis, removal of antigen prevents autoimmunity.
• The development of high affinity mutated antibodies and immune responses to clusters of anatomically related antigens, strongly imply B-cell selection of autoantigen.
• T-cell specificities in systemic autoimmunity are unknown but may be anti-idiotype.
• Autoantigens are, for the most part, accessible to circulating lymphocytes which normally include autoreactive T- and B-cells. Dominant autoantigens will induce tolerance but T-cells specific for peptides presented at low concentrations (cryptic epitopes) will be potentially autoreactive.

### The T-helper is pivotal for control

• It is assumed that the key to the system is control of autoreactive T-helper cells which are normally unresponsive because of clonal deletion, clonal anergy, T-suppression or inadequate autoantigen processing.

(Continued on p. 422)

### Autoimmunity can arise through bypass of T-helpers

• Abnormal modification of the autoantigen through synthesis or breakdown, cross-reaction with exogenous antigens, or 'piggy-back' recognition of T-helper epitopes, can provide new carrier determinants and epitope spread.

• T-helpers could also be bypassed by idiotype network interactions with cross-reactions between public idiotypes on autoantibodies and microbial antibodies or microbes themselves, or by antibodies formed to antiviral idiotypes which behaved as internal images of the virus and reacted with the cell surface viral receptor.

• Finally, B-cells and T-cells can be stimulated directly by polyclonal activators such as EB virus or superantigens.

### Autoimmunity can arise through bypass of regulatory mechanisms

• T-helper bypass alone may be insufficient to *maintain* autoimmunity and it is generally considered that, in addition, a defect in cells which normally regulate autoimmunity is required.

• This could occur through an inability of the central T-helper cell to be tolerized or to respond to or induce T-suppressors.

• It could also arise through defects in antigen-specific, idiotype-specific and nonspecific T-suppressor systems.

• Another possibility would be the derepression of class II genes giving rise to inappropriate cellular expression of class II so breaking the 'silence' between cellular autoantigen and autoreactive T-inducer.

• This would make the cell a target for activated T-cells but without costimulators such as B7, perhaps only professional APCs could prime the resting autoreactive T-cell.

• Cytokine imbalance provides the circumstances for this to occur.

### Autoimmune disorders are multifactorial

• Given the genetic predisposition, these changes could come about by some spontaneous internal dysregulation related perhaps to ageing, and/or through environmental factors, particularly microbes, which could act in an uncomfortably large number of different ways.

## FURTHER READING

Suggestions for further reading are given at the end of the following chapter.

# CHAPTER 20

# AUTOIMMUNE DISEASES
## 2—Pathogenesis, Diagnosis and Treatment

## CONTENTS

We have mentioned that despite certain exceptions as, for instance, myocardial infarction or damage to the testis, traumatic release of organ constituents does not in general elicit antibody formation. Destruction of thyroid tissue by therapeutic doses of radioiodine does not initiate thyroid autoimmunity, nor does damage to the liver in alcoholic cirrhosis result in the synthesis of mitochondrial antibodies, to give but two examples. We should now look at the evidence which bears directly on the issue of whether autoimmunity, however it arises, plays a **primary pathogenic role** in the production of tissue lesions in the group of diseases labeled as 'autoimmune'.

## PATHOGENIC EFFECTS OF HUMORAL AUTOANTIBODY

### Blood

The erythrocyte antibodies play a dominant role in the destruction of red cells in **autoimmune hemolytic anemia**. Normal red cells coated with autoantibody eluted from Coombs' positive erythrocytes (cf. figure 16.13) have a shortened half-life after reinjection into the normal subject, essentially as a result of their adherence to Fcγ receptors on phagocytic cells in the spleen. Remember also that B-1 cells in a mouse bearing a transgene encoding the New Zealand Black mouse (NZB) red cell autoantibody cause hemolytic disease (cf. p. 419). To put the case for B-1 cells beyond all reasonable doubt, any manipulation of NZB mice which eliminates these cells such as intraperitoneal injection of water, treatment with anti-interleukin (IL)-10 or introduction of the *xid* gene, prevents the development of hemolytic anemia.

Some children with immunodeficiency associated with very low white cell counts have a serum lymphocytotoxic factor which requires complement for its activity. Lymphopenia occurring in patients with systemic lupus erythematosus (SLE) and rheumatoid arthritis (RA) may also be a direct result of antibody, since nonagglutinating antibodies coating the white cells have been reported in such cases.

Although the antibodies to proteinase III (antineutrophil cytoplasmic antibodies (cANCA); figure 20.1 and table 19.2) characteristic of **Wegener's granulomatosis** are directed to an intracellular antigen associated with the primary granules of the polymorph, recent studies reveal a possible mechanism by which they might induce vasculitic lesions. Cytokine priming of polymorphs causes translocation of proteinase III to the cell surface, whereupon reaction with the autoantibody activates the cell causing degranulation and generation of reactive oxygen intermediates (ROI). A possible scenario might go something like this: tumour necrosis factor (TNF) induced by infec-

tion could activate endothelial cells to secrete interleukins IL-1 and IL-8 which attract neutrophils, upregulate their lymphocyte function associated molecule-1 (LFA-1) adhesion molecules, and prime them for reaction with the proteinase III antibody. Endothelial cell injury would then be a consequence of the release of superoxide anion and other ROI. Other authors have laid claim to endothelial membrane antibodies which upregulate adhesion molecules and increase secretion of IL-6 and 8 and MCP-1. Anti-ANCA idiotypes are demonstrable in the IgM fraction of serum from patients in remission and their removal uncovers underlying IgG ANCA activity.

Platelet antibodies are apparently responsible for **idiopathic thrombocytopenic purpura** (ITP). IgG from a patient's serum when given to a normal individual causes a depression of platelet counts and the active principle can be absorbed out with platelets. The transient neonatal thrombocytopenia which may be seen in infants of mothers with ITP is explicable in terms of transplacental passage of IgG antibodies to the child.

The primary **antiphospholipid syndrome** is characterized by recurrent venous and arterial thromboembotic phenomena, recurrent fetal loss, thrombocytopenia and cardiolipin antibodies. Passive transfer of such antibodies into mice is fairly devastating, resulting in lower fecundity rates and recurrent fetal loss. The effect seems to be mediated through reaction of the autoantibodies with a complex of cardiolipin and $\beta_2$-glycoprotein 1 which inhibits triggering of the coagulation cascade, but may also activate the endothelial cells to increase prostacyclin metabolism, produce pro-inflammatory cytokines such as IL-6 and upregulate adhesion molecules.

## Surface receptors

### Thyroid

Under certain circumstances antibodies to the surface of a cell may stimulate rather than destroy (cf. type V sensitivity; Chapter 16). This would seem to be the case in **thyrotoxicosis** (Graves' or Basedow's disease). There has long been indirect evidence suggesting a link between autoimmune processes and this disease: thyroid antibodies are detectable in up to 85% of thyrotoxic patients and histologically the majority of the glands removed at operation show varying degrees of thyroiditis; thyrotoxicosis is found with undue frequency in the families of Hashimoto patients; there is an association with gastric autoim-

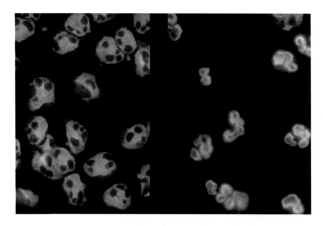

**Figure 20.1. Antineutrophil cytoplasmic antibodies (ANCA).** *Left* — cytoplasmic cANCA diffuse staining specific for proteinase III in Wegener's granulomatosis; *right* — perinuclear p-ANCA staining by myeloperoxidase antibodies in periarteritis nodosa. Fixed neutrophils are treated first with patient's serum then fluorescein-conjugated anti-human Ig. (Kindly provided by Dr G. Cambridge.)

munity in that 30% have gastric antibodies and up to 10% pernicious anemia. The direct link came with the discovery by Adams and Purves of thyroid stimulating activity in the serum of thyrotoxic patients (Milestone 19.1), ultimately shown to be due to the presence of antibodies to TSH receptors (TSH-R) which seem to act in the same manner as TSH (cf. figure 16.21). Both operate through the adenyl cyclase system as indicated by the potentiating effect of theophylline, and both produce similar changes in ultrastructural morphology in the thyroid cell, but it is one of Nature's 'passive transfer experiments' which links TSH-R antibodies most directly with the pathogenesis of Graves' disease. When thyroid stimulating antibodies (TSAb) from a thyrotoxic mother cross the placenta they cause the production of neonatal hyperthyroidism (figure 20.2), which resolves after a few weeks as the maternal IgG is catabolized.

There is a good correlation between the titer of TSAb and the severity of hyperthyroidism. Because TSAb act independently of the pituitary–thyroid axis, iodine uptake by the gland is unaffected by administration of thyroxine or tri-iodothyronine, whereas normally this would cause feedback inhibition and suppression of uptake; this forms the basis of an important diagnostic test for thyrotoxicosis.

There is reason to believe that enlargement of the thyroid in this disorder is due to the action of antibodies which react with a 'growth' receptor and directly stimulate cell division as distinct from metabolic hyperactivity (figure 20.3). In contrast, sera from patients with **primary myxedema** contain antibodies capable of blocking the mitogenic action of TSH, thereby preventing the regeneration of follicles which is a feature of the enlarged **Hashimoto goiter**. Graves' disease is often associated with exophthalmos which might be due to cross-reaction of antibodies to a 64 kDa membrane protein present on both thyroid and eye muscle.

### Muscle and nerve

The transient muscle weakness seen in a proportion of babies born to mothers with **myasthenia gravis** calls to mind neonatal thrombocytopenia and hyperthyroidism and would certainly be compatible with the transplacental passage of an IgG capable of inhibiting neuromuscular transmission. Strong support for this view is afforded by the consistent finding of antibodies to muscle acetylcholine receptors (ACh-R) in myasthenics and the depletion of these receptors within the motor endplates. In addition, myasthenic symptoms can be induced in animals by injection of monoclonal antibodies to ACh-R or by active immunization with the purified receptors themselves. Nonetheless, the majority of babies with myasthenic mothers do not display muscle disease and it may be that they are protecting themselves through production of antibodies directed to idiotypes on the maternal autoantibodies. Many myasthenics develop thymomas bearing molecules which cross-react with ACh-R although structurally not belonging to that gene family. It must be on the cards that molecular mimicry based on comparable peptide sequences may prime autoreactive T-cells which then drive genuine anti-ACh-R responses. An association with ACh-R polymorphism hints at some contribution to risk from the autoantigen.

Neuromuscular defects can also be elicited in mice injected with serum from patients with the **Lambert–Eaton** syndrome containing antibodies to presynaptic calcium channels. Autoantibodies to sodium channels which cross-react with *Campylobacter* bacilli have been identified in **Guillain–Barré syn-**

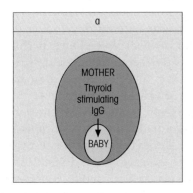
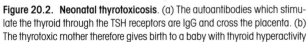
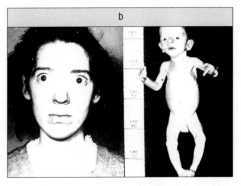

**Figure 20.2. Neonatal thyrotoxicosis**. (a) The autoantibodies which stimulate the thyroid through the TSH receptors are IgG and cross the placenta. (b) The thyrotoxic mother therefore gives birth to a baby with thyroid hyperactivity which spontaneously resolves as the mother's IgG is catabolized. (Photograph courtesy of Dr A. MacGregor.)

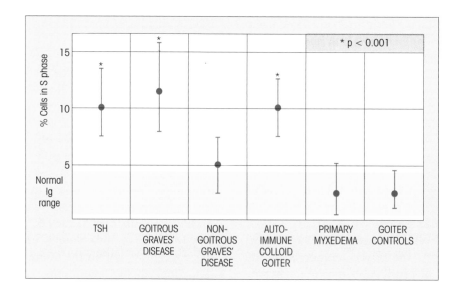

**Figure 20.3. Autoantibodies affecting thyroid growth.** Stimulating antibodies in goitrous Graves' disease and autoimmune colloid goiter shown by the increase of cells entering the DNA synthetic (S) phase of the cell cycle in thyroid fragments treated with IgG from the patient's serum. *P* values relate to differences from results with normal Ig. Blocking antibodies in primary myxedema can be revealed by the ability of patient's IgG to inhibit the growth stimulation caused by TSH. (Data from Drexhage H.A., Bottazzo G.F., Doniach D., Bitensky L. & Chayen J. (1980) *Lancet* **ii**, 287.)

**drome**, a self-resolving peripheral polyneuritis. Rather more wayout is **Rasmussen's encephalitis**, a childhood disease of relentless and intractable focal seizures with an inflammatory histopathology in the brain; these patients have antibodies capable of inducing rapid and reversible nondesensitizing inward currents in kainic acid responsive neurons through reaction with type 3 glutamine receptors. Would one uncover yet more phenomena of this kind in other neurological disorders if the search was widened and intensified?

*Stomach*

The underlying histopathological lesion in **pernicious anemia** is an atrophic gastritis in which a chronic inflammatory mononuclear invasion is associated with degeneration of secretory glands and failure to produce gastric acid. The development of achlorhydria is almost certainly accelerated by the inhibitory action of antibodies to the gastric proton pump, an $H^+,K^+$-dependent ATPase located in the membranes of the secretory canaliculi, and possibly also the gastrin receptors.

The idea that some cases of gastric ulcer may result from stimulation of acid secretion by activation through antibodies to histamine receptors is appeal-

ing and we still await the further work required to establish its validity.

*Other cellular receptors*

Some patients with **atopic allergy** have serum blocking antibodies to β-adrenergic receptors and these may represent just one of many different types of factor which could alter the baseline sensitivity of mast cells and make the individual more at risk for the development of disease. Antibodies which block insulin receptors are a rare exotic species found in patients with acanthosis nigricans (type B) and ataxia telangiectasia associated with insulin resistance.

## Other tissues

*Gut*

Some patients with **autoimmune atrophic gastritis** diagnosed by achlorhydria and parietal cell antibodies (see above and table 19.2) just meander on year after year without developing the vitamin $B_{12}$ deficiency which precipitates **pernicious anemia**. It is probable that autoallergic destruction is roughly balanced by regeneration of mucosal cells, an explanation which could account for the observation that high doses of steroids may restore gastric function in certain patients with pernicious anemia. In one such case studied, biopsy after intensive treatment with prednisone showed a diminution in the cellular infiltrate and new formation of parietal and chief cells in the gastric mucosa; acid and intrinsic factor were now produced after histamine stimulation and the ability to absorb vitamin $B_{12}$ assessed by the Schilling test was restored to near-normal values. Presumably, elimination of inflammatory cells by the prednisone allowed the regeneration of gastric mucosal cells to become dominant. However the balance would be upset were the patient now to produce antibodies to intrinsic factor in the lumen of the gastrointestinal tract; these would neutralize the small amount of intrinsic factor still available and the body would move into negative balance for $B_{12}$. The symptoms of $B_{12}$ deficiency, pernicious anemia and sometimes subacute degeneration of the cord, would then appear some considerable time later as the liver stores became exhausted (figure 20.4).

The normally acquired tolerance to dietary proteins seems to break down in **celiac disease** where T-cell sensitivity to wheat gluten in the small intestine can be demonstrated. Since gluten can bind strongly to the extracellular matrix protein, endomysium, one could hypothesize that uptake of the complex by IgA B-cells specific for endomysium would 'piggyback' the gluten into the B-cell for processing and presentation on major histocompatibility complex (MHC) class II to gluten-specific T-helpers (cf. figure 19.12). Stimulation of the B-cell would now follow with secretion of the IgA endomysial antibodies which are exclusive to patients with celiac disease. Together with the increased expression of Fcα receptors in the lamina propria and evidence of complement and eosinophil activation, it is conceivable that antibody-mediated mechanisms could be pathogenic.

## Skin

An antibody pathogenesis for **pemphigus vulgaris** is favored by the recognition of a 130 kDa autoantigen on stratified squamous epithelial cells which is a member of the cadherin family of $Ca^{2+}$-dependent adhesion molecules. Likewise, antibodies to desmoglein 1 must mediate the blistering of the epidermis in **pemphigus foliaceus**.

## Sperm

In some **infertile males**, agglutinating antibodies cause aggregation of the spermatozoa and interfere with their penetration into the cervical mucus.

## Glomerular basement membrane (g.b.m.)

With immunological kidney disease the experimental models preceded the finding of parallel lesions in the human. Injection of cross-reacting heterologous g.b.m. preparations in complete Freund's adjuvant produces glomerulonephritis in sheep and other experimental animals. Antibodies to g.b.m. can be picked up by immunofluorescent staining of biopsies from nephritic animals with anti-IgG. The antibodies are largely, if not completely, absorbed out by the kidney *in vivo* but they appear in the serum on nephrectomy and can passively transfer the disease to another animal of the same species.

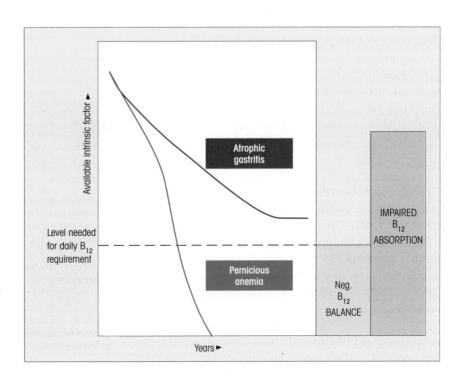

**Figure 20.4. Pathogenesis of pernicious anemia.** Patients with long-standing atrophic gastritis having parietal cell but no intrinsic factor antibodies do not go into negative $B_{12}$ balance. Pernicious anemia develops when intrinsic factor antibodies become superimposed upon the atrophic gastritis. (After Doniach D. & Roitt I.M. (1964) *Seminars in Hematology* I, 313.)

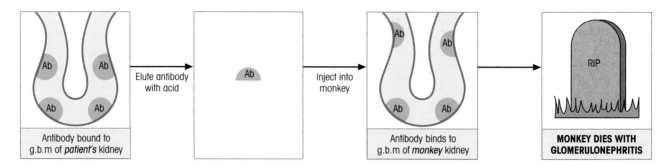

**Figure 20.5. Passive transfer of glomerulonephritis** to a squirrel monkey by injection of antiglomerular basement membrane (anti-g.b.m.) antibodies isolated by acid elution from the kidney of a patient with Goodpasture's syndrome. (After Lerner R.A., Glascock R.J. & Dixon F.J. (1967) *Journal of Experimental Medicine* **126**, 989.)

An entirely analogous situation occurs in man in certain cases of glomerulonephritis, particularly those associated with lung hemorrhage (**Goodpasture's syndrome**). Kidney biopsy from the patient shows *linear* deposition of IgG and C3 along the basement membrane of the glomerular capillaries (figure 16.14). After nephrectomy, g.b.m. antibodies can be detected in the serum. Lerner and his colleagues eluted the g.b.m. antibody from a diseased kidney and injected it into a squirrel monkey. The antibody rapidly fixed to the g.b.m. of the recipient animal and produced a fatal nephritis (figure 20.5). It is hard to escape the conclusion that the lesion in the human was the direct result of attack on the g.b.m. by these complement-fixing antibodies. The lung changes in Goodpasture's syndrome are attributable to cross-reaction with some of the g.b.m. antibodies.

Curiously, mercuric chloride produces anti-g.b.m. glomerulonephritis in Brown Norway rats and *pari passu*, as the disease remits, there is an upsurge in anti-idiotype suppressors. Nonsusceptible strains produce suppressors rather promptly.

### Heart

Neonatal lupus erythematosus is the most common cause of permanent **congenital complete heart block**. Almost all cases have been associated with high maternal titers of anti-La/SS-B or anti-Ro/SS-A. The mother's heart is unaffected. The key observation was that anti-Ro bound to neonatal rather than adult cardiac tissue and altered the transmembrane action potential by inhibiting repolarization (figure 20.6). IgG anti-Ro reaches the fetal circulation by transplacental passage but although maternal and fetal hearts are exposed to the autoantibody, only the latter is

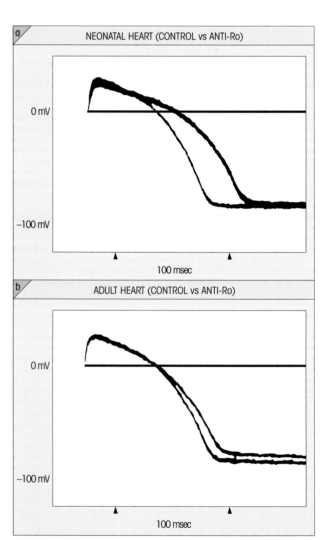

**Figure 20.6. Anti-Ro affects conduction in neonatal but not adult heart.** (a) Action potential of neonatal NZW rabbit cardiac fiber before and 20 minutes after superfusion with serum containing anti-Ro/SS-A; the repolarization phase of the action potential is reduced by 30%. (b) The same with an adult cardiac fiber showing only 5% reduction. (Reproduced from Alexander E. *et al.* (1992) *Arthritis and Rheumatism* **35**, 176.) Anti-La/SS-B can be eluted from the fetal cardiac tissue of infants with congenital heart block. It reacts with fetal but not adult laminin in the basement membrane. Autoantibodies to the endogenous retroviral envelope protein (ERV-3) appear during pregnancy and disappear after delivery except in women with autoimmune diseases where they persist, the highest levels being found in women with a history of congenital heart block children.

affected. Anti-La/SS-A also binds to affected fetal hearts reacting with laminin in the basement membrane.

## PATHOGENIC EFFECTS OF COMPLEXES WITH AUTOANTIGENS

### Systemic lupus erythematosus (SLE)

Where autoantibodies are formed against soluble components to which they have continual access, complexes may be formed which can give rise to lesions similar to those occurring in serum sickness, especially when defects in the early classical complement components prevent effective clearance (cf. figure 16.16). Thus, although homozygous complement deficiency is a rare cause of SLE (cf. figure 16.8c and d), the archetypal immune complex disorder, it represents the most powerful disease susceptibility genotype so far identified; more than 80% of cases with homozygous C1q and C4 deficiency have SLE. Up to one half of the patients carry autoantibodies to the collagenous portion of C1q but in truth there are a rich variety of different autoantigens in lupus (cf. table 19.2) many of them within the nucleus (cf. figure 19.1g), with the most pathomnemonic being **double-stranded DNA (dsDNA)**. Anti-dsDNA is enriched in cryoglobulins and acid eluates of renal tissue from patients with lupus nephritis where it can be identified, presumably in complexes containing complement, by immunofluorescent staining of kidney biopsies from patients with evidence of renal dysfunction. The staining pattern with a fluorescent anti-IgG or anti-C3 is punctate or 'lumpy-bumpy' as once described (figure 16.14b), in marked contrast with the linear pattern caused by the g.b.m. antibodies in Goodpasture's syndrome (figure 16.14; p. 340). The complexes grow in size to become large aggregates visible in the electron microscope as amorphous humps on both sides of the g.b.m. (figure 20.7). During the active phase of the disease, serum complement levels fall as components are affected by immune aggregates in the kidney and circulation. Deposition of complexes is widespread as the name implies and although 40% of patients *eventually* develop kidney lesions, the corresponding figure for organ involvement is 98% for skin (figure 20.8), 98% for joints/muscle, 64% for lung, 60% for blood, 60% for brain and 20% for heart.

Spontaneous production of anti-dsDNA is also a dominant feature of the animal models of SLE, NZB×W, MRL/lpr and BXSB mice, which involve fatal immune complex disease. The amelioration of

symptoms and reduction of renal glomerular immune complexes by treatment of NZB×W mice with DNase I provides convincing evidence for an antigen-driven complex mediated pathology. Cationic anti-DNA

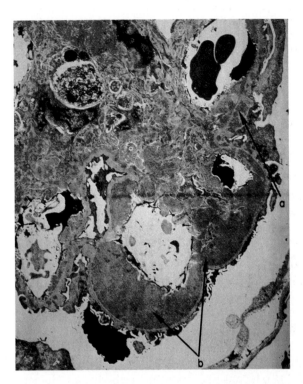

**Figure 20.7. Renal biopsy of an SLE patient with severe immune complex glomerulonephritis and proteinuria.** Electron micrograph showing irregular thickening of glomerular capillary walls by subepithelial complexes (a) and subendothelial complexes (b). The mesangial region shows abundant (probably phagocytosed) complexes. (Courtesy of Dr A. Leatham.)

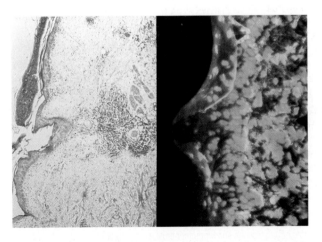

**Figure 20.8. The 'lupus band' in SLE.** *Left*—section of skin showing slight thickening of the dermo-epidermal junction with underlying scattered inflammatory cells and a major inflammatory focus in the deeper layers. Low power H & E. *Right*—green fluorescent staining of a skin biopsy at higher power showing deposition of complexes containing IgG (anti-C3 gives the same picture) on the basement membrane at the dermo-epidermal junction. (Kindly provided by Professor D. Isenberg.)

with arginines strategically positioned in locations of paratopic significance, emerges strongly as the disease progresses. IgM anti-DNA is not pathogenic and in the NZB×W model, only when the isotype switches to IgG do complex deposits become significant and mice begin to die. This isotype switch betokens T-cell control despite the observation that elimination of B-1 cells which are thought to be T-independent, essentially prevents the expression of disease. However, further support for T-cell drive is evidenced by the beneficial effects of anti-CD4 treatment and by the appearance of antibodies with somatic mutations and increased affinity, markers also of antigen selection.

It is difficult to account for the occurrence of clusters of autoantibodies directed to physically linked antigens, in particular those constituting the nucleosome and the spliceosome, without invoking antigen selection of the responding B-cells. Here one envisages the 'piggy-back' mechanism portrayed in figure 19.12 where a T-cell specific for component X of a complex XY, recognizes processed X on the surface of an anti-Y B-cell which has captured the complex; the stimulated B-cell then goes on to secrete anti-Y. Thus, a B-cell programmed to make anti-DNA can capture a histone–DNA complex from a nucleosome and be activated by a histone-specific T-helper. It could well be relevant that apoptotic cells display nucleosome ribonucleoprotein (RNP) blebs on their surface. Furthermore, it was recently discovered that anti-dsDNA would cross-react with the unfolded chains derived from the Sm and $U_1$ small RNP particles. Activated cross-reacting B-cells could capture DNA–histone complexes for example, and being activated, act as antigen-presenting cells (APCs) for resting histone-specific T-helper cells (cf. figure 19.12). There is another twist to this story in that two of these murine monoclonal high avidity anti-dsDNA cross-reacting antibodies stained the surface of fibroblast cells in culture, penetrated the cytoplasm and bound to the nucleus where they could interfere with certain normal physiological functions; unusually, these monoclonals caused kidney dysfunction *in vivo*, offering a potential pathogenetic mechanism distinct from, but presumably additional to, immune complex deposition.

We have argued at length that the production of high affinity IgG autoantibodies directed to linked-antigen clusters in human and murine SLE speaks out for both antigen selection and T-cell involvement. Of around 400 T-cell lines derived from patients with SLE, 59 induced the secretion of **cationic, i.e. nephritogenic, IgG anti-DNA** when cocultured with autologous B-cells. Of these, 49 were conventional CD4+ T-cell receptor (TCR)2 reacting with autologous APC in the absence of any added antigen and were HLA-DR restricted. Seven of the remaining 10 were CD4-8- TCRγδ and HLA unrestricted in proliferating with APCs from any lupus patients, but not normal subjects. They also induced autoantibody production when cultured with mismatched lupus patients and this interaction was blocked by antibodies cross-reacting with the ubiquitous hsp60 (don't these irrepressible heat-shock proteins just keep surfacing in the most unexpected places?). Murine T-helpers which augment pathogenic anti-DNA production induce lupus renal disease when injected into prenephritic lupus mice. Tantalizingly, the identity of the antigen(s) driving the T-cells is still elusive. The possible involvement of idiotypes was mooted in the last chapter by reference to experiments in which immunization of mice with monoclonal anti-nuclear antibodies gave rise to production of new antibodies of similar idiotype and specificity—in biblical terms, 'antibody begets antibody'. The list of antibodies has now been extended to anti-phospholipid and probably anti-collagen type II (cf. figure 20.16). One could readily envisage a scenario in which a major public idiotype network is kicked into action by say microbial infection (cf. figure 19.13); for example, the 16/6

**Figure 20.9.** (*Opposite*) **Rheumatoid arthritis** (RA). (a) Hands of a patient with chronic RA showing classical swan-neck deformities. (b) Diagrammatic representation of a diarthrodial joint showing bone and cartilagenous erosions beneath the synovial membrane-derived pannus. (c) Proximal interphalangeal joint depicting marked bony erosion and marginal erosion of the cartilage. (d) Early pannus of granulation tissue growing over the patella. (e) Histology of pannus showing clear erosion of bone and cartilage at the cellular margin. (f) Histology of the pannus stained for macrophage nonspecific esterase; note long, stained dendritic processes. (g) Chronic inflammatory cells in the deeper layers of the synovium in RA. (h) A hypervillous synovium revealing well-formed secondary follicles with germinal centers (relatively rare occurrence). (i) A high power view of an area of diseased synovium showing collections of classical plasma cells. (j) Plasma cells isolated from a patient's synovial tissue stained simultaneously for IgM (with fluorescein-labeled F(ab')$_2$ anti-μ) and rheumatoid factor (with rhodamine-labeled aggregated Fcγ). Two of the four IgM-positive plasma cells appear to be synthesizing rheumatoid factors. (k) Rheumatoid synovium showing large numbers of cells stained by anti-HLA-DR (anti-class II). (l) Rheumatoid synovium showing class II positive accessory cells (green) in intimate contact with CD4+ T-cells (orange). (m) Large rheumatoid nodules on the forearm. (n) Granulomatous appearance of the rheumatoid nodule with central necrotic area surrounded by epithelioid cells, macrophages and scattered lymphocytes. Plasma cells making rheumatoid factor are often demonstrable and the lesion probably represents a response to the formation of insoluble anti-IgG complexes.

((a) Kindly given by Dr D. Isenberg; (c), (d), (e), (g), (h) and (i) by Dr L.E. Glynn; (f) by Dr J. Edwards; (j) by Drs P. Youinou and P. Lydyard and (k) and (l) by Professor G. Janossy.)

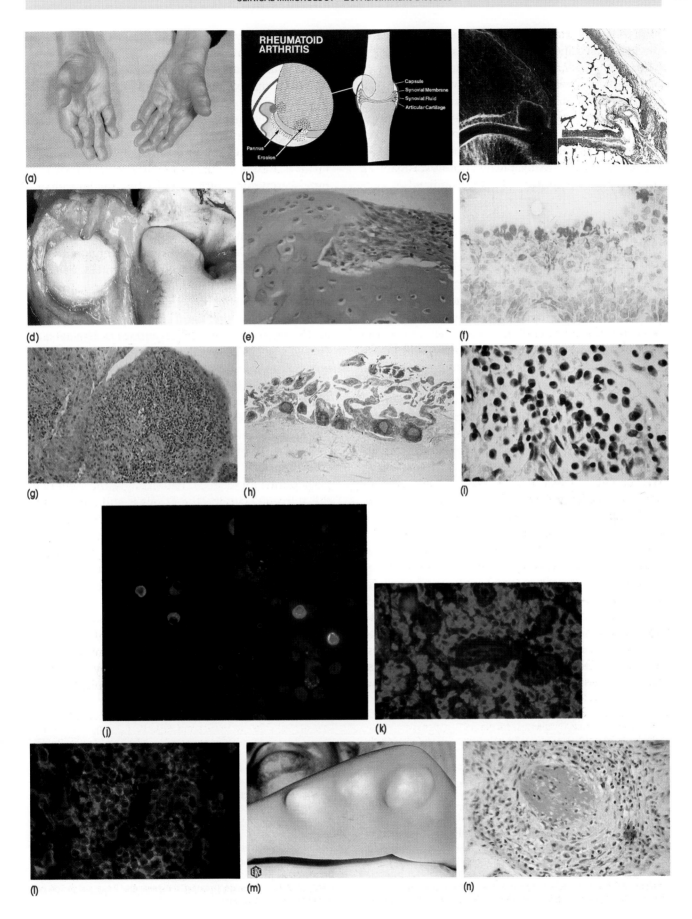

(a)

(b) RHEUMATOID ARTHRITIS — Capsule, Synovial Membrane, Synovial Fluid, Articular Cartilage, Pannus, Erosion

(c)

(d)

(e)

(f)

(g)

(h)

(i)

(j)

(k)

(l)

(m)

(n)

idiotype on a human monoclonal anti-DNA is also carried on a germ-line antibody to *Klebsiella*. A T-helper cell recognizing processed Id could selectively recruit B-cells bearing that Id (cf. figure 11.13). It could also stimulate B-cells capturing a complex of autoantigen (e.g. DNA) with Id-positive natural autoantibody (cf. figure 19.12 and p. 410). I have labored the anti-Id case just a little because I think it embodies a not unreasonable hypothesis set against a somewhat 'idiosceptical' intellectual climate.

## Rheumatoid arthritis

### *Morphological evidence for immunological activity*

The joint changes in RA are in essence produced by the **malign growth of the synovial cells** as a pannus overlaying and destroying cartilage and bone (figure 20.9a–f). The synovial membrane which surrounds and maintains the joint space becomes intensely cellular as a result of considerable immunological hyperreactivity as evidenced by large numbers of T-cells, mostly CD4, in various stages of activation, usually associated with dendritic cells and macrophages (figure 20.9l); clumps of plasma cells are frequently observed and sometimes even secondary follicles with germinal centers are present as though the synovium had become an active lymph node (figure 20.9g–i). Indeed it has been estimated that the synthesis of immunoglobulins by the synovial tissue ranks with that of a stimulated lymph node. There is widespread expression of surface HLA-DR (class II); T- and B-cells, dendritic and synovial lining cells and macrophages are all positive, indicative of some pretty lively action (figure 20.9k). The thesis is that this fiery immunological reactivity provides an intense stimulus to the synovial lining cells which undergo a Dr Jekyll to Mr Hyde transformation into the invasive pannus which brings about joint erosion through the release of destructive mediators.

### *IgG autosensitization and immune complex formation*

Autoantibodies to the IgG Fc region (see figure 20.11a), known as **antiglobulins** or **rheumatoid factors**, are the hallmark of the disease, being demonstrable in virtually all patients with RA. The majority have IgM antiglobulins which react in the classical latex and sheep cell agglutination tests (table 19.2; note 7) and both they and the 'seronegative' patients who fail to react in these tests can be shown to have elevated levels of **IgG antiglobulins** detectable by solid-phase immunoassay (cf. p. 113; figure 20.10).

If, therefore, autosensitization to IgG is an almost universal feature of the disease, one might expect plasma cells in the synovium to be synthesizing antiglobulins. In fact 10–20% bind fluoresceinated IgG, either in the form of heat-aggregated material (figure 20.9j) or immune complexes (rheumatoid factor is a low affinity antibody and good binding is only seen when multivalent IgG is used as antigen). We must take into account a strange and unique feature of IgG antiglobulins; because they are both antigen and antibody at the same time, they are capable of **self-association** (figure 20.11b) and this hides the majority of free antiglobulin valencies. Cleverly realizing that destruction of the Fc regions by pepsin would liberate these hidden binding sites, Munthe and Natvig observed that a greater percentage of the plasma cells in the synovium displayed an anti-IgG specificity following treatment with this enzyme.

IgG aggregates, presumably products of these plasma cells, can be regularly detected in the synovial tissues and in the joint fluid where they give rise to typical acute inflammatory reactions with fluid exudates. Analysis shows them to consist almost exclu-

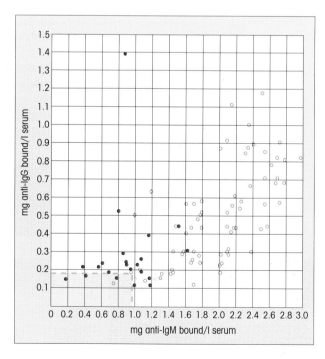

**Figure 20.10. IgM and IgG antiglobulins** determined by tube radioassay in patients with seropositive (open circles) and seronegative (filled circles) rheumatoid arthritis. The dashed lines indicate the 95% confidence limits (mean ± 2 SD) of the normal group. (From Nineham L., Hay F.C. & Roitt I.M. (1976) *Journal of Clinical Pathology* **29**, 1121.)

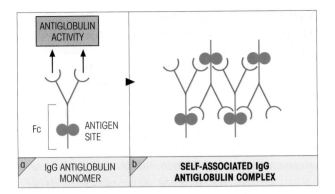

**Figure 20.11. Self-associated complexes of IgG antiglobulins.** Although of relatively low affinity, the strength of binding is boosted by the 'bonus effect' of the mutual attachment and, furthermore, such complexes in the joint may be stabilized by IgM antiglobulin and C1q which have polyvalent binding sites for IgG. Degradation of the Fc regions by pepsin, releases the 'hidden' binding sites involved in the self-association.

sively of immunoglobulins and complement, while a major proportion of the IgG is present as self-associated antiglobulin as shown by binding to an Fcγ immunosorbent after treatment with pepsin.

## Abnormal patterns of IgG glycosylation

A confession to the reader: what may seem to others in the field as an undue emphasis on agalacto-IgG in RA in the following section, really reflects my own idiosyncratic opinion that one of the most interesting events in the RA saga has been the discovery that the patient's IgG is abnormally glycosylated. The two $C_H2$ domains in the Fc region are held apart (cf. p. 51) by two asparagine-linked sugars of the general struc-

ture shown in figure 20.12a and the terminal galactose lies in a special 'lectin-like' pocket (figure 20.12b). Some chains end in *N*-acetylglucosamine and lack the terminal galactose sugars. What is extraordinary is that the percentage of sugars completely lacking galactose in the IgG of both juvenile and adult RA patients is nearly always higher than in the controls and can go as high as 60% (figure 20.13). This abnormal glycosylation could have three possible consequences:

**1** The Fc may have increased autoantigenicity.

**2** Self-associated IgG complexes (figure 20.11b) would be held together more strongly if the terminal galactose on the Fab sugar of one IgG fits into the lectin site on $C_H2$ left vacant by the lack of galactose on the Fc sugar.

**3** The interaction with inflammatory mediators may be enhanced (Figure 20.14). The exposure of *N*-acetylglucosamine in the agalacto-IgG glycoform allows recognition of immune complexes by mannose-binding protein with activation of the classical complement pathway (cf. p. 18) and stimulation of macrophages through binding of TNFα. This increased inflammatory potency is clearly seen in the superiority of agalacto-anticollagen over its normally glycosylated counterpart in the production of collagen arthritis through synergy with cell-mediated immunity (see figure 20.16).

**4** The interaction with Fcγ receptors on certain effector cells may be considerably modified. For example, feedback control of autoantibody production may be lost. An astonishing result of the collagen arthritis study mentioned above was that injection of the

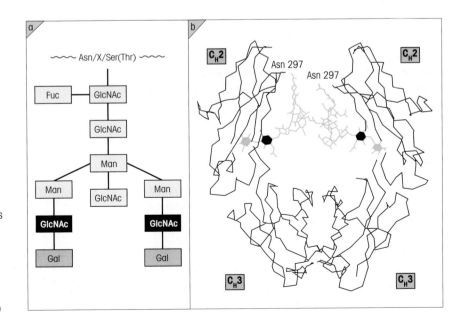

**Figure 20.12. The Fc sugars and their role in bridging the two $C_H2$ domains of IgG.** (a) Typical structure of each N-linked sugar. Some chains lack one (G1) or both terminal galactoses (agalacto-IgG; G0). (b) Structure of the $C_H2$ regions and the association between the terminal galactose on the 1,6 arm and the protein surface. The 1,3 arms, one of which must lack galactose, bridge the two domains. (GlcNAc = *N*-acetylglucosamine; Man = mannose; Gal = galactose; Fuc = fucose.)

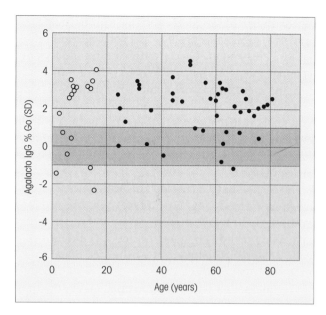

**Figure 20.13. Raised levels of agalacto-IgG (G0) in juvenile and adult forms of rheumatoid arthritis.** Because G0 varies with age in normal controls, the normal range is expressed in terms of mean ± 1SD and results for patients as SD units about the normal mean. (From review by Roitt I.M., Hutchings P.R., Dawe K.I., Sumar N., Bodman K.B. & Cooke A. (1992) The forces driving autoimmune disease. *Journal of Autoimmunity*, **5**(Supplement A), 11–26.)

agalacto-monoclonal actually led to the production of *new* anti-collagen — another example of 'antibody begets antibody' (p. 430).

Raised levels of agalacto-IgG are not seen in reactive arthritis provoked by *Yersinia* or *Chlamydia*, nor in many other chronic inflammatory states, but abnormally high levels occur during active tuberculosis infection giving further support to attempts at identifying slow-growing (mycobacterial?) organisms as initiators of disease. Spouses of patients with RA also tend to have higher agalacto-IgG values; is this evidence for some infective agent?

It is well established that pregnant women with RA have a remission of their disease as they approach term, but an exacerbation *post partum*; as the arthritis remits, the agalacto-IgG values fall and as the disease worsens after birth, agalacto-IgG becomes abnormal again suggesting intimate involvement with the disease process. Long-term studies in closed communities of Pima Indians who have an unusually high incidence of RA, have shown that changes in IgG galactose provide an early marker of future clinical disease and we know they can be of **prognostic value**.

### The production of tissue damage

As explained in the legend to figure 20.11, the complexes can be stabilized by the multivalent Fcγ-

binding molecules, IgM rheumatoid factor and C1q, and when present in the joint space they may initiate an Arthus reaction leading to an influx of polymorphs with which they react to release ROIs and lysosomal enzymes. These include neutral proteinases and collagenase which can **damage the articular cartilage** by breaking down proteoglycans and collagen fibrils. More damage results if the complexes are adherent to the cartilage, since the polymorph binds but is unable to internalize them ('frustrated phagocytosis'); as a result the lysosomal hydrolases are released extracellularly into the space between the cell and the cartilage where they are protected from enzyme inhibitors such as α₂-macroglobulin. We have already drawn attention to the enhanced inflammatory potency of complexes containing agalacto-IgG.

The aggregates may also stimulate the macrophage-like cells of the synovial lining, either directly through their surface receptors or indirectly through phagocytosis and resistance to intracellular digestion. At this point we should acknowledge that the release of cytokines such as TNFα and GM-CSF from activated T-cells provides further potent macrophage stimulation.

The activated synovial cells grow out as a malign pannus (cover) over the cartilage (figure 20.9d) and at the margin of this advancing granulation tissue breakdown can be seen (figure 20.9e), almost certainly as a result of the release of enzymes, ROIs and espe-

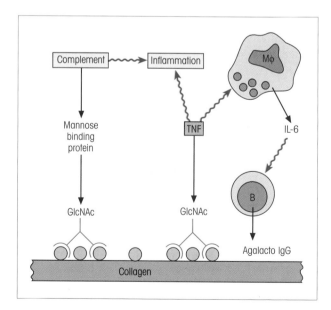

**Figure 20.14. Enhancement of inflammation by complexes containing agalacto-IgG.** Mannose-binding protein combines with the exposed *N*-acetylglucosamine (GlcNAc) and through MASP (cf. p. 18) activates classical complement pathway C2. TNFα is a lectin which also binds GlcNAc and so stimulates macrophages at the surface of the complex. The IL-6 released further promotes agalacto-IgG synthesis by B-cells.

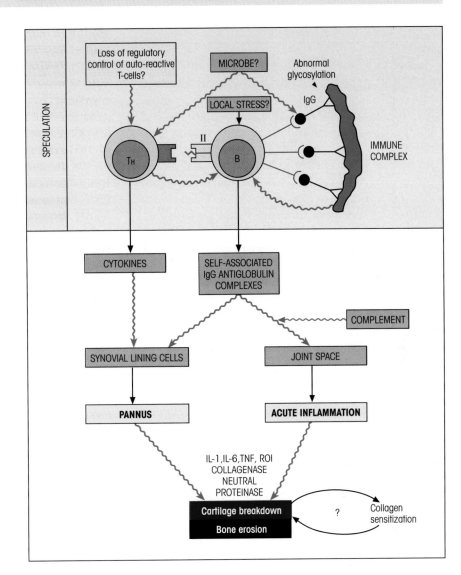

**Figure 20.15. Immune pathogenesis of rheumatoid arthritis and speculation on the induction of autoimmunity.** The defective pituitary/adrenal regulatory control on cell-mediated immunity in these patients was described in chapter 19. The identity of the peptide(s) associated with the class II molecule is unknown. There are numerous opportunities for cross-reactions between the DRβ 'shared epitope' and various microbial heat shock proteins. It has been reported that synovial fluid T-cells of juvenile rheumatoid arthritis patients respond strongly to human heat-shock protein 60, whereas adults do not.

cially of IL-1, 6 and TNFα. Activated macrophages also secrete plasminogen activator and the plasmin formed as a consequence activates a latent collagenase produced by synovial cells. Sensitization to partially degraded collagen may occur and this could lead secondarily to amplification of the lesion. The secreted products of the stimulated macrophage can activate chondrocytes to exacerbate **cartilage breakdown**, and osteoclasts to bring about **bone resorption** which is a further complication of severe disease (figure 20.9c). Subcutaneous nodules are granulomata (figure 20.9m and n) possibly formed through local production of insolubilized self-associating antiglobulins.

The contribution of these immune complexes to the pathogenesis of RA is built into the overview presented in figure 20.15, where it will be seen that a role for the T-cells must not be overlooked and will be discussed in the following section.

## T-CELL MEDIATED HYPERSENSITIVITY AS A PATHOGENIC FACTOR IN AUTOIMMUNE DISEASE

### Rheumatoid arthritis again

The chronically inflamed synovium is densely crowded with activated T-cells and their critical role in the disease process is emphasized by the beneficial effects of cyclosporin and anti-CD4 treatments, and by the increased risk of disease associated with the 'shared epitope' sequences Q(R)K(R)RAA from residues 70–74 on the DRβ chain of DR1 and certain DR4 alleles (cf. table 17.4). High levels of IL-15 within the synovial membrane can recruit and activate T-cells whose secretion of cytokines and ability to induce macrophage synthesis of TNFα and further IL-15 will drive pannus development powerfully with consequent erosion of cartilage and bone (figure

20.15). Chondrocytes themselves may also be disease targets.

Just as in SLE, the antigenic specificity of these T-cells is still unknown. But the QKRAA shared epitope sequence is throwing up some appealing clues. This five amino acid stretch lying within the 3rd hypervariable region of DR4/1 subtypes, is also present in the dnaJ heat-shock proteins from *E. coli*, *Lactobacillus lactis* and *Brucella ovis*, as well as the Epstein–Barr virus gp110 protein. This already provides an opportunity for priming of T-cells with autoreactive specificity for a processed peptide containing QKRAA presented by another HLA molecule. The plot deepens with the realisation that QKRAA binds to a second *E. coli* heat-shock protein dnaK and that HLA-DR containing the QKRAA sequence bound to the *self* analogue of dnaK, namely hsp73, which targets selected proteins to lysosomes for processing. What this all means remains to be resolved but note the hsp family yet again.

The antigenic history of **reactive arthritis** is more amenable to study since it is triggered by an infection either of the urogenital tract by *Chlamydia trachomatis* or of the enteric tract with *Yersinia*, *Salmonella*, *Shigella* or *Campylobacter*. The synovial tissue in reactive arthritis remarkably still retains antigenic descendants of the initiating bacteria many years after infection which can drive local T-cells. All the microbes are either obligate or facultative intracellular bacteria and so may escape the immune system by hiding inside cells, probably aided by high local production of IL-4.

HLA-B27 individuals are particularly at risk and the importance of the microbial component is emphasized by experiments on mice bearing the B27 transgene; if reared in a germ-free environment, lesions are restricted to the skin, but in the microbiological wilderness of the normal animal house, the skin, gut and joints are all affected. What does B27 do? Only 1 in 300 of the T-cells in the reactive arthritis synovium is CD8. It could be that a cross-reactive B27 sequence functions as a cryptic epitope perpetuating a gentle microbial stimulus with an amplifying autoimmune response.

Two experimentally induced models of arthritis are heavily dependent on T-cells. **Adjuvant arthritis** resulting from immunization of rats with just complete Freund's adjuvant (CFA) can be transferred to naive recipients with a T-cell clone specific for the mycobacterial heat-shock protein hsp60. The **collagen arthritis** model involves injection of type II collagen in complete Freund's, but here a synergy between cell-mediated hypersensitivity and antibody seems to operate: sensitization with denatured collagen in CFA-induced T-cell-mediated immunity but no arthritis unless the mice were also given IgG from animals primed with *native* collagen (figure 20.16).

Spontaneous models of arthritis are hard to come by. Up to 30% of MRL/lpr mice have arthritic lesions but this incidence varies with the animal house. If animals harbor Sendai virus, they are protected from arthritis; what is that telling us? To complete the circle, they also have raised levels of agalacto-IgG.

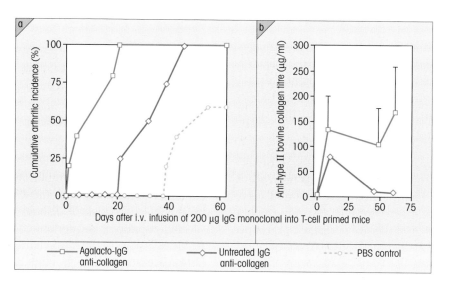

**Figure 20.16. Induction of chronic arthritis by passive transfer of agalacto-IgG.** Two injections of heat-denatured collagen type II in CFA induce delayed sensitivity but no antibody or arthritis. Subsequent i.v. injection of murine monoclonal IgG anti-native collagen produced a moderate arthritis appearing after 20 days, whereas agalacto-IgG obtained by treatment of the IgG with β-galactosidase very rapidly produced a more severe arthritis. PBS = phosphate-buffered saline. (Data kindly provided by Rademacher T.W., Jones R.H.V. & Williams P.J. from *Glycoimmunology* (1995). Alavi A. & Axford J.S. (eds) with permission of Plenum Press, N.Y.)

## Organ-specific endocrine disease

To make a fairly sweeping statement, inflammatory organ-specific diseases are generally linked to T-helper-1 (TH1) responses. Clones producing EAE or transferring diabetes from NOD mice produce IL-2 and γ-interferon (IFNγ) while in collagen arthritis, IL-12 can be substituted for the mycobacteria in the complete Freund's adjuvant. On the other hand, TH2 CD4s are responsible for the polyclonal activation in murine lupus, the glomerulonephritis and necrotizing vasculitis induced in Brown Norway rats by mercuric chloride, and the chronic autoimmunity generated during graft-vs-host disease. We will see that TH2 responses can downregulate destructive TH1 cells. Last, the TH1/TH2 polarization is not apparent in diseases such as myasthenia gravis, Graves' thyrotoxicosis, Sjögren's syndrome and primary biliary cirrhosis.

### Autoimmune thyroiditis

The inflammatory infiltrate in autoimmune thyroiditis is usually essentially mononuclear in character (see figure M19.1.1c) and, although not an infallible guide, this has been taken as an expression of T-cell-mediated hypersensitivity. Firm evidence for a direct participation of T-lymphocytes has yet to be provided, although the demonstration of class II molecules on patients' thyrocytes and the presence of antigen-specific TH1-cells in the thyroid would accord with an involvement of these cells.

We must turn to the animal models for further evidence albeit indirect. Draconian stamping out of T-cells in the Obese strain chicken by neonatal thymectomy and repeated injection of anti-T-cell serum, prevented the spontaneous development of atrophic autoimmune thyroiditis. The other model in which thyroiditis is induced by thyroglobulin in complete Freund's adjuvant (see figure M19.1.1b) can be transferred to naive histocompatible recipients with CD4+ T-cell clones specific for peptides containing thyroxine established from immunized animals. The cells infiltrate between the thyroid follicles and probably kill the epithelial cells by a combination of locally released IFNγ and TNF. We see now that there is considerable diversity in the autoimmune response to the thyroid leading to tissue destruction, metabolic stimulation, growth promotion or mitotic inhibition which in different combinations account for the variety of forms in which autoimmune thyroid disease presents (figure 20.17).

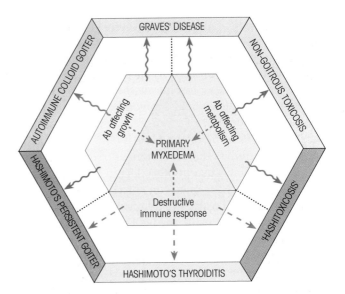

**Figure 20.17. Relationship of different autoallergic responses to the circular spectrum of autoimmune thyroid diseases.** Responses involving thyroglobulin and the thyroid peroxidase (microsomal) surface microvillous antigen lead to tissue destruction, whereas autoantibodies to TSH (and other ?) receptors can stimulate or block metabolic activity or thyroid cell division. 'Hashitoxicosis' is the down-to-earth term used by our Scots colleagues to describe a gland showing Hashimoto's thyroiditis and thyrotoxicosis simultaneously. (Courtesy of Professors D. Doniach and G.F. Bottazzo.)

### Insulin-dependent diabetes mellitus (IDDM)

Just as in autoimmune thyroiditis, IDDM involves chronic inflammatory infiltration and destruction of the specific tissue, in this case the insulin-producing β-cells of the pancreatic islets of Langerhans. The delay in onset of disease achieved by early treatment with cyclosporin A at levels which have little effect on antibody production, points an accusing finger at effector T-cells as the agents of destruction, since this drug targets T-cell cytokine synthesis so specifically. The strength of the risk factors associated with certain HLA-DQ alleles also has a strong whiff of T-cell action. *In vitro* T-cell responses to islet cell antigens including glutamic acid decarboxylase directly reflect the risk of progression to clinical IDDM.

To get further insight into the cellular siege and destruction of the islet β-cells, one has to turn to the **nonobese diabetic (NOD) mouse** which spontaneously develops diabetic disease closely resembling human IDDM in its histology and range of autoimmune responses. T-cells infiltrating the islets in diabetic mice had a TH1-type cytokine profile and could transfer disease to NOD recipients congenic for the severe combined immunodeficiency (*SCID*) mutation. The CD4/CD45RBlo memory subset of splenocytes from young nondiabetic NOD mice inhibited this transfer, but the same subset from older diabetic mice had lost its regulatory power and became pathogenic. This change to a T$_{H1}$-type response coincided with the onset of diabetes and is consistent with the observation that IL-12, which favors T$_{H1}$ responses, exacerbates disease. Just as in the human disease, MHC class II alleles hold a pivotal controlling position and introduction of a transgene in which residues at position 56 or 57 of the H-2Aβ-chain are altered, drastically inhibits the development of diabetes. One of the non-MHC susceptibility loci in NOD mapped to the *IL-1R* and *Bcg* genes on chromosome 1 associated with natural resistance to infection by intracellular parasites. As a result, the NOD mouse is resistant to *Mycobacterium avium*, but after recovery from infection the onset of diabetes is prevented. That responses to hsp65 may be involved, is implied by reports that a 24 amino acid peptide from this protein is the target of diabetogenic T-cells and treatment with this peptide downregulates spontaneous disease (why is this organ-specific?). Cohen has interpreted this as a result of dysregulation of the 'immunological homunculus' (cf. p. 209) and notes that the level of a particular idiotype associated with a TCR CDR3 consistently falls prior to the onset of diabetes, while mice reared under germ-free conditions which might inhibit the development of a natural idiotype network, are more susceptible to IDDM. Time will test the validity of this hypothesis. In the final analysis, one has to take into account the following: up to 50% of the infiltrating T-cells isolated from pre-diabetic NOD islets are insulin-specific and can transfer disease to young NOD, glutamic acid decarboxylase (GAD) specific T-cells can also be recovered and are also diabetogenic, and tolerance to either insulin or GAD prevents the onset of disease. Presumably the latter can be accommodated by an organ-related bystander tolerance mechanism described below (p. 445).

GAD in the central and peripheral nervous system produces γ-aminobutyric acid (GABA), a major inhibitory neurotransmitter, from glutamine. Autoantibodies to GAD are seen not only in early diabetes, but also **Stiff man syndrome** (sounds like a cue for a Western) where the GABA-ergic pathways controlling motor neuron activity are defective. The antibodies cannot be pathogenic because GAD is present on the inner surface of the plasma membrane, but T-cells could be. How the brain as distinct from the pancreatic islet could be specifically targeted is a conundrum but 30% of patients do develop IDDM.

### Multiple sclerosis (MS)

The idea that MS could be an autoimmune disease has for long been predicated on the morphological resemblance to experimental allergic encephalomyelitis (EAE), a demyelinating disease leading to motor paralysis (figure 20.18) produced by immunization with myelin, usually myelin basic protein (MBP) in complete Freund's. T-cell clones specific for MBP belong to restricted TCR Vβ families. They will transfer disease but this can be exacerbated by injection of a monoclonal antibody to Theiler's virus, a murine encephalomyelitis virus, cross-reacting with an epitope on myelin and oligodendrocytes. Presumably the T-cell incites a local inflammation affecting the endothelial cells at the blood–brain barrier which opens the gate for antibody to penetrate the brain tissue.

How much of this is relevant to human disease? First, the serologically determined caucasian DR2 phenotype (DRB1*1501, DQA1*0102, DQB1*0602) is strongly associated with susceptibility to MS. At least 37% of activated T-cells responsive to IL-2/4 in cerebrospinal fluid were specific for myelin components, compared with a figure of 5% for subjects with other neurological disturbances. A Leu.Arg.Gly. amino acid sequence motif found in around 40% of TCR Vβ5.2 N(D)N rearrangements in T-cells from MS lesions was present in a Vβ5.2 clone from an MS patient cytotoxic towards targets containing the MBP 89–106 peptide and in encephalitogenic rat T-cells specific for MBP peptide 87–99. One is greatly encouraged to continue with attempts to induce tolerance.

### Psoriasis

Given the evidence for T-cell mediated pathogenesis (p. 348), the isolation of clones specific for group A β-hemolytic streptococci from guttate skin lesions has fostered the thought that pathology is initiated by exotoxin (i.e. superantigen) recruited T-cells and is maintained by specific cells reacting both with streptococcal M protein and a cryptic skin epitope, possibly a keratin variant presented by cytokine-activated keratinocytes. There is extensive sequence homology between M-proteins and type I keratin. Topical cyclosporin-type ointments should work wonders.

## DIAGNOSTIC VALUE OF AUTOANTIBODY TESTS

Serum autoantibodies frequently provide valuable diagnostic markers. The most useful routine test is screening of the serum by immunofluorescence on a frozen section prepared from a composite block of

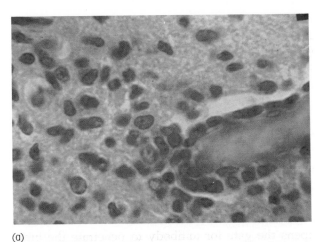

(a)

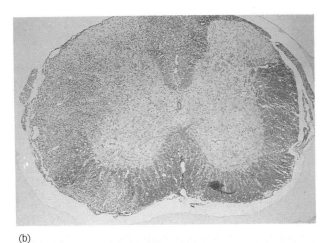

(b)

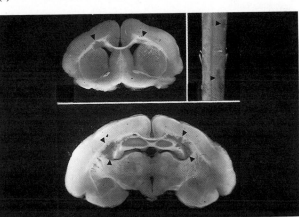

(c)

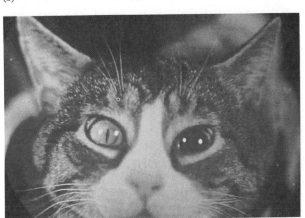

(d)

**Figure 20.18. Experimental allergic encephalomyelitis (EAE), a demyelinating model for multiple sclerosis induced by immunization with brain antigens in complete Freund's adjuvant (CFA).** (a) Early lesion of EAE in the rat at 9 days after immunization with rat spinal cord homogenate in CFA. The lesion in brain white matter, which is probably a few hours old, shows perivenous infiltration of lymphocytes and monocytes (a pure mononuclear inflammation) with cells invading the nervous parenchyma. Myelin is not stained. (b) Lumbar spinal cord of rat with chronic EAE after immunization with myelin proteolipid protein. Large demyelinating lesions in dorsal columns, in both left (large) and right (small) columns, as well as on lower left. Also gray matter involved with ongoing inflammation, in particular affecting left dorsal horn. Normal myelin is stained brown. (c) Chronic relapsing EAE in guinea-pig. Large demyelinated plaques in brain white matter (arrows) closely similar to plaques of multiple sclerosis. (d) Acute EAE in cat with optic nerve involvement. (Legend and slides provided by Dr B. Waksman; (b) originally from Dr Trotter, (c) from Drs Lassmann & Wisniewski and (d) from Dr Patterson.)

unfixed human thyroid and stomach, and rat kidney and liver. This is supplemented by agglutination tests for rheumatoid factors and for thyroglobulin, thyroid peroxidase and red cell antibodies and by ELISA for antibodies to intrinsic factor, DNA, IgG, extractable nuclear antigens and so on (see table 19.2). The salient information is summarized in table 20.1. ELISAs are taking over and tests with purified gene-cloned antigens arranged in mini-spot arrays will one day supplant the need for immunofluorescence which is time-consuming and more skilled.

The tests will also prove of value in screening for people at risk, e.g. relatives of patients with autoimmune diseases such as diabetes, thyroiditis patients for gastric autoimmunity and vice versa and ultimately the general population if the socio-logical consequences are fully understood and acceptable.

## TREATMENT OF AUTOIMMUNE DISORDERS

### Metabolic control

The majority of approaches to treatment, not unnaturally, involve manipulation of immunological responses (figure 20.19). However, in many organ-specific diseases, metabolic control is usually sufficient, e.g. thyroxine replacement in primary myxedema, insulin in juvenile diabetes, vitamin $B_{12}$ in pernicious anemia, antithyroid drugs for Graves' disease, and so forth. Anticholinesterase drugs are

Table 20.1. Autoantibody tests and diagnosis.

| DISEASE | ANTIBODY | COMMENT |
|---|---|---|
| Hashimoto's thyroiditis | Thyroid | Distinction from colloid goiter, thyroid cancer and subacute thyroiditis. Thyroidectomy usually unnecessary in Hashimoto goiter |
| Primary myxedema | Thyroid | Tests +ve in 99% of cases. If suspected hypothyroidism assess 'thyroid reserve' by TRH stimulation test |
| Thyrotoxicosis | Thyroid | High titers of cytoplasmic Ab indicate active thyroiditis and tendency to post-operative myxedema: anti-thyroid drugs are the treatment of choice although HLA-B8 patients have high chance of relapse |
| Pernicious anemia | Stomach | Help in diagnosis of latent PA, in differential diagnosis of non-autoimmune megaloblastic anemia and in suspected subacute combined degeneration of the cord |
| Insulin-dependent diabetes mellitus (IDDM) | Pancreas | Insulin Ab early in disease. GAD Ab standard test for IDDM. Two or more autoAb seen in 80% of new onset children or prediabetic relatives but no controls |
| Idiopathic adrenal atrophy | Adrenal | Distinction from tuberculous form |
| Myasthenia gravis | Muscle / ACh receptor | When positive suggests associated thymoma (more likely if HLA-B12) positive in >80% |
| Pemphigus vulgaris and pemphigoid | Skin | Different fluorescent patterns in the two diseases |
| Autoimmune hemolytic anemia | Erythrocyte (Coombs' test) | Distinction from other forms of anemia |
| Sjögren's syndrome | Salivary duct cells, SS-A, SS-B | |
| Primary biliary cirrhosis | Mitochondrial | Distinction from other forms of obstructive jaundice where test rarely +ve. Recognize subgroup within cryptogenic cirrhosis related to PBC with +ve mitochondrial Ab |
| Active chronic hepatitis | Smooth muscle anti-nuclear and 20% mitochondrial | Smooth muscle Ab distinguish from SLE. Type 1 classical in women with Ab to nuclei, smooth muscle, actin and asialoglycoprotein receptor. Type 2 in girls and young women with anti-LKM-1 (cyt P450) |
| Rheumatoid arthritis | Antiglobulin, e.g. SCAT and latex fixation / Antiglobulin + raised agalacto-Ig | High titer indicative of bad prognosis / Prognosis of rheumatoid arthritis |
| SLE | High titer antinuclear, DNA / Phospholipid | DNA antibodies present in active phase Ab to double-stranded DNA characteristic; high affinity complement-fixing Ab give kidney damage, low affinity CNS lesions / Thrombosis, recurrent fetal loss and thrombocytopenia |
| Scleroderma | Nucleolar | |
| Wegener's granulomatosis | Neutrophil cytoplasm | Antiserine protease closely associated with disease; treatment urgent |

commonly used for long-term therapy in myasthenia gravis; thymectomy is of benefit in most cases and it is conceivable that the gland contains acetylcholine (ACh) receptors in a particularly immunogenic form (? associated with HLA-D expression).

It is worth recording that maintenance therapy to replace the loss of an organ-specific molecule such as insulin in IDDM, might have the effect of subduing metabolic activity and reducing expression of the target antigen.

## Anti-inflammatory drugs

Patients with severe myasthenic symptoms respond well to high doses of steroids and the same is true for serious cases of other autoimmune disorders such as SLE and immune complex nephritis where the drug helps to suppress the inflammatory lesions.

In RA, steroids are very effective but the recognition of a defective pituitary/adrenal feedback loop in these patients has inspired a novel approach aiming to restore normal corticosteroid levels by a depot of methylprednisolone (Depomedrone) which delivers a low daily dose—the earlier in the disease the better. This treatment accelerates the induction of remission and decreases the side-effects of second-line agents such as gold salts. Selectins and adhesion molecules on endothelial cells and leukocyte integrins appear to be downregulated and this would seriously impede the influx of inflammatory cells into the joint. Anti-inflammatory drugs such as salicylates, innumerable synthetic prostaglandin inhibitors and metalloproteinase poisons are widely used. The so-called second-line drugs, sulfasalazine, penicillamine, gold salts and antimalarials such as chloroquine all find an important place in therapy but their mode of action is unknown.

Treatment with antibodies to adhesion molecules such as CD44 effectively blocks experimental arthritis but there are considerable practical and economic problems in adapting to human disease. Therapeutic blocking of other mediators directly concerned in immunological tissue damage will be feasible if cytokine and complement antagonists become available. Neutralizing TNFα with a humanized monoclonal antibody is most effective but does not achieve lasting benefit although it reveals the pathogenetic role of this cytokine. Attempts to transfect synovial cells with the natural IL-1 receptor antagonist IL-1Ra may hold out more hope for long-term effects.

## Immunosuppressive drugs

In a sense, because it blocks lymphokine secretion by T-cells, cyclosporin A is an anti-inflammatory drug and, since lymphokines like IL-2 are also obligatory for lymphocyte proliferation, cyclosporin is also an antimitotic drug. It is of proven efficacy in uveitis, early type I diabetes, nephrotic syndrome and psoriasis and of moderate efficacy in idiopathic thrombocytopenic purpura, SLE, polymyositis, Crohn's disease, primary biliary cirrhosis and myasthenia gravis. In a double-blind randomized control trial, cyclosporin demonstrated significant though not complete disease suppression over 12 months in a group of previously refractory rheumatoid arthritis (RA) patients. Unfortunately high toxic doses were used but the synergy with rapamycin is a strong indication for a trial of combined therapy.

While awaiting more selective therapy, conventional nonspecific antimitotic agents such as azathio-

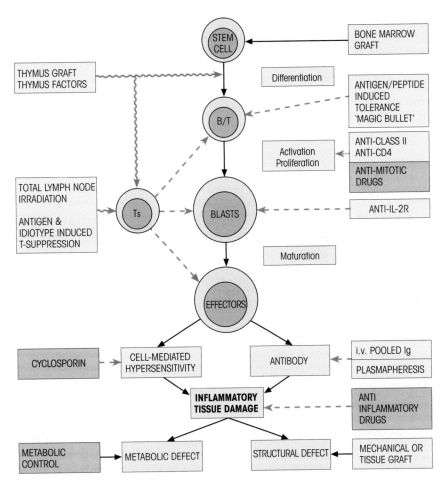

**Figure 20.19. The treatment of autoimmune disease.** Current conventional treatments are in dark orange; some feasible approaches are given in lighter orange boxes. (In the case of a live graft, bottom right, the immunosuppressive therapy used may protect the tissue from the autoimmune damage which affected the organ being replaced.)

prine, cyclophosphamide and methotrexate, usually in combination with steroids, have been used effectively in SLE, RA, chronic active hepatitis and autoimmune hemolytic anemia for example. High-dose i.v. cyclophosphamide plus adrenocorticotropic hormone (ACTH) or total lymph node irradiation through its effect on the peripheral immune system either slowed or stopped the advance of disease in approximately two-thirds of progressive multiple sclerosis (MS) patients for 1–2 years, a strong indication that the disease is mediated by immune mechanisms. This is further supported by the unfortunate finding that IFNγ exacerbates disease in the majority. The antidepressant roliprim, suppresses cytokine production and is effective in experimental allergic encephalomyelitis; it might be of value in MS.

## Immunological control strategies

### Cellular manipulation

It should one day be practical to correct any relevant defects in stem cells or in thymus processing by bone marrow or thymus grafting or perhaps, in the latter case, by thymic hormones.

Because T-cell signaling is so pivotal, it is the target for many strategies (figure 20.20). Injection of monoclonal anti-class II and anti-CD4 successfully fend off lupus in spontaneous mouse models and it is relevant to record the preliminary clinical observations that injection of immunoglobulins eluted from placentas,

and shown to contain anti-allo-class II, significantly ameliorate the symptoms of RA.

Some take the anti-IL-2 receptor approach to deplete activated T-cells (figure 20.20.1) but I would like to refer back to our discussion of the long-lasting effect of *nondepleting* anti-CD4 for the induction of tolerance (figure 20.20), particularly when reinforced by repeated exposure to antigen (cf. p. 368). Antigen reinforcement of course is an obvious continuing feature in autoimmune disease so that anti-CD4 should be ideal as a therapy in disorders where the natural 'switch-off' tolerogenic signals are still accepted by the CD4 cells; this may not be so in every case but the treatment should be a good way to test whether the CD4 read-out mechanism is still normal. Ongoing trials in RA are looking promising. Backup with nondepleting anti-LFA-I should improve efficacy even more.

We can manage perfectly well in life without a complete set of our TCR Vβ genes; after all wild mice, and presumably ourselves, delete large tracts of Vβ families during thymic differentiation and it does not seem to do them much harm. So, the argument runs, if the autoimmune T-cell clones specific for the autoantigen in a given disease happen to be restricted to membership of a particular Vβ family, we could delete all members of that family *in vivo* with the appropriate antiserum and yet not make irreparable holes in the host's defenses (figure 20.20). In PL mice immunized with the N-terminal peptide of myelin basic protein, antiVβ8 eliminated experimental autoallergic encephalitis almost entirely, so the strategy can work. Not so good with SJL mice which respond to peptide 89–101 with 50% of the T-cells using Vβ17 receptors; in this case, anti-Vβ17 did not block disease. Clearly, until we have wider knowledge of the extent of Vβ restriction for each antigen and also for each individual, we must suspend judgment on the general feasibility of the strategy.

### Manipulation of regulatory mediators

We can correct some spontaneous models of autoimmune disease by injection of cytokines: IL-1 cures the diabetes of NOD mice; TNF prevents the onset of SLE symptoms in NZB×W hybrids and transforming growth factor-β1 (TGFβ1) is known to protect against collagen arthritis and relapsing EAE. We have already reminded ourselves of the maintenance doses of steroids to restore the defective adrenal feedback control on leukocytes in RA.

If we now take it as almost gospel that the TH1 subset is pathogenic in solid organ-specific disease,

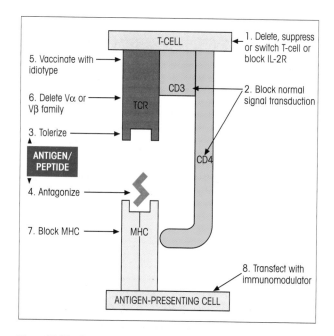

**Figure 20.20. Strategic options for therapy based on T-cell targeting.**

attempts to switch the phenotype to TH2 should be beneficial. On the assumption that a TCR signal 1 plus IL-4 can effect this switch, then treatment of an autoimmune individual with IL-4 should defuse the TH1 cells as was indeed observed in an EAE model. The exacerbation of TH1-mediated disease by IL-12 raises the possibility that the highly avid dimer of one of the IL-2 receptor chains might be a potent inhibitor. However, with the exception of steroids in RA, there is quite a gap between therapy in experimental animals and its application to human disease. It could be that transfection of the target organ with a protective cytokine like TGFβ (figure 20.20.8) will prove to be a good bet (visions of firing a biolistic gun at islets pretransplantation?).

### Idiotype control with antibody

The powerful immunosuppressive action of anti-idiotype antibodies has led to much rumination on the feasibility of controlling autoantibody production by provoking appropriate interactions within the immune network. We have focused previously on the intimate network interactions between hormone receptors, hormones and their respective antibodies (cf. p. 209) and it might be that the autoimmune disorders involving these receptors are especially amenable to idiotype control. There is a growing realization that, in general, more fundamental suppression can be achieved by utilizing the internal elements of the idiotype network rather than anti-idiotype reagents raised in other species. Thus, xenogeneic anti-idiotypes have only won transient and partial improvement in the spontaneous thyroiditis of the Buffalo rat and the autoimmune lupus of NZB×W mice, presumably due to compensation by idiotype negative clones. On the other hand, much more profound changes have been achieved by treatment with monoclonal autoantibodies (idiotypes) derived from the autoimmune strain in question.

Curiously, **intravenous injection of Ig pooled from many normal donors** is of positive benefit in a number of autoimmune blood diseases, recurrent abortions associated with cardiolipin antibodies, juvenile dermatomyositis and patients with autoantibodies to procoagulant factor VIII. The latter has been studied in some detail and the inhibitory effects of F(ab')₂ fractions from the normal Ig pool suggests that we are dealing with anti-idiotypic reactions; it is as though the normal pool was reestablishing a properly controlled network. These are intriguing observations which deserve serious consideration, although to some extent their use is marred by expense.

### Vaccination with T-cell idiotypes

It is possible to protect animals against the induction of experimental allergic encephalomyelitis by immunization with an attenuated T-cell clone specific for myelin basic protein (MBP). This must be mediated by the induction of suppressor T-cells specific for the effector cell receptor idiotype. Confirmation has come from experiments showing that the encephalitis can be prevented if mice are first immunized with synthetic peptide from the Vβ chain of the encephalitogenic clone; this procedure generates CD8 T-cells specific for the receptor peptide presented by class I MHC, and which transfer protection against induction of encephalitis.

This gambit (figure 20.20.5) has now been played in human disease. A TCR peptide vaccine embodying the Vβ5.2 sequence expressed in MS plaques and on T-cells specific for MBP was used to treat MS patients in a double-blind trial (100 μg weekly for 4 weeks and then monthly for 10 months). Lack of response to vaccination was associated with increased response to MBP and clinical progression, but successful vaccination boosted the frequency of TCR peptide-specific T-cells, reduced the frequency of MBP-specific cells and prevented clinical progression without side-effects. The reactive cells were predominantly TH2-like and directly inhibited MBP-specific TH1 responses, primarily through release of IL-10 and probably through an anti-idiotypic regulatory network. Although many of the T-cells in the lesions would not belong to the Vβ5.2 family, they could be switched off by organ-related bystander tolerance (see figure 20.22).

T-cell vaccination has been used to protect against the spontaneous development of diabetes in NOD mice and the production of arthritis following sensitization with type II collagen. It has also proved possible to switch off Freund-adjuvant-induced arthritis with an attenuated clone of T-cells generated in response to the 65 kDa mycobacterial heat-shock protein. This adjuvant model has been looked at in depth (I. Cohen). Perversely, the earliest T-cell responses preceding the adjuvant-induced arthritis were antigen-specific suppression and anti-idiotypic reactivity; responses to the antigen itself emerged a few days before the appearance of clinical arthritis. T-cell vaccination accelerated the kinetics of the antigen response, abolished antigen-specific suppression, activated anti-idiotypic T-cells and inhibited arthritis. The extremely rapid appearance of anti-idiotype and antigen-specific suppressors so soon after immunization with the 65 kDa heat-shock protein again strongly suggests a preexisting network linked to epitopes on this antigen as envisaged in the 'immunological homunculus' concept (cf. p. 209). If malfunctioning of the network produces autoimmune disease, vaccination with T-cell receptor epitopes would represent a logical attempt to reestablish natural control.

## Manipulation by antigen

The object is to present the offending antigen in sufficient concentration and in the form which will turn off an ongoing autoimmune response. Since T-cells have been accorded such a pivotal role, it is natural to devise the strategy in terms of T-cell epitopes rather than whole antigen, obviously a far more practical proposition because this reduces the problem to dealing with relatively short peptides. One strategy is to design high affinity peptide analogs that will bind obstinately to the appropriate MHC molecule and antagonize the response to autoantigen (figure 20.20.4). Since we express several different MHC molecules, this should not impair microbial defences unduly. However, we are now talking of patients not mice and this could involve repeated very high doses of peptide, although, much in their favor, peptides are well defined chemically and *relatively* cheap to produce. Antigen-specific suppression of T-cells (figure 20.20.3) would be advantageous in this respect and giving the peptide under an umbrella of anti-CD4 or using partial agonists (cf. figure 9.6) could be feasible. Injection of an MBP peptide can block EAE and a

hsp60 peptide can prevent the onset of diabetes in the NOD mouse (cf. p. 438). Awareness of the therapeutic benefit of injected insulin in the NOD model has fostered a large-scale trial in the human disease and clinical improvement has been achieved in patients with exacerbating-remitting MS given Cop1, a random copolymer of alanine, glutamic acid, lysine and tyrosine meant to simulate MBP.

We have already noted that because the mucosal surface of the gut is exposed to a horde of powerfully immunogenic microorganisms, and since enterocytes are especially vulnerable to damage by IFNγ and TNF, it has been important for the immune defenses of the gut to evolve mechanisms which deter TH1-type responses. This objective is attained by the stimulation of cells which release cytokines such as TGFβ, IL-4 and IL-10 and suppress the unwanted responses. Thus feeding antigens should tolerize TH1 cells and this has proved to be a successful strategy for blocking EAE, the collagen II arthritis model and the development of diabetes in NOD mice. Accordingly, MS patients are now being fed MBP and RA patients type II chicken collagen.

The tolerogen can also be delivered by inhalation of peptide aerosols (figure 20.21) and this could be a very attractive way of generating antigen-specific T-cell suppression in many hypersensitivity states, although it is not clear whether the suppressor mechanism is the same as for oral tolerance. Induction of anergy or active suppression may contribute to different extents. Intranasal peptides have been used successfully to block collagen-induced arthritis, EAE and

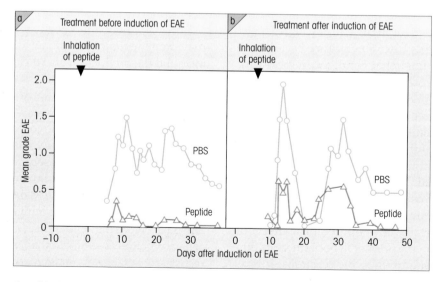

**Figure 20.21. Influence of peptide inhalation on experimental allergic encephalomyelitis (EAE) induced with pig spinal cord in complete Freund's adjuvant.** Aerosols of the peptides were inhaled (a) 8 days before and (b) 8 days after injection of the encephalitogen. PBS = phosphate-buffered saline; the peptide was an acetylated N-terminal 11-mer from myelin basic protein with lysine at position 4 substituted by alanine. (Data from Metzler B. & Wraith D.C. *Annals of the New York Academy of Science* (1996) **778**, 228, with permission of the publishers.)

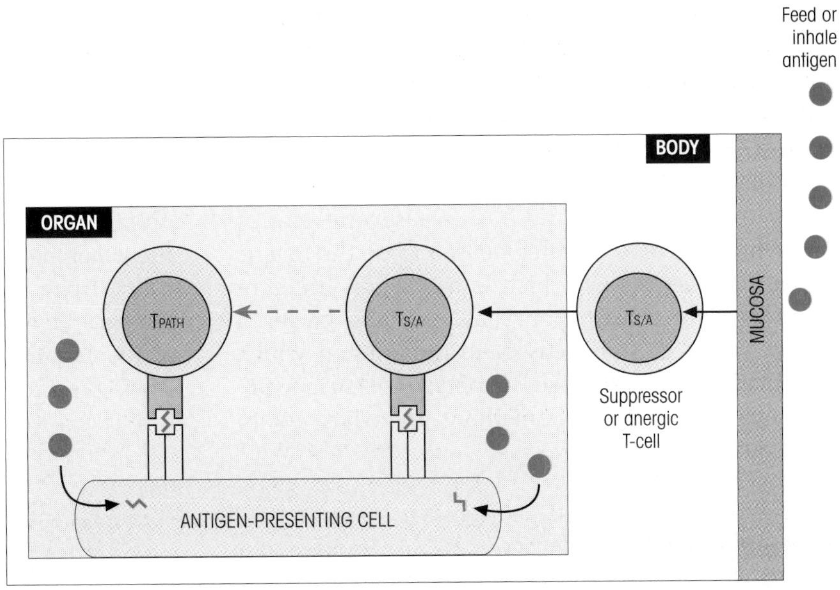

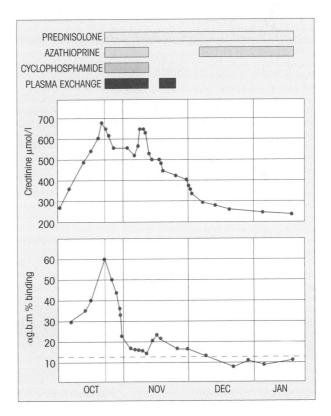

**Figure 20.22. Organ-related bystander tolerance induced by feeding or inhaling an organ-related autoantigen.** Induced suppressor or anergic tolerogen-specific T-cells enter the organ and inhibit pathogenic T-cells on the same antigen-presenting cell which processes both the tolerogen and the other organ-derived antigen recognized by the pathogenic cell. Suppressors may act by production of TGFβ, IL-4 and IL-10 which downregulate the TH1 cells. Anergic cells act by depriving the pathogenic cell of communal cytokine help required normally for stimulation (figure 12.8).

a mouse model of allergy to the house dust mite antigen Der P1. Significantly, treatment can be effective even *after* induction of disease (figure 20.21), although in established human disease this may be more difficult to achieve and might require supplementary therapy such as anti-CD4 and preliminary reduction of primed T-cells with cyclosporin or steroids. There is no shortage of strings to pull.

Now this is really important. A single internal epitope of MBP can inhibit disease induced by the *mixture* of epitopes or antigens contained within whole myelin. In other words, a single epitope can induce suppression of the pathogenic T-cells specific for other epitopes on the same or other molecules provided they are generated within the same organ or locality. I have referred to this already as **organ-related bystander tolerance**, a phenomenon best understood in terms of interactions between the regulatory cell, be it TH2 or anergic, recognizing the suppressor epitope, and the pathogenic TH1 cell recognizing a **separate epitope** processed from the same or another molecule in the same organ (figure 20.22).

Another potentially valuable approach for the future involves 'switching off' primed B-cells by presenting hapten linked to a thymus-independent carrier like the copolymer of D-glutamic and D-lysine (D-GL) or isologous IgG, particularly when given with high cortisone doses. This has certainly worked well in NZB×W hybrid mice where anti-DNA levels have been reduced using nucleosides as the haptens: we shall have to see whether man and mouse really are that different.

**Figure 20.23. Treatment of a patient with antiglomerular basement membrane (α-g.b.m) nephritis with plasma exchange, steroids and immunosuppressive drugs.** Kidney function is here monitored by the serum creatinine level. The treatment leads to loss of autoantibody (the dashed line represents the amount of g.b.m antigen bound in the assay by normal serum) and restoration of kidney function. (Courtesy of Dr C.M. Lockwood.)

Another way to manipulate antigen is to remove it. For DNA this can be accomplished by injection of DNase which splits the molecule even when complexed within the free nucleosome. Sure enough, treatment with DNase I suppressed the manifestations of lupus nephritis in the NZB×W model. And last, back to the Holy Grail business, several groups are trying to evolve a strategy based upon the 'magic bullet', the essence of which is to fashion different types of cytotoxic weaponry by coupling bacterial toxins or lots of radioactivity to the antigen which selectively homes on to the lymphocytes bearing specific surface receptors. Something good has got to come out of all this!

## Plasmapheresis

Plasma exchange to lower the rate of immune complex deposition in SLE provides only temporary benefit, although it may be of value in life-threatening cases of arteritis. Successful results have been obtained in Goodpasture's syndrome when the treatment has been applied in combination with antimitotic drugs (figure 20.23), the rationale being an increased tendency for antigen-reactive cells to divide as the negative feedback effect of IgG is lowered following removal of plasma proteins.

---

## SUMMARY

### Pathogenic effects of humoral autoantibody

• Direct pathogenic effects of human autoantibodies to blood, surface receptors and several other tissues are listed in table 20.2.
• Passive transfer of disease is seen in 'experiments of nature' in which transplacental passage of maternal IgG autoantibody produces a comparable but transient disorder in the fetus.
• Disease can also be mimicked in experimental animals by passive transfer of monoclonal autoantibodies.

Table 20.2. Direct pathogenic effects of humoral antibodies.

| DISEASE | AUTOANTIGEN | LESION |
|---|---|---|
| Autoimmune hemolytic anemia | Red cell | Erythrocyte destruction |
| Lymphopenia (some cases) | Lymphocyte | Lymphocyte destruction |
| Idiopathic thrombocytopenic purpura | Platelet | Platelet destruction |
| Wegener's granulomatosis | PMN proteinase III | PMN induced endothelial injury |
| Anti-phospholipid syndrome | Cardiolipin/$\beta$2–glycoprotein1 complex | Recurrent thromboembotic phenomena |
| Male infertility (some cases) | Sperm | Agglutination of spermatozoa |
| Pernicious anemia | $H^+/K^+$-ATPase, gastrin receptor | Block acid production |
| Hashimoto's disease | Thyroid peroxidase surface antigen | Cytotoxic effect on thyroid cells in culture |
| Primary myxedema | TSH receptor | Blocking of thyroid cell |
| Thyrotoxicosis | TSH receptor | Stimulation of thyroid cell |
| Goodpasture's syndrome | Glomerular basement membrane | Complement-mediated damage to basement membrane |
| Myasthenia gravis | Acetylcholine receptor | Blocking and destruction of receptors |
| Lambert–Eton syndrome | Presynaptic Ca channel | Neuromuscular defect |
| Acanthosis nigricans (type B) and ataxia telangiectasia with insulin resistance | Insulin receptor | Blocking of receptors |
| Atopic allergy (some cases) | $\beta$-Adrenergic receptors | Blocking of receptors |
| Congenital heart block | Ro/SS-A | Distort fetal cardiac membrane action potential |
| Celiac disease | Endomysium | Small intestinal inflammation |

(Continued)

## Pathogenic effects of complexes with autoantigens

• Immune complexes, usually with bound complement, appear in the kidneys, skin and joints of patients with SLE, associated with lesions in the corresponding organs.
• The formation of high affinity, mutated IgG antibodies to anatomically clustered antigens (e.g. nucleosome components) attests to T-cell control and antigen selection of the antibody response. These antigen clusters can appear as blebs on the surface of apoptotic cells.
• Spontaneous lupus has been observed in certain purebred animal strains and the importance of autoimmunity for pathogenesis is shown by the amelioration of symptoms whenever the immune response is suppressed.
• The IgG in RA shows defective galactosylation of the Fc sugars.
• Most patients with RA produce autoantibodies to IgG (rheumatoid factors) as a result of immunological hyperreactivity in the deeper layers of the synovium. The IgG rheumatoid factors self-associate to form complexes.
• These give rise to acute inflammation in the joint space and stimulate the synovial lining cells to grow as a malign **pannus** which **produces erosions in the underlying cartilage and bone** through the release of IL-1, IL-6, TNFα, prostaglandin E$_2$, collagenase, neutral proteinase and reactive oxygen intermediates.

## T-cell-mediated hypersensitivity as a pathogenic factor

• Suppression of disease by cyclosporin or anti-CD4 treatment is strong evidence for T-cell involvement. So is an HLA-linked risk factor.
• There is a prevailing view that organ-specific inflammatory lesions are caused by autoreactive pathogenic TH1 cells.
• Activated T-cells are abundant in the rheumatoid synovium and their production of TNFα and GM-CSF complements the immune complex stimulus for pannus formation.
• RA patients have poor corticosteroid responses to triggering of the pituitary/adrenal feedback loop and treatment with low, virtually maintenance doses of steroids is beneficial.
• Thyrocytes expressing MHC class II in autoimmune thyroid disease are direct targets for locally activated TH1-cells specific for thyroid peroxidase.
• That autoimmunity can cause thyroiditis is further shown by the deliberate induction of disease in rodents through immunization with thyroid antigens in complete Freund's adjuvant.
• The onset of IDDM is delayed by cyclosporin, HLA-DQ risk factors are prominent, and T-cell proliferative

**Table 20.3.** Comparison of organ-specific and nonorgan-specific diseases.

| ORGAN-SPECIFIC (e.g. THYROIDITIS, GASTRITIS, ADRENALITIS) | NONORGAN-SPECIFIC (e.g. SYSTEMIC LUPUS ERYTHEMATOSUS) |
|---|---|
| DIFFERENCES | |
| Antigens only available to lymphoid system in low concentration | Antigens accessible at higher concentrations |
| Antibodies and lesions organ-specific | Antibodies and lesions nonorgan-specific |
| Clinical and serologic overlap – thyroiditis, gastritis and adrenalitis | Overlap SLE, rheumatoid arthritis, and other connective tissue disorders |
| Familial tendency to organ-specific autoimmunity | Familial connective tissue disease |
| Lymphoid invasion, parenchymal destruction by cell-mediated hypersensitivity and/or antibodies | Lesions due to deposition of antigen–antibody complexes |
| Therapy aimed at controlling metabolic deficit or tolerizing T-cells | Therapy aimed at inhibiting inflammation and antibody synthesis |
| Tendency to cancer in organ | Tendency to lymphoreticular neoplasia |
| Antigens evoke organ-specific antibodies in normal animals with complete Freund's adjuvant | No antibodies produced in animals with comparable stimulation |
| Experimental lesions produced with antigen in Freund's adjuvant | Diseases and autoantibodies arise spontaneously in certain animals (e.g. NZB mice and hybrids) |
| SIMILARITIES | |

Circulating autoantibodies react with normal body constituents
Patients often have increased immunoglobulins in serum
Antibodies may appear in each of the main immunoglobulin classes particularly IgG and are usually high affinity and mutated
Greater incidence in women
Disease process not always progressive; exacerbations and remissions
Association with HLA
Spontaneous diseases in animals genetically programmed
Autoantibody tests of diagnostic value

(Continued on p. 448)

responses to β-islet cell antigens reflect prognosis of disease.

• TH1-cells from diseased NOD mice which mimic the human disorder in histopathology and autoimmunity, can produce typical pancreatic lesions in young mice of the same strain. Introduction of a transgene encoding changes at residues 56 or 57 in the H-2β-chain dramatically ameliorates disease.

• Similarity to experimental allergic encephalomyelitis, a demyelinating disease induced by immunization with myelin in complete Freund's adjuvant, has made autoimmunity the front-running hypothesis in MS. Approximately one-third of the IL-2 or 4 activatable T-cells in the CSF of MS patients are specific for myelin and the DR2 phenotype is a strong risk factor.

### Diagnostic value of autoantibody tests

• A wide range of serum autoantibodies now provides valuable diagnostic markers.

• Routine immunofluorescent screening is carried out on composite sections of human thyroid and stomach and rat kidney and liver, supplemented by agglutination tests for rheumatoid factors, thyroid and red cell antibodies, and by radioassays for intrinsic factor and acetylcholine receptor antibodies.

• Solid-phase ELISA tests are used for antibodies to DNA and other nuclear antigens and will increasingly displace fluorescence as purified autoantigens become available.

### Treatment of autoimmune disorders

• Therapy conventionally involves metabolic control and the use of anti-inflammatory and immunosuppressive drugs.

• A whole variety of potential immunological control therapies are under intensive investigation. These include antibody and T-cell idiotype manipulations and attempts to induce antigen-specific unresponsiveness particularly to T-cells using peptides.

• Organ-related bystander tolerance means that single epitopes can induce suppression of pathogenic cells within an organ reacting to other epitopes on the same or other antigens.

• Plasma exchange may be of value especially in combination with antimitotic drugs.

• The accompanying comparison of organ-specific and nonorgan-specific autoimmune disorders (table 20.3) gives an overall view of many of the points raised in these last two chapters.

## FURTHER READING

Albani S., Keystone E.C., Nelson J.L. *et al.* (1995) Positive selection in autoimmunity: abnormal immune responses to bacterial dnaJ antigenic determinant in patients with early rheumatoid arthritis. *Nature Medicine* **1**, 448–452.

Austen K.F., Burakoff S.J., Rosen F.S. & Strom T.B. (eds) (1996) *Therapeutic Immunology*. Blackwell Science, Oxford.

Bach J-F. (ed.) (1996) Symposium on autoimmunity. *Journal of Autoimmunity* **9**, 205–304.

Brostoff J., Scadding G.K., Male D. & Roitt I.M. (1991) *Clinical Immunology*. Gower Medical Publishing, London.

Celis E. (1993) T-helper cells and autoantibodies in autoimmune disease. *The Immunologist* **1**, 126–130.

Chapel M. & Haeney M. (1993) *Essentials of Clinical Immunology*, 3rd edn. Blackwell Scientific Publications, Oxford.

Gelfand E.W. (ed.) (1996) Intravenous immune globulin: mechanisms of action and model disease states. *Clinical and Experimental Immunology* **104**(Suppl. 1), 1–97.

Kingsley G., Lanchbury J. & Panayi G. (1996) Immunotherapy in rheumatic disease. *Immunology Today* **17**, 9–12.

Lachmann P.J., Peters D.K., Rosen F.S. & Walport M.J. (eds) (1993) *Clinical Aspects of Immunology*, 5th edn. Blackwell Scientific Publications, Oxford.

Lanzavacchia A. (1993) Identifying strategies for immune intervention. *Science* **260**, 937–944.

Lichtenstein L.M. & Fauci A.S. (eds) (1996) *Current Therapy in Allergy, Immunology and Rheumatology*, Mosby, St Louis.

Lokki M-J. & Colten H.R. (1995) Genetic deficiencies of complement. *Annals of Medicine* **27**, 451–459.

McInnes I.B., Leung B.P., Sturrock R.D., Field M. & Liew F.Y. (1997) Interleukin-15 mediates T cell-dependent regulation of tumor necrosis factor-a production in rheumatoid arthritis. *Nature Medicine* **3**, 189–195.

Morrow J. & Isenberg D.A. (1987) *Autoimmune Rheumatic Disease*. Blackwell Scientific Publications, Oxford.

Peter J.B. & Shoenfeld Y. (eds) (1996) *Autoantibodies*, Elsevier, Amsterdam.

Rademacher T., Williams P. & Dwek R.A. (1994) Agalactosyl glycoforms of IgG autoantibodies are pathogenic. *Proceedings of National Academy of Sciences* **91**, 6123–6127.

Read A.P. & Brown T. (eds) (1992) *Autoimmunity*. BIOS Scientific Publishers. (Easily digested didactic overview of most of the important areas of clinical development. Slim volume.)

Rich R.R. *et al.* (eds) (1996) *Clinical Immunology: Principles and Practice*. Mosby, St Louis.

Selimena M. *et al.* (1990) Autoantibodies to GABA-ergic neurones and pancreatic β-cells in stiff man syndrome. *New England Journal of Medicine* **322**, 1555. (Fun to read just for the title!)

Shoenfeld Y. & Isenberg D.A. (eds) (1993) *Natural Autoantibodies. Their Physiological Role and Regulatory Significance*. CRC Press, Boca Raton, FA.

Shoenfeld Y. & Isenberg D. (1989) *The Mosaic of Autoimmunity (The Factors associated with Autoimmune Disease)*. Elsevier, Amsterdam. (An excellent account.)

Sieper J. & Kingsley G. (1996) Recent advances in the pathogenesis of reactive arthritis. *Immunology Today* **17**, 160–163.

Song Y.-H., Li Y. & Maclaren N.K. (1996) The nature of autoantigens targeted in autoimmune endocrine diseases. *Immunology Today* **17**, 232–238.

Stites D.P., Stobo J.D. & Wells I.V. (eds) (1994) *Basic and Clinical Immunology*, 7th edn. Appleton & Lange, Norwalk, CN.

Thomas J. & Lipsky P.E. (1996) Could endogenous self-peptides presented by dendritic cells initiate rheumatoid arthritis? *Immunology Today* **17**, 559–564.

Thompson R.A. (ed.) (1985) Laboratory investigation of immunological disorders. *Clinics in Immunology and Allergy*, vol. 5. W.B. Saunders, London.

Thompson R.A. (series ed.) *Recent Advances in Clinical Immunology*.

Churchill Livingstone, Edinburgh.

Todd J.A. (1996) Human genetics: Transcribing diabetes. *Nature* **384(6608)**, 407–408.

Vandenbark A.A. *et al.* (1996) Treatment of multiple sclerosis with T-cell receptor peptides. *Nature Medicine* **2**, 1109–1115.

Weetman A.P. (ed.) (1991) *Autoimmune Endocrine Disease*. Cambridge University Press, Cambridge, UK.

Weiner H.L. & Mayer L.F. (1996) Oral tolerance: mechanisms and applications. *Annals of the New York Academy of Science* **778**, 1–453.

Wicker L. & Wekerle H. (eds) (1995) Autoimmunity. *Current Opinion in Immunology* **6**, 783–852. (Several critical essays in each annual volume).

# CD MARKERS

CD (Cluster of differentiation) markers on hematopoietic cells.

| CD | Identity | Function | Cellular distribution | Ligands |
|---|---|---|---|---|
| CD1a | | Peptide and lipid antigen presentation | Thymocyte, LC, DC | Unknown |
| CD1b | | | Thymocyte, DC | Unknown |
| CD1c | | | Thymocyte, DC, LC, B(sub) | Unknown |
| CD2 | LFA-2, T11 | T adhesion to target cells or APC | Thymocytes, T, NK | LFA-3, CD58, CD59 |
| CD3 | | Signal transduction ($\zeta$) and T activation | Thymocyte, T | Unknown |
| CD4 | | Helper activity | Thymocyte (sub), T(sub), Mo, M$\phi$ | MHC class II |
| CD5 | Leu-1, Ly-1 | Signal for T and thymocyte activation | Thymocyte, T, B(sub) | CD72 |
| CD6 | | T activation and thymocyte–stromal interaction | Thymocyte, T | CD166 |
| CD7 | | Signal transduction | SC, thymocyte, T | Fc$\mu$R? |
| CD8 | | Maturation and positive selection of T | Thymocyte (sub), T(sub) | MHC class I |
| CD9 | | Platelet activation and aggregation | Pre-B, Plt | CD41/CD61 |
| CD10 | CALLA, NEP | May limit activity of peptide hormones | BM | Unknown |
| CD11a/CD18 | LFA-1, $\alpha_L\beta_2$ | Leukocyte–leukocyte/leukocyte–endothelium interactions | Hematopoietic cells, most leukocytes, eosinophils | ICAM-1, 2, 3 |
| CD11b/CD18 | Mac-1, $\alpha_M\beta_2$, CR3 | Adhesion of Mo/neutrophils to vascular endothelium | NK, most leukocytes | ICAM-1, iC3b, fibrinogen |
| CD11c/CD18 | CR4, $\alpha_x\beta_2$, p150,95 | Adhesion of Gr to inflamed endothelium | NK, Gr | iC3b, fibrinogen |
| CDw12 | | | Mo, Gr, Plt | |
| CD13 | | Aminopeptidase | Mo, Gr | |
| CD14 | | LPS-binding protein | Mo | |
| CD15 | | ELAM receptor | Gr | |
| CD16 | Fc$\gamma$RIII | Phagocytosis and ADCC | Gr, NK, M$\phi$ | Fc$\gamma$ |

(Continued on p. 452)

CD markers (*Continued*)

| CD | Identity | Function | Cellular distribution | Ligands |
|---|---|---|---|---|
| CDw17 | | Lactosylceramide | Mo, Gr | |
| CD18 | | β-chain of CD11 | Leukocytes | |
| CD19 | B4 | B activation and proliferation | B | Unknown |
| CD20 | B1, Bp35 | Regulation of B activation and proliferation | B | Unknown |
| CD21 | CR2, EBVR, C3dR | Part of a signal-transduction complex | B, FDC | C3d, CD23, EBV |
| CD22 | BL-CAM | B adhesion interactions | B Mat (sub) | Sialyl proteins, CD45 |
| CD23 | FcεRI | B activation and IgE regulation | B, *Mφ, FDC, Plt | Fcε, CD21 |
| CD24 | HSA | Signaling and support of T growth | T, B, Gr | Unknown |
| CD25 | IL-2 Rα | T growth | Thymocytes, *T , pre-B | IL-2 |
| CD26 | DPPIV | Binds and transports adenosine deaminase to the cell surface | *T, *B, Mφ | Unknown |
| CD27 | | Costimulatory signal for T activation | Thymocyte, T | CD70 |
| CD28 | | Costimulatory molecule | T(sub), *B | CD86, CD80 |
| CD29 | VLA β chain | | Leukocytes | |
| CD30 | | Transduction of a signal for apoptosis | *T, *B | CD153 |
| CD31 | PECAM-1 | Transendothelial migration of leukocytes | Mo, Plt, neutrophils, NK, endothelial and naive T | CD31, $\alpha_v\beta_3$ |
| CD32 | FcγRII | | B, Mφ, Gr | Fcγ |
| CD33 | My9 | | Mo, Mφ, mast cells | |
| CD34 | My10 | Adhesion | Progenitor cells, endothelial cells | CD62E?, CD62L? |
| CD35 | CR1, C3b/C4b R | Inhibits complement activation | Erythrocytes, B, T(sub), phagocytes, eosinophils | C3b, C4b |
| CD36 | GPIIIb, MFGM PAS IV | Adhesion molecule | Endothelial cells, Plt, Mo, megakaryocytes | Thrombospondin, collagen |
| CD37 | | B activation and proliferation | B, T | Unknown |
| CD38 | T10 | Unknown | B(sub), *T | Unknown |
| CD39 | gp80 | | B(sub), *NK(sub), *T(sub) | |
| CD40 | | B activation, proliferation and differentiation | B, Mo, DC | CD154 |
| CD41/CD61 | $\alpha_{IIb}\beta_3$, GPIIb IIIa complex | Platelet aggregation | The major integrin on Plt plasma membrane, megakaryocytes | VWF, fibrinogen, fibronectin |
| CD42 | GP IX, (CD42a), GP Ibα, (CD42b), GP Ibβ, (CD42c), GP V, (CD42d), GP Ib–IX–V complex | Plt adherence and aggregation at sites of vascular damage | Plt, megakaryocytes, vascular tonsilar endothelial cells | VWF, thrombin |
| CD43 | Leucosialin, gp115 | Hematopoietic progenitor cell proliferation | Leukocytes | ICAM-1 (CD54) |
| CD44 | H-CAM, Pgp-1, HERMES | Cell–cell and cell–ECM adhesion | Hematopoietic cells, B and T, Mo, neutrophils, epithelial cells | Hyaluronate |

CD markers (*Continued*)

| CD | Identity | Function | Cellular distribution | Ligands |
|---|---|---|---|---|
| CD45 | LCA | Signaling in B and T | Leukocytes | CD22 |
| CD45RA | Restricted LCA | | T(sub), B, Gr(sub), Mo | |
| CD45RB | Restricted LCA | | T(sub), B, Gr, Mo | |
| CD45RC | Restricted LCA | | | |
| CD45RO | Restricted LCA | | T(sub), Gr, Mo | |
| CD46 | Membrane cofactor protein (MCP) | | Widespread | |
| CD47 | Integrin-associated protein (IAP) | Associated with vitronectin receptor | Broad | |
| CD48 | Blast-1, OX-45, BCM1 | T adhesion to target cells and APC | Hematopoietic and nonhematopoietic tissues | CD2 (rodent) |
| CD49a/CD29 | VLA-1, $\alpha_1\beta_1$ | Receptor for the E1 domain of laminin and a region of collagen I and IV | Fibroblasts, capillary endothelial cells, NK cells, activated T | Laminin, collagen I and IV |
| CD49b/CD29 | VLA-2, $\alpha_2\beta_1$ | Regulates the expression of MMP-1 and collagen type I | Fibroblasts, endothelial cells, Plt, B and T, keratinocytes | Collagen I–IV, laminin |
| CD49c/CD29 | VLA-3, $\alpha_3\beta_1$ | Cell–cell interaction | Fibroblasts, keratinocytes, epithelial cells, B | Fibronectin, collagen |
| CD49d/CD29 | VLA-4, $\alpha_4\beta_1$ | Leukocyte rolling, adhesion and migration | Widespread | VCAM-1, fibronectin |
| CD49e/CD29 | VLA-5, $\alpha_5\beta_1$ | Cell adhesion, cell migration and matrix assembly | Fibroblasts, epithelial and endothelial cells, muscle cells, Plt | Fibronectin and L1 |
| CD49f/CD29 | VLA-6, $\alpha_6\beta_1$ | Cell adhesion, spreading and migration | Widespread | Laminin |
| CD50 | ICAM-3 | Signaling and costimulatory molecule on T | Mo, neutrophils, lymphocytes | $\alpha_d\beta_2$, LFA-1 |
| CD51/CD61 | $\alpha_v\beta_3$, vitronectin receptor | Recruitment, distribution and retention of cells via ECM molecules | Endothelial cells, Mo, Plt, osteoclasts, tumor cells, some B, T | CD31, laminin, fibrinogen, fibronectin |
| CD52 | Campath-1 | | Leukocytes | |
| CD53 | MEM-53 | Activation | Leukocytes | |
| CD54 | ICAM-1 | Leukocyte adhesion to endothelium in inflammation | Endothelial cells, dendritic cells, epithelial cells, Mo, B | LFA-1, MAC-1, CD43 |
| CD55 | | Decay accelerating factor (DAF) | Most cells | |
| CD56 | NCAM, D2-CAM, Leu-19, NKH1 | Development of normal tissue architecture | Neurons, astrocytes, myoblasts, myotubes, *T, NK | CD56, heparan sulfate |
| CD57 | HNK-1, Leu-7 | MHC nonrestricted cytotoxicity after activation | NK, T(sub), B(sub), Mo | Unknown |
| CD58 | LFA-3 | Interactions of APC and target cells with T | Leukocytes, erythrocytes, endothelial cells, epithelial cells, fibroblasts | CD2 |
| CD59 | | Protects from complement-mediated lysis | Widespread | CD2 |
| CDw60 | NeuAc–NeuAc–Gal | | T(sub), Plt | |
| CD61 | Vitronectin receptor $\beta$ | | Plt | |

(Continued on p. 454)

CD markers (*Continued*)

| CD | Identity | Function | Cellular distribution | Ligands |
|---|---|---|---|---|
| CD62E | E-Selectin, ELAM-1 | Tethering and rolling of leukocytes on cytokine-activated endothelium | Endothelial cells | ESL-1 |
| CD62L | L-Selectin, Leu-8 | Tethering and rolling of lymphocytes on LN HEV and leukocytes on endothelium | Leukocytes; is downregulated on activation by endoproteolysis (shedding) | CD34, MAdCAM, GlyCAM-1, sLe$^x$ |
| CD62P | P-Selectin, GMP-140, PADGEM | Adhesion of Plt to Mo and neutrophils, and leukocytes to endothelium | Thrombin/histamine activated Plt and endothelium; stored in granules prior to activation | PSGL-1 |
| CD63 | LIMP, ME491 | | *Plt, Mo | |
| CD64 | FcγRI | | Mo | Fcγ |
| CD65 | Lew$^x$ poly-*N*-acetyllactosamine | Unknown | Mo | Unknown |
| CD65s | sLew$^x$ poly-*N*-acetyllactosamine | Unknown | Mo, neutrophils | Unknown |
| CD66 series | Carcinoembryonic antigen (CEA) gene family | | Gr | |
| CD67 | CANCELLED (now CD66b) | | | |
| CD68 | Microsialin | | Mo, Mφ, *Plt | Oxidized LDL |
| CD69 | AIM, Leu23 | Activation, signal transduction | Early *T, early *B, *Mφ | |
| CD70 | Ki-24 | | *T(sub), *B(sub) | CD27 |
| CD71 | | Transferrin receptor | *T, *B, *NK, *Mo, Mφ, SC | |
| CD72 | | B activation and proliferation | B | CD5 |
| CD73 | | Ecto-5'-nucleotidase | T(sub), B(sub) | |
| CD74 | | MHC class II invariant chain | B, Mo, LC | |
| CDw75 | | Unknown | B, T(sub) | CD22? |
| CDw76 | | | B(sub), T(sub), endothelial cells | CD22? |
| CD77 | | Globotriaosylceramide | B | |
| CDw78 | Ba | | B, Mφ(sub) | |
| CD79a | Igα, mb1 | Signal transduction as part of B receptor | B | Unknown |
| CD79b | Igβ, B29 | Signal transduction as part of B receptor | B | Unknown |
| CD80 | B7.1, BB1 | Binding regulates IL-2 gene expression | B (sub) | CD28, CD152 |
| CD81 | TAPA-1 | Cross-linking induces effects consistent with a role in signal transduction | T, B | Unknown |
| CD82 | R2 | Largely unknown (signal transduction?) | Leukocytes | Unknown |
| CD83 | HB15 | Unknown (antigen presentation?) | *T, *B, DC | Unknown |
| CD84 | 2G7 | | Mo, Mφ, Plt, B | |
| CD85 | | Unknown | B, Mo | Unknown |
| CD86 | B7.2 | Regulates IL-2 expression | B, Mo | CD28, CD152 |
| CD87 | Urokinase plasminogen activator protein | Receptor | Mo, Mφ, Gr, *T, endothelial cells | Vitronectin |

(Continued)

CD markers (*Continued*)

| CD | Identity | Function | Cellular distribution | Ligands |
|---|---|---|---|---|
| CD88 | C5a receptor | Complement receptor | Gr, Mo, Mφ, mast cells | C5a |
| CD89 | Fcα receptor | Fc receptor | Gr, Mo, Mφ, B(sub), T(sub) | IgA1, IgA2 |
| CD90 | Thy-1 | Lymphocyte recirculation and T activation | Thymocyte, T (mouse) | Unknown |
| CD91 | $\alpha_2$-Macroglobulin receptor LDLR-related protein | Receptor | Mo, Mφ | $\alpha_2$-Macroglobulin |
| CDw92 | VIM15 | | Gr, Mo, Plt, endothelial cells | |
| CD93 | p120 | | Mo, Gr, endothelial cells | |
| CD94 | kp43 | Inhibition/activation of cytotoxicity | T(sub), NK | Some HLA-class I molecules |
| CD95 | Fas, APO-1 | Transduces an apoptotic signal | Widespread | Fas-L |
| CD96 | Tactile | | *T, *NK | |
| CD97 | p74/80/89 | | Gr, Mo, *T, *B | CD55 |
| CD98 | 4F2 | Modulates intracellular $Ca^{2+}$ levels | T, B, NK, Gr | Unknown |
| CD99 | E2, MIC2 | T and red-cell rosette formation | Thymocyte, T, B | Unknown |
| CD100 | | Proliferation of PBMCs | Leukocytes | Unknown |
| CD101 | | Type I transmembrane protein | Gr, Mo, Mφ, DC, *T | Unknown |
| CD102 | ICAM-2 | Lymphocyte recirculation and trafficking | Endothelial cells, HEVs, lymphocytes, Mo, NK, Plt | LFA-1 |
| CD103 | $\alpha_E\beta_7$, M290/β7 integrin, HML-1 | Heterotypic adhesion of mucosal lymphocytes to epithelial cells | Most intraepithelial T and 50% of *lamina propria* lymphocytes, absent from PBLs | E-cadherin |
| CD104 | Integrin $\beta_4$-chain | Adhesion molecule with integrin $\alpha_6$-chain | | Laminin, epiligrin |
| CD105 | Endoglin | | *Mo, endothelial cells | |
| CD106 | VCAM-1 | Leukocyte migration and recruitment to sites of inflammation | APC, BM stromal cells, vascular endothelial cells | VLA-4, $\alpha_4\beta_7$ |
| CD107a | LAMP-1 | | *Plt | |
| CD107b | LAMP-2 | | *Plt | |
| CDw108 | GPI-gp80 | | *T | |
| CD109 | Sialo-mucin | Unknown | Endothelial cells, stromal cells, some myeloid cells | Unknown |
| CD114 | G-CSF R, IL-10R | Proliferation and differentiation of human B | Gr, Mo, Plt | IL-10, G-CSF |
| CD115 | CSF-1R | Cytokine receptor | Mo, Mφ | M-CSF |
| CD116 | GM-CSF Rα | Unknown | Mo, Gr | GM-CSF |
| CD117 | c-*kit*, SCF-R | Signal transduction, regulation of adhesion | Hematopoietic progenitors, mast cells | SCF |
| CDw119 | IFNγR | Cytokine receptor | Mo, Gr | IFNγ |
| CD120a | TNF receptor type I | Cytokine receptor | Broad | TNFα, lymphotoxin (TNFβ) |
| CD120b | TNF receptor type II | Cytokine receptor | Broad | TNFα, lymphotoxin (TNFβ) |
| CD121a | IL-1 RI | Stimulates T growth | Thymocytes, T, fibroblasts, endothelial cells | IL-1α, β, ra |
| CD121b | IL-1RII | | B, T, Mo, Mφ | IL-1α, β, ra |

(*Continued on p. 456*)

CD markers (*Continued*)

| CD | Identity | Function | Cellular distribution | Ligands |
|---|---|---|---|---|
| CD122 | IL-2 Rβ | Unknown | T, NK | IL-2 |
| CDw123 | IL-3 Rα | Unknown | Not determined | IL-3 |
| CD124 | IL-4Rα | Proliferative activity in pre-activated B and T | T and B, hematopoietic precursors, fibroblasts | IL-4 |
| CDw125 | IL-5Rα | Growth and differentiation of eosinophils | Eosinophils, basophils | IL-5 |
| CD126 | IL-6Rα | Differentiation and proliferation of hematopoietic precursors and acute phase response | Activated B, plasma cells, T, Mo, epithelial cells, fibroblasts, neural cells | IL-6 |
| CD127 | IL-7Rα | Proliferation of pro- and pre-activated B and T | Immature thymocytes, hepatocytes, pre-B, T Mat | IL-7 |
| CDw128 | IL-8R | Cytokine receptor | Gr, T(sub), Mo | IL-8 |
| CD129 | IL-9R | Growth promoting activity for T tumors | T and B, macrophages, megakaryoblasts | IL-9 |
| CD130 | gp130 | Signal transduction | Not determined | IL-6, IL-11, LIF, OSM, CNTF, CT-1 |
| CDw131 | Common β-chain | B growth | Mo, Gr, eosinophils, human B basophils, mouse B | IL-3, IL-5, GM-CSF |
| CD132 | Common γ-chain | B/T growth | T and B, hematopoietic precursors, fibroblasts | IL-2, 4, 7, 9, 15 |
| CD134 | OX40 | Adhesion of *T to vascular endothelial cells | Expressed on *T | OX40 ligand, gp34 |
| CD135 | Flt3/Flk2 | Receptor, tyrosine kinase | CD34 cells, carcinoma cells | Flt3/Flk2 ligand |
| CD136 | MSP R, RON | Receptor, tyrosine kinase | Not determined | Macrophage stimulating protein |
| CDw137 | 4-1BB | Co-stimulatory molecule for T activation | T | 4-1BB ligand |
| CD138 | Syndecan-1 | Heparan sulfate proteoglycan | B(sub) | Collagen type 1 |
| CD139 | | Unknown | B | Unknown |
| CD140a | PDGF Rα | Tyrosine kinase | Unknown | PDGF A or B |
| CD140b | PDGF Rβ | Tyrosine kinase | Endothelial cells, stromal cells, mesangial cells | PDGF B |
| CD141 | Thrombomodulin | Down-regulates coagulation | Myeloid cells, endothelial cells, smooth muscle cells | Thrombin |
| CD142 | Tissue factor | Induces coagulation | Mo, endothelial cells, keratinocytes, epithelial cells | Factor VII |
| CD143 | ACE | Peptidyl-peptidase | Endothelial cells, epithelial cells, Mφ | N/A |
| CD144 | VE-cadherin | Adhesion molecule | Endothelial cells | Unknown |
| CDw145 | | | Endothelial cells | |
| CD146 | MUC18, S-endo | Extravasation/homing of *T? | Endothelial cells, FDC, *T | Unknown |
| CD147 | Neurothelin, basigin, TCSF, EMMPRIN, M6 | Adhesion molecule? | Endothelial cells, myeloid cells, lymphoid cells | Type IV collagen? Fibronectin? Laminin? |
| CD148 | HPTP-eta, DEP-1 | Contact inhibition of cell growth | Hematopoietic cells | Unknown |
| CD149 | MEM133 | Unknown | Lymphocytes, Mo | Unknown |
| CDw150 | SLAM | Signaling molecule | T(sub), B(sub), thymocytes | Unknown |

(*Continued*)

CD markers (*Continued*)

| CD | Identity | Function | Cellular distribution | Ligands |
|---|---|---|---|---|
| CD151 | PETA3 | Signaling complex with FcR IIa? | Plt, Gr, endothelial cells, smooth muscle cells, epithelial cells | Integrins? HLA-DR? |
| CD152 | CTLA-4 | Negative regulator for T costimulation | *T | CD80, CD86 |
| CD153 | CD30L | Costimulatory for T | *T, Gr, B, Mφ | CD30 |
| CD154 | CD40L, gp39 | Costimulatory molecule | *T, *B, NK, mast cells | CD40 |
| CD155 | Polio virus R | Unknown | Mo, macrophages, thymocytes, CNS neurons | CD44? |
| CD156 | ADAM 8 | Unknown | Mo, macrophages, Gr | Unknown |
| CD157 | Bst-1 | ADP–ribose cyclase | Mo, neutrophils, endothelial cells, FDC | Unknown |
| CD158a | p58.1, p50.1 | Inhibition of cytotoxicity | T, NK | HLA-CW2, CW4, CW5, CW6 |
| CD158b | p58.2, p50.2 | Inhibition of cytotoxicity | T, NK | HLA-CW1, CW3, CW7, CW8 |
| CD161 | NKRP1A | Regulation of NK cell-mediated cytotoxic activity | NK, Mo, T(sub) | Negative charged CHOs |
| CD162 | PSGL-1 | Leukocyte rolling on activated endothelium | Mo, Gr, T, subset of B | P-selectin |
| CD163 | M130 | Unknown | Mo, some Mφ | Unknown |
| CD164 | MGC-24 | Adhesion of hematopoietic progenitor cells to stromal cells | Myeloid cells, T, epithelial cells, BM stromal cells, hematopoietic progenitor cells, certain carcinoma cells | Unknown |
| CD165 | AD2, gp37 | Adhesion of thymocytes to thymic epithelium | T, NK, Plt, thymocytes, thymic epithelium, CNS neurons | Unknown |
| CD166 | ALCAM | Activated leukocyte adhesion molecule | Activated B and T, eosinophils, thymic epithelium, fibroblasts, endothelial cells, keratinocytes | CD6 |

Abbreviations: APC, antigen-presenting cell; BM, bone marrow; T, T-cell; B, B-cell; NK, natural killer cell; Mo, monocyte; Mφ, macrophage; Gr, granulocyte; Plt, platelet; LC, Langerhans cell; DC, interdigitating dendritic cell; FDC, follicular dendritic cell; SC, stem cell; *, activated; Rest, resting; Mat, mature; (sub), subset; EBV, Epstein–Barr virus; ECM, extracellular matrix; VWF, von-Willebrand factor.

# GLOSSARY

**acquired immune response:** Immunity mediated by lymphocytes and characterized by antigen-specificity and memory.

**acute phase proteins:** Serum proteins, mostly produced in the liver, which rapidly change in concentration (some increase, some decrease) during the initiation of an inflammatory response.

**adjuvant:** Any substance which nonspecifically enhances the immune response to antigen.

**affinity (intrinsic affinity):** The strength of binding (affinity constant) between a receptor (e.g. one antigen-binding site on an antibody) and a ligand (e.g. epitope on an antigen).

**allele:** Variants of a polymorphic gene at a given genetic locus.

**allelic exclusion:** The phenomenon whereby, following successful rearrangement of one allele of an antigen receptor gene, rearrangement of the other parental allele is suppressed, thereby ensuring each lymphocyte expresses only a single specificity of antigen receptor (although this does not occur for α chains in T-cells).

**allergen:** An antigen which causes allergy.

**allergy:** IgE-mediated hypersensitivity, e.g. asthma, eczema, hayfever and food allergy.

**allogeneic:** Refers to the genetic differences between individuals of the same species.

**allograft:** Tissue or organ graft between allogeneic individuals.

**allotype:** An allelic variant of an antigen which, because it is not present in all individuals, may be immunogenic in members of the same species which have a different version of the allele.

**alternative pathway (of complement activation):** Activation pathway involving complement components C3, Factor B, Factor D, and Properdin which, in the presence of a stabilizing activator surface such as microbial polysaccharide, generates the alternative pathway C3 convertase $C\overline{3b}\overline{Bb}$.

**anaphylatoxin:** A substance (e.g. C3a, C4a or C5a) capable of directly triggering mast cell degranulation.

**anaphylaxis:** An often fatal hypersensitivity reaction, triggered by IgE or anaphylatoxin-mediated mast cell degranulation, leading to anaphylactic shock due to vasodilation and smooth muscle contraction.

**anergy:** Potentially reversible specific immunological tolerance in which the lymphocyte becomes functionally nonresponsive.

**antibody-dependent cell-mediated cytotoxicity (ADCC):** A cytotoxic reaction in which an antibody-coated target cell is directly killed by an Fc receptor-bearing leukocyte, e.g. NK cell, macrophage or neutrophil.

**antigen:** Any molecule capable of being recognized by an antibody or T-cell receptor.

**antigen-presenting cell (APC):** A term most commonly used when referring to cells that present processed antigenic peptide and MHC class II molecules to the T-cell receptor on CD4+ T-cells, e.g. macrophages, dendritic cells, B-cells. Note, however, that most types of cell are able to present antigenic peptides with MHC class I to CD8+ T-cells, e.g. as occurs with virally infected cells.

**antigenic determinant:** A cluster of epitopes (*see* epitope).

**apoptosis:** A form of programmed cell death, characterized by endonuclease digestion of DNA.

**atopic allergy:** IgE-mediated hypersensitivity, i.e. asthma, eczema, hayfever and food allergy.

**autologous:** From the same individual.

**avidity (functional affinity):** The binding strength between two molecules (e.g. antibody and antigen) taking into account the valency of the interaction. Thus the avidity will always be equal to or greater than the intrinsic affinity (*see* affinity).

**β$_2$-microglobulin:** A 12 kDa protein, not itself encoded within the MHC, but forming part of the structure of MHC class I-encoded molecules.

**B-1/B-2 cells:** The two major subpopulations of B lymphocytes. B-1 cells are Mac-1+, CD23− and most express the cell surface antigen CD5; they are self-renewing, and frequently secrete high levels of antibody which binds to a range of antigens ('polyspecificity') with a relatively low affinity. The majority of B cells, however, are B-2 which do not express CD5 and are Mac-1−, CD23+; they are directly generated from precursors in the bone marrow, and secrete highly specific antibody.

**basophil:** A type of granulocyte found in the blood and resembling the tissue mast cell.

**BCG (bacille Calmette–Guérin):** Attenuated *Mycobacterium tuberculosis* used both as a specific vaccine for tuberculosis and as an adjuvant.

**biolistics:** The use of small particles, e.g. colloidal gold, as a vehicle for carrying agents (drugs, nucleic acid, etc) into a cell. Following coating with the desired agent(s), the particles are fired into the dermis of the recipient using a helium-powered gun.

**bispecific antibody:** An artificially produced hybrid antibody in which each of the two antigen-binding arms is specific for a different antigenic epitope. Such antibodies, which can be produced either by chemical cross-linkage or by recombinant DNA techniques, can be used to link together two different antigens or cells, e.g. a cytotoxic T-cell and a tumor cell.

**bursa of Fabricius:** A primary lymphoid organ in avian species, located at the cloacal-hind gut junction; it is the site of B-cell maturation.

**capping:** An active process whereby cross-linking of cell surface molecules (e.g. by antibody) leads to aggregation and subsequent migration of the molecules to one pole of the cell.

**carrier:** Any molecule which when conjugated to a non-immunogenic molecule (e.g. a hapten) makes the latter immunogenic by providing epitopes for helper T-cells which the hapten lacks.

**CD antigen:** Cluster of differentiation designation assigned to leukocyte cell surface molecules which are identified by a given group of monoclonal antibodies.

**CD3:** A trimeric complex of $\gamma$, $\delta$ and $\epsilon$ chains which together with a $\zeta\zeta$ homodimer or $\zeta\eta$ heterodimer acts as a signal transducing unit for the T-cell receptor.

**CD4:** Cell surface glycoprotein, usually on helper T-cells, that recognizes MHC class II molecules on antigen-presenting cells.

**CD8:** Cell surface glycoprotein, usually on cytotoxic T-cells, that recognizes MHC class I molecules on target cells.

**cell-mediated immunity (CMI):** Refers to T-cell mediated immune responses.

**chemokines:** A family of structurally-related cytokines which selectively induce chemotaxis and activation of phagocytic cells and lymphocytes. They are also able to rapidly trigger integrin-mediated leukocyte adhesion.

**chemotaxis:** Movement of cells up a concentration gradient of chemotactic factors.

**chimeric:** Composite of genetically distinct individuals, e.g. following an allogeneic bone marrow graft.

**class switching:** The process by which a B-cell changes the class but not specificity of a given antibody it produces, e.g. switching from an IgM to an IgG antibody.

**classical pathway** (of complement activation): Activation pathway involving complement components C1, C2 and C4 which, following fixation of C1q, e.g. by antigen–antibody complexes, produces the classical pathway C3 convertase C4b2b.

**clonal deletion:** A process by which contact with antigen (e.g. self antigen) at an early stage of lymphocyte differentiation leads to cell death by apoptosis.

**clonal selection:** The selection and activation by antigen of a lymphocyte bearing a complementary receptor, which then proliferates to form an expanded clone.

**clone:** Identical cells derived from a single progenitor.

**colony stimulating factors (CSF):** Factors that permit the proliferation and differentiation of hematopoietic cells.

**complement:** A group of serum proteins, some of which act in an enzymatic cascade, producing effector molecules involved in inflammation (C3a, C5a), phagocytosis (C3b), and cell lysis (C5b-9).

**complementarity determining regions (CDR):** The hypervariable amino acid sequences within antibody and T-cell receptor variable regions which interact with complementary amino acids on the antigen or peptide-MHC complex.

**conA (concanavalin A):** A T-cell mitogen.

**congenic:** Animals which only differ at a single genetic locus.

**conjugate:** Covalently-linked complex of two or more molecules (e.g. fluorescein conjugated to antibody).

**Coombs' test:** Diagnostic test using anti-immunoglobulin to agglutinate antibody-coated erythrocytes.

**cortex:** Outer (peripheral) layer of an organ.

**C-reactive protein:** An acute phase protein which is able to bind to the surface of microorganisms where it functions as a stimulator of the classical pathway of complement activation, and as an opsonin for phagocytosis.

**cyclophosphamide:** Cytotoxic drug used as an immunosuppressive.

**cyclosporin A:** A T-cell specific immunosuppressive drug used to prevent graft rejection.

**cytokines:** Low molecular weight proteins that stimulate or inhibit the differentiation, proliferation or function of immune cells.

**cytophilic:** Binds to cells.

**cytotoxic:** Kills cells.

**cytotoxic T lymphocyte (Tc):** T-cells (usually CD8+) which kill target cells following recognition of foreign peptide-MHC molecules on the target cell membrane.

**delayed-type hypersensitivity (DTH):** A hypersensitivity reaction occurring within 48–72 hours and mediated by cytokine release from sensitized T-cells.

**differentiation antigen:** A cell surface molecule expressed at a particular stage of development or on cells of a given lineage.

**DiGeorge syndrome:** Immunodeficiency caused by a congenital failure in thymic development resulting in a lack of mature functional T-cells.

**diversity (D) gene segments:** Found in the immunoglobulin heavy chain gene and T-cell receptor $\beta$ and $\delta$ gene loci between the V and J gene segments. Encode part of the third hypervariable region in these antigen receptor chains.

**edema:** Swelling caused by accumulation of fluid in the tissues.

**effector cells:** Cells which carry out an immune function, e.g. cytokine release, cytotoxicity.

**ELISA (enzyme-linked immunosorbent assay):** Assay for detection or quantitation of an antibody or antigen using a ligand (e.g. an anti-immunoglobulin) conjugated to an enzyme which changes the color of a substrate.

**endocytosis:** Cellular ingestion of macromolecules by invagination of plasma membrane to produce an intracellular vesicle which encloses the ingested material.

**endogenous:** From within.

**endosomes:** Intracellular smooth surfaced vesicles in which endocytosed material passes on its way to the lysosomes.

**endotoxin:** Pathogenic cell wall-associated lipopolysaccharides of Gram-negative bacteria.

**eosinophil:** A class of granulocyte, the granules of which contain toxic cationic proteins.

**epitope:** That part of an antigen recognized by an antigen receptor (*see* antigenic determinant).

**Epstein–Barr virus (EBV):** The virus responsible for infectious mononucleosis and Burkitt's lymphoma. Used to immortalize human B-cells *in vitro*.

**equivalence:** The ratio of antibody to antigen at which immunoprecipitation of the reactions is virtually complete.

**erythema:** The redness produced during inflammation due to erythrocytes entering tissue spaces.

**erythropoiesis:** Erythrocyte production.

**exotoxin:** Pathogenic protein secreted by bacteria.

**exudate:** The extravascular fluid (containing proteins and cellular debris) which accumulates during inflammation.

**Fab:** Monovalent antigen-binding fragment obtained following papain digestion of immunoglobulin. Consists of an intact light chain and the N-terminal $V_H$ and $C_H1$ domains of the heavy chain.

**F(ab')$_2$:** Bivalent antigen-binding fragment obtained following pepsin digestion of immunoglobulin. Consists of both light chains and the N-terminal part of both heavy chains linked by disulfide bonds.

**Fas:** A member of the TNF receptor gene family. Engagement of Fas (CD95) on the surface of the cell by the Fas ligand present on cytotoxic cells, can trigger apoptosis in the Fas-bearing target cell.

**Fc:** Crystallizable, non-antigen binding fragment of an immunoglobulin molecule obtained following papain digestion. Consists of the C-terminal portion of both heavy chains which is responsible for binding to Fc receptors and C1q.

**Fc receptors:** Cell surface receptors which bind the Fc portion of particular immunoglobulin classes.

**fibroblast:** Connective tissue cell which produces collagen and plays an important part in wound healing.

**fluorescein isothiocyanate (FITC):** Green fluorescent dye used to 'tag' antibodies for use in immunofluorescence.

**fluorescent antibody:** An antibody conjugated to a fluorescent dye such as FITC.

**follicular dendritic cell:** MHC class II-negative Fc receptor-positive dendritic cells which bear immune complexes on their surface and are probably involved in the generation of antibody-secreting cells and maintenance of B-cell memory in germinal centres. (N.B. a different cell type to interdigitating dendritic cells).

**framework regions:** The relatively conserved amino acid sequences which flank the hypervariable regions in immunoglobulin and T-cell receptor variable regions and maintain a common overall structure for all V-region domains.

**Freund's adjuvant:** Complete Freund's adjuvant is an emulsion of aqueous antigen in mineral oil that contains heat-killed *Mycobacteria*. Incomplete Freund's adjuvant lacks the *Mycobacteria*.

**gammaglobulin:** The serum proteins, mostly immunoglobulins, which have the greatest mobility towards the cathode during electrophoresis.

**germ line:** The arrangement of the genetic material as transmitted through the gametes.

**germinal center:** Discrete areas within lymph node and spleen where B-cell maturation and memory development occur.

**giant cell:** Large multinucleate cell derived from fused macrophages and often present in granulomas.

**glomerulonephritis:** Inflammation of renal glomerular capillary loops, often resulting from immune complex deposition.

**graft versus host (g.v.h.) reaction:** Reaction occurring when T lymphocytes present in a graft recognize and attack host cells.

**granulocyte:** Myeloid cells containing cytoplasmic granules (i.e. neutrophils, eosinophils and basophils).

**granuloma:** A tissue nodule containing proliferating lymphocytes, fibroblasts, and giant cells and epithelioid cells (both derived from activated macrophages), which forms due to inflammation in response to chronic infection or persistence of antigen in the tissues.

**granzymes:** Serine esterases present in the granules of cytotoxic T lymphocytes and NK cells. They induce apoptosis in the target cell which they enter through perforin channels inserted into the target cell membrane by the cytotoxic lymphocyte.

**gut-associated lymphoid tissue (GALT):** Includes Peyer's patches, appendix, and solitary lymphoid nodules in the submucosa.

**H-2:** The mouse major histocompatibility complex (MHC).

**haplotype:** The set of allelic variants present at a given genetic region.

**hapten:** A low molecular weight molecule that is recognized by preformed antibody but is not itself immunogenic unless conjugated to a 'carrier' molecule which provides epitopes recognized by helper T-cells.

**helper T lymphocyte (TH):** A subclass of T-cells which provide help (in the form of cytokines and/or cognate interactions) necessary for the expression of effector function by other cells in the immune system.

**hemagglutinin:** Any molecule which agglutinates erythrocytes.

**hematopoiesis:** The production of erythrocytes and leukocytes.

**high endothelial venule (HEV):** Capillary venule composed of specialized endothelial cells allowing migration of lymphocytes into lymphoid organs.

**hinge region:** Amino acids between the Fab and Fc regions of immunoglobulin which permit flexibility of the molecule.

**histamine:** Vasoactive amine present in basophil and mast cell granules which, following degranulation, causes increased vascular permeability and smooth muscle contraction.

**HLA (human leukocyte antigen):** The human major histocompatibility complex (MHC).

**humoral:** Pertaining to extracellular fluid such as plasma and lymph. The term humoral immunity is used to denote antibody-mediated immune responses.

**hybridoma:** Hybrid cell line obtained by fusing a lymphoid tumor cell with a lymphocyte which then has both the immortality of the tumor cell and the effector function (e.g. monoclonal antibody secretion) of the lymphocyte.

**hypersensitivity:** Excessive immune response which leads to undesirable consequences, e.g. tissue or organ damage.

**hypervariable regions:** Those amino acid sequences within the immunoglobulin and T-cell receptor variable regions which show the greatest variability and contribute most to the antigen or peptide-MHC binding site.

**idiotope:** An epitope made up of amino acids within the variable region of an antibody or T-cell receptor which reacts with an anti-idiotope.

**idiotype:** The complete set of idioptopes in the variable region of an antibody or T-cell receptor which react with an anti-idiotypic serum.

**idiotype network:** A regulatory network based on interactions of idiotypes and anti-idiotypes present on antibodies and T-cell receptors.

**immune complex:** Complex of antibody bound to antigen which may also contain complement components.

**immunoadsorption:** Method for removal of antibody or antigen by allowing it to bind to solid phase antigen or antibody.

**immunofluorescence:** Technique for detection of cell or tissue-associated antigens by the use of a fluorescently-tagged ligand (e.g. an anti-immunoglobulin conjugated to fluorescein isothiocyanate).

**immunogen:** Any substance which elicits an immune response. Whilst all immunogens are antigens, not all antigens are immunogens (*see* hapten).

**immunoglobulin superfamily:** Large family of proteins characterized by possesion of 'immunoglobulin-type' domains of approximately 110 amino acids folded into two β-pleated sheets. Members include immunoglobulins, T-cell receptors and MHC molecules.

**inflammation:** The tissue response to trauma, characterized by increased blood flow and entry of leukocytes into the tissues, resulting in swelling, redness, elevated temperature and pain.

**innate immunity:** Immunity which is not intrinsically affected by prior contact with antigen, i.e. all aspects of immunity not directly mediated by lymphocytes.

**interdigitating dendritic cell:** MHC class II-positive, Fc receptor-negative, antigen-presenting dendritic cell found in T-cell areas of lymph nodes and spleen. (N.B. a different cell type to follicular dendritic cells).

**interferons (IFN):** IFNα is derived from various leukocytes, IFNβ from fibroblasts and IFNγ from T lymphocytes. All three types induce an anti-viral state in cells and IFNγ acts as a cytokine in the regulation of immune responses.

**interleukins (IL):** Designation for some of the cytokines secreted by leukocytes.

**internal image:** An epitope on an anti-idiotype which binds in a way that structurally and functionally mimics the antigen.

**invariant chain:** A polypeptide which binds MHC class II molecules in the endoplasmic reticulum, directs them to the late endosomal compartment and prevents premature association with self peptides.

**Ir (immune response) genes:** The genes, including those within the MHC, that together determine the overall level of immune response to a given antigen.

**isotype:** An antibody constant region structure present in all normal individuals, i.e. antibody class or subclass.

**ITAM:** Immunoreceptor Tyrosine-based Activation Motifs are consensus sequences for src-family tyrosine kinases. These motifs are found in the cytoplasmic domains of several signaling molecules including the signal transduction units of lymphocyte antigen receptors and of Fc receptors.

**J chain:** A molecule which forms part of the structure of pentameric IgM and dimeric IgA.

**joining (J) gene segments:** Found in the immunoglobulin and T-cell receptor gene loci and, upon gene rearrangement, encode part of the third hypervariable region of the antigen receptors.

**K (killer) cell:** Large granular lymphocyte which mediates antibody-dependent cell-mediated cytotoxicity (ADCC), is Fc receptor positive, but does not rearrange or express either immunoglobulin or T-cell receptor genes.

**kinins:** A family of polypeptides released during inflammatory responses and which increase vascular permeability and smooth muscle contraction.

**knockout:** The use of homologous genetic recombination in embryonal stem cells to replace a functional gene with a defective copy of the gene. The animals that are produced by this technique can be bred to homozygosity, thus allowing the generation of a null phenotype for that gene product.

**Kuppfer cells:** Fixed tissue macrophages lining the blood sinuses in the liver.

**Langerhans cell:** Fc receptor and MHC class II-positive antigen-presenting dendritic cell found in the skin.

**large granular lymphocyte (LGL):** Large lymphocytes which contain cytoplasmic granules and function as natural killer (NK) and killer (K) cells. Activated CD8+ cytotoxic T lymphocytes (Tc) also assume an LGL morphology.

**lectins:** A family of proteins, mostly of plant origin, which bind specific sugars on glycoproteins and glycolipids. Some lectins are also mitogenic (e.g. PHA, conA).

**leukotrienes:** Metabolic products of arachidonic acid which promote inflammatory processes(e.g. chemotaxis, increased vascular permeability) and are produced by a variety of cell types including mast cells, basophils and macrophages.

**ligand:** General term for a molecule recognized by a binding structure such as a receptor.

**linkage disequilibrium:** The occurrence of two alleles being inherited together at a greater frequency than that expected from the product of their individual frequencies.

**lipopolysaccharide (LPS):** Endotoxin derived from Gram-negative bacterial cell walls which has inflammatory and mitogenic actions.

**Ly markers:** A nomenclature based on the genetics of murine lymphocyte cell surface antigens. Nowadays largely replaced by the monoclonal antibody-based CD nomenclature as originally developed for human cell surface antigens.

**lymph:** The tissue fluid which drains into and through the lymphatic system.

**lymphadenopathy:** Enlarged lymph nodes.

**lymphokine:** Cytokine produced by lymphocytes.

**lymphokine-activated killer cells (LAK):** Killer (K) and natural killer (NK) cells activated *in vitro* by IL-2 to give enhanced killing of target cells.

**lymphotoxin:** Synonym for tumor necrosis factor-β (TNFβ).

**lysosomes:** Cytoplasmic granules containing hydrolytic enzymes involved in the digestion of phagocytosed material.

**lysozyme:** Anti-bacterial enzyme present in phagocytic cell granules, tears and saliva, which digests peptidoglycans in bacterial cell walls.

**macrophage:** Large phagocytic cell, derived from the blood monocyte, which also functions as an antigen-presenting cell and can mediate ADCC.

**mannose binding protein:** A member of the collectin family of calcium-dependent lectins, and an acute phase protein. It functions as a stimulator of the classical pathway of complement activation, and as an opsonin for phagocytosis by binding to mannose, a sugar residue usually found in an exposed form only on the surface of microorganisms.

**marginal zone:** The outer area of the splenic periarteriolar lymphoid sheath (PALS) which is rich in B cells, particularly those responding to thymus-independent antigens.

**margination:** Leukocyte adhesion to the endothelium of blood vessels in the early phase of an acute inflammatory reaction.

**mast cell:** A tissue cell with abundant granules which resembles the blood basophil. Both these cell types bear Fc receptors for IgE, which when crosslinked by IgE and antigen cause degranulation and the release of a number of mediators including histamine and leukotrienes.

**medulla:** Inner (central) region of an organ.

**megakaryocyte:** A bone marrow precursor of platelets.

**membrane attack complex (MAC):** Complex of complement components C5b–C9 which inserts as a pore into the membrane of target cells leading to cell lysis.

**memory (immunological):** A characteristic of the acquired immune response of lymphocytes whereby a second encounter with a given antigen produces a secondary immune response; faster, greater and longer lasting than the primary immune response.

**memory cells:** Clonally expanded T- and B-cells produced during a primary immune response and which are 'primed' to mediate a secondary immune response to the original antigen.

**MHC (major histocompatibility complex):** A genetic region encoding molecules involved in antigen presentation to T-cells. Class I MHC molecules are present on virtually all nucleated cells and are encoded mainly by the H-2K, D, and L loci in mice and by HLA-A, B, and C in man, whilst class II MHC molecules are expressed on antigen-presenting cells (primarily macrophages, B-cells and inter-digitating dendritic cells) and are encoded by H-2A and E in mice and HLA-DR, DQ, and DP in man. Allelic differences can be associated with the most intense graft rejection within a species.

**MHC restriction:** The necessity that T-cells recognize processed antigen only when presented by MHC molecules of the original haplotype associated with T-cell priming.

**minor histocompatibility antigens:** Non-MHC-encoded cell surface processed peptides which, in association with MHC-encoded molecules, contribute to graft rejection, albeit not usually as severe as that due to MHC mismatch.

**mitogen:** A substance which non-specifically induces lymphocyte proliferation.

**mixed lymphocyte reaction (MLR):** A T-cell proliferative response induced by cells expressing allogeneic MHC.

**monoclonal antibody:** Homogeneous antibody derived from a single B-cell clone and therefore all bearing identical antigen-binding sites and isotype.

**monocyte:** Mononuclear phagocyte found in blood and which is the precursor of the tissue macrophage.

**mononuclear phagocyte system:** A system comprising blood monocytes and tissue macrophages.

**mucosal-associated lymphoid tissue (MALT):** Lymphoid tissue present in the surface mucosa of the respiratory, gastrointestinal and genitourinary tracts.

**multiple myeloma:** Plasma cell malignancy resulting in high levels of monoclonal immunoglobulin in serum and of free light chains (Bence-Jones protein) in urine.

**murine:** Pertaining to mice.

**myeloma protein:** Monoclonal antibody secreted by myeloma cells.

**negative selection:** Deletion by apoptosis in the thymus of T-cells which recognize self peptides presented by self MHC molecules, thus preventing the development of autoimmune T-cells. Negative selection of developing B-cells is also thought to occur if they encounter high levels of self antigen in the bone marrow.

**neutrophil:** The major circulating phagocytic polymorphonuclear granulocyte. Enters tissues early in an inflammatory response and is also able to mediate antibody-dependent cell-mediated cytotoxicity (ADCC).

**NK (natural killer) cell:** Large granular lymphocyte which does not rearrange nor express either immunoglobulin or T-cell receptor genes but is able to recognize and destroy certain tumor and virally-infected cells in an MHC and antibody-independent manner.

**nude mouse:** Mouse which is T-cell deficient due to a homozygous gene defect (*nu/nu*) resulting in the absence of a thymus (and also lack of body hair).

**oncofetal antigen:** Antigen whose expression is normally restricted to the fetus but which may be expressed during malignancy in adults.

**opsonin:** Substance, e.g. antibody or C3b, which enhances phagocytosis by promoting adhesion of the antigen to the phagocyte.

**opsonization:** Coating of antigen with opsonin to enhance phagocytosis.

**PAF (platelet activating factor):** An alkyl phospholipid released by a variety of cell types including mast cells and basophils, which has immunoregulatory effects on lymphocytes and monocytes/macrophages as well as causing platelet aggregation and degranulation.

**paracortex:** The part of an organ (e.g. lymph node) which lies between the cortex and the medulla.

**perforin:** Molecule produced by cytotoxic T-cells and NK cells which, like complement component C9, polymerizes to form a pore in the membrane of the target cell leading to cell death.

**periarteriolar lymphoid sheath (PALS):** The lymphoid tissue which forms the white pulp of the spleen.

**Peyer's patches:** Part of the gut associated lymphoid tissue (GALT) and found as distinct lymphoid nodules mainly in the small intestine.

**PHA (phytohemagglutinin):** A plant lectin which acts as a T-cell mitogen.

**phage antibody library:** A collection of cloned antibody variable region gene sequences which can be expressed as Fab or scFv fusion proteins with bacteriophage coat proteins. These can be displayed on the surface of the phages. The gene encoding a monoclonal recombinant antibody is enclosed in the phage particle and can be selected from the library by binding of the phage to specific antigen.

**phagocyte:** Cells, including monocytes/macrophages and neutrophils, which are specialized for the engulfment of cellular and particulate matter.

**phagolysosome:** Intracellular vacuole where killing and digestion of phagocytosed material occurs following the fusion of a phagosome with a lysosome.

**phagosome:** Intracellular vacuole produced following invagination of the cell membrane around phagocytosed material.

**phorbol myristate acetate (PMA):** A mitogenic phorbol ester which directly stimulates protein kinase C and acts as a tumor promoter.

**plaque forming cell (PFC):** Antibody-secreting plasma cell detected *in vitro* by its ability to produce a 'plaque' of lysed antigen-sensitized erythrocytes in the presence of complement.

**plasma cell:** Terminally differentiated B lymphocyte which actively secretes large amounts of antibody.

**pokeweed mitogen (PWM):** A plant lectin which is a T-cell dependent B-cell mitogen.

**polyclonal:** Many different clones, or the product of many different clones, e.g. polyclonal antiserum.

**poly-Ig receptor:** A receptor molecule which specifically binds J-chain containing polymeric Ig, i.e. dimeric secretory IgA and pentameric IgM, and transports it across mucosal epithelium.

**positive selection:** The selection of those developing T-cells in the thymus which are able to recognize self MHC molecules. This occurs by preventing apoptosis in these cells.

**precipitin:** Precipitate of antibody and multivalent antigen due to the formation of high molecular weight complexes.

**primary immune response:** The relatively weak immune response which occurs upon the first encounter of naive lymphocytes with a given antigen.

**primary lymphoid organs:** The sites at which immunocompetent lymphocytes develop, i.e. bone marrow and thymus in mammals.

**prime:** The process of giving an initial sensitization to antigen.

**prostaglandins:** Acidic lipids derived from arachidonic acid which are able to increase vascular permeability, mediate fever, and can both stimulate and inhibit immunological responses.

**proteasome:** Cytoplasmic proteolytic enzyme complex involved in antigen processing for association with MHC.

**protein A:** *Staphylococcus aureus* cell wall protein which binds to the Fc region of IgG.

**protein tyrosine kinases:** Enzymes which are able to phosphorylate proteins on tyrosines, and often act in a cascade-like fashion in the signal transduction systems of cells.

**prozone effect:** The loss of immune precipitation or agglutination which occurs when antibody concentration is increased to an extent that the antibody is in such excess that it is no longer able to effectively cross-link the antigen. A similar phenomenon may occur in antigen excess.

**Qa antigens:** 'Non-classical' MHC class I molecules of mice.

**respiratory burst:** The increased oxidative metabolism which occurs in phagocytic cells following activation.

**reticuloendothelial system (RES):** A rather old term for the network of phagocytes and endothelial cells throughout the body.

**rheumatoid factor:** IgM, IgG and IgA autoantibodies to IgG, particularly the Fc region.

**rosette:** Particles or cells bound to the surface of a lymphocyte (e.g. sheep erythrocytes around a human T-cell).

**scFv:** A single chain molecule composed of the variable regions of an antibody heavy and light chain joined together by a flexible linker.

**SCID (severe combined immunodeficiency):** Immunodeficiency affecting both T and B lymphocytes.

**secondary immune response:** The qualitatively and quantitatively improved immune response which occurs upon the second encounter of primed lymphocytes with a given antigen.

**secretory component:** Proteolytic cleavage product of the poly-Ig receptor which remains associated with dimeric IgA in sero-mucus secretions.

**secretory IgA:** Dimeric IgA found in sero-mucus secretions.

**somatic hypermutation:** The enhanced rate of point mutation in the immunoglobulin variable region genes which occurs following antigenic stimulation and acts as a mechanism for increasing antibody diversity and affinity.

**stem cell:** Multipotential cell from which differentiated cells derive.

**superantigen:** An antigen which reacts with all the T-cells belonging to a particular T-cell receptor V region family, and which therefore stimulates (or deletes) a much larger number of cells than does conventional antigen.

**surface plasmon resonance:** A technique based upon changes in the angle of reflected light which occur upon ligand binding to an immobilized target molecule on a biosensor chip. This permits the observation of protein–protein interactions (such as antibody binding to an antigen) in 'real-time', i.e. by continuous monitoring of the association and dissociation of the reversible reaction.

**switch sequences:** Highly conserved repetitive sequences which mediate class switching in the immunoglobulin heavy chain gene locus.

**syngeneic:** Genetically identical, e.g. a fully inbred strain of mice.

**TAP:** The Transporters associated with Antigen Processing (TAP-1 and TAP-2) are molecules which carry antigenic peptides from the cytoplasm into the lumen of the endoplasmic reticulum for incorporation into MHC class I molecules.

**T-cell receptor (TCR):** The heterodimeric antigen receptor of the T lymphocyte exists in two alternative forms, consisting of α and β chains, or γ and δ chains. The αβ TCR recognizes peptide fragments of protein antigens presented by MHC molecules on cell surfaces. The function of the γδ TCR is less clearly defined but it can recognize native proteins on the cell surface.

**T-dependent antigen:** An antigen which requires helper T-cells in order to elicit an antibody response.

**T-independent antigen:** An antigen which is able to elicit an antibody response in the absence of T-cells.

**thymocyte:** Developing T-cell in the thymus.

**titer:** Measure of the relative 'strength' (a combination of amount and avidity) of an antibody or antiserum, usually given as the highest dilution which is still operationally detectable in, for example, an agglutination assay.

**tolerance:** Specific immunological unresponsiveness.

**tolerogen:** An antigen used to induce tolerance. Often depends more on the circumstances of administration (e.g. route and concentration) than on any inherent property of the molecule.

**toxoid:** Chemically or physically modified toxin that is no longer harmful but retains immunogenicity.

**tumor necrosis factors (TNFα and TNFβ):** Two related cytokines originally named for their cytotoxic effects on certain tumor cells but which also have immunoregulatory functions.

**variable (V) gene segments:** Genes that rearrange together with D (diversity) and J (joining) gene segments in order to encode the complementarity-determining variable region amino acid sequences of immunoglobulins and T-cell receptors.

**vasoactive amines:** Substances including histamine and 5-hydroxytryptamine which increase vascular permeability and smooth muscle contraction.

**xenogeneic:** Genetic differences between species.

**xenograft:** A tissue or organ graft between individuals of different species.

# INDEX